• Maintain breathing • Prevent further injury • Prevent shock • Send for a physician

DON'T

- Do not move the victim unless absolutely necessary to remove from danger.
- Do not wait or look for help.
- Do not stop to loosen clothing or warm the victim.
- Do not give up.

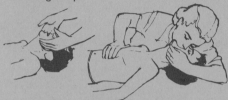

MOUTH-TO-MOUTH BREATHING FOR INFANTS AND SMALL CHILDREN

DO

- Put child in a face-up position.
- Tilt child's head backward.
- Lift child's lower jaw with fingers of both hands so that it "juts out."
- Keep child in this position so that the tongue will not fall back to block the air passage.
- Take a deep breath and place your mouth over the child's MOUTH AND NOSE.
- Blow your breath gently into the child's mouth and nose until you see the chest rise and you feel the lungs expand. The air you blow into the child's lungs has enough oxygen to save his life.
- Remove your mouth and let the child exhale.
- As soon as you hear the child breathe out, replace your mouth over his mouth and nose and repeat procedure.
  REPEAT 15 TIMES PER MINUTE.
- When possible, place your hand over the child's stomach. Use moderate pressure to keep the stomach from becoming inflated.

MOUTH-TO-MOUTH BREATHING FOR ADULTS

DO

- Place victim half-way between a face-up and a side position.
- Lift victim's neck with one hand and tilt his head back by holding the top of his head with your other hand.
- Pull the victim's chin up with the hand that was lifting the neck so that the tongue does not fall back to block the air passage.

- Take a deep breath and place your mouth over the victim's nose **or** mouth, making a leak-proof seal. Pinch nostrils. See illustration.
- Blow your breath into the victim's mouth or nose until you see the chest rise. The air you blow into the victim's lungs has enough oxygen to save his life.
- Remove your mouth and let the victim exhale while you take another deep breath.
- As soon as you hear the victim breathe out, replace your mouth over his mouth or nose and repeat procedure.
  REPEAT 15 TIMES PER MINUTE.

    Mouth-to-Nose Breathing: Make leak-proof seal by holding the victim's lips closed with your thumb. Be sure your lips do not close the victim's nostrils.

    Mouth-to-Mouth Breathing: Seal your lips around the victim's mouth. Pinch his nostrils closed with your thumb and finger.

MANUAL METHOD OF ARTIFICIAL RESPIRATION

    The manual method of artificial respiration should be used if for any reason the mouth-to-mouth method cannot be used.

DO

- Place victim in a face-up position.
- Place something under victim's shoulders to raise them and allow the head to drop backward.
- Kneel above victim's head, facing the victim.
- Grasp victim's arms at the wrists, crossing and pressing victim's wrists against the lower chest.
- Immediately pull arms upward, outward, and backward as far as possible.
  REPEAT 15 TIMES PER MINUTE
- If a second rescuer is present, he should hold the victim's head so that it tilts backward and the jaw juts forward.

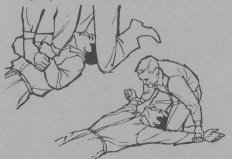

TODAY'S
HEALTH
GUIDE

TODAY'S HEALTH GUIDE

A manual of health information & guidance for the American family

Published by the
American Medical Association

Edited by
W. W. Bauer, M.D.
Director Emeritus
Department of Health Education
American Medical Association

First Printing, June 1965
Second Printing, September 1965

Library of Congress Catalog Card Number: 64-8095

Manufactured in the United States of America

FOREWORD

This HEALTH GUIDE is the product of the combined knowledge and experience of many doctors and allied scientists. It is a logical outgrowth of the purpose of physicians, expressed through their membership in the American Medical Association, to serve their patients in every possible way.

Doctors have always been teachers—that is the original meaning of the title "doctor." Throughout the long history of medicine, from Aesculapius to modern Osler, the great physicians have also been teachers.

True to this tradition, the American Medical Association has devoted much of its energy since its establishment in 1847 to the cause of education—first the education of medical students, and more recently the education of the public toward a better understanding of what modern medicine offers for better health and longer life.

This is not a "doctor" book in the old-fashioned sense, nor an encyclopedia. It is an effort to select, from the enormous mass of information about health, topics which will be most helpful to the family in making the best and most economical use of the sources of health information, preventive medical services, treatment of illness, and adequate meeting of emergencies.

The American Medical Association, on behalf of its more than 200,000 members, hopes that this book will be helpful to you.

F. J. L. BLASINGAME, M. D.
Executive Vice President

CONTRIBUTORS
&
CONSULTANTS

THE AMERICAN MEDICAL ASSOCIATION expresses its deepest gratitude to the more than 200 practicing physicians and specialists, dentists, veterinarians, clergymen, chemists, physicists, nurses, educators, engineers, safety experts, writers, and reviewers who have made possible the assembling of this GUIDE. None has been compensated in any way, except through this expression of appreciation.

The names of these distinguished participants follow in alphabetical order. In addition, there has been wide participation by many members of the headquarters staff of the AMA both as contributors and consultants.

CONTRIBUTORS
to TODAY'S HEALTH GUIDE

Allman, David B., M.D.
General Surgeon, Atlantic City, New Jersey

Anderson, Jackson M., Ph.D.
American Association for Health,
Physical Education and Recreation (NEA),
Washington, D. C.

Apgar, Virginia, M.D.
National Foundation-March of Dimes,
New York, New York

Barr, Robert N., M.D.
Minnesota Department of Health,
Minneapolis, Minnesota

Barrett, Morris, M.P.H
Lankenau Hospital,
Philadelphia, Pennsylvania

Beaton, Lindsay E., M.D.
Vice-Chairman, Council on Mental Health,
AMA, Tucson, Arizona

Bethel, Millard B., M.D.
Department of Public Health
Raleigh, North Carolina

Bland, John H., M.D.
University of Vermont College of Medicine,
Burlington, Vermont

Block, Marvin A., M.D.
State University Medical School at Buffalo,
Buffalo, New York

Brady, J. Morrison, M.D.
Medical Consultant, Muscular Dystrophy Associations of America, Inc.,
New York, New York

Buck, McKenzie W., Ph.D.
University of Florida, Gainesville, Florida

Burke, Jack W.
National Safety Council, Chicago, Illinois

Burney, Leroy E., M.D.
School of Medicine, Temple University,
Philadelphia, Pennsylvania

Calderone, Mary S., M.D.
Planned Parenthood Federation of America,
Inc., New York, New York

Carlson, Reynold E.
Indiana University, Bloomington, Indiana

Clark, William S., M.D.
The National Foundation,
New York, New York

Colwell, Arthur R., Jr., M.D.
Northwestern University Medical School,
Chicago, Illinois

Crile, George, M.D.
Cleveland Clinic, Cleveland, Ohio

Crook, William G., M.D.
Jackson-Madison County General Hospital,
Jackson, Tennessee

Crosby, Edwin L., M.D.
Director, American Hospital Association,
Chicago, Illinois

Doll, Edgar A., Ph.D.
Bellingham Public Schools,
Bellingham, Washington

*Deceased

Dykstra, Phil, B.A.
National Safety Council, Chicago, Illinois

*****Fabricant, Noah D.,** M.D.
Chicago, Illinois

Fahy, Agnes, A.B.
National Tuberculosis Association,
New York, New York

Falls, Frederick H., M.D.
Illinois State Department of Public Health,
River Forest, Illinois

Fleming, John P.
National Safety Council, Chicago, Ilinois

Gardner, George E., Ph.D., M.D.
Harvard Medical School,
Cambridge, Massachusetts

Gebhard, Bruno, M.D.
Cleveland Health Museum, Cleveland, Ohio

Grant, Roald N., M.D.
American Cancer Society, Inc.,
New York, New York

Hale, Donald E., M.D.
Cleveland Clinic, Cleveland, Ohio

Hill, Paul F., B.A.
National Safety Council, Chicago, Illinois

Hillman, Robert W., M.D.
State University of New York College of Medicine, Brooklyn, New York

Hogan, Michael J., M.D.
University of California School of Medicine,
San Francisco, California

House, Leland R., M.D.
Loma Linda University School of Medicine,
Loma Linda, California

Johnson, Harry J., M.D.
Life Extension Foundation,
New York, New York

Johnson, Wendell, Ph.D.
University of Iowa, Iowa City, Iowa

*****Johnson, Wingate M.,** M.D.
Bowman Gray School of Medicine
of Wake Forest College,
Winston-Salem, North Carolina

Klinghoffer, Max, M.D.
Elmhurst, Illinois

Larimore, Granville W., M.D.
New York State Department of Health,
Albany, New York

Lehman, Jean Utley, Ph.D.
California State College,
Los Angeles, California

Lichter, Max L., M.D.
Melvindale, Michigan

McCulloch, William F., D.V.M.
State University of Iowa College of Medicine,
Iowa City, Iowa

March, Cyril H., M.D.
New York University Postgraduate Medical
School, New York, New York

Morrey, Lon W., D.D.S.
American Dental Association,
Chicago, Illinois

Page, Irvine H., M.D.
Cleveland Clinic Foundation, Cleveland, Ohio

Page, Malcolm I., M.D.
Communicable Disease Center, Public Health Service, Atlanta, Georgia

Perkins, James E., M.D.
National Tuberculosis Association, New York, New York

Quigley, Thomas B., M.D., B.A.
Harvard Medical School, Cambridge, Massachusetts

Rappaport, Ben Z., M.D.
University of Illinois, Chicago, Illinois

Rasor, Robert W., M.D.
Public Health Service Hospital, Lexington, Kentucky

Richmond, Julius B., M.D.
State University of New York, Upstate Medical Center, Syracuse, New York

Rusk, Howard A., M.D., A.B.
New York University Medical Center, New York, New York

Ryan, Allan J., M.D.
Meriden Hospital, Meriden, Connecticut

Seifert, Martin H., M.D.
Northwestern University, Evanston, Illinois

Shipman, Sidney J., M.D.
University of California Medical School, San Francisco, California

Simmons, James Q., Jr., M.D.
National Multiple Sclerosis Society, New York, New York

Smith, Austin, M.D.
Pharmaceutical Manufacturers Association, Washington, D. C.

Tenney, H. Kent, M.D.
University of Wisconsin Medical School, Madison, Wisconsin

Tenney, Horace K., III, M.D.
University of Wisconsin Medical School, Madison, Wisconsin

Vickery, Dorothy S., A.B.
American Heart Association, Inc., New York, New York

"W.", Bill
Co-founder, Alcoholics Anonymous, New York, New York

Wakerlin, George E., M.D., Ph.D.
American Heart Association, Inc., New York, New York

Westberg, Granger E., D.D
University of Chicago School of Medicine, Chicago, Illinois

Winick, Charles, Ph.D.
American Social Health Association, New York, New York

Wright, Willard A., M.D.
Chairman, AMA Council on Medical Services, Williston, North Dakota

Yahr, Melvin D., M.D.
College of Physicians and Surgeons, New York, New York

CONSULTANTS

to TODAY'S HEALTH GUIDE

Allison, Alexander B., M.A., D.D.
Wilmette, Illinois

*Deceased

Auerbach, John, B.S.
Bicycle Institute of America, Inc., New York, New York

Baer, Rudolf L., M.D.
New York University School of Medicine, New York, New York

Bell, Julius N., M.D.
Chicago Medical School, Chicago, Illinois

Bortz, Edward L., M.D.
Lankenau Hospital, Philadelphia, Pennsylvania

Burket, Lester W., D.D.S., M.D.
University of Pennsylvania School of Dentistry, Philadelphia, Pennsylvania

Cecil, Russell L., M.D.
Arthritis & Rheumatism Foundation, New York, New York

Chapman, Albert L., M.D.
Pennsylvania Department of Health, Harrisburg, Pennsylvania

Cleere, Roy L., M.D.
University of Colorado Medical School, Denver, Colorado

Cohen, Seymour J., Rabbi, Ph.D.
Synagogue Council of America, Chicago, Illinois

Cole, Warren H., M.D.
University of Illinois College of Medicine, Chicago, Illinois

Crotty, Carol M.
Division of Speech Correction, Board of Education, Chicago, Illinois

Crownhart, Charles H., LL.B
Madison, Wisconsin

Culpepper, John P., Jr., M.D
Hattiesburg, Mississippi

Davidsohn, Israel, M.D
Chicago Medical School, Chicago, Illinois

Davis, M. Edward, M.D.
University of Chicago School of Medicine, Chicago, Illinois

Denison, George A., M.D.
Former Health Commissioner of Birmingham and Jefferson County, Birmingham, Alabama

Dzenowagis, Joseph G., Ed.D.
Michigan State University, East Lansing, Michigan

Feinberg, Samuel M., M.D.
Northwestern University Medical School, Chicago, Illinois

Ferree, John W., M.D.
National Society for the Prevention of Blindness, Inc., New York, New York

Finnerud, Clark W., M.D.
University of Illinois College of Medicine, Chicago, Illinois

Fister, George M., M.D.
Past President, American Medical Association, Ogden, Utah

Fleming, Willard C., D.D.S.
University of California School of Dentistry, San Francisco, California

Florida State Board of Health (individual credits declined)
Jacksonville, Florida

Frazier, Robert G., M.D.
American Academy of Pediatrics,
Evanston, Illinois

Friermood, Harold T., Ed.D., Ph.D.
National Board of Young Men's Christian Associations, New York, New York

Gastineau, Clifford F., M.D.
Mayo Foundation-Mayo Clinic,
Rochester, Minnesota

Gordon, Edgar S., Ph.D., M.D.
University of Wisconsin, Madison, Wisconsin

Gray, A. L., M.D.
Mississippi State Board of Health,
Jackson, Mississippi

Gundersen, Gunnar, M.D.
Past President of the American Medical Association, LaCrosse, Wisconsin

Heise, Herman A., M.D.
Milwaukee, Wisconsin

Horwitz, Essie L., Mrs., B.S.
Chicago Board of Education, Chicago, Illinois

Hull, Thomas G., Ph.D.
Former Director of Exhibits, AMA,
Yarmouth Port, Massachusetts

Jahn, Richard P., M.D.
Marquette University School of Medicine,
Milwaukee, Wisconsin

Jenkins, Gladys G., M.A.
Iowa City, Iowa

Keown, Kenneth K., M.D.
University of Missouri School of Medicine,
Columbia, Missouri

Krumbiegel, Edward R., M.D.
Commissioner of Health,
Milwaukee, Wisconsin

Lamont-Havers, Ronald W., M.D.
Arthritis & Rheumatism Foundation,
New York, New York

Larson, Leonard W., M.D.
Past President, American Medical Association, Bismarck, North Dakota

Leadbetter, Wyland F., M.D.,
Massachusetts General Hospital,
Boston, Massachusetts

Levy, Inez B., B.S.
Chicago Board of Education, Chicago, Illinois

Lifson, Sol S., M.P.H.
National Tuberculosis Association,
New York, New York

Lueth, Harold C., M.D.
Evanston, Illinois

McAfee, Ruth G., M.A.
Evanston, Illinois

McMahon, Alphonse, M.D.
St. Louis University School of Medicine,
St. Louis, Missouri

Mainwaring, Rosser L., M.D.
Wayne State University School of Medicine,
Detroit, Michigan

Mann, Marty
National Council on Alcoholism, Inc.,
New York, New York

Masserman, Jules H., M.D.
Northwestern University School of Medicine,
Chicago, Illinois

*Deceased

Maxwell, Cyrus H., M.D.
National Heart Institute, U.S. Public Health Service, Bethesda, Maryland

Mendel, Levitte B., M.P.H.
National Health Council,
New York, New York

Miller, Seward E., M.D.
University of California,
Los Angeles, California

*Moore, Josiah J., M.D.
Chicago, Illinois

Newhouser, Lloyd R., M.D.
University of Miami School of Medicine,
Miami, Florida

Oberteuffer, Delbert, Ph.D.
Ohio State University, Columbus, Ohio

Paul, Oglesby, M.D.
Northwestern University School of Medicine,
Chicago, Illinois

Pearson, Homer L., M.D.
Miami, Florida

Piszczek, Edward A., M.D.
Suburban Cook County Tuberculosis Sanitarium District, Forest Park, Illinois

Potthoff, Carl J., M.D.
University of Nebraska College of Medicine,
Omaha, Nebraska

Powers, Margaret Hall
Bureau of Physically Handicapped Children,
Board of Education, Chicago, Illinois

Prendergast, Joseph, LL.D.
National Recreation Association,
New York, New York

Ramsey, Herbert P., M.D.
Washington Hospital Center,
Washington, D. C.

Robins, R. B., M.D.
Camden, Arkansas

Root, Howard F., M.D.
Boston, Massachusetts

Rose, Norman J., M.D.
Illinois Department of Public Health,
Springfield, Illinois

Rouse, Milford O., M.D.
Southwestern Medical School of University of Texas, Dallas, Texas

Schmuck, William
Medical Department, Pan American Airways,
Chicago, Illinois

Seevers, Maurice H., M.D.
University of Michigan, Ann Arbor, Michigan

Shacter, Helen S., Ph.D.
Clinical Psychologist, Chicago, Illinois

Shaffer, Thomas E., M.D.
Ohio State University College of Medicine,
Columbus, Ohio

Sheldon, C. Hunter, M.D.
Pasadena, California

Sheridan, William J., M.D.
Chattanooga, Tennessee

Sherman, William B., M.D.
Columbia University, New York, New York

Sill, Van Rensselaer, B.S.
U.S. Public Health Service, Washington, D. C.

Snider, Charles H., D.V.M.
 Assistant Surgeon General for Veterinary Services, Bethesda, Maryland

Stare, Frederick J., M.D.
 Harvard University,
 Cambridge, Massachusetts

Stubblefield, Robert L., M.D.
 Southwestern Medical School, Dallas, Texas

Stovall, William D., M.D.
 University of Wisconsin, Madison, Wisconsin

Sulzberger, Marion B., M.D.
 U.S. Army, Washington, D. C.

Sutter, Richard A., M.D.
 Washington University School of Medicine, St. Louis, Missouri

Vail, Derrick T., M.D.
 Northwestern University Medical School, Chicago, Illinois

*Deceased

Vandam, Leroy D., M.D.
 American Society of Anesthesiologists, Inc., Park Ridge, Illinois

*Welsh, Ashton Leroy, M.D.
 Cincinnati, Ohio

Wheatley, George M., M.D.
 Metropolitan Life Insurance Company, New York, New York

White, Paul Dudley, M.D.
 Boston, Massachusetts

Williams, Huntington, M.D., Dr. P.H.
 Baltimore, Maryland

Wiprud, Theodore
 Medical Service of District of Columbia, Washington, D. C.

Woodbridge, Philip D., M.D.
 Greenfield, Massachusetts

Yoder, Franklin D., M.D.
 Illinois Department of Public Health, Springfield, Illinois

Zollinger, Robert M., M.D.
 Ohio State University, Columbus, Ohio

CONTENTS

PART IV

SAFEGUARDING YOUR HEALTH

PART V

MENTAL AND EMOTIONAL HEALTH

PART VI

RECREATION AND RELAXATION

SURGERY TODAY

THE PROPER USE OF DRUGS

PHYSICAL HANDICAPS

COMMUNITY HEALTH

KEEPING POSTED

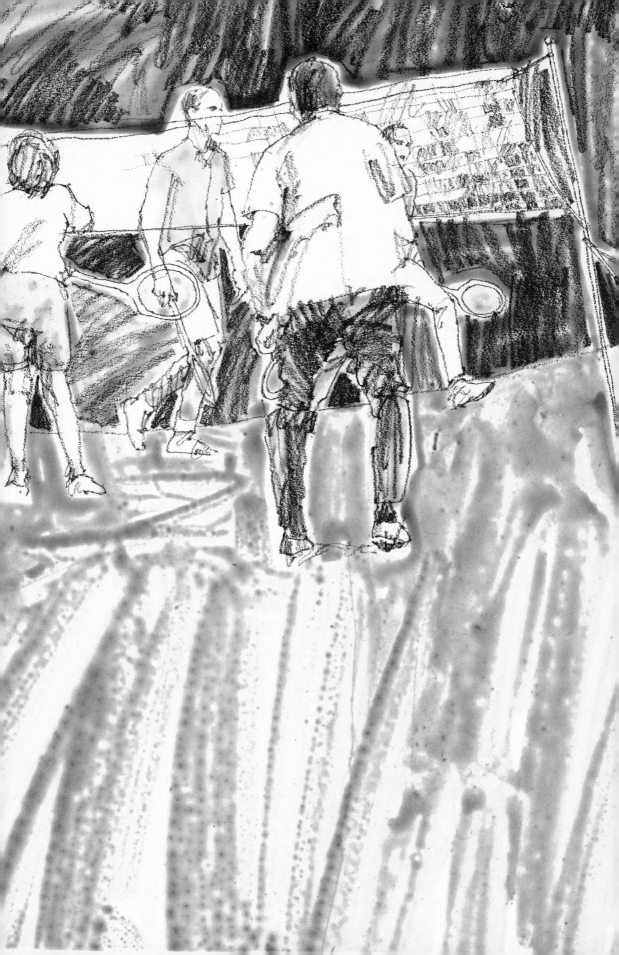

PART I

The Home
As a Health Center

THE HOME is the center of the family's health for a number of reasons. It is a place where the same people constantly congregate and where these people and their living practices may be handled as a unit. Home is also the place where the individuals in the family react upon one another, so that the actions of one necessarily influence all. It is or should be a place of rest, comfort, love, and refuge. It is the family's castle. But home is more than a place. It is a concept and an ideal, where love and loyalty rule.

THE HOME AS A HEALTH CENTER

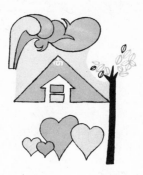

As FAR BACK as historical records go, the home and the family have constituted the center of human living. Homes have existed alone or have been grouped together in villages or cities. Patterns of community organization have varied, but the home has been essentially the same throughout the centuries.

In modern times, importance of the community has been emphasized above that of the home. Many observers regard this attitude to be contrary to the welfare of the individual, of the community, and ultimately of the nation. Strong communities and strong nations have always been based on strong homes. It is for that reason that this book about healthful patterns of living at home is directed to the homemaker and to the members of the family.

The home is usually centered in some form of dwelling. Historically, this may once have been a cave or a tent. During an important portion of American history the home was often the covered wagon. It may still be a shack, a modest house, an apartment, a mansion, or in these days, a trailer. Regardless of where or what the home is as a dwelling, it serves as a shelter and a center for all the activities of the family group. It should therefore be a safe, convenient, comfortable, livable place, and we shall have more to say about that.

As a natural convenience the family eats together. For this reason the home becomes the center for nutrition, either good or bad. In many homes, the main meal of the day is the only one shared by all. It can be the occasion for mutual planning.

Because of the reactions within the family group upon the various members, the home influences personalities. It also affects manners and interrelationships. A wholesome home influence is a help to its individual members; the reverse is a detriment.

Persons of exceptionally strong individual character can overcome disadvantages due to inadequate homes, but often they do so with difficulty. They would have been better off under a better environment. Conversely, even the best home may fail to turn out individuals with good character and personality and good health. Despite these individual deviations, it is generally true that a happy home and family life favor the development of efficient, healthy, well-integrated individuals and lack of these advantages works in the opposite direction. Statistics bear this out—married persons tend to live longer than do the single, widowed, or divorced persons.

In this book we are concerned primarily with the influence of the home upon health. If we follow the American Medical Association's idea of "Seven Paths to Fitness," we can readily see that the home is important in reaching all these goals. These seven paths are: Good medical care; adequate nutrition; good dental care; satisfactory working conditions; a sensible activity program; rest, relaxation, and recreation; and good emotional adjustment.

Health is probably the most personal factor in human living. It is therefore extremely important that the home shall contribute to keeping the family members healthy. The primary responsibility for health maintenance must therefore be centered in the home. The home is also regarded as the necessary center for many other phases of living, and there are many who believe that the integrity and the capability of the home are essential to the maintenance of a free and independent society and the way of life which we Americans cherish.

The individual should look to the home first for health. The home may need help from outside its own resources, and therefore the family group has a right and an obligation to look to the community for such health safeguards as cannot be provided by the home unaided, such as a safe water supply and sewage disposal. The organization of modern American life and its increasing urbanization have made the home more dependent upon the community than was formerly the case, and perhaps have encouraged a tendency to make it too dependent.

The pioneer home in the wilderness had to provide every necessity for living. Until recently the same was true to a great extent of most rural homes. Today, the pioneer home is practically a thing of the past, and the rural home is greatly changed. Today's city home is different from what it was only a few years ago. An increase in the number of apartments and the increasing mobility of our population also affect the home. Nevertheless, in spite of all the influences which seem to be leading individuals away from the home, we still must regard the home as the necessary center and basis for a good pattern of living. And this is particularly true in regard to health.

Community Health Services

The modern community has grown much more sensitive to health needs within the past few decades. Community helps now abound, but no matter how available, they are of little use unless their existence is known to the homemaker and unless the homemaker knows how to make the necessary contacts and how to use these facilities to the best possible advantage.

In general, community health service facilities cover such things as water purification, sewage disposal, control of air pollution, estimation of radioactive fallout, pollen distribution count, reduction of needless noise, inspection and control of food production, handling and disposal of garbage and wastes, and pest control. Included also are health education and educational leadership in attacks upon medical quackery, in the health of infants and children, the diseases of advancing age, and the leading causes of death: principally heart disease, cancer, hardening of the arteries, diabetes, arthritis, and stroke.

It is not the community's role to provide medical, dental, or hospital care free of charge, except to the needy who cannot meet this responsibility themselves. Community resources are of two kinds, governmental and voluntary.

Governmental services, supported out of taxation, are defined by legislative enactments, and administered by elected or appointed public officials. Some of these resources are at the local level and are usually available in cities, towns, and counties, or through the state capital. Others are at the federal level, available either in Washington or at regional offices in the larger cities. Through these governmental resources liaison is made for international health arrangements, such as quarantine and the exchange of information about communicable diseases and public health experiences, and to some extent direct international control of the diseases which threaten the welfare of civilization and of the human race.

Many problems exist which have not been attacked, or at least not successfully attacked, through governmental channels. The United States is almost alone among the nations in having a highly developed system of voluntary health agencies. A voluntary health agency is a group that may include physicians or laymen and usually includes both. It is organized with or without government cooperation by individuals having a vital interest in a particular health problem. This interest is professional in the case of physicians, nurses, and related groups, and personal from the standpoint of patients and non-medical participants.

These voluntary health organizations are supported by various means, such as the sale of stamps or seals, by memberships, by sale of their publications, by "drives" such as the March of Dimes or similar devices, and by personal solicitation through the mail or house-to-house visitation. They also receive grants-in-aid, gifts, trust funds, and bequests. Much of their support comes from philanthropic foundations established by wealthy and public-spirited citizens. Most of these agencies are organized on a basis of local chapters, state organizations, and a national office. The addresses of the various voluntary health agencies can usually be ascertained through the local health department or through the local chapter of any one of them, since they are all well-known to each other and cooperate closely through membership in a National Health Council, which has its offices in New York.

Importance of Family Doctor

The most important step which the homemaker can take toward safeguarding the health of the family is to have a continuing and friendly contact with a family physician and a family dentist. These professional persons should be consulted regularly while one is healthy in order to forestall disease. It is much cheaper—and more pleasant—to prevent than to treat and cure. In addition, some preventable diseases are not curable if they are permitted to develop too far, and some are not curable at all. The details of developing good relationships between the family and its physician or dentist will be elaborated in a later chapter. Here the point is emphasized because there is nothing more important. The family physician or dentist can be and should be a guide and a judge whenever health matters arise about which there is any doubt.

Another important factor in keeping the home and its members healthy is the making of a definite place in the family budget for all necessary costs of living, including health care. Some families budget in a very formal manner; others informally; too many fail to budget at all. It is the latter group that usually has trouble paying its bills. Benjamin Franklin said that any man can save no matter what he makes, by spending just a little less. Under some modern conditions this may be difficult to do, but despite the exceptions the principle is sound.

If there is anything certain in life besides death and taxes, it is illness. Since life has been so greatly extended, many persons now fear disability as much as they do death, or even more. Practically no one as an individual, and certainly no family, ever totally escapes illness. The severity of illnesses, their frequency, and their duration vary widely, and some families are much more fortunate than others.

While illness is practically certain, the time of its arrival is indefinite and unpredictable; so are its severity and its duration. Later on in this book you will find a full discussion devoted to budgeting for health, including the means for paying the costs of minor illnesses out of income and providing for the more serious or even catastrophic illnesses through appropriate forms such as savings, reserves, bonds, and health insurance. Every family owes it to all its members to budget for the maintenance of health and for the cost of illness.

Parental Responsibility

Despite the passing of the old-time autocratic "head of the house," the fact remains that parents must still exercise leadership in the home. This is true in all phases of living, but it is particularly true with regard to health. Whether it be nutrition, care of the teeth, proper cleanliness, the procurement of immu-

nizations, adequate convalescence after illness, promptness in procuring medical care, or any of the other important factors in maintaining good health and developing sound personalities, the responsibility rests upon the parents.

When the children are small they are incapable of assuming these responsibilities. As they grow up, they are unlikely to assume them unless they have witnessed a good parental example. It is important therefore that homemakers should be well oriented in leadership, guidance, and influence as they pertain to health. Such orientation is the purpose of this health guide.

Health is generally regarded as an asset. There have indeed been slogans which have emphasized this, often inaccurately. It is not true as sometimes claimed that "health is wealth." There are many healthy people who are not wealthy and many wealthy persons who are not healthy. Another slogan is to the effect that life is not worth living without good health. Certainly it is true that good health contributes greatly to the joy of living and should be preserved and cherished. At the same time there are many handicapped persons who have been able to make a good life for themselves and to set a notable example to their fellow human beings by the courageous way in which they have faced and conquered disability, disease, and suffering. Obviously it is foolish to sacrifice health needlessly. It is just as unwise to lie down and give up when your health is impaired. The modern attitude toward the handicapped is to observe not what they can no longer accomplish, but what they are still able to do. A sensible attitude toward health therefore is that it is an asset which should be preserved, but that all is not necessarily lost when health is impaired.

This is not a "doctor book" in the old-fashioned sense. When large areas of this country were undeveloped and many persons lived removed from community facilities, the household doctor book was a useful item, indeed a necessity. The state of medical knowledge has advanced more in the past hundred years than in all the rest of recorded history and thus many of the time-honored home remedies have become outmoded and should be replaced by more modern methods. All this new knowledge has added to the complexities and technicalities of modern medicine and has influenced home care of the sick in a similar manner. Also, the development of rapid transportation and advanced communication by telephone and other media has brought people closer together in point of time. For all these reasons the old-fashioned doctor book is no longer necessary and in many ways the home is better off without it.

When we speak of the inability of the non-medical person to make a diagnosis and to provide treatment for an illness, we do not in any way intend to reflect upon his intelligence. It is not a matter of intelligence but of education and experience. Many diseases are deceptively similar, and symptoms can be gravely misleading. A diagnosis involves not only the observation of a symptom or what doctors often call the principal complaint, but getting medical history from the patient. Such questions may not appear to be leading to immediate relief of the chief complaint, but they serve an important purpose. Often they give the first inkling of what may be the underlying cause for the principal symptom.

After a good history has been taken, an adequate physical examination must be made. Frequently the direction and the extent of this examination are guided by the information derived from the health history.

Next comes the appropriate use of laboratory tests. Most are relatively new and they are frequently regarded as much more infallible than they really are. These tests have tended to overshadow other phases of medical diagnosis in the mind of the patient. Actually, the test is merely a confirmation and an accessory to a diagnosis which the doctor has already made. There are so many tests that if the doctor were to order all of them, both the patient and his pocketbook would be exhausted. The doctor must at least have a tentative diagnosis in order to know which confirmatory tests are needed.

When all this procedure has been accomplished, the doctor must then sum up the points that he has derived from the history, the examination, the laboratory tests, and perhaps most important of all, he must put together and summarize all available facts pertaining to the patient. Sir William Osler, perhaps the most famous of all modern physicians, observed that it is much less important what disease the patient has than what kind of a patient has the disease. This observation is the basis of successful medical treatment. The doctor treats the patient not the disease.

The homemaker, no matter how intelligent or how highly educated in the arts and crafts, in other professions, or in other branches of science, is unable to bring modern medical procedures into the home by possessing and reading a book. She is lacking in experience, especially in the observation of patients, which helps the doctor develop that sixth sense which he needs to aid his other five senses. The homemaker also lacks the wide background of technical knowledge which is required to interpret so "simple" a thing as a headache, a feeling of numbness, a pain, an itch, a weakness, or a trembling.

Hippocrates, the father of medicine, 400 years before Christ made the statement that "time is short, the art long, the occasion instant, decision difficult." This is the problem that faces the physician. This is why no "doctor book" can take the place of the doctor. It is our hope, however, that while we cannot put a substitute for your physician into your home, we can help you to understand and appreciate healthful patterns of living.

Aside from the many things which the homemaker cannot do and for which she must rely upon professional assistance, there are innumerable things which the homemaker can do. Beginning with the location of the home, its design, its maintenance, and its safety and proceeding on to the numerous other phases of healthful living, the homemaker can create an atmosphere, a "climate," in which health will be favored, disease discouraged, life prolonged, and above all enriched.

It is this prolongation and enrichment of life for which this book is intended. We hope that you will find it useful.

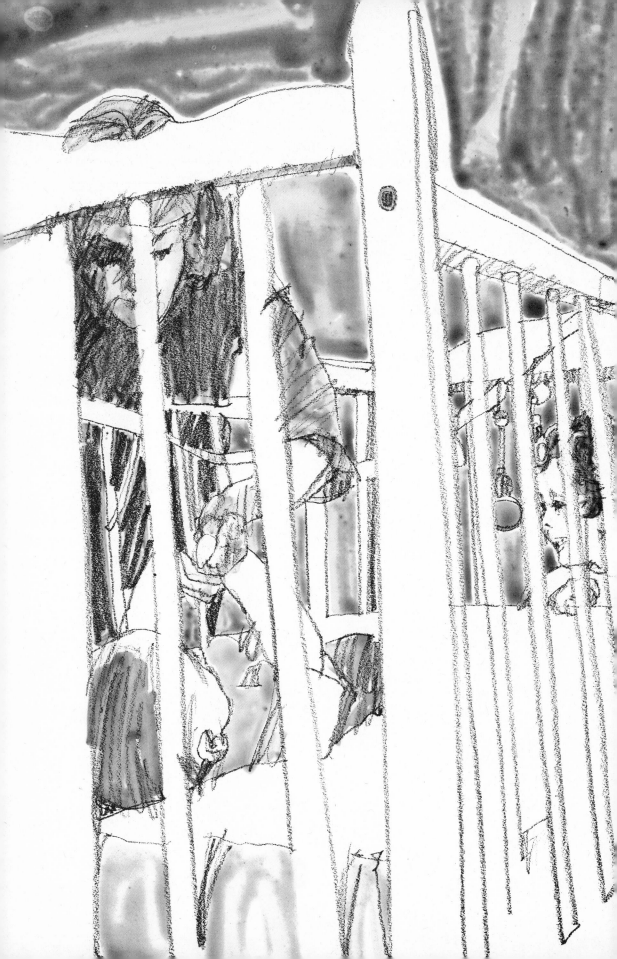

PART II

Health
and Your Family

CHAPTER ONE

HEALTH FACTORS IN THE HOME

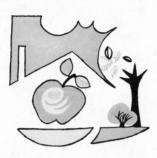

AMERICANS LIVE in everything from houseboats to tree houses and from shanties to mansions. Some cherish the isolation of the desert hut or the mountain cabin while others love their cliffhouse apartments in the city. Rural, suburban, and urban living all have their advocates by the scores of millions.

If Ben Franklin were living today, he might well urge "costly thy *house* as thy purse can buy." This is merely to say that a good home is worth what it costs. What you can afford to spend, you should spend; for the good home pays dividends far beyond its value in shelter. The enjoyment of family and community living, the pleasures of gracious entertaining, and sheer physical comfort are but a few examples of the benefits to be gained from life in a superior dwelling.

While no two homes are alike, all good homes share certain common characteristics. Your home may have them all and you may still seek a better dwelling. If on the other hand your home lacks some of these features, perhaps you can add them.

For the Sake of Comfort

Nearly all homes protect their tenants' lives by sheltering them from bitter cold or blazing heat. The good home goes a step further by providing comfort as well as protection. Thus does man strive to alter his environment rather than to adapt to it.

The ideal house can be readily warmed in winter and kept reasonably cool in summer.

Indoor temperatures in winter should be fairly steady, around 70° for active, healthy people (measured at knee height), higher for people at rest and for the infirm, and lower for sleeping. Winter comfort within a home is determined mostly by air and wall temperatures. (Humidity and air circulation are somewhat less important factors.)

Air temperature can be controlled only by heating devices—fireplaces, stoves, or furnace—and by ventilation. Wall temperatures result from outdoor temperatures and from the wall's construction. Everyone knows that it feels cooler in front of a window than next to an insulated wall. In front of the window we lose our own body heat faster and thus tend to chill more readily. Too rapid loss of body heat makes us uncomfortable.

Temperatures within the home normally vary more in summer than in winter. In summer, humidity and air circulation are the most important factors in body comfort because low humidity and moving air help us to lose body heat. Summertime discomfort stems from too little loss of body heat.

Insulation tends to make the home more comfortable the year around and helps cut winter heating costs. Thermostats likewise make for comfort by helping to maintain uniform temperatures.

Cross-ventilation is a must for summertime comfort. Air conditioning remains beyond the reach of a great many people, comfortable though it is. Air delivered by the fans of air conditioners is actually purer than "fresh" outdoor air, because it is filtered or washed.

Air free from dust and unpleasant odors is much to be sought. Fumes, gases, and vapors such as carbon monoxide, artificial, and natural gas are dangerous or even deadly.

Within the home, the most common sources of unpleasant odors are the human body and cooking. Both can be kept to a minimum by the reasonable practice of personal cleanliness and by adequate ventilation. During the summertime odors can enter from the outside from improperly stored garbage and rubbish and from animal droppings on the premises.

In winter enough ventilation is secured—even in well constructed homes—from air leakage through porous walls and ceilings and around doors and windows. Just as we may safely occupy a home in daytime in winter with windows closed, so is it healthful to sleep at night with closed windows. In the winter air does not need to be cold to be fresh. On the other hand, night air differs in no way from daytime air. Those who like to sleep in a cold room with windows open are free to do so, but should recognize that it is a matter of individual preference and not a question of health. Cold air advocates should also remember they are running up their heating costs.

In summer, with windows and doors normally open, fresh air has free play. Here the rural dweller is best off, the suburban resident is a close second, and the urbanite a poor third. Fumes, odors, soot, and grime are the lot of the latter the year around, and usually are worst near the center of a city and in areas of heavy industrial activity.

Proper Lighting

At the latitude of Washington, D.C., window glass area in a good home should equal about 15 per cent of its floor area. In general, more glass is needed farther north and somewhat less will do farther south.

Every occupied room, bathrooms included, should have at least one window providing the greatest possible illumination and this, insofar as possible, without glare or shadow. Glare is controllable by drapes and shades, of which the venetian blind is probably the best for this purpose. Rooms that are shaded by trees, tall buildings, or porches need proportionately more window space.

Direct sunlight is often advantageous, especially in winter and particularly for the ill or infirm. It is physically and psychologically stimulating and, if properly admitted, a remarkable fuel saver.

Even when the best natural illumination has been obtained, glare-free artificial lighting must be added. There is no substitute for electric lighting, generously applied, especially for reading, studying, sewing, and similar tasks. Whether you use incandescent or fluorescent lighting is a matter of choice; fluorescent is more economical.

Noise takes its toll in tension, frayed nerves, and short tempers. Here again the rural and suburban dwellers are apt to have the better of it. Their urban cousins would do well for their health to block out screeching factory whistles, sirens, raucous traffic, and related sounds as much as possible. Air conditioning in city apartments is as useful for keeping noise out as for bringing cool fresh air in.

In a house with children, space is as much a matter of comfort as of health. A rainy day in crowded quarters can become as nerve-wracking for the children as for their mother.

Play areas should also include outdoor space as well as room inside the home. If the home is on a farm or a ranch there is obviously room for all. In towns or cities, small yards may be compensated for by adequate nearby parks, especially if they are well equipped. Such facilities must be considered among the rights, as well as the delights, of childhood.

For the Sake of Mental Health

The human spirit being what it is, people need both privacy and generous portions of companionship. Too much solitude requires relief through the company of others. Too much of the world's noise and tension, plus normal bits of family bickering, entitle parent and child alike to the release and relaxation that privacy alone can provide.

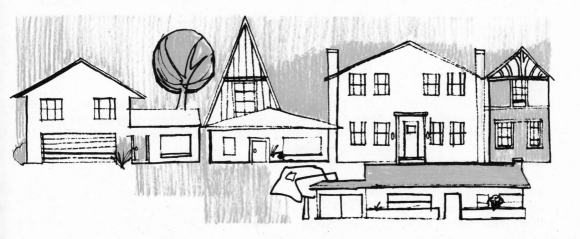

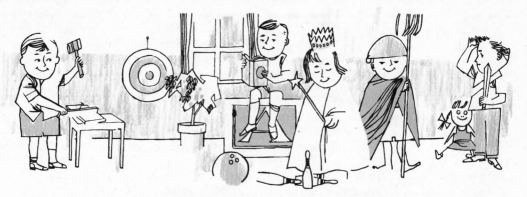

In the interest of privacy "a room of my own" is ideal. A room shared with but one other person is next best, of course. Except for married couples and young children, rooms should be shared only by persons of the same sex. Separation of sexes should occur by age eight or by age ten at the latest. For sleeping, young children should be separated from their parents early, and certainly by the age of two.

Toilets, bathrooms, and bedrooms should be directly accessible without the need to pass through other bedrooms.

Normal family life provides those social contacts expected in the home and in the community. People cannot be mentally healthy without them. Even prisons no longer isolate felons except in emergencies.

A suitable dwelling should have a living room or family room, one or more gathering places, plus kitchen, dining room or area, and whatever bedrooms and bathrooms the family may need and can afford. The need for companionship as well as for privacy, as moods change from time to time, can thus be satisfied to help keep the family happy.

Some modern apartment structures provide much in the way of building-wide services that are usually expected in the average home. In addition to heat, there may be laundry rooms, recreation or "family" rooms for giving parties, even nurseries, workshops, and spare bedrooms that families may rent when they have guests.

Some families may occupy one dwelling for a lifetime, enduring a measure of crowding as the family increases in size and later enjoying perhaps too much space as children leave home. Others move to larger or smaller houses or apartments according to the space they need. Each method has points in its favor. The first accepts a bit of crowding at times in return for community stature and stability. The second more nearly assures enough space at all times.

It goes without saying that the good home, in addition to providing space for its young children, must afford opportunity for youth to meet persons of the opposite sex under wholesome circumstances.

Some opportunity shades over into community responsibility also. Recreational facilities and libraries plus the usual marks of our culture—the shopping district, the church, and the school—all should be reasonably close at hand. And, though commuting is the lot of many, it is desirable that the bread-winner's job should not be too far away.

Cleanliness and Orderliness

The mentally healthy, well-adjusted person can abide extremes of cleanliness and tidiness for short periods and can put up with disorder and disarray when necessary. But most persons prefer to live in a state between these extremes.

The good home will have facilities to ease the fatigue of the housewife's 60 hour week. Direct and easy access to storage, cooking, dishwashing, laundering, ironing, garbage and refuse disposal are a few examples from among dozens of regular tasks. It is unreasonable to have to carry supplies up and refuse down three to seven floors, as it is necessary in some older apartments.

Circulation within the home, the ability to move with ease and purpose, is of primary importance to the whole family. Such things as narrow doors or halls, crooks and turns and unexpected step-downs reduce the home's liveability.

Cleanliness demands water, in plenty, at the right places, much of it hot, and under proper pressure. Water so supplied makes the home a different world from one where water must be carried and heated on a stove. Plenty of water inevitably means cleaner people in a cleaner

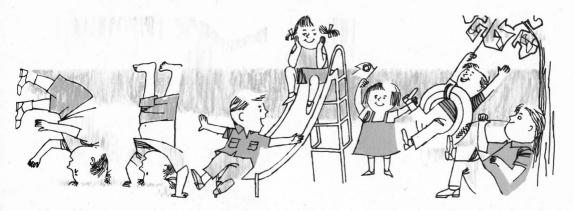

home. No harm can come from getting dirty, either in honest labor or zestful play. Staying dirty is quite another matter. Oddly, to be always filthy or always spotlessly clean marks one as being abnormal, perhaps emotionally disturbed. (See Part V, Chapter One.)

The appeal of beauty is so universal that the good home will exhibit many attempts to create the beautiful. What succeeds in one home may fail in another, but the attempt will usually be made and should be encouraged. Success and satisfaction along these lines are emotionally stimulating and uplifting. Beauty for the sake of beauty needs no justification.

In like manner, a home marked by lack of beauty, poorly maintained and not in keeping with those around it, is an ever-present cause of feelings of inferiority and of emotional stress, particularly in children. While we generally deplore the tendency to keep up with the Joneses, we should not be too remarkably unlike them.

The Control of Contagious Diseases

Though contagious and infectious diseases no longer play the major role they once did in American life, their combined toll is still significant. The kind of homes people live in, their size, design, and quality have a great deal to do with the amount of illness caused by communicable disease.

No house can be built that will entirely prevent contagious diseases among the occupants, but it goes without saying that well built homes give better protection than do jerry-built huts.

Safe Water and Proper Sewage Disposal

Enough good, safe water is a priceless heritage for a nation and a treasure in any home. Ideally it will be under pressure, as in a municipal supply, or through an automatic pump arrangement. It must not be subject to contamination by disposal of waste materials. Hopefully it will be free of objectionable tastes, odors, and chemicals.

With the nation becoming more and more densely populated, pure water—safe for domestic use—is becoming harder and harder to find. It is necessary, therefore, to protect, insofar as possible, all water supplies, whether for the giant city or for the single rural or suburban dwelling.

The greatest threat to a good water supply is raw, untreated sewage. In many areas of the country industrial wastes run a close second as a threat. Again, this is true whether speaking of a large city or an isolated home.

Sewage and industrial wastes therefore should be carefully collected and treated before being discharged into our waterways. Water, in turn, should be given adequate treatment before being used for domestic purposes. The drinking of water of unknown quality is a clear and present danger, an open invitation to attack by any of a number of serious diseases.

Fortunately, mankind has been able to devise methods of treating sewage and industrial wastes successfully. Also, it is completely feasible to use and reuse treated water as it passes to the sea. Some cities and some homes, drawing their water from safe deep wells, are spared some of the tremendous expense of treating it to bring it up to drinking water standards. Even good water should be chlorinated to assure safety.

All domestic water supplies, whether public or private, should be tested periodically for purity. Every consumer is entitled to know there is no risk of contamination.

In spite of the tremendous knowledge built up in this field there is much water of questionable quality in daily use in this country. The old-time pit privy has not disappeared from the

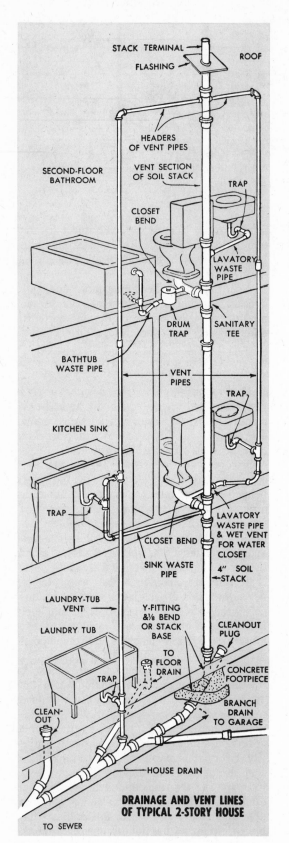

STACK TERMINAL

FLASHING — ROOF

HEADERS
OF VENT PIPES

SECOND-FLOOR
BATHROOM

VENT SECTION
OF SOIL STACK

TRAP

CLOSET
BEND

LAVATORY
WASTE
PIPE

DRUM
TRAP

SANITARY
TEE

BATHTUB
WASTE PIPE

VENT
PIPES

KITCHEN SINK

TRAP

TRAP

LAVATORY
WASTE PIPE
& WET VENT
FOR WATER
CLOSET

CLOSET BEND

SINK WASTE
PIPE

4" SOIL
STACK

LAUNDRY-TUB
VENT

Y-FITTING
&⅛ BEND
OR STACK
BASE

LAUNDRY TUB

CLEANOUT
PLUG

TO
FLOOR
DRAIN

TRAP

CONCRETE
FOOTPIECE

CLEAN-
OUT

BRANCH
DRAIN
TO GARAGE

HOUSE DRAIN

**DRAINAGE AND VENT LINES
OF TYPICAL 2-STORY HOUSE**

TO SEWER

face of the land. Such practice contaminates the ground water and the wells in some rural areas. Subdivisions in rapidly-growing areas outside city or village boundaries are sometimes provided only with septic tanks instead of sewer systems. Sooner or later this is likely to cause trouble and expense.

Just as water must be protected before it is brought into a home and as sewage must be properly handled as it leaves, so must care be exercised within the home. This involves having correctly installed, leak-proof plumbing, with no possible cross-connection between water pipes and sewer lines. The possibility of such an occurrence seems beyond belief, but cross-connections do occur with distressing frequency, and have been responsible for many outbreaks of water-borne disease.

Protection Against Vermin

Man's most health-endangering enemies around the home are rats, flies, and mosquitoes. Other vermin, such as roaches, may not be implicated in the spread of disease, but should be eliminated for general health reasons. All can under given circumstances cause disease, so that necessary measures to keep them out, or to destroy them, are implicit in the good home. Sound construction and screening are the principle weapons. Rats and flies are attracted primarily by food. Thus, you can generally keep them away by storing all garbage and rubbish in containers that are fly-tight and rodent-proof.

Pets and fleas go together like macaroni and cheese. Lice cannot always be avoided, particularly head lice encountered at school. Some ticks are to be expected, particularly by persons who love forest and field.

Feces from large pets such as dogs, deposited on the dwelling premises, are frequently causes of odor and fly infestation. During the summer months, such conditions account for the majority of citizens' complaints reaching health departments. Such nuisances are an abuse of neighborliness as well as a menace to health and an affront to decency. Complaints to public authority are usually a last resort and are seldom effective. The real solution is neighborly observance of the Golden Rule.

All vermin are to be combatted on general principles, whether they are of disease-producing or merely nuisance varieties. Reliable poisons exist to rid the home if they are applied successfully at the time of invasion. These poisons must be properly used.

Food Protection

American industry, on the whole, provides us fresh foods and milk beyond compare. Most of it requires good refrigeration to keep it so. Every home should be able to keep foods at 50° or lower. Failure to do so is to invite trouble from any of a number of disease-producing agents.

Removing food from the refrigerator, using part of it, and allowing the remainder to stand and grow warm, is a particularly bad habit to acquire. Unused portions should be returned promptly so they will stay cold.

Contact Infection

It is obvious, and experience has proved time and again, that crowding promotes the spread of certain infectious diseases. Influenza and the common cold are typical examples. While no house can be built big enough to guarantee the occupants protection against contact diseases, overcrowded homes definitely are harmful in this respect. Sleeping space seems to be particularly important.

Bedrooms should provide 50 or more square feet per person and beds should be 3 or more feet apart, especially in case of illnesses of a communicable nature. Thus, tiered bunks or double-deck beds are undesirable.

For the Sake of Safety

Home safety implies a sound structure, reasonably fire-resistant, and not likely to collapse under the impact of the locality's most rigorous weather. In urban and suburban communities, building codes serve to insure these conditions. Rural dwellers, despite the many compensations of rural living, probably would profit by the application of some of the rules required under city building codes.

Different areas of our immense nation decree different building methods. Much of Florida long ago went to hurricane-proof housing. Earthquakes must be considered on the West Coast. Most Texas roofs, on the other hand, do not need the strength to withstand the weight of snowfall measured in feet.

Homes have varying degrees of fire-resistance. Whether in the magnificent urban apartment housing hundreds of people, or in more modest domiciles, reasonable fire-resistance and accessible exits to be used in case of fire are essential.

Involved in fire protection also are such things as construction of chimneys and flues, furnaces, stoves, and electrical wiring. Automatic circuit breakers are coming to replace the older style of fuse box, but the dangers of the penny inserted behind the burned out fuse still exist, as do many other hazards created by carelessness or ignorance.

We may or may not approve of the trends in American family living which tend to attract members away from the home. We still spend a lot of time there. In industry, despite its safety precautions and close supervision, we have accidents. On the highway, in spite of the best of engineering, policing, and regulation, we have accidents. But at home we have even more accidents than anywhere else. Perhaps we are less wary, our guard is down, and we are freer to do as we please.

Some of the worst home booby traps are:
- poor lighting;
- stairways that are too narrow, too steep, too crooked;
- winding stairways with inadequate tread on the inner side of the curve and no handrail along the wall;
- toys, stools, chairs, or ladders out of place, left where the unwary may trip over them;
- low window sills that lead to falls by careless leaners, especially children;
- bathrooms with slick floor, tub, or shower surfaces, and inadequate holds or grab-bars;
- electrical fixtures or outlets that can be reached while standing in water;
- two-way swinging doors;
- sharp turns that can lead to collisions;
- carbon monoxide from inadequate stove, heater, or fireplace flues or from a leak of either natural or artificial fuel gas;
- burns, from an endless number of causes;
- electrical shocks;
- toxic vapors, as from cleaners and solvents, as well as insecticides improperly and too extensively used;
- explosions;
- poisonings.

Merely to catalog the diversity and perversity of American home accidents would consume a whole volume, but the National Safety Council has done it and will provide information, aid, and advice to all who seek it. (See Part VII for further information on safety.)

Safe living and maintaining good health involve the same basic principles whether one lives in the city or on a farm. However, there are problems and hazards peculiar to rural living not experienced elsewhere. The proper handling of toxic farm chemicals such as insecticide sprays, the safe use of dangerous farm machines, the utilization of techniques to prevent spread of animal diseases to humans, provision for pure water, and adequate sewage disposal for the farm home are but some of the many areas which should be of special concern to farm families. (See Part VII, Chapter Six.)

The Rural Home

If unnecessary illnesses and accidents are to be prevented on the farm, a thorough knowledge of the dangers and how to prevent unfortunate results is essential. Knowledge of the toxic potential of the many chemical products used in the home and on the farm is needed. The majority of farm chemicals are adequately labelled as to proper precautions in using. It is failure to follow instructions or not even reading the instructions which most often give rise to serious consequences. Proper storage of chemicals away from children is important.

On the farm, petroleum products are often swallowed by young children. Keeping the fuel supply under lock and inaccessible to children would save many needless instances of serious or fatal poisonings. The use of the various pesticides about the farm is becoming increasingly a part of good farming techniques. Certainly these products should be used with the utmost caution including the use of the protective clothing when advocated by the manufacturer.

There are said to be some 40 diseases transmitted from animal to man and vice versa in the United States. Many cause serious disease in humans. These diseases are largely preventable through good animal husbandry.

Disease testing programs in animal herds are important in the eradication of diseases such as bovine tuberculosis and brucellosis. If milk produced on the farm is to be used by the farmer's family, it should be pasteurized in order to kill the disease germs. Certainly the veterinarian should be called upon whenever disease becomes apparent in an animal herd; his advice will protect the herd and guard in the control of diseases which can be transmitted to humans.

Farm accidents are almost entirely preventable. Constant use of the safety mechanisms provided by the manufacturers of farm equipment, keeping hands and feet away from moving parts on a machine at all times, using tractors for their intended purpose in the farm operation rather than as a means of locomotion —oftentimes over a rough and hazardous terrain—would save many limbs and many lives. Long hours in operating a piece of farm equipment in the field without periods of adequate rest results in undue fatigue which can also be responsible for farm machine accidents.

Water used on the farm for human consumption can carry serious disease germs. Certainly the water supply should be tested for harmful ingredients, both chemical and bacterial. Your local health officer or your family physician will inform you as to where containers may be obtained and placed to collect samples of water for testing. This water testing service is provided by most state departments of health.

Proper disposal of sewage and other wastes is important to good health on the farm. Information pertaining to safe sewage disposal can also be obtained from your department of health, either local or state. Your family physician will be able to provide you with the information as to whom you should contact.

Physicians, the AMA, state and local medical societies, the various farm organizations, the extension services, and others, are to be commended for the improved health status that has already been achieved in rural areas. However, new problems are constantly arising. Through the coordinated efforts of all who are interested, improved rural health can be obtained. County health departments in growing numbers are a source of valuable information, advice, and assistance in meeting health problems in rural areas.

A Good Home is Worth Working For

Having touched upon some, but by no means all, of the things that can work for good or ill around our homes, it seems hardly necessary to urge Americans to seek always to improve their lot in this regard. It is an American habit to make it better, build it bigger, or render it more attractive and useful. Almost nowhere could this outlook on life be more profitably applied than in the development of our homes. If the labor is great, the benefits are greater—and not the least of these is the blessing of better health.

CHAPTER TWO

HEALTH AND THE EXPECTANT MOTHER

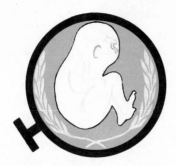

THE IMMINENT ARRIVAL of a baby in a home (especially the first) presages many changes in the home and in family life. But the first and most important consideration is the health of the mother-to-be and the unborn child.

If the expectant mother has a family physician, the task of choosing a doctor is relatively easy. Thousands of family physicians successfully care for millions of mothers and babies every year. Thus the family physician himself may well care for the mother during pregnancy and childbirth, and later for the baby. If, however, he chooses not to do so, he will help the family choose an obstetrician and pediatrician. Good medical care is available in either case. In the event of complications, obstetrical consultation may be necessary, but for the most part, childbirth is usually an uncomplicated procedure.

Prenatal Care

The proper care of unborn generations of Americans is one of the most important projects facing our nation. It is vital that we provide the best facilities and protection available for this important group of our society.

This should begin with proper instruction in our schools, especially for the girls. It should be impossible for a girl to graduate from high school without having learned the fundamental facts about her own body and its functions, and about how to care for a newborn child.

It is further important to realize that the child is father to the man and that the boy in his teens will soon be heading his own home, responsible for the health and welfare of three or more people. The more he knows about the reproduction of his species, the better off he and his marital partner and their offsprings will be.

Many states require couples to have a medical examination within 15 days before marriage to determine the absence of venereal infection.

However, a proper premarital medical examination should cover much more. The couple should have a complete physical examination including examination of heart and lungs, and/or the genital tract to see if any abnormalities or deformities of these organs are present. The blood pressure should be taken to determine if it is higher or lower than normal. The urine must be tested for albumin or other evidence of kidney damage, and for sugar. After such an examination a physician can usually give reassurance that there are no abnormalities.

If abnormalities are found, especially with the bride-to-be, their significance in the light of possible pregnancies should be frankly discussed. The possible dangers, and how they should be treated, may be outlined.

Minor abnormalities can be treated immediately. For example, a tough or thick hymen may be dilated slightly or incised if it is thought to be necessary. Cervical polyps, if present, can be treated. These precautions will help to prevent needless apprehension, pain, and embarrassment after marriage.

When is Pregnancy Most Likely

The details of the origin of human life are given in Chapter Five of this section which discusses the immediate factors in pregnancy and childbirth. Among the first questions is, "When is pregnancy most likely to occur?"

Assuming that the woman has a normal menstrual cycle of 28 days and that this is reasonably regular, the date of ovulation (when the ovum is discharged from the ovary) can be calculated with fair accuracy. When the cycle is irregular, this becomes more difficult, and the greater the irregularity, the less likely it is that the period of greatest fertility can be estimated.

Since fertilization depends on the meeting of the ovum with a living sperm, the most likely time for fertilization to occur is at the time of

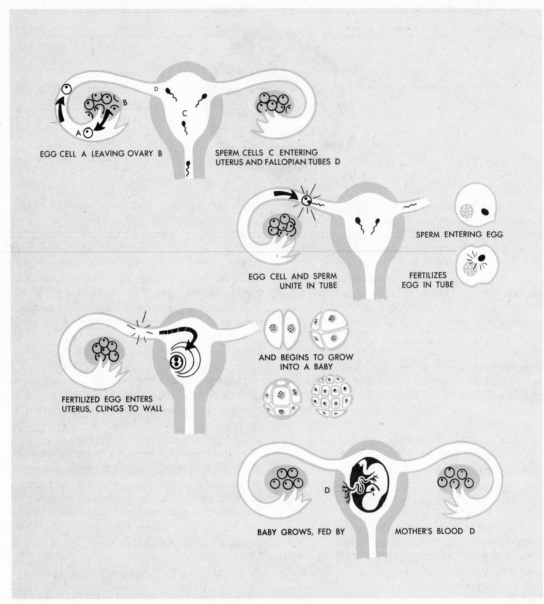

EGG CELL A LEAVING OVARY B   SPERM CELLS C ENTERING
                                    UTERUS AND FALLOPIAN TUBES D

EGG CELL AND SPERM   SPERM ENTERING EGG
UNITE IN TUBE

                            FERTILIZES
                            EGG IN TUBE

AND BEGINS TO GROW
INTO A BABY

FERTILIZED EGG ENTERS
UTERUS, CLINGS TO WALL

BABY GROWS, FED BY   MOTHER'S BLOOD D

ovulation. The life-span of the unfertilized human ovum is unknown, but is perhaps less than 24 hours. Fertilized ova require four to five days to progress from the end of the fallopian tube to the uterus. The sperm likewise lives for about 36 to 48 hours after being discharged into the vagina. The most fertile time therefore comes midway between the first days of two successive menstrual periods in a regular cycle. The least fertile periods are normally those times most remote from the central point in time when the ovum is discharged. Pregnancies, however, have been known to occur at all stages of the menstrual cycle, so there is no time when a pregnancy may be regarded as out of the question.

Knowledge of the normal fertility cycle is useful in planning the family—when children are desired as well as when they are not. Family planning is discussed in Chapter Five.

Signs and Symptoms of Pregnancy

The signs and symptoms of pregnancy vary greatly in different women and at different states of pregnancy. During the early weeks they are vague, but become more clear in time.

The missing of a menstrual period is probably evidence that pregnancy exists if periods have previously been regular. However, some women menstruate more regularly than others because of their physiological and psychological constitutions. A period may be delayed a week or more as a result of such simple causes as nervous shock, bad news, change of climate, or acute infections. If, however, added to this symptom there is a feeling of nausea on arising in the morning or at various times during the day, especially if this is associated with the odor of cooking, the presumption of pregnancy is strong. In early pregnancy, the breasts become larger and there is more tingling and soreness of the nipples. The pressure of the enlarging uterus upon the bladder may result in greater frequency of urination. Nervous instability and an abnormal desire for unaccustomed foods such as sour pickles is normal.

After the second missed period, a special test (Friedman) can be made using an immature female rabbit and injecting into her vein 10 cc. of the patient's filtered urine. After 48 hours the rabbit is killed, the abdomen opened, and the ovaries exposed. If there are certain changes in the rabbit's ovaries which are characteristic of pregnancy, it can be correctly assumed in 85 per cent of cases that the woman is pregnant.

Another test using frogs as the test animal gives about the same percentage of correct diagnoses. Thus, these tests can be depended upon only to supplement other findings in diagnosing pregnancy.

There is also a tablet test in which the patient is given hormone pills when she has missed a period. If she is not pregnant, she menstruates within two or three days.

More recent simple tests for pregnancy are based on the immune reaction of the woman's body to the hormones secreted by the placenta (afterbirth). These are detected by skin tests which require only a few hours, and are very simple to perform. Tests based on chemical estimation of hormones in the urine are also in use and, by making an internal examination, the doctor can usually tell whether the uterus is enlarged and softened and whether the other local changes characteristic of pregnancy have taken place.

The Months of Pregnancy

The early diagnosis of pregnancy is of great importance. In the 1930's and earlier, pregnancy and childbirth accounted for 60 or more deaths of mothers for every 1,000 babies born alive. Currently this loss is only about 3 mothers per 10,000 babies born alive—a reduction of 95 per cent. This tremendous improvement has made pregnancy safer—literally—than crossing a busy street. The progress is due to two principal factors: recognition that most pregnancies are normal and that labor should be allowed to progress without interference unless there are complications; and the growing practice of maternal supervision during the entire pregnancy.

If the expectant mother sees her doctor regularly at the intervals which he suggests, she gives him an opportunity to observe her progress, control her weight, and take prompt measures to correct any abnormalities which may appear. Through observation, examinations, urinalyses, and blood pressure readings, he is able to detect threatened toxemias due to liver or kidney failure and to watch the growth of the baby and its position in the uterus. The usual schedule of visits is once a month for the first seven months; thereafter at such intervals as the mother's condition requires.

Obstetrical History

When taking the patient's health history the doctor will inquire about illnesses which the patient has experienced involving heart, lungs, and abdomen, especially rheumatic heart disease, diabetes, German measles, surgical operations, and their dates and circumstances. He will wish to know about diseases in the patient's family and that of her husband. The menstrual history as regards amount, duration, regularity, and type of blood, and whether she has leukorrheal (whites) discharge will be discussed, together with any known pelvic abnormalities or disease. Previous pregnancies, if any, their dates, and outcome will be recorded.

Physical Examination

When pregnancy seems likely, a thorough examination is in order. Many young women look upon this with considerable apprehension. This is one of the difficult mental hazards to be overcome. In reality, it is a very simple and very necessary procedure. The doctor must know certain anatomical and physiological facts which he can obtain only by making a complete examination. This will determine if there are any physical defects which must be considered in connection with the management of the pregnancy. The heart, lungs, teeth, nervous system, kidneys, blood, and blood pressure are investigated. Defects, if found, are re-corded and treatment recommended to remedy them before the onset of labor.

A careful pelvic examination is made to dis-close if bony deformities or tumors are present which might obstruct the passage of a baby. For a patient to be examined thoroughly, she must remove sufficient clothing so that the doc-tor may have ready access to the organs being examined, thus saving time and permitting a more accurate diagnosis. The examination find-ings are carefully recorded on a chart, by the nurse, for later comparison.

Laboratory examinations which are impor-tant in pregnancy are:

1. *Urine analysis* which determines the abil-ity of the kidneys to do their work properly. This is very important; the patient will be asked to bring one or two ounces of urine to the doc-tor in a clean bottle each time she comes for a prenatal examination. Urine should be col-lected according to the specific directions of her physician.

2. *Blood count and hemoglobin estimation.* This is especially important because many women are anemic before becoming pregnant or become anemic during pregnancy, and all are faced with the possibility of blood loss dur-ing labor and after delivery. Since this cannot be anticipated in most cases, it seems logical to estimate the amount of blood a patient has and how much she is apt to lose. Typing her blood will greatly assist the doctor. Similar blood can then be made available for transfusion and cross-matched with hers at a few minutes' no-tice, if necessary.

Blood tests are also important to determine the Rh factor to prevent a possible severe trans-fusion reaction or even injury to the unborn baby. The Wassermann or Kahn test is also done routinely. If positive, it usually means that the patient has syphilis, and if treatment can be started before the 16th week of preg-nancy, the baby will not be infected and the mother will get the benefit of immediate medi-cal treatment.

3. *X-ray examinations* may be necessary in exceptional circumstances to determine the presence of the developing baby, and its pre-sentation and position. When recommended, such examinations are entirely safe for mother and baby. Deformity in the pelvic bones, tumor masses which might prevent normal delivery, and the presence of twins or triplets can also be determined by x-ray.

4. *Blood pressure* is taken to detect any sig-nificant rise above normal that might indicate a possible toxic condition in the mother which could be dangerous.

Growth of the Fetus

The baby begins to move within the uterus with sufficient vigor to be felt by the mother at about the 20th week, if it is her first pregnancy, and at about the 18th if she has previously had a baby. This is called "quickening" or "feeling of life." At first the movement is a weak flutter, but later vigorous kicks are felt. Along about the time the fourth period has been missed or a few weeks earlier, the size of the abdomen be-comes markedly greater and continues to in-crease as time goes on. The stretching of the skin of the abdomen gives rise to streaks of a silvery or pink color. These never completely disappear after pregnancy, but the color be-comes silvery after a few weeks or months.

The baby grows at a regular rate so that the degree of development is an index to the length of the pregnancy. The length of the fetus in centimeters equals the square of the month of pregnancy; one month equals 1 cm., two months equals 4 cm., three months 9 cm. After the 5th month of gestation the fetus grows 5 cm. in length every month until the 10th lunar month. During this period the nervous system, lungs, liver, kidneys, heart, and other vital or-gans develop and become functional so that a baby born after the 28th week can usually sur-vive if properly cared for. However, every week that the baby spends in the uterus until the full 280 days have passed is so much clear gain as far as its strength, maturity, and ability to sur-vive is concerned. For this reason it is advisable to try to prevent the onset of premature labor whenever possible.

Diet

Except for limitation of the daily calorie in-take, the diet of the expectant mother does not differ from that of any adult who pays proper attention to the intake of all essential food-stuffs. A good general diet includes proteins, meat, eggs, and fish. Red meats are particularly important during pregnancy because they fur-nish hemoglobin which will be stored in the liver, spleen, and bone marrow, and used to make new blood cells and thus protect from the dangers of anemia due to hemorrhage if this oc-curs. Necessary minerals such as calcium, phosphorus and manganese are also supplied

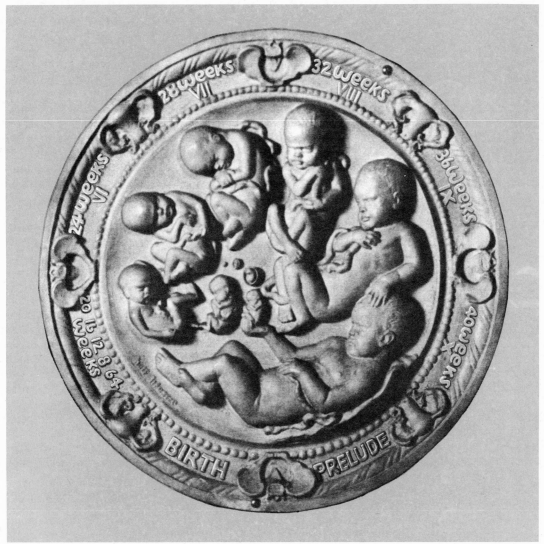

Ten fetal and embryonic stages are shown above. Largest fetus is holding three-month embryo in his hand.

through foods and transferred from the blood through the placenta to the baby. Fruits, vegetables, dairy products, cereals, and some meats contain vitamins necessary for the health of both mother and child.

Weight control is of the greatest importance to the pregnant woman, both during her pregnancy and afterward. Excess weight puts an extra burden on the liver and kidneys, which already carry an overload. It adds to her discomfort, especially in the later months when the abdomen becomes enlarged. It increases the likelihood of permanent marking on her skin. It also impairs her figure after the baby is born.

Most physicians limit a woman's gain during pregnancy to 20 pounds. The need for careful control of diet under the doctor's supervision cannot be emphasized too strongly. (See Part IV, Chapter Three for a full discussion of diet and nutrition.)

Digestive Disturbances

Most women have some nausea with or without vomiting in the early weeks of pregnancy—due probably to the adjustment that has to be made in the function of the thyroid and other glands of internal secretion. Certain changes in their functions are important in the initiation and maintenance of pregnancy. Constipation bothers many pregnant women, but it can usually be controlled by the eating of sufficient fruits and vegetables and by the avoidance of a diet that seems to produce constipation. The doctor will suggest additional measures for bowel stimulation if necessary.

Diarrhea is usually due to some indiscretion in the diet and should be checked promptly if severe because it may stimulate uterine contractions and even bring on miscarriage, especially in the early months. For this reason all severe reactions of this type should be reported to the doctor, who may prescribe medicine or other measures to control it. A bland diet of custard, milk, and cheese is helpful. If the nausea persists the doctor will probably advise hospitalization for further study and treatment.

"Heartburn" or sour stomach is frequently present in the early months. Ordinarily this occurs about one hour after meals and can usually be controlled by taking one-half teaspoonful of baking soda in a glass of water or a few soda mint tablets.

Exercise and Rest

Every pregnant woman in normal health should take some form of exercise. Walking, swimming, rowing, and other comparable activities are advised in moderation. Diving, horseback riding, and other sports in which the hazards of blows or falls are great are best avoided. The amount of exercise taken depends on how the woman reacts to it. If she feels refreshed after a rest, the exercise has been beneficial. Any spotting, bleeding, or uterine cramps, however, indicate she should stop exercise until she has consulted her doctor.

A rest period of 20 minutes or so before noon will help the pregnant woman get through the day more comfortably. She should try to get eight hours of sleep at night if possible, and more if necessary. Fatigue is the enemy of the pregnant woman.

Back pains may be caused in later pregnancy by loosening of the sacroiliac joints. This condition can be helped by the use of a properly fitted maternity corset which supports the joints. Dry or moist heat applied to the lower back on retiring is very soothing.

Dental Hygiene

Dental hygiene during pregnancy is particularly important. Pregnancy puts a drain on the body's calcium supply, and this may cause tooth decay. It was formerly believed that a woman had to lose "a tooth for every child."

An old wives' tale obviously, but it stresses what can happen during pregnancy. The best practice is to have teeth put in order in anticipation of a pregnancy. Dental work can be done during pregnancy, but is best done at a date removed from that at which menstruation would have been expected in the absence of pregnancy.

Dress

The most important item in a pregnant woman's dress is her shoes, both for comfort and safety. These should be well fitted, with low heels. "Wearing out" old and delapidated shoes during pregnancy is not only uncomfortable but dangerous, since they may cause falling.

In early pregnancy, up to the fourth month, one may wear ordinary clothing except for stockings. These should support the superficial veins of the legs because they tend to dilate during pregnancy. If veins remain dilated after pregnancy, varicose veins may result, which may require an operation for their correction. Good-looking supporting hose are available at drugstores and women's shops.

About the fifth month the distension of the abdomen by the pregnant uterus requires some form of girdle support. A well-fitted maternity corset with sacroiliac belt attachment can be obtained at any store handling women's apparel. This will help to prevent or relieve low backache when under physical strain and will furnish additional protection against cold weather.

It is particularly important for the pregnant woman to avoid chilling and to be well-protected against colds, sore throat, influenza, and other infections. Heavy underwear (pants) and stockings and overshoes to avoid cold and wet feet are recommended. Round garters are not desirable because they impede circulation and cause varicosities—particularly in the later months of pregnancy.

The Breasts

Much of the later health and well-being of the baby may depend on the mother's ability and willingness to nurse it. There is, in most cases, no other food which is quite as good. The primary reason for this is that immune substances transmitted to the baby from the mother protect it from the diseases which she has had and recovered from.

An additional reason for nursing the baby is

that many authorities believe it helps establish a sense of security in the baby and develops an emotional closeness which may help to prevent behavior problems as the baby grows up. Nursing is also a help in restoring the uterus to normal. Nursing the baby, however, is not a means of preventing conception, as is commonly believed.

During pregnancy nipples should be kept clean and made longer and softer by massage and *gentle* pulling using a cold cream or cocoa butter in the last three months to prevent inversion (turning inward). Rough handling must be avoided during pregnancy and while nursing the baby. Small breasts may undergo considerable development during pregnancy; if they become tender, a well-fitting brassiere gives considerable comfort. Occasionally they leak fluid near the time of delivery, and it may be necessary to wear a protective pad.

Miscarriage and Premature Labor

Most pregnancies end ten menstrual months (nine calendar months or about 280 days) after the first day of the last period or a few days sooner or later. If the end comes two or three weeks or more earlier, we speak of a premature labor; if two weeks to four weeks later, a postmature labor. If labor occurs before the 28th week it is called a miscarriage, unless it occurs before the 20th week in which case it is termed an abortion.

The symptoms of threatened abortion are cramps, a varying amount of bleeding, backache, and sometimes nausea. Some women have repeated abortions without any apparent cause. These may be associated with anatomical abnormalities in the uterus. A woman with such a history should have special tests made to determine this possibility so that she may have special treatment and advice. The doctor may start preventive treatment in anticipation of a planned pregnancy or before any signs of abortion have occurred. If these symptoms appear in a first pregnancy, the woman should go to bed, call the doctor, and follow his advice. If the bleeding is severe, it is best to call the doctor and then go to the hospital. The doctor can meet you there or telephone his instructions to the hospital staff, pending his own arrival. Many abortions may be prevented if proper treatment is started soon enough.

Predisposing factors to abortion should be especially avoided by women prone to this complication. These include violent exercise, heavy lifting, sexual intercourse, long automobile trips, overwork, excessive fatigue, painful dentistry, and exposure to infections.

Toxemia

One of the serious dangers that may develop during pregnancy is toxemia, medically called eclampsia, due to liver and kidney breakdown in the mother. This occurs because the additional waste products produced by the baby must be neutralized and passed out through the mother's kidneys. These organs may already be overworked because of the complex changes the pregnant woman undergoes and the additional metabolism necessary to carry through a pregnancy. This load gets heavier towards the end of pregnancy; and when the kidneys and liver cannot compensate for the strain, symptoms of an intoxication appear, such as a rise in blood pressure, sudden increase in weight, headache, and swelling of the feet and face and hands. If these are not relieved by treatment, convulsions and even death may occur. This is why the doctor insists on checking for these signs and symptoms at least once a month in the first six months and every two weeks or more often in the last three months. Women who have a history of kidney disease should be especially careful to observe symptoms and carefully follow out the doctor's instructions, especially toward the end of pregnancy. The onset of this toxic condition may be quite sudden in some cases. Fortunately, almost all cases can be handled by medical management. Cesarean section may have to be performed in severe cases.

Hospital Versus Home Delivery

In recent years, women have increasingly gone to hospitals to have their babies. This is especially true in the cities where home conditions are such that proper privacy and facilities for obstetrical care may be lacking and good hospital facilities are fairly close. Hospitals are prepared to take over the management of a case as soon as the patient arrives. Emergency deliveries can be carried out safely outside the birthroom, if necessary. Expert help can be mobilized rapidly to deal with any kind of complications. Nurses are on duty to assure proper administration of the doctor's orders and aides assist with diet, drinking water, clean linen, and moral support. If trouble should suddenly develop, trained people are available to make proper preparations so that when the doctor arrives he can devote his full time to caring for the mother. Safety factors involved in unexpected developments are very high in hospitals and very low in homes.

Home delivery does, however, have some advantages. There is no traveling to be done during labor. The nurse who cares for the patient at home has no other patients on her mind and so can devote all of her time to one mother and baby. There is a sentimental value attached to the home as the birthplace of a baby. The baby is not in contact with other babies, and therefore epidemic diseases are not as common. The choice lies largely with circumstances. What facilities can be provided in the home and what are available at the hospital? The doctor can advise best in this regard.

Home Delivery

In some communities, especially in rural areas, certain agencies—including hospitals—have instituted a home delivery service. A home delivery is probably best suited to a mother who has had previous uncomplicated deliveries. A mother who is delivering her first born or who has shown signs of complications is usually delivered in a hospital where the conveniences of a modern delivery room and services of a full staff are readily available.

If the doctor decides that a home delivery is suitable, certain preparations made well in advance can contribute immeasurably to a well-managed delivery. Many doctors provide lists of necessary equipment. More frequently, they depend on the nursing staff of the home delivery service to initiate planning with the mother soon after the latter makes her first visit to the clinic or doctor's office. In fact, one of the nurses will either visit the home or request a visiting nurse to do so in order to assess the facilities of the home and to make complete plans for the time of delivery and for care of the mother and baby immediately following delivery. The nurse in the clinic and in the home will not only advise on equipment but also elaborate on the doctor's instructions relative to the onset of labor, dietary needs, rest, exercise, and the like.

The first decision to be made is the choice of the room to be used. There should be enough space so that the bed can be approached from either side and enough light for the delivery team to see what they are doing. A bathroom with running water should be nearby.

Specific information can best be obtained from the doctor and nurse who are responsible for the management of the prenatal period, labor, delivery, and postnatal period. As previously mentioned, in most instances the family will be provided with a list of essentials as well as with assistance in the preparation of materials. The physician and the nurse will also bring certain supplies and equipment with them at the time of delivery. It is most important that all these preparations be made well in advance of the expected time of arrival of the baby.

A great impetus to the hospitalization of obstetrical cases has come from the various hospitalization insurance plans that have been offered in the past few years. By these plans, at a cost of only a few cents a day, the complete cost of obstetrical care can be covered, including the hospital and birth-rooms, and nursery care of the baby. Hospital insurance and medical care are covered in Part VIII, Chapter Six.

Estimating the Time of Delivery

The doctor will calculate the expected date of delivery if the date of the first day of the last menstrual period is known. He does this by counting back three months from this date and adding seven days—unless one of these three months is February in which case ten days are added.

A woman having her first baby "feels life" 20 weeks before delivery. If she has had living babies she adds two weeks because she recognizes quickening two weeks earlier. This date may be noted for future reference.

About 40 weeks from the first day of the last menstrual period is usually picked as the expected date of confinement. It is not uncommon for patients to deliver normally either before or after the expected date.

Labor

Noticeable contractions of the uterus (labor pains) begin when it is time for birth to occur—usually 280 days after conception in the average pregnancy. At first these may be a half hour or more apart and are not painful. When discomfort occurs with the contractions and they come every 10 to 15 minutes, labor has begun. Gradually the cramps and backache become more frequent; if there is a watery discharge or if bleeding occurs, the doctor should be notified at once. If he is not available, call the hospital and ask for advice regarding enter-

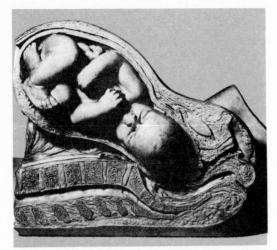

1. *Just before birth, baby rests head downward. Delivery has started, but not necessarily labor pains.*

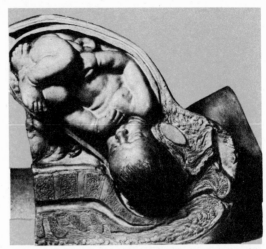

2. *Labor has begun. Cervix is dilating; baby's head is pressing downward through the opening.*

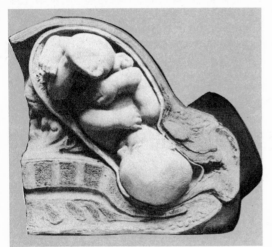

3. *Cervix has dilated and head rests on pelvic floor. Membrane around the fetus has not yet ruptured.*

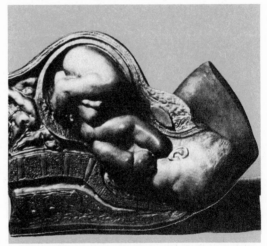

4. *The mother's "tail bone" or coccyx is bent back. Baby's body is streamlined to make the exit easier.*

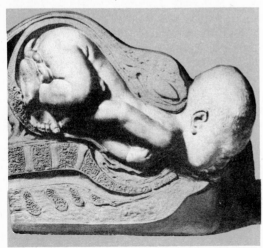

5. *The head emerges and turns upward, accentuating the lengthening of the baby's head.*

Photos: Cleveland Health Museum

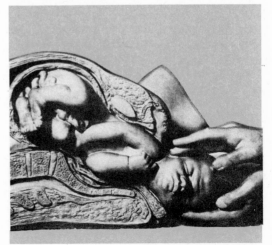

6. *While shoulders emerge, doctor's hands support head. Baby's cry indicates it has started to breathe.*

ing the hospital. In case of doubt, it is better to go to the hospital a little early rather than too late. Transportation should be arranged three months before the expected date of delivery. The woman should know where to report at the hospital and where the delivery rooms are located. Each doctor has standing orders which will be put into effect upon his patient's arrival. She will be thoroughly examined to see if labor is advancing, if her blood pressure is normal, and if her heart and lungs are functioning properly. A urine specimen examination to show any abnormal kidney function is also made. The lower bowel is often emptied with an enema to reduce the obstruction to the birth canal and improve cleanliness during delivery. The baby's heart beats are counted to determine if it is in good condition.

When the contractions get stronger and more frequent, the doctor will order the proper amount and kind of sedation to relieve discomfort without stopping labor. Many factors enter into his decision and it varies with different patients and with the same patient under different conditions. An occasional patient may decline any relief.

When the contractions gradually get stronger and more sedative is required, inhalation anesthesia is given with the contractions. Complete anesthesia is given in most cases when operative delivery becomes necessary. This must not be too deep or too prolonged because the anesthetic goes from the mother's blood through the afterbirth to the baby's blood, and may so depress the baby's respiratory center that it will not begin to breathe after birth.

Some women wish to have their babies by the so-called "natural method," in which preparation for labor is made throughout the pregnancy by exercises, and the baby is born with the mother fully conscious and able to observe the entire procedure. This is not suitable for all women. The same may be said for hypnosis, which is applicable only in selected instances and which must be used only by experienced and qualified physicians.

While childbirth is theoretically a normal function, there are many deviations from normal. Emphasis on "natural childbirth" should not obscure the need for medical alertness and supervision during any pregnancy, nor the importance of getting advice from medical sources only.

Physicians differ as to the advisability of allowing the father to witness his baby's birth. Birthrooms must be kept infection-free, and the doctor has enough responsibility without being faced with a father who might become ill or emotionally upset or who might unintentionally violate important precautions against infection. The physician's preference should be respected in this matter.

When the baby is born, its care is usually taken over at once by the family doctor or a pediatrician. Practices differ in the matter of keeping babies in a hospital nursery or having them in the mother's room from the start. Where hospital facilities permit a choice, the attending physician is the person to decide this, in conjunction with the baby's doctor.

A Few Words for the Father

Being associated with the care of a woman having a baby is a great responsibility and a privilege. A husband should realize that his wife is undergoing an emotional trial based on complex changes in her glands of internal secretion over which she has no control. You should also know that she needs, and rightfully expects, your full support to bolster her confidence in herself and you and the baby for the future. Little things that you do for her mean very much. A box of candy, a short vacation trip, overlooking some obvious mistake, or outlining some cherished plan for the future will do much to enrich the sacred experience of founding a family.

CHAPTER THREE

CHILDREN IN THE FAMILY

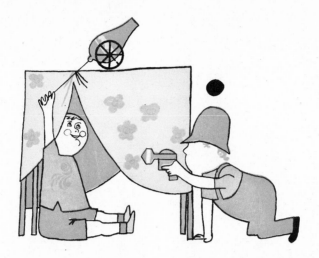

AND THEN THE BABY CAME! This dramatic experience in the life of a young husband and wife changes their whole outlook on life and living. The loving twosome, interested until now only in each other, has been invaded by a little stranger. To be sure, there have been nine months of anticipation. Pregnancy has brought many adjustments already in the family routine. But it is not until the first of their heirs actually arrives that the physical and emotional relationships that previously existed take on new dimensions. Not only are the immediate living patterns disrupted by baby's arrival, but things will never again be the same. Never!

In this chapter, we will try to learn the meaning of "children in the family." We will see that changes take place in the inter-relationships of the family group—see what influences children have upon the family's health patterns as well as the influence of the family upon the child's health. And we will briefly review the patterns of growth and development a child experiences during his first five years.

Family Structure

The chief reason for the family group in any society is to protect children until they can care for themselves, to give them an opportunity to learn the social responsibilities of the particular culture in which their family lives, and to learn the basic information about life and living that will allow them ultimately to establish a new family of their own. Children who, for one reason or another, are deprived of both natural parents should be placed as early as possible into a suitable family situation so that they may

have the experience of developing in a family and benefiting from the supervision and guidance of foster parents. Those who must grow up deprived of one of their parents are often seriously affected by this deprivation.

When most young people get married, having children is not their immediate concern. They are concerned primarily with each other's happiness and with learning the give and take that is basic to the marriage relationship and to family life in general. These two people are creating their own little world, whether it be in a rooming house, an apartment, or a house of their own. Their home is their castle and no others may enter without their expressed permission.

The probabilities nowadays are that each will have a job. Two incomes establish a fairly substantial level of living. Each person enjoys a measure of freedom within a pattern of restriction which they themselves develop to suit their own particular needs. They may come and go as they will, their hours may be irregular, their entertainment is of their own selection to be had whenever they wish it. This is the period in which they are getting acquainted, learning each other's interests, establishing their compatibilities, and building strength into their family through common interests and the recognition that each has interests that the other may never share.

In due time, whether through accident or deliberate design, conception occurs and the wife becomes pregnant. During this period of expectancy new adjustments must take place. The family that never before thought of the need for a physician now must have one to make the prenatal examinations and provide the necessary care during pregnancy. These examinations, spanning the period of pregnancy, enable the doctor to keep close watch on the health of the expectant mother and her child.

Frequently young families neglect to consider the financial aspects of health. Working on the assumption that not having been sick they are not likely to get sick, they often neglect to make the preparations that are essential to protect against major medical expenses. This may be the first time this couple has been aware of the need for hospital and medical insurance. Today, many of the corporations for which one or both of these young people might be working have insurance programs that provide protection against the reasonable costs of hospitalization and physician services.

If such health insurance is not a part of their compensation where they work, they should have been considering this need before now, because most hospital insurance programs will not provide care for the birth of a baby that takes place within 10 months of the purchase date of the policy. Nevertheless, if up to now the need for medical care has not been anticipated, certainly now is the time to establish the means for properly caring for their own health in the future, as well as the health of this very important first child.

During this period thought must be given also to the family estate. This child will need care and support from now to the end of his education period, anything from 18 to 25 years. It is high time that money be set aside either in regular savings or through the purchase of insurance to assure that, should something happen to the breadwinner of the family, there would be funds available to care for the mother and child.

Another financial problem will soon be facing the couple when the wife is no longer able to carry on her job outside the home. Some mothers do return to employment a few weeks after delivery, but many feel that it is desirable to stay at home. When they do, the only income is that of the husband.

If, during the earlier period of their marriage, they have been spending all of both salaries for living, this abrupt lowering of the standard of living is likely to be very uncomfortable. Not infrequently this change in the standard of living builds up resentments against the child whom they subconsciously feel is responsible. Feelings of rejection are very easy for the youngster to detect, and his whole fu-

ture personality can be affected by this antagonism, subconscious as it may be. The parents should recognize the situation and accept in good grace the fact that the mother will have a limited opportunity to contribute to the family income for many years to come.

Preparing for the Child's Arrival

During pregnancy there are likely to be many minor emotional conflicts between husband and wife. This is a very emotional period. Each must make an effort to understand that even though pregnancy is a perfectly normal physiological condition and that even though these emotional irritations are as normal as pregnancy, they do occur, they do require consideration, and the individuals involved must be careful that they do not mar the relationship that has been so carefully developing since the days of courtship.

Preparation for this addition to the family involves more than being seen by the doctor once in a while and trying to keep emotionally balanced. As the time of delivery approaches, the things needed in the hospital should be packed and the trip planned and rehearsed. The clothes that this new member of the family will need on his way from the hospital to his new home must also be provided. Many of these will be gifts of friends who know no better than you whether it will be a boy or a girl. Consequently, out of the accumulation of things that are likely to be presented, the most useful for this short trip will be a shirt, a diaper, and a blanket.

There must also be a place for this baby in the home. Here we have a difference of opinion among the authorities. Some are quite convinced that the baby should be in a room by himself where he has a minimum of disturbance from the people around the household. Others are equally adamant that the child's crib should be in his mother's room and that it should be movable so that it can be wherever in the house that the people are. This is one subject which it would be well to discuss with the doctor who is going to help you take care of your baby during his infancy and childhood.

The Baby Arrives

And then the baby came home! This is an exciting occasion under any circumstances; yet each time the circumstances are somewhat different. As a rule the major care of the baby will fall to Mother, and she will be so busy as a mother that she may forget to be a wife. Unless Father is a very well-adjusted personality, he is going to resent this neglect. Not only will he be resentful toward his wife, but he may also harbor subconscious antagonism toward this third person that has invaded their happy home. The apparent monopoly that the mother has over her child may offer little time during these early days for father to even get acquainted with his new child.

Obviously a whole new pattern of relationships and scheduling of time must be worked out. A child has 2 parents and he needs his father's attention at 3 weeks as much as he will at 3 years or 13. In fact, getting acquainted with father is as much a baby's job as getting acquainted with mother. A father who accepts his offspring, shares in his care, and enjoys his companionship will not only have a rewarding experience, but will also contribute much to the child's personality development and adjustment to social living.

Dad's Role

The father role is not that of an aloof male who condescends to hold the youngster for a few minutes after he's fed and dry. It involves helping with feeding. It involves changing diapers and giving an occasional bath. It, in fact, involves some share in all of the tasks of baby care, partly to relieve mother of some of the chores, but more important, to let the youngster know that he has two parents, both of whom love him.

To develop an adequate personality, this youngster is going to have to have a feeling that he is loved by both parents. Children, even at this tender age, are quick to sense the resentment, rejection, and frustration that are sometimes experienced by the new father and mother. It is only when parents are able to handle their youngsters with a comfortable outgoing feeling that children can experience the security which is the foundation for a well-developed personality.

Bringing Up Baby

Even in his first weeks of life, the child must begin to learn some of the lessons of living. Styles of child rearing change. There was a time of great rigidity in which youngsters ate at a certain time no matter what, and if they didn't develop bowel and bladder control by a certain age, they were literally forced into a control pattern. Then came a period of permissiveness that was known as the demand period, in which the youngster was allowed to set his own schedule for food and other services. He soon learned that when he made his demands his parents, or any other adults within earshot, jumped. He soon found out that by the loudest demand he was getting the most attention, and children like attention. The result has been a generation of demanding children.

The pendulum is now swinging in the other direction. More discipline is being introduced into child rearing at this early stage, and it is making life much more comfortable. With some regularity in the various factors of child care, family life can also operate according to a reasonable schedule. One group of physicians is quite convinced that instead of picking youngsters up when they cry and make demands, they should merely be checked to make sure they are not wet or in pain and then left to cry alone. They should be picked up when they are happy and smiling. If they associate the pleasant experience of attention with the smile and the laugh, they are much less likely to put on tantrum-like demands, particularly if the tantrums do not get them the attention that they are seeking.

Modern child rearing practices recognize that the infant has little or no emotional control. Only as he lives with people and learns from them does he develop his own personality and a pattern of reactions to his environment. He can be spoiled by lack of or inconsistency in discipline, as well as suppressed by a too demanding program based on rigid schedules. It is now believed that a natural development in a loving and supporting family which accepts the baby as an individual with his right to be himself is most beneficial. At the same time he is taught the skills of social living and how to accept the restrictions that are necessary in our present world.

Apropos of this discussion of discipline is an anecdote of the late Dr. Thurman B. Rice, professor, author, speaker, and at one time Health Officer of Indiana. After speaking on the sex education of children he was asked at what age one starts such instruction. "Immediately," he answered, "while the baby is still in the cradle." His questioner objected, "After all, Doctor, you can't teach much sex information to a week-old baby." To which the Doctor replied, "Listen—the minute that kid learns that he can't have what he wants when he wants it, he's laid the foundation for a satisfactory sex life." And very likely for many other facets of successful living with other people.

Subsequent Arrivals

Before too long, another child may be on the way. When the first child crossed the threshold, his parents had difficulty rearranging their lives, readjusting their schedules, and realigning their affections to include a third person. Even father reacted to the diversion of attention from him to the youngster. Now, when a second youngster comes, imagine what must go on in the small head of the first one who has little or no understanding of what is happening. He sees a considerable portion of the love and attention which he has learned to accept as his right being spent on somebody else whom he considers an intruder, while he himself is unwanted and unloved.

Before this second youngster comes home from the hospital, there should have been a long period of preparation and anticipation for the reception of "our" baby. Under no circumstances should the first youngster be surprised by the arrival of the second one. He should be aware of the meaning of the changes in the shape of his mother, even though he may be too young to understand the words that are used. The tone of voice and the attitude during presentation are far more important than what is said. By counting him in on the joy that goes with an addition to the family he will acquire security from this feeling of acceptance.

According to his age and ability, the first child should be given the opportunity to help out. If he can do little helpful things that show that he has a responsibility toward this new baby, that the new baby is as related to him as to other members of the family, and that the love and acceptance which he has enjoyed from his parents have not diminished by the addition of this baby, he probably will accept it and go on from there.

It is most unfortunate when through lack of preparation, a new brother or sister intrudes into the life of a first child unannounced and without warning. It is extremely frightening to a youngster to feel that this stranger has usurped the love and the attention that he has received previously, and that he now is an outcast, no longer within the family circle.

As the third and subsequent children come into the family much the same pattern develops, though we will find the older child is now more understanding. That is, he *can* be more understanding if he is made to feel that he is still loved and accepted in spite of the fact that others have been added who also are loved and accepted. Somehow, by tone of voice and attitude, the idea must carry over that love within the family is one of the unlimited things of which there is always enough to go around with plenty to spare, regardless of how many must divide it.

The occasion of an addition to the family is an excellent opportunity to help older children understand family relations and reproduction. Obviously youngsters of two or three will not understand all that can be said to them about sex, reproduction, family relations, and related activities. But they can be given the feeling that this process and relation is a very necessary and legitimate part of life, that it is as accepted as eating or sleeping or any other of our physiological activities, and that there are a great many normal kinds of interpersonal relationships within the family that are a necessary part of family life. If the child can develop a healthy attitude toward the men and women and boys and girls within his experience, and if he learns to identify with the sex to which he belongs, he is well on his way toward sound personality development and has laid a foundation on which he can learn more about sex and life.

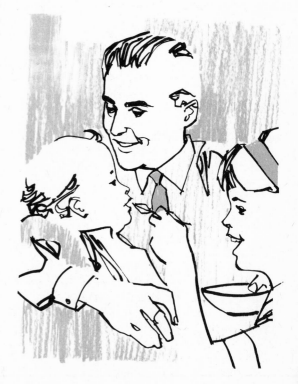

How Children Grow

The development of a newborn child from an uncoordinated reflex organism into a well coordinated, informed, and purposeful adult is a truly remarkable process. Even more remarkable is the series of developmental changes that lead to the individualized personality that this child will ultimately become. These two phenomena are developmental tasks that evolve in parallel, and each influences the other.

Most parents use the ability to do things as an index of their child's growth. Unfortunately they compare the age of each accomplishment with the age at which an earlier child or the neighbor's youngster accomplished the same task, not realizing that each child develops at his own individual rate.

The Newborn

A full-term, average-sized boy will weigh seven pounds eight ounces, while a girl will average five or six ounces less. Many factors affect birth weight: the parents, the mother's diet and health, and the exact length of gestation. The average length of a newborn child is 21 inches. This again is affected by heredity, stage of maturity, diet, and other factors. On the average, a normal-sized newborn will double his weight in the first five months and triple it in the first year. It is easy to see that the rate of growth, which started nine months before birth when this child was a single microscopic cell that doubled its mass every few minutes, has slowed down considerably by the time birth occurs.

Movements at birth are random and unorganized. A few complicated reflexes operate, such as grasping and sucking. A baby hears well and starts at a loud sound and is soothed by a gentle one. He cannot see well, but soon follows a light. Touch, taste, and smell are better developed. Essentially, the newborn baby cannot think, he only feels, and this state characterizes the first three months. He protects himself with a cry when wet, cold, hungry, frightened, or uncomfortable.

The First Year

Coordination and voluntary action begin in the third month. Smiling is one of the child's first voluntary actions. Soon he learns to turn his head to follow movement and sound. A short time later he reaches toward things that attract him. He learns to anticipate things within his experience and soon opens his mouth when he sees a bottle or nipple. Soon the development of tongue and throat control will permit him to swallow foods other than liquids, and his feedings will become rather regular and effective, even though a bit messy.

In the fourth month he may try to turn over by himself. He will probably succeed during the fifth month. During this period he increasingly enjoys being held in a sitting position. The really dramatic changes which make this baby a social person start during the fourth to sixth month. He begins to enjoy people, responds to other children in the family as well as to his parents, and babbles and coos a great deal. He smiles freely and may laugh. If he is well cared for, he will lie for long periods happily watching things and playing with his hands. He tends to cry less for attention than he once did. Improved muscle coordination will permit the baby to sit alone during his sixth month and he may sit for short periods in his high chair. He knows the difference between people who are familiar to him and those who are strangers, and he knows his mother and father well. His first teeth—the lower central incisors—may arrive this month or the next.

Efforts to crawl begin. Since there are many ways to crawl, he will probably invent his own method sometime in the ninth month. At this time he wants to touch and handle everything. The most useful tool for exploration is his mouth, into which he puts everything he can reach. He learns to bring his thumb and index finger together to pick up objects sometime during his 9th or 10th month. Since he now can find and pick up rather small things, all of which go into his mouth, and since he now gets around on his own, it is essential that the whole family be careful about leaving little things "within his reach"—pins, buttons, pills,—anything that could attract the attention of an inquisitive youngster.

By the 9th or 10th month the youngster gets into the sitting position whenever he wants to. He can stand with support and may pull himself into the standing position, but has difficulty getting down again. Very few children walk at 10 months, but some experiment with walking movements.

By now a child identifies approval and disapproval by the inflection of his mother's voice. He makes the proper response to "no," and may be ready to be taught the first lessons on how to live with others. Because he is easily distracted, he can be turned from some forbidden or undesirable activity by the offer of a more attractive substitute.

He now can drink from a cup, but may not be emotionally ready to be separated from his bottle at bedtime or during periods of stress. He probably will suck his thumb if not satisfied. He can feed himself with his fingers and may try to use a spoon, but because of his short attention span mother must take over when his interest begins to lag.

The One-Year-Old

By the end of his first year our helpless, uncoordinated baby has become a child. He is rapidly developing his own personality and learning how to fit his physical, emotional, and intellectual activities into appropriate patterns of behavior. He is very responsive to other people, especially his mother. Motion attracts him and he likes to watch passing cars and people, birds, animals—anything that moves. He can amuse himself as long as he can watch others. Though he likes to romp and play, he also likes being held on a lap. He will throw his toys and laugh. He enjoys putting things into boxes and loves pots and pans. He is a great explorer and will crawl all over his small world to investigate everything he can reach. He also likes rhythms and such games as pat-a-cake and peek-a-boo.

Individual children show different rates of development. These variations among children may or may not be significant. Often a child who is attentively waited upon by the adults in his family has no need to crawl or walk or develop language to get what he wants, so he does not develop these skills till later. For example, some children begin walking as early as 10 months, others may make little or no effort to walk until they are as old as 17 months. Some children begin to use recognizable words by 12 months, others may be 18 months or older before they pronounce meaningful words.

The Toddler

The period from 15 or 18 months of age to 2 or 2½ years is known as the "toddler" period. Our youngster is no longer earthbound. He can walk and climb rather than crawl. However, he has neither the maturity nor the stability of the "runabout" he will become in a year or so. At 15 months he stands alone or walks with a broad base but can neither run nor turn corners. By the end of this period he not only walks "grown up" but walks backwards and runs. At 15 to 18 months he still learns about his world by touching, feeling, and mouthing everything within his range—and his range is increasing since he no longer likes his playpen and may have learned to climb out of it.

A two-year-old (more or less) has finger co-

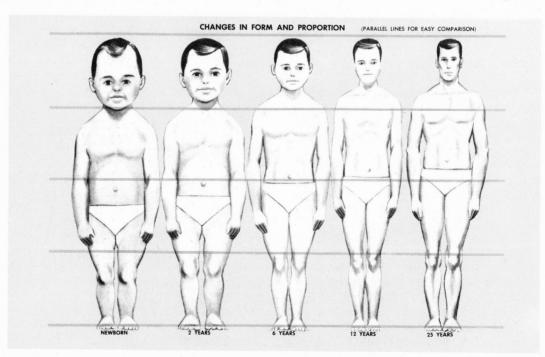

CHANGES IN FORM AND PROPORTION (PARALLEL LINES FOR EASY COMPARISON)

NEWBORN   2 YEARS   6 YEARS   12 YEARS   25 YEARS

ordination that lets him put big pegs in a peg board, build a pile of blocks, and turn the pages of a book made of heavy papers. He lifts, pulls, tries to dance to music, may try to turn on the radio and thoroughly enjoys playing rhythm games. He likes to play in sand and water and enjoys a roughhouse. He likes to "keep" mother and wants her near, but he also likes to be near other children. At this age he has not learned to play "with" them. Fellow toddlers play independently more than they play together. However, he still enjoys their company. He holds his possessions close and cries when they are taken away, but may accept a suitable substitute.

As our youngster begins to become part of the world of people, there are so many developmental tasks to complete that priorities must be recognized. Up to 18 months concentration on learning to walk has caused a neglect of language. Now language becomes important. A two-year-old may have a considerable vocabulary and uses sentences of three words. Variations that occur will be due to his family's use of words, his own need to use words, and the presence of older children to talk with him.

So far he has no sense of time, so he sees no reason to hurry. However, he wants to do things for himself at age two, such as dress, undress, and eat. With no sense of time, the resulting parental pressure to get the job done may discourage him from further trying. Even a child who has mastered the removal of shoes, sox, and shirts, or even putting them on, may demand service in getting dressed or undressed if he is tired or if he feels the need for attention and the security of an adult's presence.

You will recall that during the first year the baby tripled his birth weight, adding 15 pounds more or less. In his second year he will gain only four to seven pounds. Obviously he will not need the volume of food he needed earlier. This may be well, because his poor eye and finger coordination coupled with his "I want to do it myself" attitude make him a messy eater. It takes him a while to master these skills, with parents constantly interfering, and he may not get much food in the meantime.

The child may develop fears and be frightened by loud noises and large objects. General apprehensiveness and timidity can be due to his parents' expecting of him more control than he can muster. He needs less scolding and more reassurance. This is particularly true in relation to toilet training. If mother is relaxed, the youngster may develop control as soon as he is

physically ready. A tense, anxious mother may delay his toilet training considerably. Bowel training is accomplished several months before urinary control is possible. Both are reasonably well established by three years, with only an occasional accident.

A child begins to discover himself in the toddler period. He asserts himself and is not easily distracted. Often his temper tantrums and crying are due to having too few words to express himself. Because of his tendency to say "no" to everything, parents should avoid his negativism by not giving the child too many chances to say "no." This difficult age requires the light touch. He is too young for severe discipline, but requires more control than was used during his first year. Consistency of parental behavior toward the toddler is difficult, but when parents are consistent the toddler has a firm base on which to grow.

The Runabout

The "runabout" years span the period from two and one-half to five years of age. This will vary with individuals, but it is essentially the period between the end of the toddler period and the beginning of formal schooling—kindergarten or first grade, as the case may be. Many quite startling changes occur during the runabout period which makes a self-reliant person out of what was still a cuddly baby, even at two and one-half.

Large muscle coordination improves rapidly. The three-year-old likes to climb, slide, use a trapeze, and ride a tricycle. At four he hangs by his feet and swings. Up to four sand and water play are fun, but after four he prefers active, noisy play.

Small muscle coordination also improves. At two and one-half a child can thread large beads, at three he enjoys a small peg board, and at four he can handle cutting and sewing cards.

Language now develops rapidly. Most children add 500 to 600 words a year to their vocabulary between two and six years and understand many more. The runabout's problem of having so much to say and not enough words to say it leads to repetition that is usually outgrown. The two and one-half may be hard to understand, but the four-year-old usually speaks clearly. At four it is fun to play with words and sounds. "Bad words," whether or not their meaning is understood, have a peculiar fascination, largely because they attract the attention of adults. These words will be forgot-

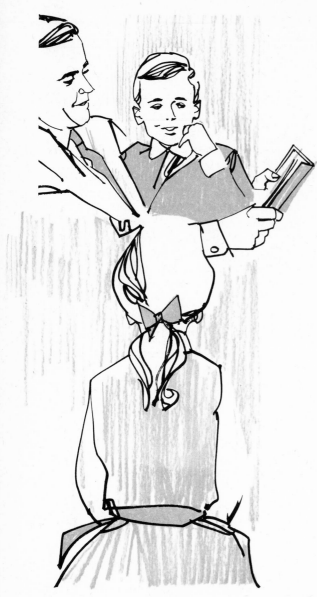

can identify. Movies are a form of story telling, but often offer experiences which are beyond the runabout's understanding. Runabouts believe what they see to be real, and movies containing frightening situations can be quite disturbing, since the child cannot separate fantasy from fact or cinema from real life.

This is the age of curiosity, the endless question. Adults should answer questions, but, more important, they should encourage the "let's find out" approach which helps the youngster learn to find answers for himself. At this age he still needs to touch most things but he no longer mouths them. It is important that he be given time to see and feel things since his perception is neither as rapid nor as experienced as an adult's.

Parallel or simultaneous play is the pattern when the runabout period begins, but by three the other child is definitely in the picture. He soon learns to play *with* others, to share and to take turns, and to ask for something he wants rather than snatch it. A common pattern is to select one person as a playmate and ignore the group, though this person may be a different one each play period. Boys and girls of this age play the same games and either is as likely to select a boy as a girl for companionship.

Life with a runabout child is difficult at best. At two and one-half he is learning to assert himself and insists that things be done his way. His constant "no" to every request and his resentment of interference with his physical activity and possessions is characteristic of this stage of personality development.

A three-year-old is already less negative. He seems to want to do things the right way and he can be given reasons for doing things a certain way because he understands words better. Nevertheless, he still likes things to be done his way even though he is less resentful of adult interference.

At four he becomes noisier, stormier, and more active. The tendency of parents to expect more of a four-year-old than he is physically or emotionally able to deliver contributes to the misunderstanding between child and adult. "Running away" is common. Generally this is not naughtiness or disobedience or even a wish to get away from home. He simply has become interested in things a few blocks away or wants to visit a friend and thus takes off. By now he has learned to cross a quiet street safely and probably knows his neighborhood quite well. This is the period when safe pedestrianism must be taught, because he will continue to

ten if ignored. Sometimes an unemotional explanation of the word's meaning and why it should not be used will solve the problem. An emotional prohibition tends to fix these words in a youngster's vocabulary. Since speech patterns are learned by imitation, simple, clear speech by parents is valuable to a child's language development. Baby talk should be avoided.

Stories are important at this age. They should be about the real world as the child knows it. He will not be ready to cope with the supernatural world of fairies and magic until he understands the real world more clearly. He likes stories about other children with whom he

cross streets without adult guidance.

The runabout likes to do things by himself. At two and one-half he may try to wash himself when in a tub and will struggle to put on his sox and shirt. By four he is fairly efficient at dressing and undressing. He likes to take over and surprise mother by appearing fully dressed. The job may be done poorly by adult standards, but the effort deserves praise.

The ability to feed himself improves during this period. His table manners are not good, but will improve by imitation of others at the table. It is important that the child feed himself effectively. He will enjoy doing it if not discouraged by adult insistence on what he considers unimportant detail.

A child of runabout age likes to help mother though he is often more bother than use. At two and one-half he may try to set the table, dust, or make beds. A four-year-old can efficiently empty waste baskets or dry silver. However, interest fades quickly, the attention span is short, and he cannot be responsible for finishing a job. These early efforts must not be judged by adult standards, since adverse criticism may easily destroy the desire to help. Understanding parents will give the child help when he wants it even if he knows how to do the job. They also will be understanding when the job is done poorly or not finished.

The Five-Year-Old

At the end of the runabout period we have a five-year-old. In three short years he has developed from a cuddly, soft, uncoordinated baby to a reasonably sure person. He has developed a personality of his own and is beginning to show the kind of person he will be. The characteristics that make him unique are already evident. The baby is now an independent person, able to be away from home for two or three hours each day.

Physical growth has been slowed, even more than in the earlier periods. At five a boy will measure 42 to 45 inches in height and weigh 38 to 48 pounds. A girl will be 42 to 45 inches tall and weigh 36 to 48 pounds. The five-year-old can be expected to gain two to three inches and three to six pounds this year.

The five-year-old can use his body quite purposefully and skillfully. He can jump, skip, dance, and climb. Though the large muscles are better developed than those of fingers and hands and he does better with large muscle movements, he is beginning to learn more effective hand use. At this stage hand and eye are not well coordinated and the child is probably farsighted, so he should spend little time on close work with small things. Big muscle activities are still his forte. Handedness is determined by five, and 90 per cent will be right-handed. Lefthanded children should be taught to use their left hands and not be changed to righthandedness.

A five-year-old is noisy and vigorous but his activity has definite direction. He needs equipment for purposeful, planned activity. He is learning to throw and catch. He may try roller skates or rope jumping. These are all large muscle activity. But a five-year-old tires easily and voluntarily withdraws to watch or seek quieter activity. Often he may need a nap to balance his violent activity.

Where Do We Go From Here

At this stage we will leave the detailed description of what happens from here on through childhood and adolescence. The foundation has been laid on which will be built his physical, emotional, and intellectual life. He has become an independent personality and much of his future has been determined by what has happened to him so far. Has he had understanding parents? Has he been protected from unnecessary fears and frustrations? Has he had the support of parental love? Have his questions been answered? Has he been guided into muscular skills that help him learn about his world? Has he absorbed from his association with his parents and peers the sense of integrity and fair play so necessary in life? Has he a sense of trust, of feeling secure in his world? Does he feel that he is a person, different from other persons but related to them? Has he, in fact, been helped to meet the challenge of each developmental task as his understanding and physical ability has expanded?

If so, he is ready for the next step—school. This new experience leads to increasing separation from home and parents. It leads to an increasing influence on his personality by adults and children outside of the home. If these five years, and the few that preceded them, have seen established a home in which family life is at its best, these new experiences will be taken in stride and will contribute to the further development of a sound, healthy person with a pleasant personality.

CHAPTER FOUR

THE CARE AND FEEDING OF BABIES

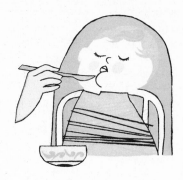

THE REALIZATION that the care of babies is a medical problem was given its greatest spur in about 1900 when the appalling death toll that malnutrition and intestinal disorders were taking among our infant population became widely known. This resulted in the establishment of "infant feeding stations" for the poor, and this activity helped so much to correct the situation, that infant feeding problems are today fewer.

As more and more diseases have fallen into the category of "preventable" and as our recognition of the vital role that mental health plays in the over-all health of the individual has grown, our emphasis on the care of babies has broadened to include the prevention of many infectious diseases by immunization and to the prevention of emotional problems through family counseling.

Let us follow a baby along through periodic visits to the physician and see some of the things that parents frequently ask about, and some of the things the physician wants the parents to know.

What about the baby who tends to "spit up" some of his feeding with great regularity?

Most of the time this is of no importance and can be ignored. However, if the "spitting up" becomes forceful vomiting and the baby fails to gain weight, or loses weight, then careful observation is necessary to rule out an obstruction at the outlet of the stomach. This spitting up almost always occurs in the first two months of life. After that time it may be a great nuisance when baby's food comes back, but it is not usually a nutritional problem. Incidentally, the sour smell that so often clings to the baby's (or mother's) clothes can be eliminated by using a little baking soda in the "mop-up" water.

What about constipation in babies?

The breast-fed baby will not be constipated. He may have a movement only once a week, but it will be normal in character. Regularity of movement in the bottle fed baby is not necessary either. However, the stools of such babies are more likely to become dried out and cause difficulty in passage so that changes in formula or the introduction of some fruits into the diet may be called for.

How fast should a baby gain weight?

This is probably the first question by parents that will bring forth the answer that "no two children are alike." In other words, some children are destined by heredity to be large-framed and husky adults, others to be small and light, and the rest to be in between. These varying patterns of growth are obvious quite early in the child's life. Therefore, it is unwise to expect any two infants, even in the same family, to follow the same pattern. Nevertheless, there are some guideposts that you can observe which will give you an indication of your baby's nutritional progress. The weekly gain should not be less than four ounces. This will result in at least doubling the birth weight in six months and trebling it at one year. Many babies, in fact perhaps most babies, will gain more than this without being obese—but less gain than this should call for close observation.

What about immunization?

Until the past few years it was a generally accepted practice to wait until about six months of age before starting immunizing procedures. This was due to the belief that the very young infant could not develop immune antibodies.

Recent studies, however, show that at an age even as early as two months satisfactory responses are obtained. The schedule suggested by the American Academy of Pediatrics for basic immunization is found in the accompanying chart.

The schedule for "booster" injections after this is subject to some variation in practice among different physicians. This is true except for tetanus, where there is general agreement that the interval between injections should not be greater than four years. It is also agreed that, in order to keep up our present record of virtually no smallpox in the United States, we should all be vaccinated every four or five years. (See Part VI, Chapter Six for foreign travel requirements.)

Although immunization of all children against tuberculosis is not generally advocated, we should say something about the present status of the attempts to control this disease in children.

We now have available drugs that are effective in killing the tuberculosis organisms and methods for early detection of their presence in the body. We should thus be able to attain a greater degree of control of tuberculosis than we have so far. The part of a control program that should be included in the medical supervision of babies is early detection of infection. The tuberculin test is an entirely harmless test and is our most reliable method of detecting tuberculous infection. For this reason the American Academy of Pediatrics advises that the test be given at one, two, four, and six years of age.

The tuberculin test may be performed in a number of ways; in each case the principle is the same. The physician selects the testing method that is best adapted to the existing circumstances.

The tuberculin test determines whether or not tuberculosis germs have entered the body. If the result is positive, it does not indicate that the child actually has tuberculosis. It merely means that he should be watched to be sure that the germs have not been able to establish themselves and grow, thus developing into an actual tuberculous infection.

If we are ever to achieve real control and, hopefully, eradication of tuberculosis, it can only be by the continuing cooperation by all of

IMMUNIZATION SCHEDULE FOR CHILDREN*

Diseases		Age at Time of First Dosage	Material (Antigen)	No. Doses	Interval	Age at Time of Booster (Recall) Doses
Diphtheria Tetanus Whooping Cough		2 months	Triple Preparation	3	Not less than one month nor more than three months	12 months after third dose; again at 4 years and 8 years Tetanus and diphtheria toxoids (adult type) 12 years and 16 years Tetanus toxoid every 5 years thereafter
Poliomyelitis		2 months	Inactivated (Salk)	4	One month intervals; 4th at 15 months	Every 2 years after 4th dose
		2 months	Oral (Sabin) vaccine Type I Type III Type II	1 dose each	6-8 weeks	12-15 months, Types I-II-III combined
		2 months	Oral (Sabine) trivalent vaccine (3 vaccines combined)	3	6-8 weeks	4th dose 12-15 months
Smallpox		6-12 months	Cowpox virus	1		Every 5 years, when going overseas, or in presence of epidemic
Typhoid-paratyphoid-fevers		Only when needed	Typhoid—paratyphoid vaccine	3	1-4 weeks	Upon advice of physician or public health authorities
Measles (4 Plans)	1	9 months	live, attenuated vaccine	1		No recommendations; immunity may be permanent
	2	9 months	Same + gamma globulin	1		
Choice rests with physician	3	9 months	Inactivated vaccine	3	Monthly	One or more booster doses; intervals undetermined; not for routine use
	4	9 months	Same, followed by live attenuated vaccine			Recommendation pending

*Adapted from Table One, The Red Book, American Academy of Pediatrics, 1964, modified by Supplementary Statement October 25, 1964.

us in known and proved public health measures directed toward this goal.

At what age should children learn and be able to do certain things?

Here, again, you will encounter and must believe the dictum that "no two children are alike." If we were to give you a listing of certain motor and intellectual skills that your child should acquire at a certain age, you would most probably develop either an unwarranted pride in the precociousness of your child or an unwarranted pessimism over his slowness.

Therefore, as was the case with weight gain, it would seem best to give a few liberal but reliable mileposts and then go on to some of the effects of development on behavior.

1 month—Can lift chin off table.

2 months—Can lift chest off table.

3 months—Reaches for objects but without success. (It is interesting to note that, as Dr. Arnold Gessell phrased it, "He reaches with his eyes well before he can reach with his hands.")

4 months—Can sit with support.

5 months—Can sit on lap and can grasp small objects.

6 months—Can sit in high chair and grasp a dangling object.

7 months—Can sit alone.

8 months—Can stand with help.

9 months—Can stand by holding on to pieces of furniture.

10 months—Can creep.

11 months—Can walk if led by one hand.

12 months—Can pull himself up and stand with the help of furniture.

13 months—Can climb up a few stairs.

14 months—Can stand alone.

15 months—Can walk alone.

In addition to these motor skills, by two months the baby will smile at anyone who speaks to him. By one year he should participate in such games as "peek-a-boo," and by 18 months or 2 years he should make a stab at naming at least 6 objects.

What are some of the behaviorial problems that may accompany these increasing physical skills?

This is the age at which new experiences can be initiated by the child. Simultaneously he has an awakening awareness of himself as an individual person. He begins to view himself not as a more or less compliant receptacle for the feedings you have mixed for him, not as a "clothes horse" to display the cute little suits you have made for him, but as a thinking, feeling human being entitled to have his feelings understood and respected by those he respects the most—you, his parents. This does not mean that we can sanction every move he makes. But it does mean that we must remove from his sphere of influences as much of the forbidden fruit as possible, and that we try to limit our prohibitions to those acts that are dangerous.

Children *must* learn that some things are prohibited, but we must remember that their ability to learn this is limited by the stage of their maturity. Thus, we cannot expect a 2-year-old to behave like a 10-year-old; conversely, we must not allow a 10-year-old to act like a 2-year-old. The transition from the irresponsibility of the 2-year-old to the beginning responsibility of the 10-year-old and on to the greater responsibility of the adult is initiated and hastened by the feeling of success and approval that a child gets from his parents. In other words, we must try to encourage his successes while helping him to overcome his failures. So, when a child's behavior seems to be a violent rebellion against authority, remember that in reality it is not a true rebellion against authority, but rather a manifestation of an increasing awareness of "self."

Infant Feeding

Breast feeding is the natural way to feed a baby, and when it can be accomplished, it is satisfying to both mother and baby. The reasons behind the mother's choice between breast and bottle feeding are often complex, but regardless of what the reasons are, here are a few facts about breast feeding that are often misunderstood:

●The size of the breasts has no influence on the success or failure of nursing.

●Nursing a baby will not make the breasts sag if they are supported properly.

●The quality of breast milk is always good. It always agrees with the baby.

●Nursing a baby is not a sure way to prevent another pregnancy.

During pregnancy, the glandular tissue in the mother's breasts enlarges and, toward the end of pregnancy, begins secreting a creamy yellow fluid called colostrum. After delivery, when the baby is put to the breast, this protein-rich fluid is all that he gets until about the third to fifth day (sometimes later), when the milk comes in. There is often more milk produced than the baby is able to take at first and the mother may be uncomfortable, but soon supply and demand are equalized.

The mother's milk supply will change from day to day and will increase as the baby grows older and requires more milk. Probably the most important factors in the regulation of the mother's milk supply are: a vigorous baby who is able to suck hard and empty the breast, thereby stimulating milk production; and a relaxed mother who is not under emotional strain and who really wants to nurse her baby. The health of the mother, her diet, the amount of housework she has to do, her husband's attitude, and other factors also play a role in determining success, but are not as important as the first two.

Many mothers who are nursing their babies want to know how long they should continue to do so. This decision is entirely up to them. There is no physiological reason why an infant cannot be fed at the breast into the second year, as long as he gets some other foods containing iron, vitamin D, and vitamin C. In this country, social pressure is such that it is rare for a woman to want to nurse this long, but it is acceptable from a medical point of view. However, many women find it convenient to nurse their babies for about 8 to 10 months and then to wean the infant directly to the cup, thus eliminating the stage of bottle feeding.

Some women find they must supplement the breast supply by giving the baby a daily bottle, while others begin breast feeding and then switch to all bottle feeding when the child is a few months old. Such varied schedules are at the discretion of the mother, since the baby's only concern is that he be fed an adequate amount by a warm, loving individual.

Some mothers cannot or do not choose to nurse, and thus must give their babies milk from a bottle. Cow's milk serves as the basis for all baby formulas, except in the rare cases of specific milk allergy. Since breast milk is the ideal food for babies, formulas are made similar in composition to breast milk in amounts of carbohydrate, fat, and protein. The most inexpensive way of doing this is in your own kitchen using whole or evaporated milk as a basis, and adding water and carbohydrate (corn syrup) according to the formula supplied by your physician. There are also many ready-made formulas on the market which are easy to use and which resemble breast milk in composition.

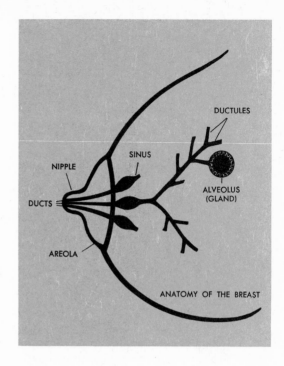

ANATOMY OF THE BREAST

Your physician is in the best position to advise what type of milk is best for your baby.

Many new products have been recently introduced to help feed babies. These include disposable nipples and bottles, ready-to-use formulas that do not need diluting, and plastic bottles of various kinds. All these products make it easier to care for the baby—the disposable bottles and nipples are especially good on a trip—but they do add to the cost of feeding.

Psychological Aspects of Feeding

Since the majority of an infant's day is spent eating or sleeping, his conscious contact with the world and the people in it comes at mealtime. Thus feeding is not merely a matter of supplying him with nutrition for his growth and activity; it also has a great influence on his personality development. When a young infant is hungry he screams loudly because he is in extreme discomfort and feels frightened. When he is saved from this situation by being fed, he feels comfortable again and begins to associate this feeling with the person who has saved him. Because this process is repeated many times, the baby learns to trust this person—or people in general—and to consider them desirable parts of his environment.

During the feeding period there is a communication between the infant and the person feeding him. If this communication conveys a sense of love, warmth, and acceptance, the infant will develop a feeling of security. If the baby is being breast fed the communication will be between infant and mother; if the baby is bottle fed, the feeder may be mother, father, sister, or grandmother, but regardless of who it is, the same feeling can be conveyed to the infant. Hopefully, however, the "feeder" will not often be a pillow or other impersonal means of propping the bottle, since there is no communication in such a situation. At times it may be necessary to prop a bottle during a feeding, but since this does not permit any social contact for the baby, it should be done rarely.

Other Foods

Any food other than milk, such as cereal or fruit, is considered a solid even though its consistency may be very fluid. Foods of this type are given to babies as a source of iron—which milk lacks—and also to get the baby accustomed to eating with a spoon. Cereal is often started first, since it is bland and smooth and not apt to cause allergies, but other foods such as fruits, vegetables, or meats may be given first.

Practices regarding the age at which solid food is started have been changing in the past few years. At one time it was standard practice to start spoon feeding at about four to six months of age, but now it is not unusual to have a mother giving her baby solids at three weeks of age. This is sometimes done with the idea that it will allow the baby to sleep through the night, but a recent study on this subject indicates that there is no relationship between the time of starting solids and sleeping through the night. The average age at which the babies in this study gave up their 2:00 a.m. feeding was nine weeks regardless of whether or not they

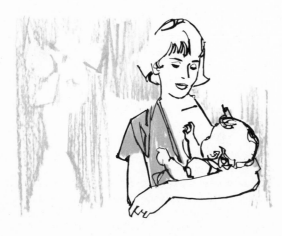

had started eating cereal. It is much easier to give the baby just milk for the first two to four months and then start cereal. However, there are some babies who are growing so rapidly that they must be started on solids sooner. Again, your physician is in the best position to decide what should be done for your baby.

Publicity has been given to the ability of babies to accept cold feedings without bad effects. This may comfort some parents when they are compelled to give a feeding that has not been heated. However, the natural temperature for baby's food is that of breast milk, and this should also be the temperature of the artificial feeding whenever possible.

Some time after the baby is six months old he will be willing to accept coarser food even though he has no teeth. Samples of table food, mashed vegetables, chopped meat, etc., may then be tried and increased in amount if he accepts them. Almost anything that the family eats can be given to a baby if one avoids highly seasoned or overly fat food and sweet desserts. When the family meal does not contain suitable food, jars of junior food may be purchased at the grocery store for an easy quick meal.

Vitamins

Vitamins A, D, and C are always necessary for babies to insure their proper growth, but they do not necessarily have to be given in liquid form. Most manufactured baby formulas have vitamins already added and extras should not be given. Also, much of the milk available from dairies in the United States has enough vitamin D added to prevent rickets during summer months up to the age of one year. In the winter, the physician's advice should be sought about giving additional amounts, especially in northern latitudes. Orange juice as a source of vitamin C can be added to the child's diet at an early age, and as he grows older foods containing the B vitamins will be in the diet. It is best to let your doctor decide whether the child's diet contains enough vitamins, or whether these should be added.

Infant feeding consists of supplying a child with essential nutrients for bodily growth and social stimulation for personality growth. Milk is the chief food of infants and this is best supplied by the mother's milk if possible. As the child grows older, simple solids are added when he is ready for them. Perhaps the most important item on his menu should be large servings of common sense.

CHAPTER FIVE

FERTILITY AND INFERTILITY

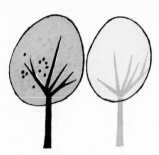

OF ALL THE TOPICS of special interest to families, none holds a more important place than a baby. A baby represents for almost everyone all that is most beautiful, most precious, most wonderful in life. A baby in a happy, healthy family means that two people who have joined their lives together in love and respect have created out of their devotion a new human being who, while embodying a part of each of their bodies, minds, and spirits, yet has been given a personality and make-up that is all his own and unique in the world. A baby, then, is in a sense our own vision of ourselves carrying on our love and work and life into the future, eventually to be passed on by him to his own children.

Infertility

Conceiving and bearing a baby presents for most families no problems at all. Medical advances have been such that pregnancy, in itself a normal process, is more comfortable and safer than ever before in history. The same thing is true of delivery. There are couples, however—about 1 out of every 10—who do have trouble conceiving. Modern science has found several reasons for this which are about equally divided between husband and wife. Sometimes it may be a simple, easily-corrected, anatomical defect in one or the other that prevents the sperm from reaching the egg. Sometimes it is a defect that causes the husband's sperm either not to develop at all, or to develop in numbers too small or in quality too poor to make fertilization possible. Whatever the cause, medical science has made it possible for more than half of the apparently infertile couples to be helped to achieve pregnancy, provided their problems are properly diagnosed and correctly treated.

There are several important things for a couple to remember if they seem to have an infertility problem:

- Just because you have not achieved pregnancy, don't jump to the conclusion that you are infertile. Only a specialist in infertility can make such a diagnosis.
- The best way to find a specialist qualified to handle infertility problems is to call your county medical society for a list of names of such specialists in your area. The Planned Parenthood - World Population Organization has a list of its own, and other centers specialize in infertility, either with direct services or by referral to qualified specialists in the area. In addition, if you live near a medical school or large hospital, call the office of the head of the obstetrics department. There you can find out if the institution has infertility services or obtain the names of physicians who have a special background for diagnosing and treating infertility problems.
- Because the causes of infertility are about equally divided between husbands and wives, it is vital that both partners be studied together. This is particularly important because the identification of problems involving the husband is more easily, quickly, and less expensively done than is the case with the wife.
- Fertility is highest among the young and tends to diminish with years. Therefore, a newly-married couple in their twenties should not postpone their first pregnancy for more than two years. Modern medical contraceptive measures, as approved by the U.S. Food and Drug Administration, have never been known to affect fertility adversely. Indeed, some of them may actually increase it. Nevertheless, if unknown to themselves the couple has an infertility problem, they will not discover this fact until they stop the use of contraceptive mea-

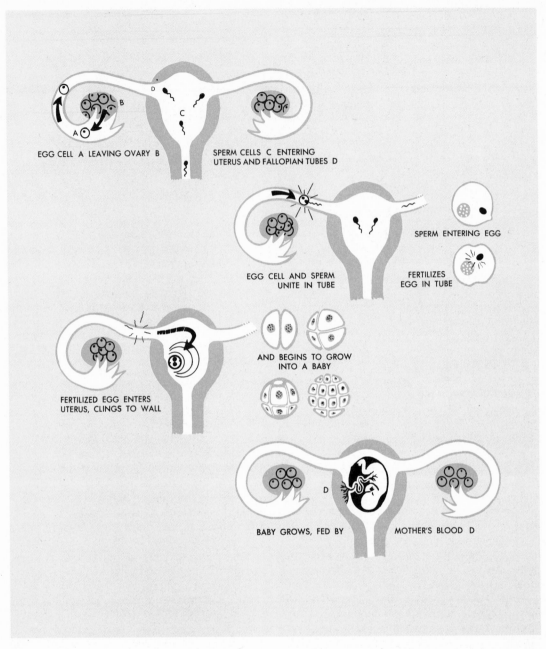

EGG CELL A LEAVING OVARY B   SPERM CELLS C ENTERING
                                  UTERUS AND FALLOPIAN TUBES D

SPERM ENTERING EGG

EGG CELL AND SPERM
UNITE IN TUBE

FERTILIZES
EGG IN TUBE

AND BEGINS TO GROW
INTO A BABY

FERTILIZED EGG ENTERS
UTERUS, CLINGS TO WALL

BABY GROWS, FED BY   MOTHER'S BLOOD D

sures and try to become pregnant. Because of the age-time factor, it is thus wise not to postpone trying for a pregnancy for more than two years.

•Newly-married couples who are in their thirties are advised not to postpone efforts for a first pregnancy at all, or at least not for more than the two or three months that it will take them to establish their home. Here the age-time factor increases in importance, and pregnancy should be sought as soon as possible.

•The young teen-age marriages, however,

belong in a very different category. These young couples must do a good deal of growing up at the same time that they are establishing their married life. Because of the very high divorce rate among these young marriages, many persons consider it wise for them to postpone attempts at a first pregnancy until both are in their twenties. This will give them time to mature, to finish their education, and to establish themselves in life as adult people with a well-developed marital relationship, before they become parents.

One last word about infertility: Worrying about it does more harm than good, and feeling guilty does the most harm of all. Infertility is not anyone's fault, and is common enough so that there need be no reason to be ashamed of it or to hide it. Furthermore, worrying about it can often seriously affect the couple's marital relationship. Do not worry about possible infertility; but if you have tried for pregnancy for a reasonable time, seek and follow competent advice, and the chances will be in favor of having the baby you dream of.

Fertility

Fertility was never a problem in the tragic days when a couple was likely to lose one out of every two or three of their babies. Indeed, before 1900, a couple expected to have eight or nine babies in order to be able to raise four or five. Advances of medical science, such as the sanitation of water and milk supplies, the control of communicable diseases, and better prenatal and infant care, have made this no longer true, not only in the United States but increasingly in all parts of the world. Thus in the United States most couples can reasonably expect that babies born to them will survive to grow up.

This happy state of affairs means, therefore, that many families will consider themselves to be large enough while the husband and wife are still in their early twenties. If they continued bearing children until the wife's menopause, they could theoretically end up with a family of 15 to 18 children. Some families do reach this number, but it can truthfully be said that the mothers and fathers of such families seldom wanted so many children.

Despite, or perhaps because of, our high level of living in the United States, many mothers and fathers wish to limit the size of their families for economic reasons. It is estimated that it costs a minimum of $15,000 to $18,000 to rear a child to adult life simply in terms of shelter, food, clothes, medical, and dental care. This does not include those cultural advantages that most mothers and fathers want their children to have: good education, recreation, travel, and music and dancing lessons. Society as a whole is concerned with the implications for the future of the present "population explosion."

Our great urban areas, in which it is estimated 60 per cent of our people will be living by 1980, are getting more and more crowded.

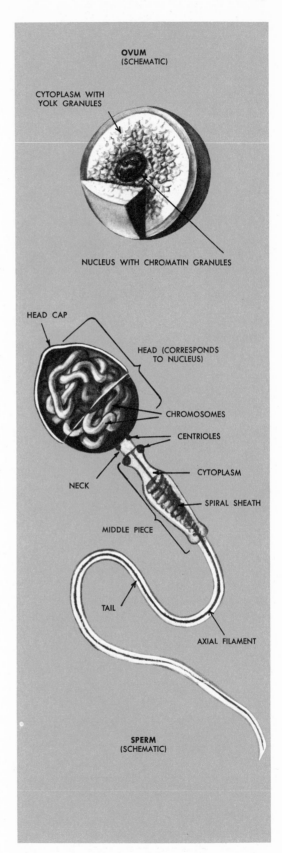

OVUM
(SCHEMATIC)

CYTOPLASM WITH YOLK GRANULES

NUCLEUS WITH CHROMATIN GRANULES

HEAD CAP

HEAD (CORRESPONDS TO NUCLEUS)

CHROMOSOMES

CENTRIOLES

CYTOPLASM

NECK

SPIRAL SHEATH

MIDDLE PIECE

TAIL

AXIAL FILAMENT

SPERM
(SCHEMATIC)

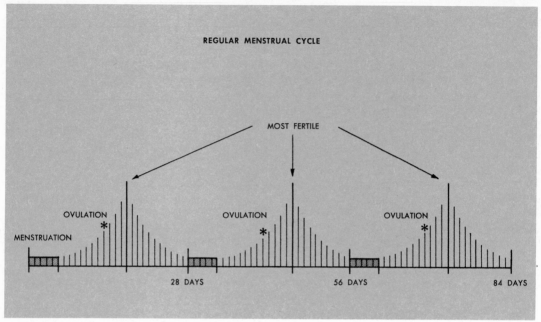

In a regular menstrual cycle, eggs are released from the ovaries once every 28 or 30 days. Conception is most likely within a few days before or after ovulation; conception is possible at any phase of the menstrual cycle.

There is less road space as the number of cars increases, less play and recreation space as the number of children increases, less desk space as the schools become more and more crowded. All of this means not only rising taxes, but rising tensions as people have to adjust to living under these increasingly crowded and difficult conditions.

Our religious and scientific leaders, therefore, have begun to think in terms of what parenthood means in the light of these changing times. Responsible parenthood, family planning, and planned parenthood are terms used interchangeably by Catholic, Protestant, and Jewish clergymen as they counsel couples not to enter parenthood lightly but to be aware of the heavy responsibilities that parenthood places on them. The three faiths just as strongly condemn those who avoid parenthood for selfish and frivolous reasons.

To prevent conception for good and sufficient medical or social reasons has been widely discussed by many groups. Protestant and Jewish church bodies have, in general, approved the use of artificial means to this end. The Catholic is not opposed to spacing families as long as it is done naturally, by abstention or rhythm, both of which he regards as in accordance with nature.

Most husbands and wives want children and will have them. Thus, "responsible parent-

hood" means simply that husbands and wives take stock of themselves, the kind of people they are, and the kind of parents they want to be, and take care to space their children accordingly. In this way, each baby can enjoy his babyhood to the full, and not be deprived of what is important for his future development by being pushed out of his crib and his mother's arms too soon by a new baby.

By the time a mother and father have two children, they will be well aware that having children today means joy. But most realize that it is also necessary to assure a warm, well-ordered family atmosphere in which children can grow and develop normally and well, with a father and mother who are devoted and happy both as husband and wife and as parents. Because by this time too the father should be well started on his life's work, this will be a good moment for the couple to plan together the number of children they would like to have.

Some families already have two or three children by the time the mother and father are in their early twenties. These thoughtful families then plan to regulate their child-bearing so that this first group of children can grow up with the kind of life that their parents want them to have. In many homes, the mother has a vocation to which she plans to return when her children are in school. Thus a couple in their early twenties with two or three children could plan for the mother to return to work when her youngest child enters school. Her salary could then pay for domestic help as well as add to the bank account for the future education of the children.

Some youthfully-married couples, when their children have reached high school or college age, may decide to add one or more babies to their families in their middle and late thirties. These families are likely to enjoy circumstances that make the new baby an especially happy and rewarding experience for all concerned. They are a splendid example of what religious leaders mean when they use the term "responsible parenthood." Their "first" family has been well started in life, and they can now feel secure in enjoying a "second" family.

Modern science has developed many methods that make it possible for parents to plan their families effectively, and more will be forthcoming. Only medically-approved methods should ever be used for spacing children, and the advice of one's doctor should always be sought. Roman Catholics, who may use only the rhythm method, should know that to reach its highest effectiveness it should be learned under someone qualified to teach it. Many non-Roman Catholic as well as Roman Catholic doctors have the special background to do this

teaching, and some centers where the rhythm method may be learned are being set up under Roman Catholic scientific and religious auspices. Furthermore, an Institute for Population Research has recently been established at Georgetown University, Washington, D.C., a Catholic institution, with the first project being research to perfect the rhythm method.

Eminent Catholic and Protestant clergymen as well as the National Academy of Sciences have expressed the hope that generous support will develop for increased studies in all phases of human reproduction. If, for instance, a method could be developed by which a woman could herself detect the exact moment when her egg is released, this would greatly increase the effectiveness and the ease with which the rhythm method could be practiced.

As the world is moving now, it is obvious that for too long a time the privilege of knowing how to plan one's family has been available to far too few families. Religious and scientific leaders in all parts of the world now are realizing that means of family planning acceptable to individual religious faiths and consciences must be made available to *every* mother and father, to help them regulate their fertility in a way that will be good for their family, good for their community, and good for their country.

CHAPTER SIX

SEX EDUCATION

SEX EDUCATION involves much more than relating the facts of life. It is only as good as the attitudes it develops in young people about family life, and marriage, about babies, their own bodies, the way love is expressed, and toward members of the other sex. Sound attitudes in such matters encourage sexual conduct that brings the rewards of self-respect, the likelihood of mutual happiness in marriage, and healthy family life.

The attitudes that parents and other adults in contact with children have about sex are catching. Whether grown people look upon sex as a great creative force in life, or as something not to be talked about, or as a topic for dubious jokes, the children in their care are likely to reflect the same point of view. In sex education the sharing of attitudes and feelings is fully as important as the sharing of information. Consequently, adults need to be alive to their own feelings about sex as they guide the youngsters for whom they are responsible.

The home is the ideal place for telling the story of life, for parents have a continuing relationship with their children on this subject. They are the ones who care most about their children, and who provide a buffer between them and the outside world. In many homes, parents provide excellent guidance in the sex education of their children. Other parents want to give such guidance, but seem unable to do so; these parents say they need the help of the school, the church, or the community.

In one such case, the parents, the school principal, and the fifth grade teacher were troubled by an unwholesome undercurrent of sex talk in that group. Boys made improper remarks about girls; girls gathered in little groups for whispered, furtive conversations. In this school, the parents had requested for several years that the film *Human Growth,* dealing with human growth and reproduction, be shown annually to the sixth grade. After careful preparation on the part of teachers, parents, and children, this was done and with good results.

One mother said afterwards, "The picture proved to be what the fifth grade needed, and all the dirty talk stopped. One little boy even came to the teacher and thanked her for giving him the chance to find out many things that he had wanted to know and couldn't talk to his folks about." This boy had been one of the leaders in stirring up trouble.

Feelings and attitudes that are significant in the child's sexual development begin to form very early in life, almost at birth. The child's parents and his home environment influence such attitudes first of all; playmates, the life of the neighborhood, and school and community exert their influence as he grows older. These attitudes usually last over many years and will affect his own approach to love, marriage, and family life.

Love is Basic

Parents and other adults who are seeking a sound approach to sex education need to know that there is no one approach or method that is always right for all children. Yet there is a basic core to sex education. It is the continued, reassuring love or friendship that parents, teachers, and youth leaders give to the children under their guidance.

The love of a husband and wife for each other and for their children is the very essence of good sex education. In a home where such love is abundant, the baby or young child soon takes the first steps toward being able to give love in return. First loving his mother and father and other members of the family, he later learns to love playmates, teachers, special friends, and finally is ready for the love that leads to marriage and parenthood. But if the baby or young child is not loved, it will be difficult for him to learn to give love.

In a large industrial city, a panel of high school students named lack of love and affection as one of the four causes of delinquency which they considered most important, the others being poor home upbringing, overly strict parents, and a bad choice of friends. "You should have a relaxed home without your mother getting mad at you and yelling all the time," said one of them.

Adults should realize that a dependable, useful love does not mean that they must never direct or control the children or youth in their care. For example, a mother shows her love for her young child by teaching him to eat a variety of good foods, instead of indulging him in a diet of sweets.

Through this mature kind of love, adults should help young people to form standards of good conduct and to develop the inner resources to live by those standards. It does not mean indulging every wish or whim but rather helping youth to form values which will enable them to make wise choices.

Some adults may feel anxious about their own ability to show their affection to children and young people. If the affection is sincere, there is usually little reason for concern. The essential thing is to cultivate this ability. As a rule the young are quick to recognize a genuine liking for themselves, and they readily learn that friendliness may be expressed in many different ways.

Many Approaches to Sex Education

Many adults who wish to help children form sound ideas about sex are uncertain how to go about it. An awareness of the fact that daily life is full of natural opportunities for sex education may make their task easier. Many opportunities occur at home, others arise from the child's own experiences at school or in the community, or from events in the news.

Nowadays, the world outside the home may intrude its point of view on the child's mind when he is still very young, through television, radio, motion pictures, newspapers, and picture magazines. Matter that is presented through these channels and is intended chiefly for adults may also find a large audience among children and youth. Along with their elders, they may view programs about family life, look at photographs of a mother's labor and her baby's birth, or read about sex crimes or sensational divorces.

To meet the impact of these experiences, it is more important than ever for children and youth to have the support that comes from happy family life, from sound sex attitudes and information at home, at church, and at school, and from wholesome opportunities to work and play with companions of both sexes.

Sex Education for Today

Apart from the effects of war and national unrest, standards of family life and sex conduct have changed markedly since the beginning of this century. The divorce rate has increased.

Young people have greater freedom, and there are many more opportunities for the two sexes to be together without adult supervision. This present-day freedom imposes upon adults an obligation to educate young people to use their freedom wisely, so that youth will accept greater responsibility for basing their own actions on sound ethical principles.

Some persons believe that the present-day widespread knowledge of contraception has tended to lessen restraints on sexual conduct, since young people may conclude that they can have sexual intercourse before marriage without risk of pregnancy. This would be unfortunate, if true, because there is always a risk of pregnancy in such circumstances. Young couples who indulge in premarital intercourse usually obtain their contraceptive information from unreliable sources. And in secret or hurried relations, they are likely to be careless in their precautions, or else fail to take any.

However, available information indicates that neither knowledge about contraception nor a lack of it is the determining factor in the increase of illegitimacy. Rather it is only one of several factors involved in an era where uncertainty and confusion about sexual conduct are widespread.

A number of aspects of present-day life distinctly favor effective sex education. One such factor is the tendency toward a companionable relationship between the adults and the young people in a family. Such a relationship makes it natural to talk about daily happenings related to sex and to move from general conversations to the questions or matters of interest that the children and young people of the family may have on their minds. This gives status to the young people, for it makes them feel that they have an accepted and important part in the exchange of ideas in the family.

Most young parents are also increasingly eager to provide for the sex education of their children, and better prepared to do so than earlier generations of parents. The increasing opportunities for the study of child development and family life that are available to parents have been most helpful in this respect.

In general, there are more opportunities today than in the past for boys and girls to work, play, and study together, and thus to learn to understand each other. In many communities, good recreational facilities offer wholesome social contacts for boys and girls and young men and women, all of which are important in their sexual development. Not the least of the encouraging elements of today's situation is our growing knowledge of human behavior, including its sexual aspects, and the use of such knowledge in counseling by physicians, either in their private practice or through counseling centers in a community. The growing number of ministers, priests, and rabbis who are specially prepared in this field is also encouraging. For help in finding a reliable individual or agency to give such counsel, you may go for information to your county medical society or to a council of local social agencies.

Approaching the Subject

As an adult who has a responsible stake in sex education, you may approach the task with more confidence if you first take stock of your assets. You should find such a task helpful, whether you are a parent, youth leader, teacher, minister, physician, or nurse.

First, you have a store of experiences accumulated during your own sexual development through your childhood and youth. Both painful memories and the pleasant ones should give you greater understanding and sympathy for the young whom you wish to help.

Even though you will not expect your children to repeat the same experiences, your memories can give insight into your children's needs if you reflect on the place of such events in your own growing up.

As you exercise your responsibilities in sex education, it will be helpful to be aware of your own feelings about sex, and to try to understand why you feel the way you do. An older physician who had been the helpful counselor of many young people wrote, "I was brought up in a world where human sex was just plain nasty. Pregnancy was something to hide, and to this day, human sex is not for me an entirely natural phenomenon. I know the feeling is wrong, but nevertheless it still exists. A bit

more freedom of discussion could have made a difference in my own life. Certainly keeping things under cover answers no problems."

You have a great advantage if you like children and young people, and are able to win their confidence, so that they feel free to exchange ideas, ask questions, and discuss their problems with you. The ability to talk easily with young people may be cultivated, and may grow with experience, as many a teacher has learned who faced her first pupils with some diffidence.

As parent, teacher, or youth leader you also can count as an asset your knowledge of how individuals grow and develop. Especially valuable is your knowledge of the particular boys and girls in your care, and of the age group to which they belong. You know how they are growing physically, how intelligent they are, what things interest them, what sort of questions they ask, what their friendships are like, what their problems are.

The example you set is another important factor in sex education. Children are likely to copy their parents or other adults whom they love and respect. In homes where the parents' love for each other and for their children is expressed by mutual consideration and respect, the children are likely to learn to give such love. If parents avoid the mention of sex, or consider it something "dirty," their children are likely to be prudish. At the other extreme, if parents use coarse language in speaking of sex, or often make vulgar references to it, their children probably will speak of sex in the same way. When parents make light of irregular sexual conduct, it is not surprising that the sex conduct of their children reflects the parents' attitudes. Wherever adults set an example of integrity and thoughtfulness for others, young people are helped to form friendships based on those qualities. These attitudes are as important in relations between the sexes as in other areas of human relationships.

Knowing the Basic Facts

There is no doubt that you need to know the basic facts about sex. You do not need to know *all* the facts, but you do need the information most likely to be required by the children and youth in your care. You need to know where to go for information that you do not have, for there will be occasions when it is best to say, "I don't know; let's look that up."

You need a vocabulary which you can use

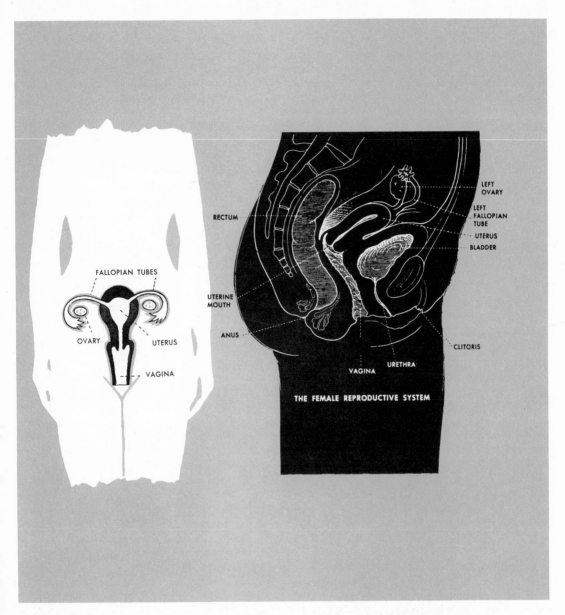

FALLOPIAN TUBES

OVARY UTERUS

VAGINA

RECTUM

UTERINE MOUTH

ANUS

LEFT OVARY

LEFT FALLOPIAN TUBE

UTERUS

BLADDER

CLITORIS

VAGINA URETHRA

THE FEMALE REPRODUCTIVE SYSTEM

with ease. Knowledge of correct terms for parts of the body associated with sex and reproduction, such as navel, penis, vagina, and so forth, can help you to be more objective and unemotional about sex education. Ease in using such terms can be acquired gradually, through practice. Fathers and mothers should use them with each other in talking about the development of their children. Teachers and youth leaders may find such opportunities in study groups or in professional groups where child development is discussed.

Some parents, teachers, and youth leaders have found that a practical way of refreshing their own knowledge and vocabulary about sex is to help in previewing films or in selecting books or pamphlets that are to be used in sex education by children or youth.

The Human Plan for Reproduction

The human plan for reproduction is far superior to most other forms of plant and animal reproduction in the protection it gives to the young. Moreover, the experience of human beings is greatly enriched by the family life that has developed around the human variety of procreation.

The life of every person begins with the union of two special sex cells—the sperm cell, or spermatozoon (*sper-ma-to-zo-on*) of the father, and the egg cell, or ovum (*o-vum*) of the mother. The male and female bodies are intricately formed to make such union possible. The sex organs of the male are well designed to place the sperm cells inside the body of the woman, where they begin their journey to find an egg cell. The female body makes remarkable provisions for supplying the egg cells, for giving shelter and food to the unborn baby through the nine months of its development, and for helping the baby to be born.

The Female Reproductive System

Egg cells are produced in the ovaries (*o-va-ries*), which are the female sex glands. The ovaries also produce hormones. A hormone is a chemical substance, formed in one organ or part of the body, that is carried in the blood to another organ or part of the body which is thereby stimulated to some activity. The hormones of the ovaries affect growth and development and help to provide for the welfare of the baby during prenatal development. Girls and women have two ovaries, one on each side of the body, in the lower part of the abdomen. Each ovary is about the size and shape of an almond during childhood.

The ovaries of a baby girl contain immature egg cells, but it is not until puberty that egg cells begin to mature. After that, one egg cell matures, or ripens, each month as a rule, in a process called ovulation (*o-vu-la-shun*). Ovulation occurs in most women until about the age of 45 or more years, when the menopause (*men-o-paws*) takes place.

When ovulation occurs, the egg cell leaves the ovary and is drawn into the opening of one of the two Fallopian (*fal-o-pea-an*) tubes. One of these tubes opens near each ovary and provides a passageway through which the egg cell is carried to the uterus (*u-te-rus*) by the motions of the fine, hairlike cilia which line the tubes.

The uterus, or womb, is located in the lower abdomen of the female, with an ovary on each side. It is a hollow, thick-walled, muscular organ that in size and shape is something like a pear with the larger end up. The developing baby lives in the uterus during the nine months of its life before birth. The lower end of the uterus, called the cervix (*sir-viks*), opens into the vagina (*va-jeye-na*).

The vagina is an elastic canal which connects the uterus with the outside of the body. It is the passageway through which sperm cells enter, as well as the opening through which the baby leaves its mother's body at birth. The outside opening of the vagina is between the legs, where it is protected by folds of skin and flesh that are known as the vulva (*vul-vah*). Where the folds of the vulva meet in front, there is a sensitive tip of tissue called the clitoris (*klit-o-ris*).

The opening of the vagina is partly covered by a membrane known as the hymen. At one time it was thought that a broken hymen meant that a woman had had sexual intercourse, but we now know that the thickness of the hymen varies widely among women, even at birth, and that it may become torn without a woman's knowing why or when.

The outside opening of the vagina lies between two other body openings. In front is the opening of the urethra (*u-ree-thrah*), for the passage of urine from the body. Some distance behind the vagina opening, is the anus (*a-nus*), for the discharge of waste from the intestines.

More must be said now about the process of ovulation. First, an egg cell becomes surrounded by a small sac known as a follicle (*fol-ik-l*) and goes to the surface of the ovary. There the follicle opens, releasing the ripened egg cell. The follicle then fills the cells called the corpus luteum, (*kor-pus lu-teum*), or yellow body. The corpus luteum produces a hormone that causes the soft lining of the uterus to build up some new lining, providing an increased supply of blood. If an egg cell should be fertilized, the lining of the uterus would then be ready to receive and nourish it as it develops into a baby.

Most of the 300 or 400 egg cells that leave the ovaries during a woman's life are not fertilized. These disintegrate and disappear after reaching the uterus. Then the corpus luteum shrinks, and stops making its hormone. As a result, the inner layer of the thickened lining of the uterus comes off and, along with the extra blood, passes out of the body through the vagina. This discharge is called menstruation (*men-stru-a-shun*).

The Male Reproductive System

The principal sex organs of the male are the two testes (*tes-teez*), or testicles (*tes-tik-kls*), and the penis (*pee-nis*). The testes are the male sex glands. Like the ovaries, they make a hormone which affects the boy's growth and sexual development. They also produce the spermatozoa, or male sex cells, from the time a boy reaches puberty.

The male sex organs make complex, delicately adjusted provisions for the growth, storage, and discharge of the sperm cells. The two testes are suspended between the legs in a pouch, or sac of skin, called the scrotum (*skro-tum*). Each testis is about the size of a plum, being about an inch thick and one and three-quarter inches long. The testes are filled with hundreds of fine, threadlike tubes, or tubules, tightly coiled, in which the sperm cells grow.

The spermatozoa are extremely small, only about 1/85,000 the size of the egg cell, which is one of the larger cells of the human body.

There may be from four to five hundred million sperm cells in a teaspoonful of the semen (*see-men*) in which they are discharged from the body. When seen under a powerful microscope, a sperm cell looks something like a tadpole, with a larger head at one end and an active tail at the other which enables it to swim in body fluids.

The penis hangs in front of the testes. It is shaped something like a thumb, but is usually larger. It varies in size, but its size has nothing to do with sexual virility or fertility. The urethra runs the length of the penis and provides a channel through which sperm cells leave the body. The urethra is also the outlet for the discharge of urine from the bladder, but sperm

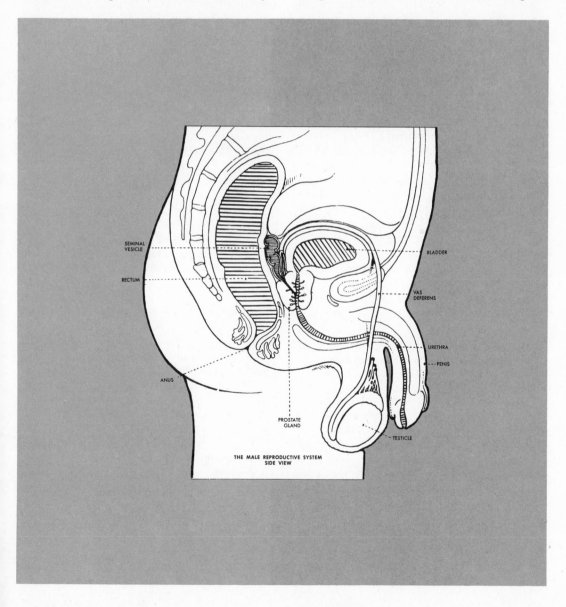

THE MALE REPRODUCTIVE SYSTEM
SIDE VIEW

cells and urine do not normally pass through it at the same time.

The sperm cells reach the urethra after a complex journey. All of the small, coiled tubules in one testis open into one larger tube, through which the sperm cells leave the testis. Behind each testis, in the scrotum, this larger tube forms a mass of coils which may serve as a temporary storage space for the sperm cells. This organ, known as the epididymis (ep-ih-did-ih-mis), is about two inches long and a fourth of an inch wide. The lower end of each epididymis is joined to a tube, or duct, called the seminal (sem-in-al) duct, or vas deferens (vahs def-er-ens). Each duct rises into the groin, and finally opens into the urethra. Before opening into the urethra, each duct is connected with an organ known as the seminal vesicle (ves-i-kl) which, as one of its functions, serves as a storage sac for sperm cells. After the seminal ducts unite with the urethra, the combined channel passes through the prostate (pros-tate) gland and into the penis. The secretions of the epididymis, the seminal vesicles, and the prostate gland mingle to form the whitish fluid known as semen.

The end of the penis at birth is partly covered by loose skin which is often removed by a physician in a minor operation known as circumcision.

Although usually limp and soft, the penis, under mental or physical sexual excitement, fills with blood so that it becomes firm and an erection occurs. In a man, or in a boy whose sex organs have matured, semen may then be discharged from the erect penis as a result of the contraction of certain tissues. This is an ejaculation. The penis then becomes limp again.

Conception, Prenatal Development, and Birth

Various technical or semi-technical terms, such as coitus (co-i-tus), copulation (cop-u-lay-shun), sexual intercourse, or mating, may be used to describe the sex act in which sperm cells are deposited in the female. Such terms may be an aid in discussing reproduction and the sexual relations between husband and wife, although they give no picture of the love that brings husband and wife together, or of the strengthening of the marriage bonds which may grow out of this intimate relationship.

The caresses of husband and wife may arouse sexual desire and thus cause an increased flow of blood to the sex organs and an increase in the secretions that moisten them, as well as other body changes that are a preparation for intercourse. The husband's penis becomes erect and then can fit into the wife's vagina. With rhythmic movements this union can give pleasure to both husband and wife. At the climax of intercourse, there is an ejaculation of semen from the penis. After intercourse, both husband and wife may feel the relaxation of deep satisfaction.

When sperm cells are released into the vagina, they swim from that passage into the uterus and on into the tubes. If there is an egg cell in one of the tubes, one sperm cell may unite with it to make a fertilized egg cell. This is the moment of conception, and after that, the woman is pregnant. From then on, during pregnancy, ovulation and menstruation will not normally occur.

The child's sex is determined at the moment the egg cell and the sperm cell unite, as are the hereditary traits that are passed on to him from both his mother and father. There are two kinds of sperm cells which apparently are formed in equal numbers. When one kind unites with an egg cell, the child will be a girl; union of the other kind with the egg cell produces a boy.

Soon after the egg cell is fertilized, it divides into 2 cells; then 4, 8, 16—and on and on. About eight days after conception, the mass of growing cells, about 1/50 of an inch in diameter, reaches the uterus and nestles into the lining that is now ready to receive it. The cells arrange and rearrange themselves in many ways, and eventually form into three layers from which will develop all the different parts of the body. The skin, for example, will develop from the outer layer, the digestive tract from the inner layer, and the skeleton and nervous system from the middle layer.

The developing baby is spoken of as an embryo (em-bree-o) during the early weeks of life, but from about three months until birth, it is called a fetus (fee-tus).

At first, the unborn child looks little like a human being. At the end of the second month, it is about an inch long, its head is developing, hands and feet are forming, and the external sex organs have begun to appear. However, it is not possible to tell one sex from the other at this state, since male and female organs look the same at first.

At the end of the third month, the main parts of the body have appeared. The mother may

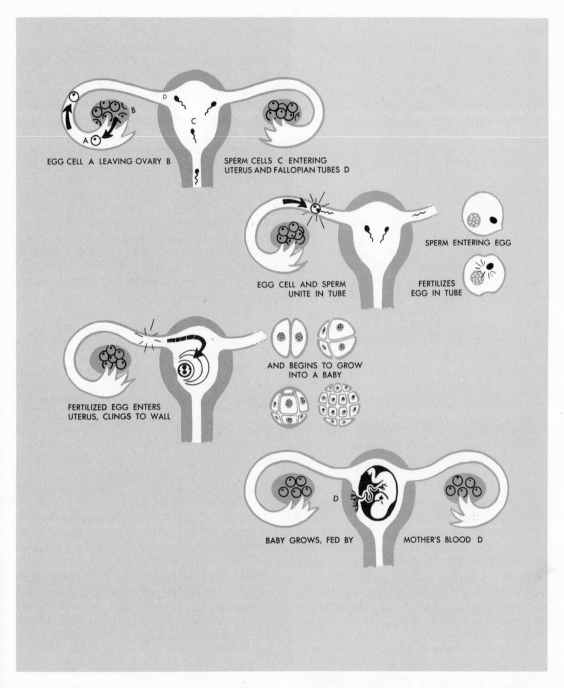

EGG CELL A LEAVING OVARY B   SPERM CELLS C ENTERING
                                UTERUS AND FALLOPIAN TUBES D

SPERM ENTERING EGG

EGG CELL AND SPERM   FERTILIZES
UNITE IN TUBE   EGG IN TUBE

AND BEGINS TO GROW
INTO A BABY

FERTILIZED EGG ENTERS
UTERUS, CLINGS TO WALL

BABY GROWS, FED BY   MOTHER'S BLOOD D

feel the baby's movements around the fourth or fifth month, and by five or six months the developing baby looks rather as he will at birth, except that he is only about a foot long and is very lean. In the last two or three months before birth, he grows plumper and longer and his internal organs develop enough so that he is able to live in the outside world. At birth, the baby is usually 20 inches long and weighs about 7 pounds.

Some babies are born before the full term of nine lunar months. Some such babies may be mature at their birth, even though their period of prenatal development has been shorter than usual. Frequently, however, babies born before full term are immature. These babies are commonly spoken of as "premature babies" and they weigh less than 5½ pounds and are less than 18 inches in length from head to toe. When these babies survive, they develop as other children do, but at first they may need special care at the hospital in an incubator that provides the same even temperature as the mother's body.

The unborn child can live in the fluid within the mother's uterus because he receives food and oxygen by certain special arrangements. Early in his development, a cord containing some of the baby's blood vessels attaches him to the lining of the uterus. The cord, known as the umbilical (*oom-bil-i-kl*) cord, is attached to the baby's body at his navel.

Where the cord is attached to the uterus, there is a special network of blood vessels called the placenta (*pluh-sen-tuh*). In the placenta, the blood vessels of the mother and of the baby mingle closely, but the mother's blood does not flow through the baby's blood vessels. Instead, food substances and oxygen in her blood filter through the blood vessel walls into the blood of the baby, and are carried throughout his body in his bloodstream. Wastes are carried in the baby's bloodstream to the placenta. There they filter out through the vessel walls into the mother's blood and her body gets rid of them. Thus the mother eats, breathes, and gets rid of waste substances for the unborn baby.

By the last few weeks of pregnancy, the baby usually has taken a position head down in the uterus. At the end of pregnancy, the muscles of the uterus stop stretching (as they have been doing throughout pregnancy), and begin to contract instead. This process, called labor, pushes the baby, usually head first, into the vagina. The opening from the uterus into the vagina stretches wide and the vagina also stretches tremendously, and thus the baby can be born.

When the baby first appears, the cord is still attached to his navel and to the placenta. The doctor cuts and ties the cord a short distance from the baby's body. Soon the bit of cord that is left will dry up, and the place where it was attached will appear as the baby's navel. Neither mother nor child feels any pain when the cord is cut, because there are no nerves in it. After the baby is born, muscular contractions separate the placenta from the uterus and force it out, along with the rest of the cord, which is about two feet long. This discharge is called the afterbirth.

When a physician examines a pregnant woman, he sometimes finds that her birth passages are too small to allow the baby to pass through. He then plans to remove the baby from the uterus by an operation on the abdomen when it is time for the birth. This is called a caesarean birth, because Julius Caesar is supposed to have been born in that way. Babies born by the caesarean method grow up in the same manner as other children do.

After the baby's birth, the uterus and other parts of the mother's body return to much the same size as before pregnancy, except that the birth passages remain somewhat larger.

During pregnancy the mother's breasts prepare to supply milk for the baby. They become larger and firmer, and the area around the nipples grows darker. Physicians frequently advise a mother to breast-feed her baby if possible. Many mothers are able to supply milk from their own breasts as long as the baby needs it. After the mother stops nursing her baby, her baby is said to be weaned from the breast. Her breasts then gradually stop producing milk.

Sexual Development

You realize that little children develop mentally through many steps of learning, and that the first grade will be followed by the second, and the third, and so on, in a process of learning that need not stop when school days are over. You assume that children develop emotionally too, as when you say, "You're a big boy now, too old to cry about a little cut on your finger, even if it does hurt."

It should be equally easy for you to accept the facts that sexual feelings and sexual activity do not occur suddenly in an individual when his sex organs are ready for reproduction, and that sexual maturity is reached through various stages.

You will understand the meaning of the sexual behavior of children and young people best when you relate it to the stage of development they have reached, instead of judging it by adult standards. For example, the child of three or four years may repeat sex words he has heard, but his use of them would not have the same significance as their use by an older child who understands their meaning.

Although it is useful to understand the rather general pattern of sexual development, you have probably observed that individual children show great differences. Your knowledge of these differences will help you to provide the kind of sex education that is needed by the particular children or young people in your care. For example, the girl who menstruates early, say at 11, probably will have shown other signs that she is maturing sexually before menstruation occurs.

The following pages suggest some of the phases of sexual development through which children pass, as well as common differences you are likely to see in the children you know. The information is given in four groupings, covering development in infancy, and up to age 8 or 9 years; boys and girls of about 9 to 12; young teenagers of about 12 to 15 years; and older teenagers and young adults, of about 16 to 21 years.

Infancy and Early Childhood

The baby's rapid growth does not affect all parts of his body evenly. For example, at birth his head is large and his legs short in comparison with adult proportions. The various parts of the body later go through periods of rela-

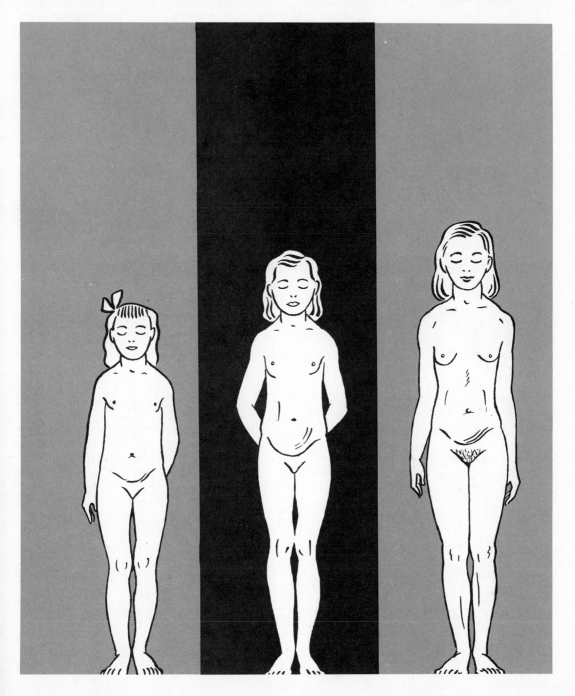

tively rapid growth at differing times, until adult size and proportions are reached.

In both sexes, the organs of reproduction are completely formed at birth. The ovaries of a baby girl contain thousands of immature egg cells, but neither the ovaries of the baby girl nor the testes of the baby boy are yet capable of discharging sex cells. The sex organs increase a little in size during the first three or four years of the child's life, but even then are only a small fraction of their adult weight.

However, even a young baby boy can have an erection of the penis. This is especially likely to happen when the baby has a full bladder. It does not mean that anything is the matter with him, and parents need not fear that such a sex manifestation is unnatural.

During the prenatal development of a baby boy, the testes first develop rather high in the abdomen. At birth, one or both testes may have descended from inside the baby's body into the scrotum, or at least may be in the process of

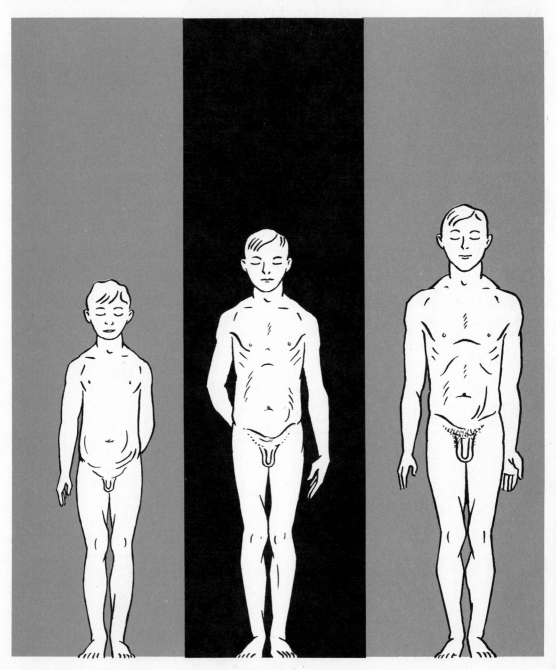

descending. It may be a few years before they have both descended into the scrotum. In the higher temperatures in the abdomen, conditions are not right for the complete formation of sperm cells. For this reason, a doctor should be consulted if one or both testes fail to descend properly.

Although the young child's sex organs do not function by producing sex cells, the child's experiences in these early years are important in his sex education. In these years he can begin to form healthy relationships with other people and to develop healthy attitudes about sex.

It has already been pointed out that children who receive abundant love at home are more likely to be able to give love and friendship generously as they grow up. In the early years, little children may pass through several phases in their feelings toward their parents. For a time, perhaps at the age of four, five, or six, there may be a period of romantic attachment when the boy may say to his mother, or the girl to her father, "I'm going to marry you." This sentiment passes and the first or second grade child may go through a phase when he may not be able to accept hugs or kisses, although he still wants and needs to be loved. The important thing to remember is that the child's need for love is always there, through all phases of development.

During the pre-school years, children do not usually show much preference in their friendships, and they play happily with either sex. The first year or two of school may see the beginning of a period when the child will prefer playmates of his own sex.

In homes where mother and father regard each other's work and duties with respect, children are likely to reflect these attitudes. But if the father looks down on homemaking as "woman's work," or considers it a slur on his earning ability when his wife works, the children are quick to realize it. Confusion about the role of father and mother need not arise if families share responsibilities amiably and interpret fairly to children any activities which are at variance with neighborhood or community standards.

Another factor which may affect the little child's sex attitudes is the family attitude toward bodily excretions. To a baby, there is nothing disgusting about bowel movements, and it is not uncommon for the child of two or three to play with his own excretions. The little child's feeling about the excretory parts of the body may affect his attitudes toward the repro-

ductive organs because they are near each other, and if he learns to feel disgust toward the one, it may affect his feelings toward the other. The mother who can diaper her child and keep him clean in a matter-of-fact, cheerful way avoids emphasizing such an unfortunate association of ideas and feelings.

Answering Questions

In his early years, the child is full of curiosity and is eager to learn. His questions are likely to be about the mother's part in reproduction. Children of about three to five years may ask, "Where did I come from?" or "Where did the new baby come from?" Many children are not ready to learn of the father's part in reproduction until the age of eight or nine, although some six-year-olds may ask for this information and be able to understand it.

You should not give all of this information to a young child at once unless his questions show that he is ready for it, and this is unlikely. It is better to tell the story a little at a time, giving an answer to all the questions the child asks, but making sure the answer is one he can understand.

For example, when the three-year-old asks where the new baby came from, it is usually enough to say "the baby grew inside his mother." The child will ask the same questions about sex over and over, in different ways, as he grows older. In answering the questions, or in conversations about birth that come up naturally, you can add gradually to the child's store of knowledge.

About Sex Play

It is difficult for an adult to realize how many kinds of facts the baby and the little child must learn, about size, color, texture, space, time, people, bodies—their own and other people's. It is not surprising that little children may explore their own bodies as a result of their natural curiosity.

Babies often handle their sex organs in a casual way, just as they often play with their toes or their ears. This casual bodily exploration should not disturb parents.

Older children sometimes discover that they receive pleasure from manipulation of their sex organs. When this is only occasionally observed in a little child, it is probably best to overlook it. If such sex play seems excessive, consult with the family physician.

It is also rather common for children of about four to nine years to take part in various kinds of sex play (perhaps under the guise of playing "doctor"), in which they remove all or part of their clothing, and perhaps touch each other. Sometimes they secrete themselves in the bathroom and giggle about toilet functions.

An adult facing such a situation at home, school, camp, or club, can handle it best by keeping calm, and promoting some other type of play activity without shaming the children. The children themselves often feel uneasy about such sex play, and usually feel relieved when an adult puts an end to it, lending a friendly hand in starting some other kind of in-

friend grows faster. Boys of 11 and 12 may be distressed when girls of their own age pass them in height, as is often the case.

The spurt of growth in height and weight is the forerunner of puberty, the time of life when sex organs mature and the sex glands begin to discharge sex cells. In girls, the period of rapid growth in height usually begins from two and a half to three and a half years before the first menstruation. The year of most rapid growth in height usually occurs within two years before the first menstrual period, while the greatest gain in weight may come only a few months before that event. Earlier, faster growth is usually associated with earlier menstruation. There is

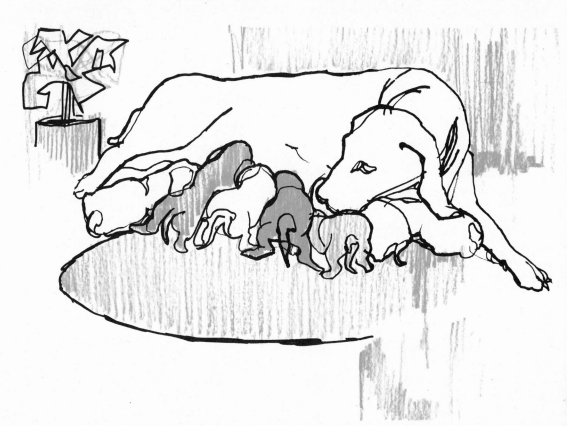

teresting activity. It may be that the child's unanswered questions about sex and the urge to find the answers have led him into sex play, even though he has not put his questions into words. This is the adults' cue to answer the unspoken questions.

From 9 to 12 Years

Each child follows his own pace in growing. A child sometimes may worry because a best

also reason to believe that boys have their greatest gain in height at about the time they reach puberty. If a child's growth records are kept throughout his childhood, they can reveal a good deal about his progress in physical development.

In a group of girls from 9 to 12 years, some will have begun to menstruate at 11 or even 10 years, although menstruation most often begins at about 13, and may begin as late as 15 or 16. The secondary sex characteristics also begin at varying ages, earlier for girls who menstruate early, and later for those who mature late.

One of the earliest signs of the approach of puberty in boys is an increase in the size of the penis and the testes. This increase may occur at 11 or 12, usually a year or more before pubic hair appears on the lower abdomen. While such hair usually appears at 13 or 14, it may sometimes appear as early as 10 or 11. It is followed by the growth of hair under the arms and later on the face. The change of voice usually takes place at 14 or 15. The proportions of the boy's body also change, with a widening of the shoulders; his hips do not widen and round out as do a girl's.

In a group of boys from 9 to 12 years, only a few will have matured sexually to the point of having ejaculations of semen.

Children who have not been informed before they experience these changes often worry for fear something is wrong with them. The young child who matures early may have special need for information, with reassurance that he is normal and the changes natural.

Curiosity About Sex

Although boys and girls of 9 to 12 years are not usually interested in each other, they are not necessarily uninterested in sex. Often their curiosity about sex is strong, especially if their questions have not been adequately answered. By this time, they need to know about both the mother's and the father's role in reproduction.

From 12 to 15

Along with the maturing of the reproductive organs, there comes an upsurge of sexual feelings. Masturbation—manipulation of the sex organs aimed at physical gratification—becomes common, especially in boys, although it also occurs frequently in girls.

It is now known that masturbation occurs at some time or other in the majority of children, and that it does not cause insanity or bodily harm. In extreme cases where a child seems to be masturbating continually or frequently, the advice of a physician or child guidance clinic should be sought, for the masturbation may be the symptom of some deep-seated unhappiness. In this connection it should be remembered, however, that the parent's anxiety can increase the child's problem.

Parents facing this problem will be most helpful to the child if they provide a happy, re-laxed, loving home atmosphere, with a daily routine that offers the child interesting and absorbing things to do and avoids situations that might encourage masturbation. They should not shame or punish the child for it, threaten him with dreadful consequences, or confine him in any way to try to stop him from touching his genitals.

Parents or teachers who observe masturbation in a child in their care might well ask themselves whether he has been put under undue strain, perhaps by striving to achieve what is beyond his ability, or otherwise has been forced to find satisfaction within himself rather than in his experiences with others. They may also consider whether there has been too much enforced inactivity in his life, and whether he has had enough opportunity for satisfying play activities.

In general, if adults are able to understand masturbation as a stage in child development that will pass, they can be more relaxed in dealing with it.

Adults need to remember that with boys and girls in their teens, as with younger children, the most serious damage from masturbation rises from feelings of shame and guilt about it. The teenager who asks his parents or some other older person about it should be given straight answers: It is very common among young people. It does not cause insanity or bodily harm. Most people get over the practice as they grow older.

Young teenagers need specific help in developing sound attitudes about sex conduct. As part of their groping for independence, they sometimes rebel against social conventions. They do not yet have enough experience to know how sex conduct during their teens may affect their happiness in marriage. And so they need the information about sex that underlies the standards which adults sometimes insist upon without explanation. And they need guidance in applying standards of ethics to relations between the sexes. Sometimes they will accept this guidance either in group discussions or private conversations from a teacher, church leader, or group worker in a youth organization when they will not accept it from parents.

Boys and girls from 12 to 15 years are almost never ready for complete freedom from adult controls. Actually, they feel more secure if adults have set reasonable boundaries. This is especially true when the boundaries have been developed as the result of free discussion between the young people and the responsible adults. Clear understanding of the bounds of behavior is certainly important in situations where boys and girls are together, whether the setting is the home, school, or youth center.

Young people do not learn to act with complete freedom all at once. Adults have the delicate task of granting as much freedom and responsibility as the boys and girls can use safely, without letting them be harmed by the immaturity of their actions. Adult guidance and controls should diminish gradually as young people become more responsible.

When Dating Begins

Each boy and girl has his own pace in developing interest in the other sex; some begin to have dates very early, but others may not be interested until they are past their teens. The more socially-mature boys and girls in junior high school will be interested in having dates and going to dances, but in some junior high schools as many as half of the ninth grade boys have no interest in dating. Girls are likely to be interested in dating and dancing a year or so earlier than boys. Differences are normal and it is unwise to keep comparing a boy or girl with his friends and urging him to act in a similar fashion.

Even though your teenager may be impatient if you express concern about his dates, there are ways for adults to help him and his friends. Parents, as well as schools and community agencies, can make it possible for boys and girls to acquire skill in such activities as tennis, swimming, and dancing that help young people to be considered desirable companions by their group.

You can provide meeting places where boys and girls can be together under desirable circumstances. The first of such places is the child's own home, where the parents' genuine welcome may be the most important element in making the home attractive to the young friends of the children of the house.

Parents and other counselors may be troubled when young teenagers begin to "go steady." There is no one answer to the question whether this custom is good or bad. As a rule, the teen-age years should bring an opportunity for young people to know a considerable number of friends of the other sex, so that experience will enable the young man or woman to choose friends and eventually a marriage partner with wisdom. If "going steady" means that the young boy or girl is confined to the company of one friend—and particularly the first friend of the other sex—for a long time, it is often unwise. However, in some communities, the teenager who does not "go steady" is likely to be left out of social activities and to lose out on making friends for that reason. In other places "going steady" among young teenagers is not very serious because partners change rather often. Parents and youth leaders must take their stand in the light of what seems best for the social development of the particular boys and girls in their care. Parents need to be very sure they are right before they insist that their child should be different from all his friends.

There are many questions about dating that can best be answered by the joint consideration of the problem by youth and adults. Many of these are family questions, to be solved by parents and the young people of the family together, as equitably as possible. Who is responsible for the expense of entertainment when your boy takes a girl out? What places are permitted and what places are out of bounds? Who shall have the use of the living room on Saturday night? Who shall use the family car on such and such dates? Where families have the habit of taking counsel together, the questions may be solved more satisfactorily than where decisions are arbitrary.

Many of the questions revolving around the social activities of young people can be resolved more satisfactorily if a neighborhood or community tackles them together. Since doing what the crowd does is so important to a teenager, being different may be so painful that the youngster prefers to disobey adult authority. If adults and leaders among the young people can agree on a proper course of action, such a conflict may be avoided.

In a number of communities, parents, teachers, and young people have worked together on the preparation of a code of conduct to which all could agree. Codes have covered such diverse points as: the closing hours of social events for boys and girls in different grades; agreement that adults should be present and available when young people entertain; there should be no "party crashing"; arrangements about transportation to and from social events; the respect of property; agreement that alcoholic beverages should not be served at young people's parties; being sure that all members of a family can be reached at any time in case of emergency.

There is no magic in such codes, and they

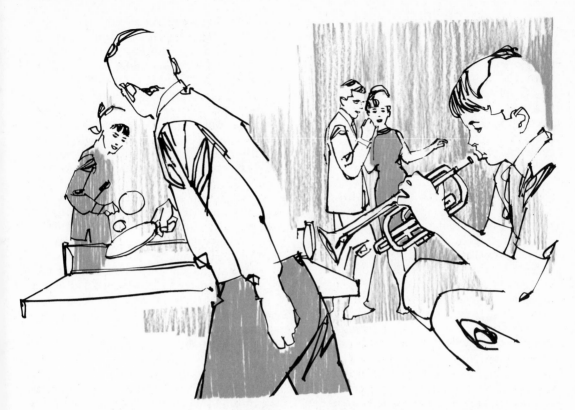

do not relieve adults of their responsibilities. Teenagers only gradually achieve enough maturity to govern their own actions, and while they are growing up they need the safeguard of knowing that adults are willing to be firm when restrictions are necessary.

Older Youth 16 to 21

Young people from 16 to 21 are considered to be young adults. In these years, most young people reach full height and complete their physical growth. As a rule, they have reached sexual maturity before entering this period, so far as the physical development of the reproductive organs is concerned. Sex urges are likely to be at their peak in young men.

The experiences and circumstances of young people in their late teens and early twenties vary widely. Some are already self-supporting, married, and raising a family, many while still in college. In fact, the average age of marriage now is a few months over 20 for young women, and about a year older for young men. Many marriages occur in the teens. Other youths in their late teens and early twenties are going to school or working while living with their parents, or attending school away from home or serving in the armed forces.

Young people must make increasingly important decisions as they pass through this period, and they should be encouraged to make them with increasing independence as they develop the capacity for mature judgment. Perhaps you are among the fortunate parents whose sons and daughters at this age continue to turn to you for counsel and to take you into their confidence, although they prefer to make their own decisions and do so rather well. This consultation is more likely to happen if, through the earlier years, your children have learned that their opinion has a valued place in family deliberations.

However, your nearly-grown sons and daughters may still need to prove their independence to themselves and you. If they are critical of you, or if they turn to other adults to discuss their problems, you need not feel that you have failed them as parents. Young people usually need, and often welcome, the widening of adult relationships that comes from discussing their concerns with respected teachers, group leaders, or other older friends outside the family.

As parents, youth leaders, or teachers, you will want to keep in mind that you need to trust your young people, for they are away from home, on their own, much of the time.

A frequent matter of concern to parents is the tendency of young people to be absent from home without the parents' knowledge of where they are. In families where adults come and go with no communication about where they are or when they will return, they may naturally expect young people to follow the same pattern. In many homes, however, it is expected as a matter of common courtesy that all members of the family make sure that some one at home knows their whereabouts.

Sex education, of course, should have begun long before young people reach 16. It should continue in relation to matters that particularly concern this age group, although there will be many young people who now consider their sex education complete and will not bother to seek further information.

The late teens and early twenties are years when many young men and women fall in love, years when questions of sexual conduct are urgent. Young people must make decisions about how intimate they will be. Knowing that some youths indulge in premarital intercourse, they are faced with decisions about their own course of action.

There can be much valuable preparation for marriage at this age, if youth have opportunities to discuss and learn what is necessary for a successful marriage. Many young people need to grow beyond their rather immature preoccupation with the glamorous aspects of being engaged. They need to learn, beforehand, that marriage's happiness and permanence can be strengthened if the young marriage partners are able to make adjustments about such matters as finances, jobs, and relationships with each other's friends, relatives, and children. Some young people need to learn that sexual adjustments, important as they are, are not the whole of happiness in marriage. Others may need to face up to the differences of potential mates in regard to age, religion, education, and social background. Young people will be fortunate if, in these years, they achieve a greater understanding of themselves and their relationships with other people.

Young men and women need some flexibility in their ideas of what is the proper role of women and men. Nowdays, when so many women work because they need to, both the young man and the young woman should be able to think clearly about how this affects the relationship of husband and wife, and how a young wife may be a successful mother if she continues to work.

While some young adults may seem to shirk responsibility, most are self-sufficient and capable of building the kind of life that will make them happy and successful parents.

When Special Help is Needed

Perhaps you have wondered at times whether the children in your care were really normal, for the whims and notions of even the most normal children sometimes seem bizarre to older people!

If you are concerned about the normality of sex conduct, it may be helpful to realize that the individual who has good physical, mental, and emotional health is always able to make healthy sexual adjustments. And if a child seems to have difficulties, it is often illuminating to find out whether he has any health problem. The family is fortunate that enjoys the services of an understanding physician who has watched the children grow up. Then he can reassure parents that certain problems will be outgrown or decide that others need attention. Some communities have child guidance centers where children with emotional problems may be helped, but many more such facilities are badly needed.

Of course, you should not conclude that a child is abnormal merely because he is different, whether the difference is in height and weight or in sexual development or conduct. Wide variations may be expected in healthy sexual growth and behavior.

A child or youth whose sexual behavior presents serious problems is likely to have other emotional difficulties, too. The promiscuous adolescent, for example, is not usually in trouble just about sex; often he is in difficulty because his basic emotional needs have not been satisfied, as when his parents do not give him enough love, or when he is failing to achieve the recognition which he needs and wants.

The child who needs special help may sometimes give you a clue if his behavior seems to be quite unsuitable for his age and state of development. It may be easier to recognize faulty sexual development in a physical way than to know when the child has a mental or emotional problem about sex. There may be such a physical problem, for example, when testes do not descend or when a girl has not menstruated by the late teens.

At some stage in his life nearly every child quite normally prefers friends of his or her own sex. This is likely to be true in the several years just before or during the earlier teens. Such young friends may experience a fine and loyal devotion to each other.

However, a same-sex friendship sometimes develops into a "crush," in which case all other friends are jealously excluded. Occasionally the two young friends fall into the same kind of fondling and embracing that accompanies sexual relations. As a rule, they outgrow the relationship and move on to an interest in the opposite sex, although unfortunately this is not always the case.

For this reason, young people need to understand that an intense, exclusive friendship with the same sex may keep a boy or girl from developing into a young adult who is able to fall in love and marry. The term "homosexual" is usually applied when friends of the same sex express their attachment in caresses of a sexual nature.

In any large community, there are likely to be adults who seek out young boys or girls to establish a homosexual relationship. Responsible men and women should be aware of this problem, and should protect the children and youth in their care by appropriate instruction. For the little child, the customary instructions against talking or going away with strangers may be enough, or a warning may be added to stay away from places known to be unsafe for children or from lonely places when the child is by himself.

Older boys and girls will need a fuller explanation of homosexuality. Occasionally youth may be approached by a homosexual adult who occupies a respected place in the community. Such a situation is difficult, but young people can be advised to avoid all situations when they are likely to be alone with the individual. Young people need to know that such things do happen and what to do in such an event, but warnings should be given in such a way as to avoid creating a general attitude of fear and distrust.

Keeping Communication Open

Although modern life is not always conducive to leisurely talk, some of the best opportunities for sex education may be found in unhurried conversations between adults and children or young people. Such discussions about sex are most likely to develop if the younger generation has discovered that it is easy to exchange ideas with mother or dad or

with this teacher, club leader, family doctor, or minister. If young folk have learned that parents or older friends always have time to talk about the new puppies next door, or shooting stars, or who won the swimming races, or what friends are going steady now, they are likely to feel free also to ask their questions about sex. Always provided, of course, that they haven't been shushed or embarrassed for doing so.

Perhaps you know certain people who have never learned that good conversation is a two-way street; when they are on the scene, all the talk seems to flow from one direction. Even adults who give other adults the courtesy of a listening ear, sometimes take over the conversation with children and youth to such an extent that the ideas of the young people are never expressed.

This is especially unfortunate from the point of view of sex education, since it is necessary for adults to know what puzzles children and what young people are thinking. With young children, it is important to hear about the fantasies that often persist even when sound information has been given them—for example, when a child keeps believing that he was born through the navel, or was adopted, though he has been told the truth.

As has been pointed out, youth in their teens may need guidance in reaching decisions about sexual conduct. At this age, when they are testing and often challenging the ideas of their elders, young people need to know adults who will listen to their views and discuss them on

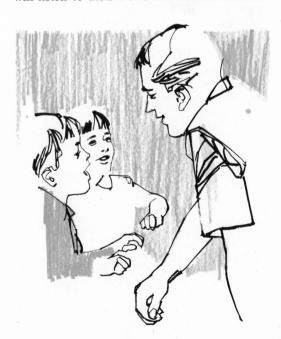

their merits instead of dismissing them on the grounds that "older people know best."

In guiding the sex education of children, you need to learn to listen, not only to what they say, but what they do not say. "My little girl never asks about sex," some parents may observe. Possibly her curiosity has been satisfied by what playmates have told her or by conversation she has overheard. How will her parents know what peculiar misinformation she may have accepted unless they make it easy for her to talk with them?

"This group of junior high school youngsters showed no interest in the family life education materials when they sat in with our church school teachers to choose the units of study for next year. I don't know why—those units are usually in demand," said the director of religious education in a large church. There could be a dozen explanations. The teachers and youth leaders may find the reasons why if ears are tuned to listen and if the channels of communication run two ways.

A Cooperative Task

There is need for the cooperation of many groups in a community if its atmosphere is to be favorable for the sex education and development of its children. First of all, do parents do all they can to carry their responsibilities? And do the parents of the community receive help from whatever appropriate agencies are available in a locality? Do parents have the help they need from schools and churches? Are the recreational facilities adequate? Do the courts and the police have specially-trained persons to work with children and youth, such as psychologists, social workers, psychiatrists? Does a community film council report on motion pictures in terms of their values for children and young people? Is a representative community group alert to the situation about pornographic publications, and is there a program of education in the community to help parents deal with the problem? Does the health department have an active and adequate program of health education and a program for the control of venereal diseases? Is prostitution a problem; if so, what is being done about it? Is there an adult education program and does it offer young parents the chance to study child development and to learn how to guide the sex education of their children? Are there marriage counseling facilities in the community? Guidance facilities for children and youth who are emotionally disturbed? Is there a local health council and is it interested in sex education?

The increase in the number of voluntary agencies and of county, state, or federal agencies concerned with health, education, and social welfare—along with the extension programs of universities—is gradually bringing such services to many communities for the first time. But in both city and country, citizens may need to learn how to make more effective use of available facilities through better teamwork.

In the preceding list of community factors that may be important in a child's experiences with sex, there is room for the efforts of every adult who hopes that young people may grow up in happy families, establishing in turn their own families based on the firm love of parents for each other and their children.

CHAPTER SEVEN

MENOPAUSE

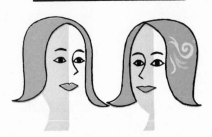

FORTUNATELY, in spite of a wide variety of superstitions and old wives' tales, most women experience the menopause serenely and in good health. The average age for the menopause is 44.5 years, but a wide variation from this is perfectly normal. Twelve per cent of women reach the menopause between 36 and 40, 15 per cent between 51 and 55, and another 6 per cent earlier or later. Many factors influence the time of the menopause, among them the woman's heredity, her general state of health, and the climate in which she lives.

Most women are aware when the menopausal changes are occurring and find little cause for alarm. Others may go through a period of one to four years when discomfort and uncertainty regarding their health play havoc with their daily lives. Since it is well known that disturbing symptoms are intensified by excitement and nervous tension, it is well to learn something about what happens during the menopause and approach it with understanding.

Women are beginning to realize that many symptoms commonly regarded as menopausal are due in part merely to the aging process. Conditions which affect men as well as women are obviously not due to the female change of life. Arthritis, diabetes, hardening arteries, high blood pressure, heart and kidney diseases, digestive disturbances, and bronchitis—all common in the middle and later years—are due to causes other than the diminished activity of the sex glands. They are coincidental with, rather than due to, the menopause.

Menopause means simply the gradual lengthening of time between menstrual periods or a diminished amount of bleeding at each period until finally a woman realizes that menstruation has ceased. This may happen slowly, or rather quickly. As the ovaries grow older, their function declines. Women vary greatly in their response to this. A number of factors, not yet fully understood, are involved when disturbing symptoms appear during menopause. The rapidity of decline in ovarian activity, the

state of a woman's nervous system, and her emotional stability seem to be important.

Decreasing ovarian activity begins several years before the cessation of the menses and continues for a time thereafter. These periods before, during, and after menopause are called premenopausal, menopausal, and postmenopausal. Together they are the climacteric.

The signs and symptoms of each period are as follows:

•Premenopausal: skipped menstrual periods and scanty or lessened menstrual periods.

•Menopausal: menstruation ceases; this cessation may be accompanied by a variety of systemic disturbances.

•Postmenopausal: these years are normally characterized by good health, assurance, and more stability of thought and action.

There is not, as many women fear, any decline in sexual desire in women who had normal responses earlier in life. A happy love life is not only possible for older people, but good for them as well. Marriage for love and companionship late in life has the full approval of psychiatrists. In one respect, at least, menopause may enhance the enjoyment of marriage in later years: many couples welcome release from the possibility of pregnancy. But it is interesting to know that there are rare cases of pregnancy after apparent menopause. A British woman gave birth to twin boys more than a year after a typical menopause and cessation of menstrual periods.

Women sometimes feel that life is unfair to their sex in that men do not have the equivalent of a menopause. There is debate as to whether they do or not. Certainly men as well as women experience a diminution in sex hormone secretions and a lessening of sexual activity. Continual sexual enjoyment may be possible for women after it has ceased to be so for men.

The severity, mildness, or complete absence of distressing symptoms during menopause apparently depends on the withdrawal of the ovarian hormone. In other words, if cessation of ovarian activity is abrupt, the woman may suffer severe withdrawal symptoms. On the other hand, if the cessation is gradual, there may be little or no disturbance.

Because for most women the complaints during this period are relatively minor, many are reluctant to visit their family doctor at a time when they need advice and guidance the most. It is all too common to blame the menopause for conditions which at another time would be considered alarming. Any unusual symptoms should be reported to the doctor so they can be diagnosed and treated if necessary.

Some of these symptoms are any abnormal vaginal discharge, spotting between periods, excessive or too frequent periods, and periods that last too long. Unusual irritation or ulceration of the genitals should be reported. Any urinary or bowel disturbances, abdominal pain, distention or swelling, bearing down sensations in the lower abdomen, or continued backache should be called to the attention of the doctor.

Cancer is a major cause of fear and worry in the minds of many women approaching menopausal age. It is wise to fear cancer enough to have periodic physical examinations. Some of the checks a doctor may use for this purpose include palpation, or pressing the abdomen with the fingers; direct examination with instruments that let the doctor see the vagina and cervix or neck of the womb; microscopic examination of cells wiped from the vagina or uterine cervix or samples of tissue removed from the inner walls of the uterus; x-ray examination; or other tests the doctor may feel necessary. When a doctor suggests these tests, he is doing so to be sure the patient does not have cancer, not because he thinks she does.

In some women it becomes necessary to remove the uterus (a hysterectomy). In such a case, every effort is made to keep the ovaries intact, if they are normal, to avoid premature menopause, sometimes called "surgical menopause." This, when it occurs, requires the same medical treatment as would the normal menopause, but it may create more difficulties because removal of the ovaries causes more abrupt changes than does their gradual aging. Since this may occur in relatively young women, the psychological aspects of the situation may be aggravated, particularly in relation to the sexual aspects. The removal of the uterus, of course, banishes any possibility of more children.

The exaggerated emotional reactions suffered during the menopause by women of past

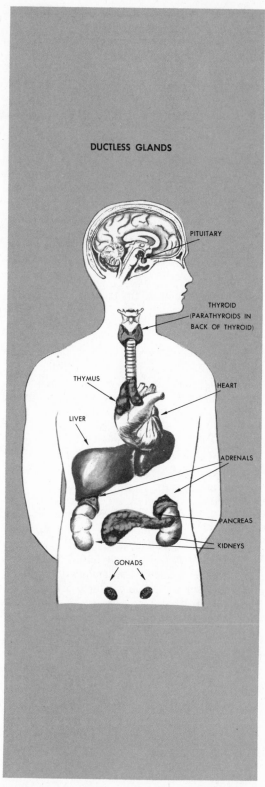

During menopause there is reduced action of the ovaries. This sometimes reacts on the other glands, producing symptoms which can usually be overcome.

generations are less common today. Despite the persistence of many superstitions, women in general understand their body functions, including those related to sex, better than formerly. They eat, dress, and exercise more sensibly. They are less reluctant to seek medical care than they were 50 or a 100 years ago, and there is more and better medical knowledge. They are not encouraged to the same extent to fear the menopause by the spreading of old wives' tales. There is less reading of romantic fiction in which the heroine always suffered from severe emotional problems related to the "change." Women have more interests in life as they grow older, and less time to feel sorry for themselves. All this adds up to a much more calm, sensible, and practical approach to the menopause.

What kinds of therapy are available for the few women who don't pass smoothly through the change of life? A wide range of treatments is available today. For some, mild sedatives are enough.

Many others who experience distressing symptoms are in need of hormone replacement therapy. This type of treatment supplements the reduced supply of estrogen. By making the transition more gradual, it removes the cause of the symptoms. Careful and frequent follow-up, including laboratory and other examinations, are essential during the early treatment period.

The need for replacement therapy, the dosage, and the methods of administration will depend on the physician's appraisal of the patient's condition as well as her response to the treatment. Where vasomotor disturbances such as hot flushes (having to do with the dilation and contraction of the surface blood vessels) are severe—occurring 15 to 20 times during the day and so frequently at night as to disturb sleep—hormonal therapy may be extremely beneficial.

In a few instances, the menopause may be accompanied by shrinking of the genitals, causing annoying itching. The doctor can sometimes alleviate such itching with medical treatment or surgery.

The responsibility for a serene menopause and later life rests first and foremost with the woman herself. Medical science, through the doctor, can alleviate menopausal symptoms and produce a gratifying sense of well-being. But it can't bring back youth to anyone. The aging processes must go on, but we can stay young in spirit. A healthy outlook is earned through intelligent effort.

Daily routines are important. More rest and relaxation are necessary during the menopause. Many women push themselves to keep up full-scale activity. Many have families and are apt to place the needs and interests of family ahead of their own health. As their families grow up, many women branch out into social and welfare activities which may become mentally and physically tiring. One of the first considerations, then, is to learn to say a polite but firm "no" whenever any activity threatens to become too much of a good thing. But a woman who has lived a full life need not suddenly start babying herself or go into so-called "retirement." There is a happy medium, and the trick is to find it and stick to it.

CHAPTER EIGHT

YOUR FAITH AND YOUR HEALTH

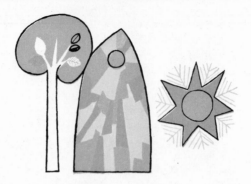

THE HAPPY FAMILY is the one that lives in total health. Total health involves the spiritual, the emotional, and the social aspects of life as well as the physical. The emotional component of illness can—and often does—lead to a physical problem. The strain, the stress, the tension of this world both inside and outside of the home demand and require that we seek help and assistance from others to maintain our total health.

Our normal reaction in times of illness is to seek out those professional persons who are trained and prepared to meet our problem. We turn to practitioners of medicine, dentistry, social work, psychology, occupational therapy, psychotherapy, and the other fields—in fact all of those who constitute the health team. There is an area underlying all of this which has serious effect upon our well-being. This is encompassed by that strange and almost undefinable word—faith. Centuries ago one writer defined faith as "the substance of things hoped for; the evidence of things not seen." Though individually we may not be able to define it, yet we do recognize that in our life—not only in our physical but in our emotional, social, and spiritual life—we do have a faith.

The physician is a man of faith. He has faith in many things. He has faith in his God-given talents, his skill, his ability; in the nurses, the drugs, the facilities; but more than this he knows well that it is more than himself, it is more than the pill, the drug, or the surgery that makes for total health and the cure of illness. His faith may not be the particular faith of your family, but as a man of compassion he understands and comprehends the importance of your faith.

As your physician it is his desire that he treat and care for you within the faith which you hold. In some cases he may need information from you as to what your faith directs so far as

treatment is concerned. Speak freely with him as to what you desire or what your faith requires. He is a man of understanding. He desires to treat and care for you within your faith so that he may make your total health possible.

A strong determined faith, not only of the individual but within the family, creates mental and emotional security and helps allay the anxieties within the family as well as those strains and pressures outside it. The world is big. Man's knowledge has become so vast that no one of us can thoroughly understand it all. We find ourselves frequently in the position of seeming so small in comparison to all there is about us and all there is to know. Faith creates for us a bulwark, a strength, a hope, a power that gives to us the courage to cope with many of the major difficulties that can strike at family life. The family that has a faith is a family that has strength.

The faith of the individual plays an important part in times of serious illness, when meeting those periods in our lives when tragedy strikes our family. Your doctor understands and recognizes the importance of faith in such times. Your faith gives you patience in long illness and suffering, gives courage to face the unknown, gives confidence in the care and treatment of your illness. Your faith gives assurance and hope in the moments of weakness.

Fear of the unknown ofttimes creates an illness within the family that is far deeper and more serious than the existing physical circumstances. In surgery, in medical treatment that involves the unknown, in moments of tragedy that strike our home—in these moments grief fills our hearts. We need not only physical care and treatment. In moments such as these our spiritual life can bring us that "treatment" of which we are in need.

Your clergyman, knowing your faith, can be a real colleague of your doctor in meeting the needs and the requirements of your family. The two complement each other in your care and treatment. A period of illness is not the time to separate yourself from your faith. It is not the time to hide your faith in secret in the belief that perhaps the physician is not concerned. In such circumstances no simple treatment or pill will quickly solve the problem or relieve the grief or sorrow that has filled your heart. Only the confidence that you have in your physician and his treatment and the strength which comes from your faith make possible a return to total health.

The father of modern surgery, Ambroise Paré, a Frenchman of the 16th century, said in a simple phrase what is meant here: "Je le pansay, Dieu le guerit." Freely translated it means, "I treated him, God healed him."

Together, men of the ministry and men of medicine share responsibility for the spiritual and physical well-being of all who seek their help.

> John L. Parks, M.D.
> Obstetrics and Gynecology
> Washington, D.C.

We need no less of the science of medicine, but more of the art, and a large measure of the art lies in the spiritual capacity of individual physicians.

> Milford O. Rouse, M.D.
> Internal Medicine
> (Gastroenterology)
> Dallas, Texas

THE CHURCH IS PRIMARILY CONCERNED WITH THE PATIENT'S SPIRITUAL WELFARE, AND THE PHYSICIAN WITH THE PATIENT'S PHYSICAL CONDITION, BUT ALL OF US ARE AWARE OF THE COMPLEXITY OF THE INDIVIDUAL AND OF THE IMPORTANCE OF TREATING THE WHOLE PATIENT.

> EDWARD H. RYNEARSON, M.D.
> INTERNAL MEDICINE
> MAYO CLINIC
> ROCHESTER, MINNESOTA

The barriers of demarcation which once separated religion from science are no longer strictly drawn. These two serving and dedicated arts complement and buttress each other.

> Rabbi Julian B. Feibelman, Ph.D.
> Temple Sinai
> New Orleans, Louisiana

There are no diseases; there are only sick people.

> Most Rev. Fulton J. Sheen, Ph.D.
> Bishop, Archdiocese of New York
> New York City, New York

AMONG ALL THE ALLIANCES IN EFFECT TODAY, NONE WILL PROVE TO BE MORE PRODUCTIVE AND BENEFICIAL TO HUMAN WELFARE THAN THE ALLIANCE OF MEDICINE AND RELIGION.

> THE REV. ROBERT P. VARLEY, TH.D.
> ST. PETER'S EPISCOPAL CHURCH
> SALISBURY, MARYLAND

CHAPTER NINE

AGING IN THE HOME

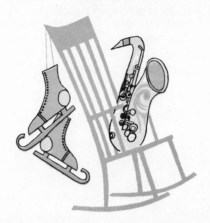

THERE ARE AT PRESENT in the United States more than 18,000,000 persons over 65 years of age. With the increasing life span due to medical advances, with expanding health knowledge in the possession of the layman, and with better living standards, this number is expected to increase in the future—and all must have somewhere to live.

While the number of older persons living with their children has declined in recent years, there is still a substantial percentage who, for varying reasons, are living in a three-generation household. Many of us can look forward either to having an older person in our homes or to living with our children when we ourselves become older.

The Need for Adjustment

There are adjustment problems involved when several generations live together. However, with adequate preparation, mutual understanding, and recognition of the needs and capabilities of those involved, problems can be avoided or minimized and the experience can be a rewarding venture in family living.

What do we mean by adequate preparation?

Ideally, preparation should begin in childhood. If, as a number of authorities in the field of aging maintain, "intelligent application of existing knowledge should produce an average life expectancy of 90 to 100 or more years," today's children must be educated to the realization that a major portion of their lives will be lived as "senior citizens." In the process of orienting them for their future role as seniors they will become aware of the needs and desires of today's seniors.

This education can be applied in two basic settings; in the school and in the home. In this latter setting, perhaps the best approach is exemplified by a variation on the "golden rule:" *Do unto your parents as you would have your children do unto you.* To put it another way, the attitude of today's parents toward their own parents and the memories which they retain of their own childhood will largely determine what they can expect from their children.

When grandparents maintain their own household, of course, conflict and strain are usually at a minimum since each generation is free to do things in its own way. The right of the older woman to be mistress of her home, the right of the older man to pursue his hobbies, the pleasure of inviting friends in for an evening, the enjoyment of indulging their grandchildren, all these seem perfectly natural and they are natural to the older person or couple living alone. But these everyday activities can produce irritation and stress if not properly handled when the older couple lives with their children.

The melding of two households into one can be difficult, but it doesn't have to be. If the pleasures and the pitfalls are frankly faced and planned for before the move is made—or even after the two or three generations are under one roof—the pitfalls can be avoided and the pleasures enjoyed. An examination of some of the problems involved—the factors which can make this a difficult situation instead of the warm, rewarding experience it should be—will be worthwhile.

The typical older woman moving in with her children has for many years been the mainstay of her own household with many demands upon her time. At first, being the older generation in her son's or daughter's household, her additional leisure is enjoyable, but gradually days without meaningful activity become long and empty. In an effort to be helpful and participate constructively in family life, to overcome this feeling of "uselessness," she may try to assist the younger woman with some of the household chores. However, if this is done in a haphazard manner rather than carefully planned and scheduled, the younger woman may interpret such actions as an unspoken criticism of her housekeeping ability with resulting strain and bad feelings.

Avoiding Friction

Older couples obviously enjoy and indulge their grandchildren—even to the extent that the young parents are sometimes frustrated in their attempts at discipline. This, too, can be a potential source of friction.

On the other hand, now that the younger couple have "built-in baby sitters," it sometimes becomes too easy to abdicate parental responsibility to the grandparents, especially when the children become irritating. This can be a particularly disturbing situation when it occurs without inquiry as to the plans of the older couple, that is when the younger couple assumes that the oldsters will *always,* at any time of the day or night, be eager and willing to care for the children.

The older man especially may have great difficulty in adjusting to his new role, since at first his opportunities for meaningful participation in family life may seem even more limited than those of his wife.

He may wish to do some work in the garden, to care for the lawn or, perhaps, to lend assistance in some minor repairs around the house. But he feels hesitant about stepping into the younger man's domain. A considerable portion of the activities of their earlier years in their own home probably revolved around entertaining friends. Now, however, they may feel reluctant to continue these relationships in this new environment for fear of imposing on their children.

While these specific situations will of course not occur in every three-generation home, they do serve to illustrate some of the general areas where stress and friction may arise.

The need for companionship, privacy, separate friendships, mutual consideration, tolerance, courtesy, and usefulness are not limited to older people but rather are universal needs. With proper understanding and planning these needs can be satisfied in a three-generation as well as two-generation household, and stress—

a normal part of any relationship—can be kept to a minimum.

It is obvious that senior citizens are eager to contribute and to participate in family life to the fullest extent possible. Their relationships with children and grandchildren are usually good and they take pride in their family. The problem arises in determining just what avenues this participation and contribution should follow.

One of the best approaches to a solution is a frank discussion between the members of the household in regard to the preferences, desires, and obligations of each. A flexible schedule of activities can be developed. For example, it could be agreed that the older woman watch the children and cook two afternoons a week, thus enabling the younger woman to have time to shop and visit with friends. Or perhaps the garden could be declared the province of the older man. If at all possible, the older couple should assume a share of the financial obligations of the household—not so much for the budget's benefit as for their own.

It could also be arranged that when mutual friends are to be entertained, both couples will be present, but the particular friends of each will be entertained separately on evenings when the other couple has an outside engagement.

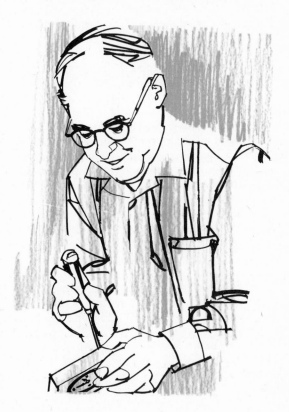

It should be recognized that older people in the home are a real asset in terms of what they can contribute in experience and help, but certain guidelines should be followed. The younger couple, for example, has primary responsibility for raising their children and, while the grandparents can certainly be of help in this area, the final decision in disciplinary matters must rest with the younger generation. Each generation has a need for both privacy and companionship, and achieving a proper balance between the two will create the most enjoyable family climate.

Good Grooming and Order

Personal neatness and grooming is, of course, essential for every individual, whatever his age. With an increase in the number of persons in a household, personal living habits become even more important. It may not be too irritating if one person throws his coat on the chair as he comes into the room but if four or five people have this habit, it could become a major bone of contention. It has been well said of marriage that while the big problems are usually discussed and solved, it is the little ones that lead to disruption. The same holds true for the two or three-generation household.

While many adjustments must be made by the younger generation, it is perhaps the oldster who must make the major ones because he or she is entering an already established household with a well entrenched routine. The following are a few suggestions for the older adult which may make life more pleasant for everyone concerned.

From his vantage point of added years and experience, the senior is in a unique position to provide valuable advice and counsel in many matters. However, he should try to avoid offering such counsel indiscriminately and arbitrarily. Waiting until one is asked before venturing an opinion on someone else's problem is the best way of insuring that such opinions will be well received and sought in the future.

Too, younger family members will not actively seek the advice or consultation of the senior if he tends to be over-talkative or harps upon the past. Of course a person of any age can be a "tedious talker." When such a person is younger, he is called a bore, but when one is older, people are ready to seize upon this as proof that he is senile. Any good conversationalist realizes that the present is related to the past—but he is not excessively concerned with

it. Those who dwell too much on the past usually do so because they are not sufficiently active or engaged in the events of the day.

It is evident that if the senior is to be an integral part of the family, he must participate in its affairs. But just as he values his privacy, so do the other members of the family value theirs. While it is natural that the senior have an interest in family affairs, he must be careful not to carry such interest to the point at which it becomes an invasion of privacy. One who goes beyond this point may become a meddler rather than a participant in the eyes of younger family members.

Another pitfall to be avoided is that of demanding preference and sympathy merely because of one's age. One who constantly complains or indulges in self-pity—regardless of his age—is engaging in a demonstration of self-centered concern that cannot help but set him apart from other family members. It is extremely difficult for young people to maintain a kindly attitude, no matter how deep their love, when the oldster concerned constantly seeks special attention. Attention and affection will stem naturally from the contributions the older individual makes to family life, but not from demands for special considerations.

Perhaps the major injunction is that special efforts should be made to insure that one does not demonstrate the unpleasant characteristics that some people associate with great age. Probably the best way to avoid either overprotectiveness or rejection by the family is to strive to do things with the same ease as when one was younger. It can help modify or may eliminate the tendency of younger members to set the older ones apart.

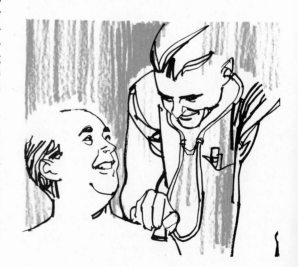

Younger and older generations have much to offer each other. Both can enrich the home in many tangible and intangible ways. The key to successful living is to exploit these ways and encourage each family member to make his own unique contribution to a more healthful and happier home.

Health Maintenance

Physicians generally agree that chronic complaints develop more frequently when a person is idle and without interests to occupy his time. It is easy for the idle oldster to overconcern himself with physical troubles—real or imagined. The human personality abhors a vacuum. For some people an easy way to fill the vacuum is with excessive attention to their aches and pains. The physical and mental health of the older person can be affected by loss of status, lack of meaningful activity, and by isolation.

Thus one of the first priorities in health maintenance for the older person is participation to the fullest extent possible in home and family activities, along the lines suggested.

Another, and one of the most important "health assets" an older person, or any individual young or old, can develop is a good working relationship with his physician. The older individual should be encouraged to visit his physician at regular intervals for a periodic health appraisal. Such an appraisal should include not only a physical examination or re-examination, but also examination of such areas as mental and emotional well-being, nutrition, physical exercise and recreation, sensitizations and allergies, and any social-psycho-somatic problems which may be present or impending.

Nutrition for the Elderly

Older persons require the same basic nutritional elements as do those of other age groups. These requirements can be satisfied by a daily diet consisting of certain amounts of the four basic food groups: the milk group; the meat group, which includes such protein food as fish, poultry, eggs, and cheese, with dried peas and peanut butter as occasional substitutes; the vegetable and fruit group; and the cereal group, including whole grain and enriched bread, cereal, and potatoes.

However, because in later adulthood certain physiological requirements lessen and a person usually is not as active physically as in his younger years, he does not need to consume as many calories. Thus it is important that the older individual make an effort to cut down on those high calorie foods which do not also provide needed protein, vitamins, minerals, and other nutrients. Conscientious watching of weight trends and periodic consultation with one's personal physician as to dietary practices will help insure correct nutrition.

Keeping Active

In later years the individual often has more time for regular exercise. This can be an important foundation stone of good health. The amount and type of exercise will, of course, vary with the strength, aptitude, and preference of the individual, and may consist of anything from a brisk walk to an hour of doubles at tennis. The important thing is that it be *regular*. Anyone contemplating a very strenuous program should discuss it with his physician before beginning. A regular exercise program can lead to: improvement in general tone and strength of the muscles involved, including the heart muscle; increased efficiency of arterial and venous blood circulation; improved respiratory function and efficiency; improved digestive and bowel function; assistance in maintaining ideal body weight; and dissipation of mental and physical tensions.

Safety in the Home

A very important factor in maintaining the health of the older individual is home safety. Because bones tend to become brittle and knit more slowly in later years, fractures may require longer hospitalization and convalescence, and a fall can have serious consequences. Home safety basically means common sense. Precautions which should be in effect, no matter what the age of household members, include well-lighted stairways with firm railings and free from toys and other clutter, firmly-tacked rugs and runners, grab bars in bath and shower, kitchen floors free of grease and from excessive waxing. (See also Part VII, Chapter One.)

Finally, it should be re-emphasized that physical health and family harmony are closely interwoven for the older person in the home.

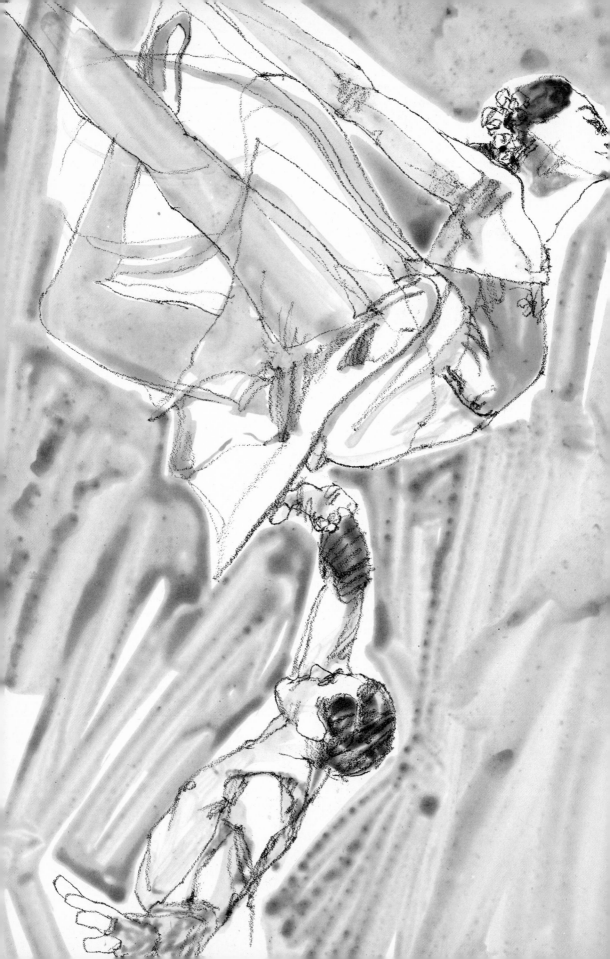

PART III

The Wonderful
Human Body

CHAPTER ONE

THE SKELETON

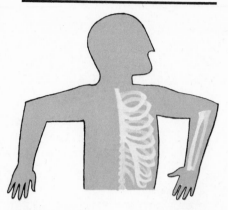

WE SOMETIMES THINK of our modern buildings and machines as "engineering marvels." But many of the ingenious devices you see in bridges, buildings, and machinery first appeared in the skeletons of animals.

The primary purpose of the skeleton is, of course, to support the rest of the body. It must be strong enough to resist great pressures, yet flexible enough to absorb a certain amount of shock without shattering.

Because the skeleton is inside the body, man and other vertebrates can grow rapidly and reach a larger size than most animals that carry their bones on the outside like a suit of armor.

Since the human skeleton is inside and grows with the rest of the body, we have constant protection of the heart, brain, and certain other vital organs by the rib cage, skull, spinal column, and pelvis.

Let's take a close look at one of the long bones of our bodies—the kind of bones in the arms and legs. The femur, the long bone between the hip and the knee, is in the general shape of a hollow cylinder—the design that gives the maximum amount of strength for a minimum amount of material.

The long bones have the general shape of tubes, but they are modified at their ends and sides, and they aren't empty inside. The bulges at the end of the femur fit into surfaces of neighboring bones to form the joints. Ridges at various points along the surface of the bone are for attachment of tendons and the muscles that move the bone.

The ends of the long bones are filled with a meshlike network of cancellous, or spongy, bone. The open areas of the spongy bone are filled with red marrow. The inside of the shaft is filled with yellow marrow.

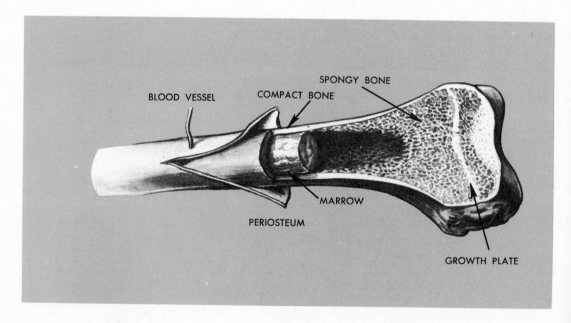

BLOOD VESSEL COMPACT BONE SPONGY BONE

MARROW

PERIOSTEUM

GROWTH PLATE

The network of spongy bone in the femur may appear to be a mixed-up pattern of thin, rigid walls. The medical scientists have found that the pattern follows exactly the lines of stress and strain that occur in the femur when you are standing, walking, or jumping. The weight of your body is transmitted along these lines to the walls of bone on the femur shaft.

How Strong is Bone?

There are points along the outside of the femur that resist pressures of over 1,200 pounds per square inch when a weight of 100 pounds is placed on the head of the bone. Generally, bone is as strong as cast iron, but it has the advantage of being several times lighter and much more flexible.

More than 20 per cent of the weight of living bone is water. Of the remainder, about two-thirds is mineral and one-third organic matter. The organic matrix is chiefly collagen, a type of protein fiber that also is found in tendons, skin, and connective tissue. The minerals are salts or compounds of calcium, phosphorus, magnesium, and other elements.

The collagen fibers, the minerals, and a cement-like substance are combined in the bone in a manner that may be compared to reinforced concrete. The organic matrix and mineral components of bone are mixed so thoroughly that if the organic matter is burned away or the minerals dissolved by acids, the remaining material will have the shape of the original bone.

So far we have talked about the skeleton in terms of granite and girders, concrete and cylinders. But the bones in our bodies are not simply well-designed pieces of inert material. They are filled with a variety of living cells and permeated by blood vessels.

The cells are of three types, each assigned to a special job in building and maintaining the bone. One is the osteoblast, which is associated with the construction of new bone material and the repair of broken bones. A second, the osteoclast, is a combination bone demolisher and efficiency expert. The osteoclast appears to have the task of dissolving bits of bone that are not important to the efficient design of the skeleton. The third, the osteocyte, is a former osteoblast that has been trapped in a tiny space within the bone. The osteocyte is assigned the job of maintaining the bone around it, using repair materials it gets from the blood flowing through nearby capillaries.

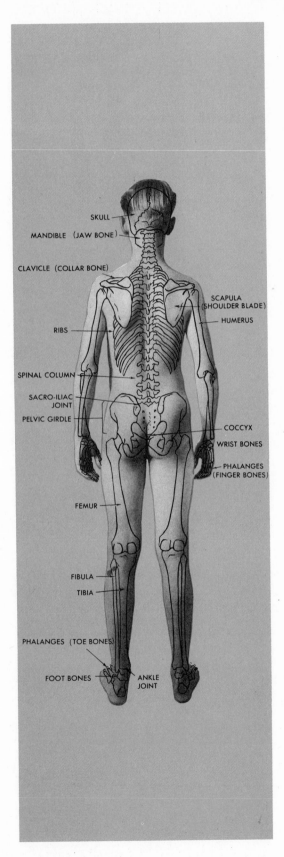

When A Bone Breaks

When a broken bone begins to heal, a sticky material is secreted by the blood. It forms a bulgy deposit, or callus, around the break to hold the broken ends together. The callus at first is cartilage and later becomes bone. Then, after the callus has served its purpose, osteoclasts slowly shave it away.

The bone minerals are constantly being torn down and rebuilt through the blood flow between the skeleton and the rest of the body. Most of the calcium in the body is found in the bones, but the chemical is also needed for the contraction of muscles, the beating of the heart, and blood clotting. When the amount of calcium available for the heart and other parts of the body drops below a certain level, the blood takes some of the calcium from the bones.

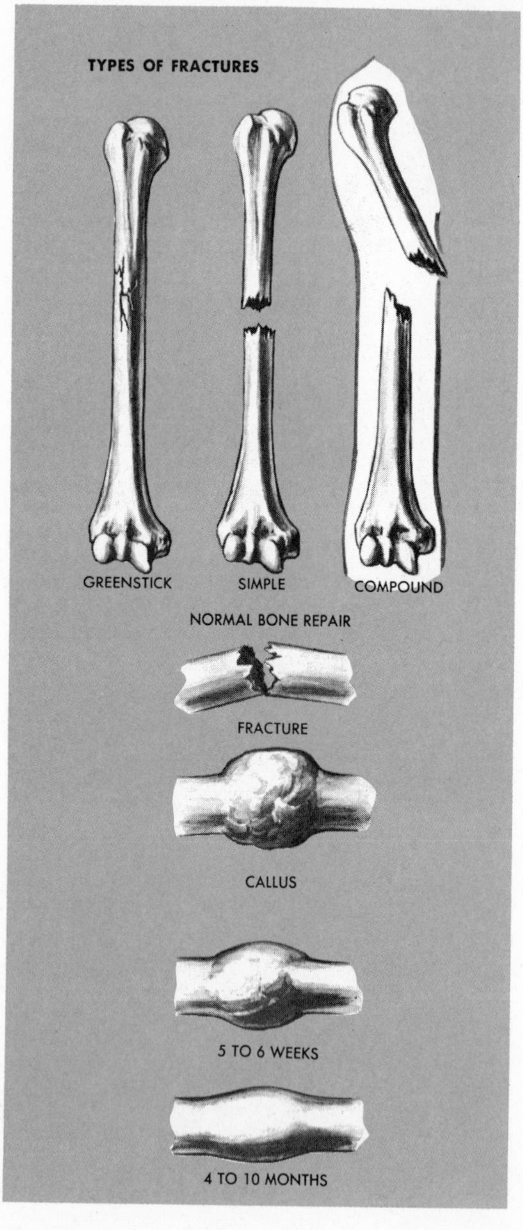

This "feedback" process is an engineering marvel that rivals in its efficiency the most complicated machines yet invented by man. It is a fully automatic method of controlling the balance of calcium in the bones, blood, and muscles.

The Bone Marrow

The red blood cells of the body are produced in the spongy area of the long bones, the ribs, and the vertebrae. They develop from the red marrow at the rate of millions per minute. The red cells must be produced at this rapid rate because the body requires billions of them and they live only a few weeks. The shafts of the long bones contain a different kind of marrow, called yellow marrow. It consists mainly of fat cells, except when the body needs more red blood cells than the red marrow can deliver. Then, some of the yellow marrow may become red marrow.

A tough, multi-layered membrane, the periosteum, covers the surface of nearly all parts of the bone. Tiny blood vessels course through the periosteum to bring nourishment to the bone. The bone matrix is pierced by a network of Haversian canals, or tunnels, through which blood can pass. Nerves also reach into the bone interior through the Haversian canals. And larger blood vessels pass directly into the spongy bone.

When you are born you have about 270 bones in your body. But after you have reached adulthood, some of the separate bones have fused together and eventually you have only 206. For example, five vertebrae fuse into the sacrum and four fuse into the coccyx of the spinal column. Thus, everyone is born with 33 vertebrae but has only 26 in later life.

The Spinal Column

The flexible stack of vertebrae in the spinal column serves as a pillar of bone to support the head and trunk of the body. The column also protects the spinal cord that extends downward from the bottom of the brain. Each vertebra is shaped like a circle of bone with a solid cylinder of bone forming the back side of the circle.

TYPES OF FRACTURES

GREENSTICK   SIMPLE   COMPOUND

NORMAL BONE REPAIR

FRACTURE

CALLUS

5 TO 6 WEEKS

4 TO 10 MONTHS

The spinal cord runs through the hollow part of the circle and sends nerve branches to various parts of the body through openings on the sides of the vertebrae. The cylinders of bone that form the supporting pillar are separated by cushions of cartilage. The cartilage, sometimes called gristle, permits you to twist or bend your back. It also helps the spinal column absorb the shock it receives when you walk, run, or jump.

The Skull

At the top of the spinal column is the skull, which is composed of 22 flat or irregular bones. Eight of the bones form the cranium, which is designed to protect the brain.

The 14 facial bones include the bones of the cheeks, jaws, and the upper bridge of the nose. The lower part of the nose is not bone but car-

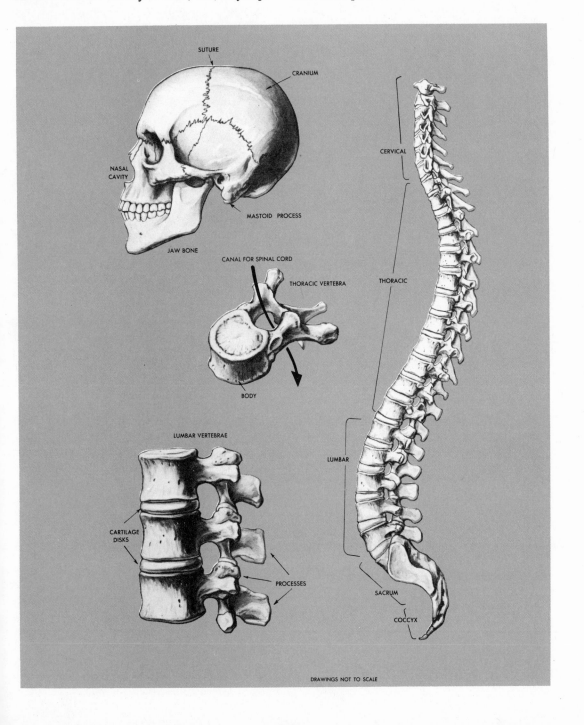

tilage. Many of the facial bones contain air spaces, or sinuses. These air spaces reduce the weight of the skull.

Several additional small bones in the head area include the hyoid, a U-shaped bone attached to the muscles that move the tongue, and the auditory ossicles. The ossicles—known commonly as the hammer, anvil, and stirrup—are located in the middle ear. They form one of the many lever systems within the body. The hammer is attached in the inner surface of the eardrum. When sound waves vibrate the eardrum, the hammer pushes the anvil which, in turn, moves the stirrup. This lever action then transmits the sound to the membrane of the inner ear.

Attached to the spinal column below the neck are the 12 pairs of ribs. The top 10 pairs are attached by strips of cartilage to the dagger-shaped sternum, or breast bone, at the front. Thus, they form a cage that is smaller toward the top. Because of the loose connection of the ribs to the spinal column and the flexible cartilage attachments at the sternum, the ribs can move when we inflate our lungs. The 11th and 12th ribs on each side—called floating ribs—are attached to the spinal column but not to the sternum.

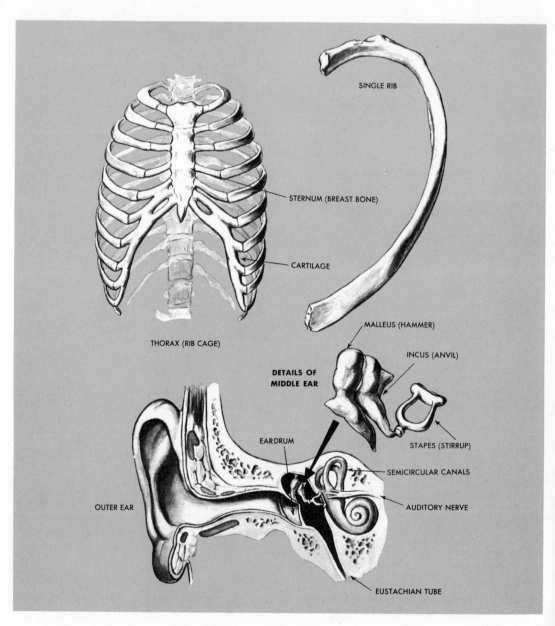

SINGLE RIB

STERNUM (BREAST BONE)

CARTILAGE

THORAX (RIB CAGE)

MALLEUS (HAMMER)

INCUS (ANVIL)

DETAILS OF MIDDLE EAR

STAPES (STIRRUP)

EARDRUM

SEMICIRCULAR CANALS

OUTER EAR

AUDITORY NERVE

EUSTACHIAN TUBE

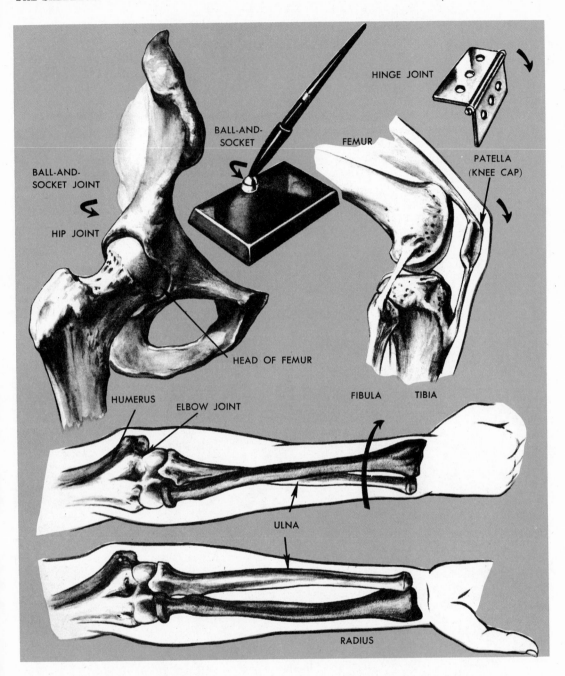

BALL-AND-SOCKET

HINGE JOINT

BALL-AND-SOCKET JOINT

FEMUR

PATELLA (KNEE CAP)

HIP JOINT

HEAD OF FEMUR

FIBULA   TIBIA

HUMERUS   ELBOW JOINT

ULNA

RADIUS

The spinal column, along with the skull and the rib cage, is called the axial skeleton. The arms and hands, legs and feet, plus the bones of the shoulder and pelvis, form the appendicular skeleton. It is in this part of the skeleton that many of the engineering feats of nature are most easily demonstrated. The joint of the femur and the hip, for example, is the ball-and-socket copied in desk pens and other devices. A similar ball-and-socket joint is found where the upper arm and shoulder meet. And levers like door hinges are found in the knees, elbows, and fingers.

A more unusual kind of bone linkage appears in the forearm, where the radius and ulna are parallel when the palm of the hand is up. When the palm is turned down, the radius crosses over the ulna. This action is controlled by pivot-joint arrangements of bones at the elbow and the wrist. The elbow's hinge action is independent of the radio-ulnar twist although the same bones are involved.

Still other bone movements occur in the wrists and ankles. The curved surfaces of facing bones in these joints permit angular motion.

Arches in the Feet

We frequently hear people speak of the arch of the foot. And a close look at the skeleton of a foot shows the 26 bones form a nearly perfect arch—the basic type of arch used for centuries in bridges and aqueducts. In fact, there are two main arches in the foot. One is the inner, or longitudinal arch. The other is the transverse arch, at right angles to the first.

Many of the bones of the body begin as bone-shaped pieces of cartilage and gradually spread throughout the cartilage "mold."

Proper nutrition is important in supplying the body with calcium and other minerals needed for bone growth and repair.

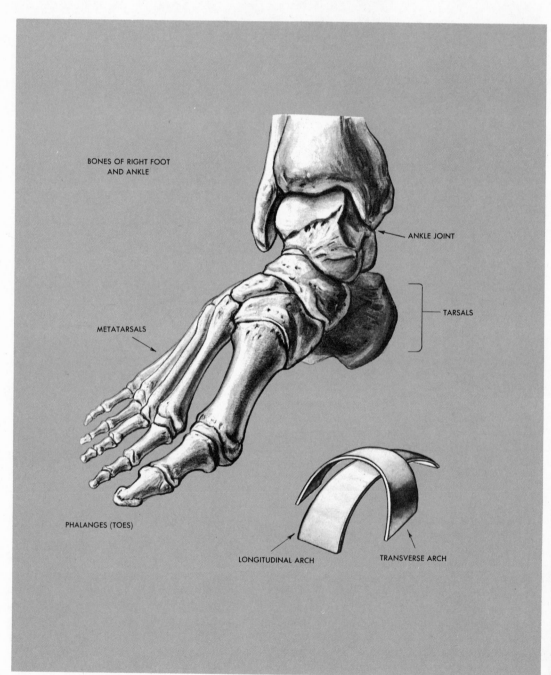

BONES OF RIGHT FOOT
AND ANKLE

ANKLE JOINT

TARSALS

METATARSALS

PHALANGES (TOES)

LONGITUDINAL ARCH

TRANSVERSE ARCH

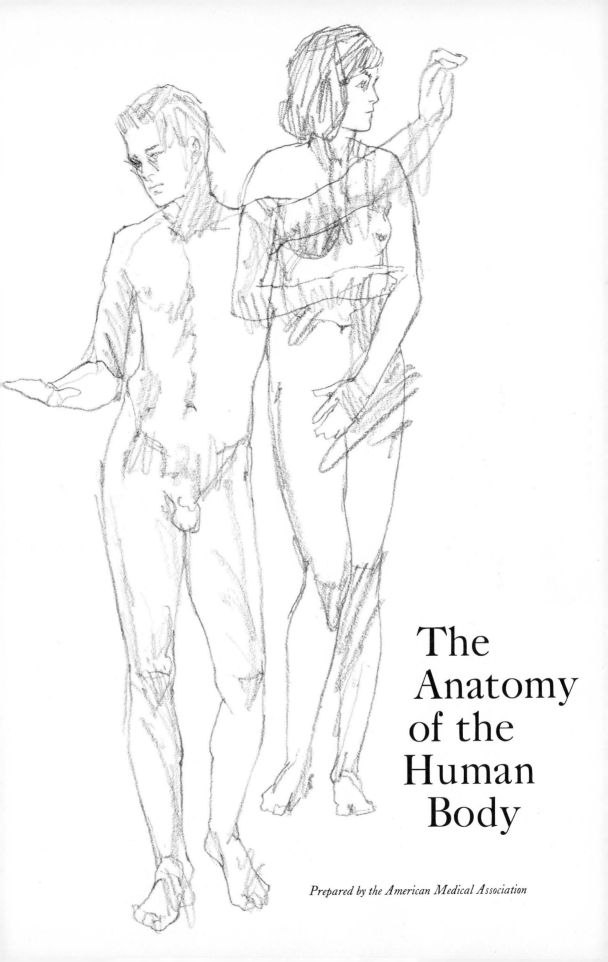

The
Anatomy
of the
Human
Body

Prepared by the American Medical Association

PLATE I

Back View

The skin of an average size adult has over 3,000 square inches of surface area, weighs about six pounds and varies in thickness from 1/50 of an inch on the eyelids to as much as 1/3 of an inch on the palms and soles. Skin is composed of three distinct layers: epidermis, dermis and subcutaneous fatty tissue.

The skin protects against the invasion of bacteria; receives and uses radiation from the sun; acts as a temperature regulator and cooling mechanism; serves as an organ of perception for the nervous system through its many specialized nerve endings; keeps blood and tissue fluids from escaping.

One-third of all blood circulating throughout the body is received by the skin.

PLATE I shows the subcutaneous layer as seen from the underside revealing some of the networks of veins. The larger veins are cut at points where they penetrate to deeper levels to join other veins returning blood to the heart.

2. Abdominal venous plexus
9. Basilic vein
23. Cephalic (upper arm) vein
37. Cubital vein
41. Epigastric artery and vein, superficial
82. Mammillary venous plexus
129. Saphenous vein, great
153. Thoracoepigastric vein

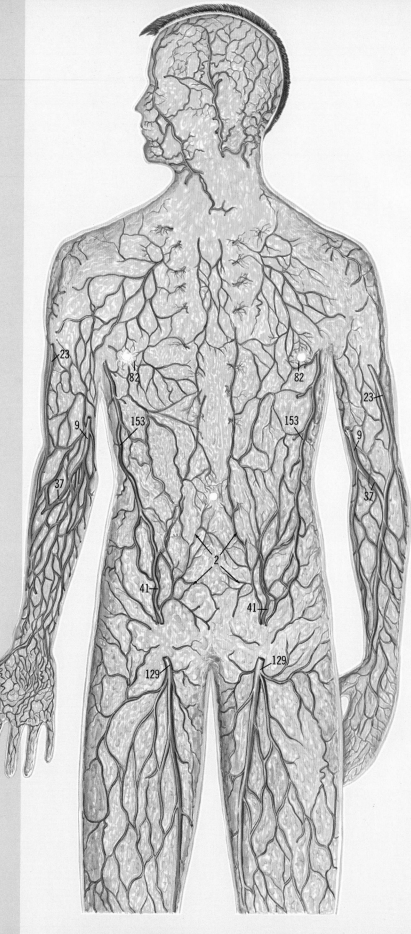

Illustrations by **ERNEST W. BECK**

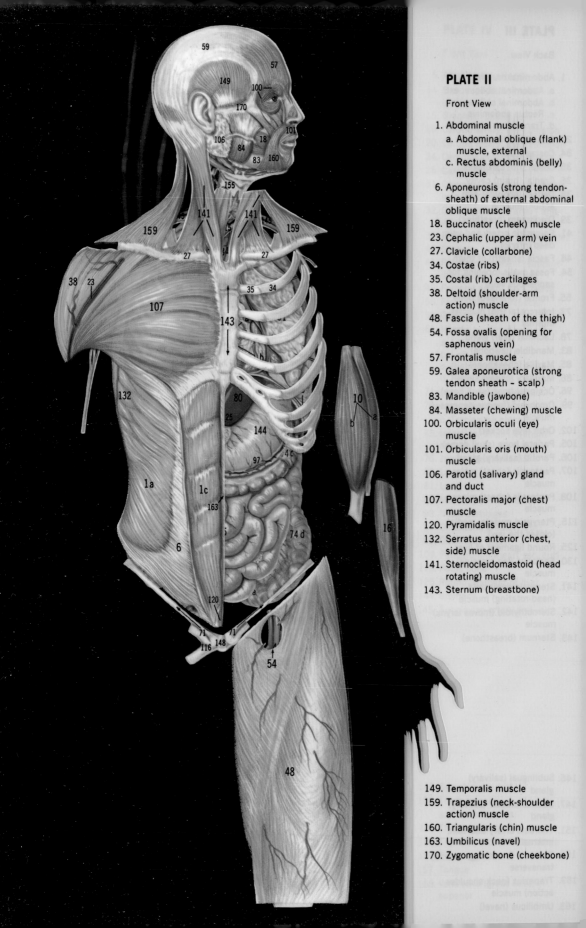

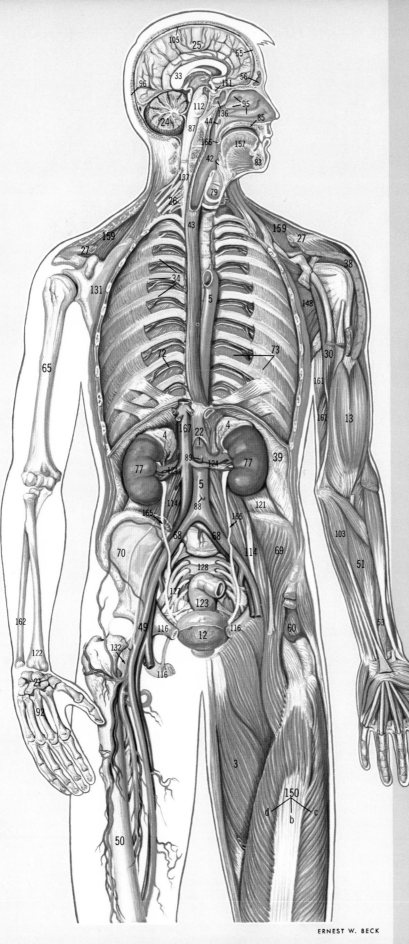

PLATE VIII

Front View

3. Adductor muscles of thigh
4. Adrenal (suprarenal) gland
5. Aorta (great artery)
12. Bladder, urinary
13. Brachialis muscle
21. Carpal (wrist) bones
22. Celiac artery
24. Cerebellum (hindbrain)
25. Cerebrum (forebrain)
26. Cervical nerves
27. Clavicle (collarbone)
30. Coracobrachialis muscle
33. Corpus callosum
34. Costae (ribs)
38. Deltoid muscle
39. Diaphragm (breathing muscle)
42. Epiglottis (windpipe valve)
43. Esophagus (gullet)
44. Eustachian tube opening
49. Femoral, artery, vein
    and nerve
50. Femur (thigh bone)
51. Flexor carpi radialis muscle
53. Flexor digitorum sublimis
    muscle (bends fingers)
55. Frontal (forehead) bone
56. Frontal sinus (airspace)
60. Gluteus medius muscle
65. Humerus (upper arm bone)
68. Iliac artery and vein, common
69. Iliacus muscle (bends thigh)
70. Ilium (hip bone)
72. Intercostal (rib) artery,
    vein and nerve
73. Intercostal (rib) muscles,
    external and internal
77. Kidney
79. Larynx (voice box)
83. Mandible (jawbone)
85. Maxilla (hard palate)
87. Medulla oblongata
88. Mesenteric artery, inferior
89. Mesenteric artery, superior
92. Metacarpal (hand) bones
95. Nasal turbinates
96. Occipital bone (skull base)
103. Palmaris longus muscle
105. Parietal bone (skull dome)
111. Pituitary ("Master") gland
112. Pons (connecting bridge)
114. Psoas muscles
116. Pubic bone
121. Quadratus lumborum muscle

122. Radius (lower arm bone)

123. Rectum
124. Renal artery and vein
127. Sacral nerve plexus
128. Sacrum
131. Scapula (shoulder
     blade)
132. Sciatic nerve
136. Sphenoid sinus
137. Spinal cord
148. Subscapularis
     muscle

150. Thigh muscle
     b. Vastus intermedius
     c. Vastus lateralis
     d. Vastus medialis
157. Tongue
159. Trapezius (neck-shoulder
     action) muscle
161. Triceps brachii muscle
162. Ulna (lower arm bone)
165. Ureter
166. Uvula
167. Vena cava (great vein),
     inferior

ERNEST W. BECK

PALMAR VIEW OF THE RIGHT HAND

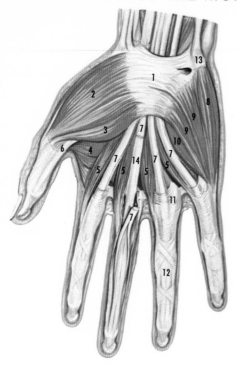

BACK OF THE RIGHT HAND

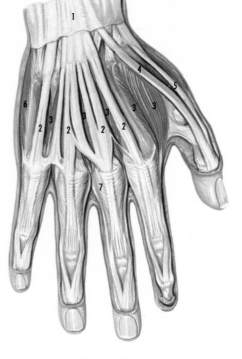

1. Transverse carpal ligament
2. Abductor pollicis brevis m.
3. Flexor pollicis brevis m.
4. Abductor pollicis m.
5. Lumbrical muscles
6. Flexor pollicis longus m.
7. Tendons of flexor digitorum
   sublimis m.

8. Abductor digiti V m.
9. Flexor digiti V brevis m.
10. Opponens digiti V m.
11. Digital ligaments
12. Annular ligaments
13. Pisiform bone
14. Tendon of flexor digitorum
    profundus muscle

1. Dorsal carpal ligament
2. Tendon of extensor digitorum
   communis muscle
3. Dorsal interosseus muscles
4. Tendon of extensor pollicis longus m.
5. Tendon of extensor pollicis brevis m.
6. Abductor digiti V m.
7. Digital ligaments

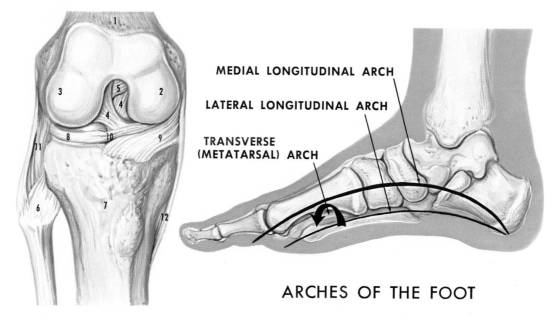

MEDIAL LONGITUDINAL ARCH

LATERAL LONGITUDINAL ARCH

**TRANSVERSE
(METATARSAL) ARCH**

ARCHES OF THE FOOT

THE RIGHT KNEE JOINT

1. Femur
2. Medial condyle
3. Lateral condyle
4. Anterior cruciate ligament

5. Posterior cruciate ligament
6. Head of fibula and ligament
7. Tibia
8. Lateral meniscus

9. Medial meniscus
10. Transverse ligament
11. Collateral fibular ligament
12. Collateral fibular ligament

CHAPTER TWO

THE SKIN

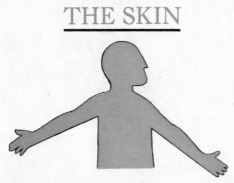

THE SKIN performs a number of important jobs. Among these are protecting the body against invasion by bacteria, against injury to the more sensitive tissues within the body, against the rays of the sun, and against the loss of moisture.

The skin also serves as an organ of perception for the nervous system. If we could see one square inch of skin under a microscope, we would find it contained about 72 feet of nerves. We also would be able to count hundreds of pain receptors, plus pressure, heat, and cold receptors.

Temperature regulation is still another job performed by the skin. That one square inch of skin also contains about 15 feet of blood vessels which dilate (grow larger) when the body needs to lose heat or constrict (become narrower) when the body must reduce the amount of heat loss through the skin.

When the surrounding air is comparatively warm, the skin is cooled by moisture secreted by the sweat glands. There are about 2,000,000 sweat glands over the surface of the body; they occur in the greatest concentration on the palms of the hands and the soles of the feet. The sweat glands are controlled by a heat regulator in the brain. The moisture secreted by the sweat glands cools the body by evaporation.

The surface of your skin may look smooth, but if you examine it under a magnifying glass, you'll see countless ridges and valleys. You also will see different patterns of skin texture on the palm of your hand and on the back of your hand.

The skin generally is soft and flexible, and more elastic in younger people. It varies in thickness from about 1/50 of an inch on the eyelids to as much as 1/3 of an inch on palms and soles.

The Skin Layers

Three layers of tissue make up the skin: the epidermis, the dermis, and the subcutaneous layer. The subcutaneous layer contains many fat lobules, blood vessels, and nerves. It links the dermis, or middle layer of the three, with tissue covering the muscles and bones. It also serves as a smooth and springy base for the skin.

As persons grow older, the fatty tissue is absorbed. This causes the outer layers of the skin to form uneven folds, or wrinkles.

The dermis, sometimes called the "true skin," is atop the subcutaneous layer. It varies in thickness in different parts of the body and contains blood vessels, nerves, nerve receptors, hair follicles, sweat glands, and oil glands.

At the top of the dermis is a layer of tiny cone-shaped objects called papillae. There are perhaps 150 million papillae scattered over the body. They are more numerous in areas such as the fingertips, where the skin appears to be more sensitive. Nerve fibers and special nerve endings are found in many of the papillae. As a result, the sense of touch is best developed in areas where papillae with nerve endings occur most frequently.

The papillary layer fits snugly against the outer layer of skin, the epidermis, which has ridges corresponding to those of the papillae. The ridges prevent the various skin layers from slipping.

The ridges on the surface of the fingertips form whorls and other patterns, which we call fingerprints. Similar ridges appear on the soles of the feet. Because it is unlikely that two persons will have exactly the same pattern of ridges, fingerprints are used by the police to identify criminals and footprints by hospitals to identify babies. The possibility that two persons would have the same set of fingerprints or footprints has been estimated to be one chance in 24,000,000,000.

The top layer of the epidermis, sometimes called the horny layer, is made of scales that actually are dead skin cells. They gradually flake off, or soak off when wet. The horny layer is constantly being replaced by cells pushed

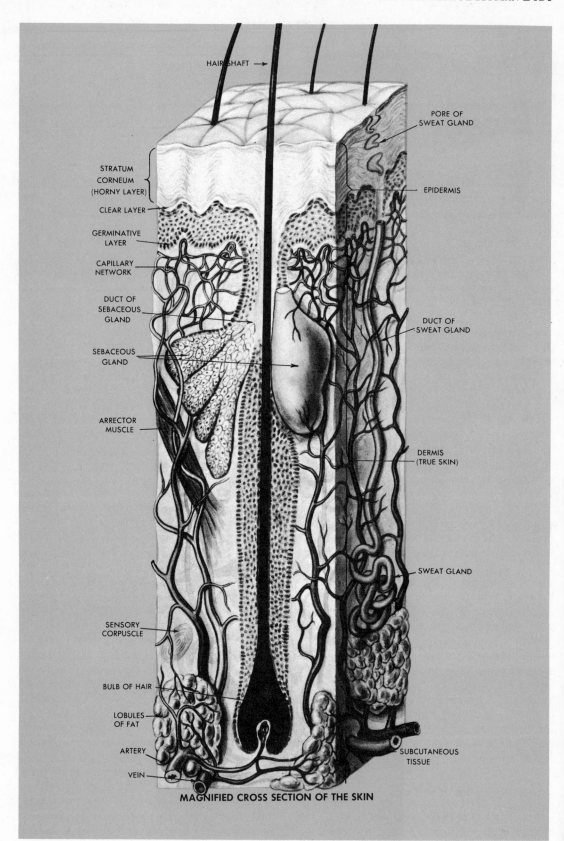

HAIR SHAFT →

PORE OF
SWEAT GLAND

STRATUM
CORNEUM
(HORNY LAYER)

EPIDERMIS

CLEAR LAYER

GERMINATIVE
LAYER

CAPILLARY
NETWORK

DUCT OF
SEBACEOUS
GLAND

DUCT OF
SWEAT GLAND

SEBACEOUS
GLAND

ARRECTOR
MUSCLE

DERMIS
(TRUE SKIN)

SWEAT GLAND

SENSORY
CORPUSCLE

BULB OF HAIR

LOBULES
OF FAT

ARTERY

SUBCUTANEOUS
TISSUE

VEIN

MAGNIFIED CROSS SECTION OF THE SKIN

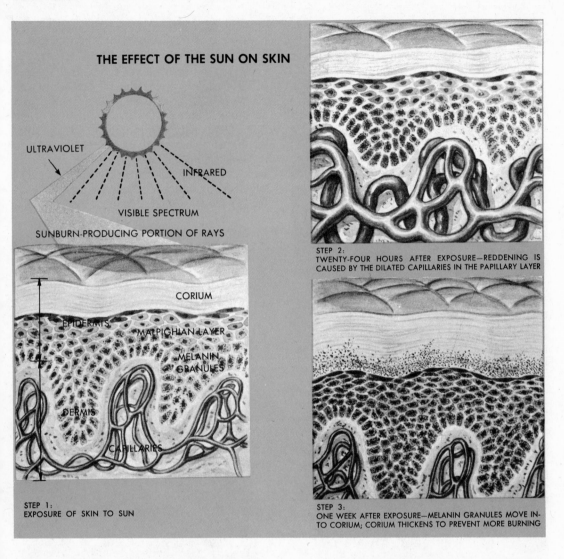

THE EFFECT OF THE SUN ON SKIN

ULTRAVIOLET

INFRARED

VISIBLE SPECTRUM

SUNBURN-PRODUCING PORTION OF RAYS

CORIUM

EPIDERMIS

MALPIGHIAN LAYER

MELANIN GRANULES

DERMIS

CAPILLARIES

STEP 1:
EXPOSURE OF SKIN TO SUN

STEP 2:
TWENTY-FOUR HOURS AFTER EXPOSURE—REDDENING IS
CAUSED BY THE DILATED CAPILLARIES IN THE PAPILLARY LAYER

STEP 3:
ONE WEEK AFTER EXPOSURE—MELANIN GRANULES MOVE IN-
TO CORIUM; CORIUM THICKENS TO PREVENT MORE BURNING

toward the surface as new cells are formed in the deeper layer of the epidermis. As the skin cells move toward the surface, their jellylike living substance—protoplasm—is converted into horny material.

In the deeper layer where the new cells are being formed, the skin may be colored by a pigment called melanin. Its purpose is to prevent the more dangerous rays of the sun from damaging tissues. Skin color also is influenced by a second, yellow pigment and by the presence of blood vessels in the dermis layer.

Tan and Sunburn

We're all familiar with the changes in the skin produced by exposure to sunlight. The effects of sunlight vary with the time of the year, the geographical area, and the hour of the

day. Generally, the skin shows a reddening due to enlargement of small blood vessels in the deeper layers of skin after about 20 minutes' exposure to the summer sun at midday. The reddening, called erythema, may not appear until several hours after exposure to the sun. If the dose of sunlight is intense, the reddening may be followed by blistering and peeling of the outer layer of epidermal cells.

If the erythema is not severe, it will fade in a few days and the skin will gradually acquire a brown coloration that we call suntan. The brown color is produced by the melanin pigment which usually is present at the bottom of the epidermal layer.

When skin is exposed to the sun, it is believed that melanin pigment moves toward the surface of the skin and is replaced by new melanin in the lower cell layer. One or two weeks may be required to develop a suntan by moderate daily doses of sunlight. The tan will begin to fade if occasional exposure to sunlight is not continued.

Freckles are caused by small areas of melanin pigment. They usually fade somewhat during winter months and increase in prominence during the summer.

Glands in the Skin

Two main types of glands are located in the dermis. One, already mentioned, is the sweat

gland. Under the microscope it appears as a tightly coiled tube deep in the dermis with a corkscrew like tubule that rises through the epidermis to the surface of the skin.

The second type is the sebaceous, or oil, gland. The oil glands usually occur in or near a hair follicle and are located in all parts of the skin except on the palms of the hands and soles of the feet. They are particularly common in the skin of the face and scalp. The glands are flask-shaped and contain an oily substance that is constantly being produced by the glands as the fat globules change into oil droplets and

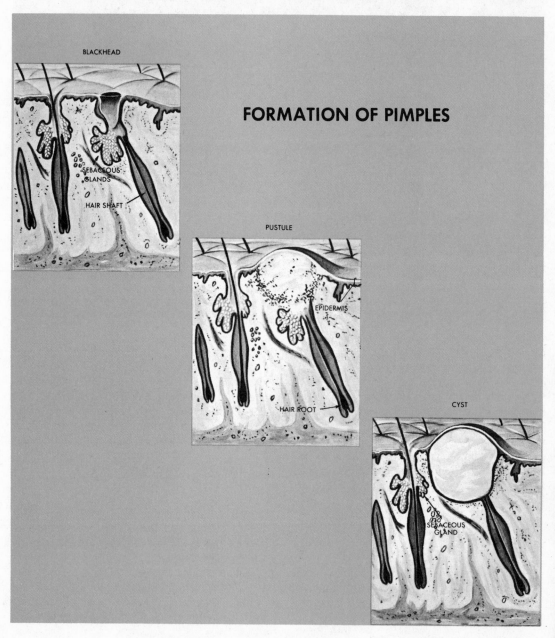

FORMATION OF PIMPLES

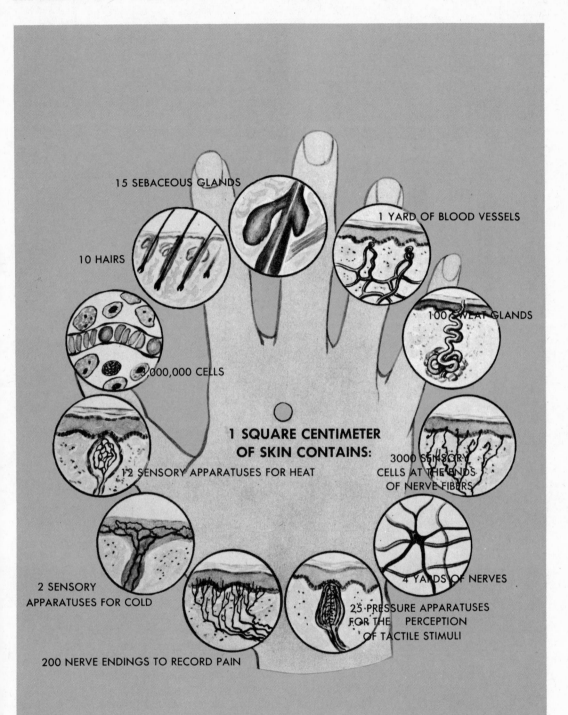

15 SEBACEOUS GLANDS

10 HAIRS

1 YARD OF BLOOD VESSELS

100 SWEAT GLANDS

3,000,000 CELLS

1 SQUARE CENTIMETER
OF SKIN CONTAINS:

12 SENSORY APPARATUSES FOR HEAT

3000 SENSORY
CELLS AT THE ENDS
OF NERVE FIBERS

2 SENSORY
APPARATUSES FOR COLD

4 YARDS OF NERVES

25 PRESSURE APPARATUSES
FOR THE   PERCEPTION
OF TACTILE STIMULI

200 NERVE ENDINGS TO RECORD PAIN

STRUCTURES IN THE SKIN

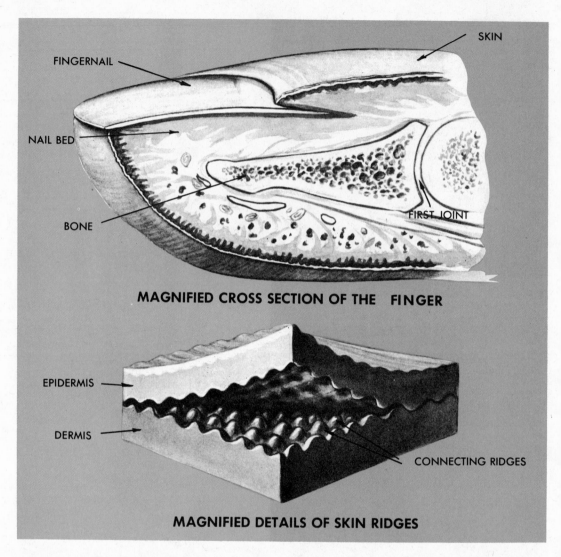

FINGERNAIL

SKIN

NAIL BED

BONE

FIRST JOINT

MAGNIFIED CROSS SECTION OF THE FINGER

EPIDERMIS

DERMIS

CONNECTING RIDGES

MAGNIFIED DETAILS OF SKIN RIDGES

move toward the surface of the skin. The purpose of the oil is to keep the hair and skin from becoming dry and brittle. The ceruminous glands of the ear, which produce ear wax, help to protect the ear canal.

Hair

Several kinds of hair are part of the skin. They range in texture from the soft, almost invisible hair on the forehead to the long hairs of the scalp and the short, stiff hairs on the eyelids. Like the oil glands, hair occurs on all parts of the skin except the palms and soles.

Each hair has a root, which is anchored at the bottom of a microscopic shaft called a follicle. It also has a shaft which extends past the top of the follicle. The follicle enters the epidermis and passes deep into the dermal layer at an angle. The follicles of long hairs may extend into the subcutaneous layer. Oil, or sebaceous, glands empty into the follicle. At the root of the hair is a cone-shaped papilla that is similar to the peg-like papillae that underlie the ridges of the fingers, palms, and soles.

The shaft of the hair is covered with tiny, overlapping scales. An inner layer of cells in the hair shaft contains pigment that gives the hair its color; in white hair the cells contain air. Curly hair appears flattened when seen in cross section under a microscope. Straight hairs appear round or oval-shaped in cross section.

Attached to each hair follicle is a small bundle of involuntary muscle fibers. Under the influence of cold or emotions, the muscle fibers contract and the hair becomes erect. The action of the tiny muscles also produces "goose flesh."

The hair follicles develop as downgrowths

of the layers of the skin. The hair then grows outward from the bottom of the follicle. Thus, the body hair actually is a special form of the skin itself.

Nails

The fingernails and toenails like hair, are a specialized form of skin. The thin layer separating the dermis and epidermis, known technically as the stratum lucidum, becomes thick and hard as the fingers and toes develop. The fully developed nail then overlays a modified part of the dermis that is the bed of the nail. The base portion of the nail is covered by epidermis.

The nail bed contains ridges rich in tiny blood vessels. The blood vessels give the area under the transparent nail its red coloration. Near the base, or root, there is less blood circulation and the nail is not so firmly attached to the nail bed. This explains why the lunula, or half-moon, area of the nail has a whiter coloration than the rest.

The rate of growth of nails varies and depends upon such factors as the age of the person and the season of the year. For example, nails grow faster in young people and during the summer months.

Blushing and Flushing

The skin is richly supplied with small blood vessels. We already noted that the blood supply in the skin accounts for the reddening of sunburn and the coloration of the fingers beneath the nails. The blood vessels also account for the reddening of the skin when we blush.

Many of the so-called birthmarks get their coloration from the tiny blood vessels concentrated in a small area of the skin. Other birthmarks are caused by patches of pigment in the skin and are similar to freckles. Moles also are pigmented patches.

Humans with little or no pigment in their skin are called albinos. Their skin color is whitish or pink. The hair is white. Some persons have streaks or patches of white hair due to partial albinism. True albinos cannot expose their skin to summer sunlight and their eyes are unusually sensitive to intense light. Normally pigmented skins range from pinkish yellow (peach) through yellow and brown to black, depending on race.

CHAPTER THREE

THE MUSCLES

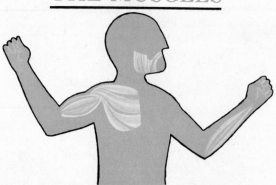

To UNDERSTAND how a muscle performs, let's take a look at a piece of muscle tissue as it would appear under a microscope. Each bit of muscle, we will see, is made of a bundle of fibers. Each fiber is about the size of a human hair but it can support 1,000 times its own weight. We probably have about 6,000,000,000 fibers in the more than 600 muscles scattered through the body.

There are three kinds of muscle tissue, as it appears under the microscope. One kind has dark and light bands across the fibers and is called striped muscle. It also may be called skeletal muscle because it is attached to some part of the skeleton. And it is known as voluntary muscle because we have some control over it—we use it to throw a ball, lift a book, or walk up a hill.

The second kind is smooth, or involuntary, muscle. Compared with the striped muscle, its cells are small and delicate, and it lacks the dark and light bands of the skeletal muscle. This type of muscle handles the work of all the internal organs except the heart. Smooth mus-

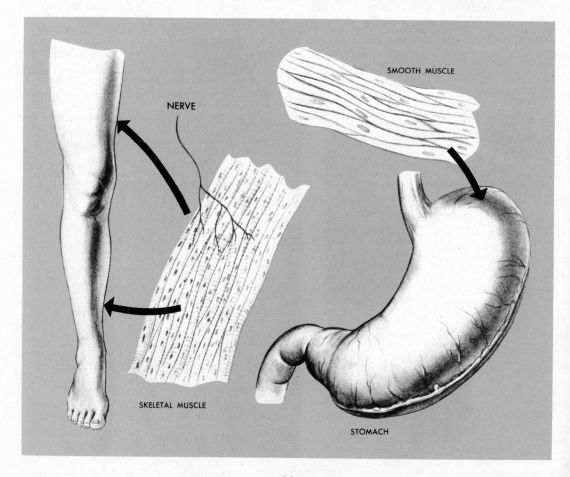

SMOOTH MUSCLE

NERVE

SKELETAL MUSCLE

STOMACH

cle is known as involuntary because we do not have direct control over its action, for example, movements of the stomach and intestines.

The third kind of muscle tissue, found in the heart, is called cardiac. Cardiac muscle fibers are striped, but they are not separated from each other by sheaths as the skeletal muscles are. Instead, they are joined in a continuous network. Since we do not have direct control over the contractions of cardiac tissue, it too is involuntary in action.

When a muscle contracts, it becomes shorter by as much as a third to a half. And as it gets shorter, it becomes thicker.

Like a regiment of soldiers on parade, each fiber reacts in the same manner when the "contract" signal is given. The signal, in the case of voluntary muscles, is sent from the brain through the central nervous system. The message is relayed instantly through a network of nerves that reach each of the fibers involved.

The smooth, or involuntary, muscles receive their signals from a different network of nerves, the autonomic system. These muscles function automatically and we usually are not even

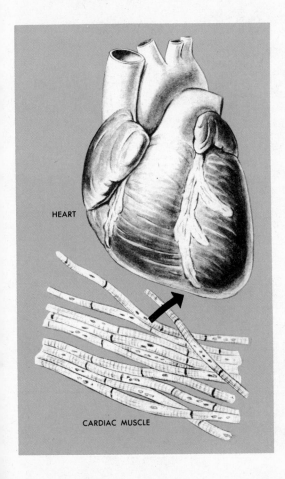

HEART

CARDIAC MUSCLE

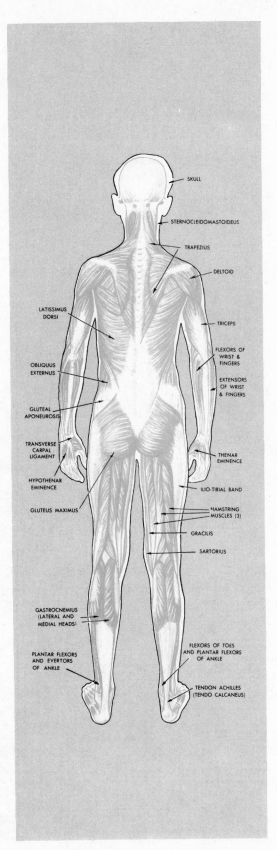

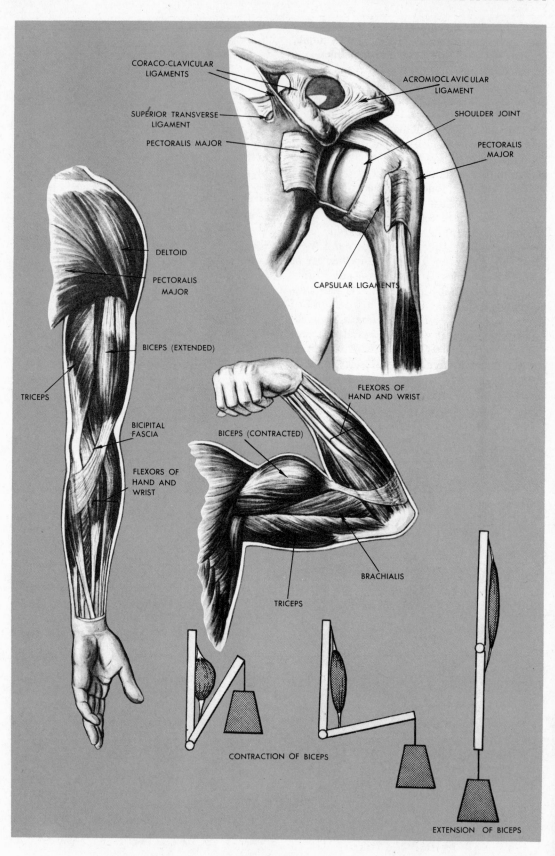

CORACO-CLAVICULAR
LIGAMENTS

ACROMIOCLAVICULAR
LIGAMENT

SUPERIOR TRANSVERSE
LIGAMENT

SHOULDER JOINT

PECTORALIS MAJOR

PECTORALIS
MAJOR

DELTOID

PECTORALIS
MAJOR

CAPSULAR LIGAMENTS

BICEPS (EXTENDED)

TRICEPS

FLEXORS OF
HAND AND WRIST

BICIPITAL
FASCIA

BICEPS (CONTRACTED)

FLEXORS OF
HAND AND
WRIST

BRACHIALIS

TRICEPS

CONTRACTION OF BICEPS

EXTENSION OF BICEPS

aware of their action. But without the automatic work of the smooth muscles we would not be able to digest food or continue breathing when asleep.

Actually, you do not consciously make any muscle contract on "command." You don't tell your biceps to contract. You decide to bend your elbow and your brain and central nervous system translate the message and route it to the muscle fibers concerned.

The biceps is a part of a team that moves the arm. It can bend the elbow, but it cannot by itself move the forearm back to its former position. To straighten the arm, the triceps must contract. The members of such a muscle team are called the flexor and the extensor. The flexor bends the joint and then the extensor straightens it.

Skeletal Muscles

Skeletal muscles are of various shapes and sizes appropriate to the jobs each must perform. Some are spindle-shaped, wide at the center and tapered at the ends. Some look like big feathers with filaments spreading out from a center line.

The skeletal muscles are attached to bones, through the periosteum. Actually, muscles taper into tough fibrous tissues called tendons which in turn are attached to rough surfaces on the bones.

Tendons are so strong that doctors sometimes find cases in which a bone breaks before the tendon attached to it gives way. Ligaments are like tendons, but ligament fibers will stretch and they join bone to bone instead of muscle to bone.

When muscles join bones, one of the bones usually serves as an anchor to help move the other bone. The point where the muscle joins the "anchor" bone is called the origin. The attachment to the bone that moves is called the insertion.

Two of the powerful biting muscles that move the jaw are the temporalis and the masseter. When these muscles contract, with the help of other muscles along the jaw, we are able to chew and grind our food.

The sternomastoid muscles on either side of the neck make the head nod when they contract at the same time. If one contracts, the head is turned to the opposite side.

At the shoulder are the deltoid, the trapezius,

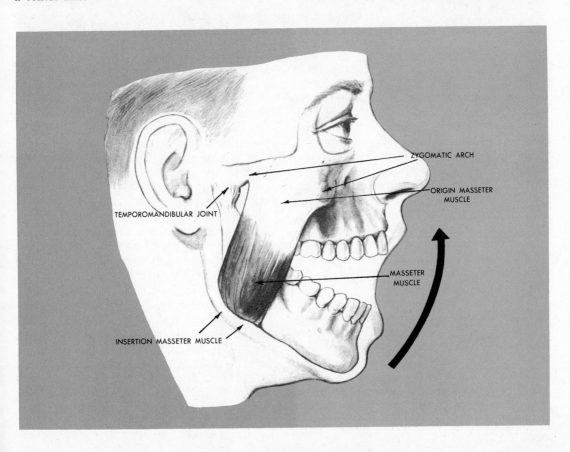

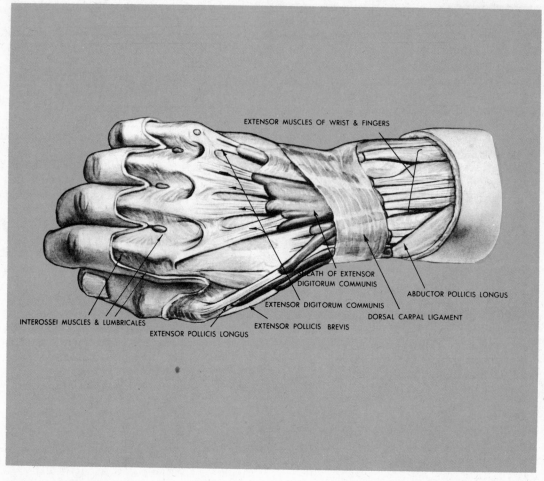

EXTENSOR MUSCLES OF WRIST & FINGERS

SHEATH OF EXTENSOR
DIGITORUM COMMUNIS

ABDUCTOR POLLICIS LONGUS

EXTENSOR DIGITORUM COMMUNIS

DORSAL CARPAL LIGAMENT

INTEROSSEI MUSCLES & LUMBRICALES

EXTENSOR POLLICIS BREVIS

EXTENSOR POLLICIS LONGUS

and the pectoralis major. The deltoid is the muscle that gives the top of the arm its "rounded" shape at the shoulder. The trapezius, among other duties, shrugs the shoulders when it contracts and lets the shoulders sag when relaxed. The pectoralis is the muscle that spreads over the chest, in front of the armpits, and attaches to the humerus. This muscle helps bring the arm across the chest.

Below the insertions of the biceps and triceps, on the forearm, are a series of muscles that help move the fingers. These muscles divide into tendons which extend down to the fingertips.

The tendons pass through sheaths in the wrist, hand, and fingers. The sheaths are tunnels that keep the tendons close to the bones they move and serve to protect them.

Many of the muscles, like the bones of the skeletal system, do double duty—they protect the nerves, blood vessels, and vital organs as well as support and move the various parts of the body.

The big muscles of the lower extremity include the gluteal muscles on the buttocks, the quadriceps and sartorius in the thigh, and the gastrocnemius and soleus in the calf.

The gluteal muscles contract to move you from a sitting to a standing position, help you walk upstairs or on the level. The sartorius is the longest muscle in the body and pulls the thigh into the cross-legged position.

The quadriceps is actually four muscles that help you keep your balance when standing. They also are used to kick. The muscles in the calf help you to stand on tiptoes and give you the "push" from the ground when dancing, walking, or running.

The thickest and strongest tendon of the human body connects the soleus and gastrocnemius muscles with the "heel bone" of the foot. It is called the Achilles tendon.

The mass of muscles extending along each side of the spinal column also should be mentioned. The mass is made up of dozens of bundles of muscle. These groups of muscles help maintain an erect posture and assist in walking by contracting as the foot on the same side is lifted. They also bend the body backward to balance the trunk when a heavy object is carried, or help turn the head or body to one side.

Inside the body at about its middle is the main muscle of breathing—the diaphragm. The diaphragm is a dome-shaped collection of muscle tissue and tendons. The tendons are attached to the spinal column, the cartilage ends of the ribs, and the lower tip of the breast bone. When the muscle fibers contract, the diaphragm moves downward. This helps our lungs to fill with air. The diaphragm is also used in coughing, sneezing, and laughing.

There is one important organ of the body that we do not always think of as a muscle. It is the tongue, which really is a group of four muscles covered by mucous membrane and other tissues. With the help of the muscles in the cheeks, the tongue presses against the roof of the mouth and forms a chute. The chewed food is forced down this chute and into the esophagus, which leads to the stomach.

Smooth Muscles

In the esophagus the muscles concerned with eating change from striped, voluntary fibers to smooth, involuntary cells. The upper part of the esophagus contains voluntary muscle and the lower portion involuntary, although the smooth muscle cells take over gradually.

The walls of the lower esophagus, intestines, and most of the stomach contain two layers of muscles that work as a team to help push the food along the digestive path. One layer is circular and contracts to make the tube narrower. The other layer is longitudinal and contracts along the length of the tube. Part of the stomach has a third layer of muscle fibers. The stomach needs a good muscular system because it must break up food particles which were not chewed completely. The muscles contract in a wave action called peristalsis.

Between the esophagus and the stomach, and at several other points along the digestive tube, there are special thick rings of muscles called sphincters. The sphincters pinch shut at irregular intervals, permitting intermittent passage of food or liquid. Smooth muscle fibers have the ability to remain contracted for longer periods of time than skeletal muscles. Smooth muscles of the digestive system can remain contracted for hours, if necessary.

Most skeletal muscles are partly contracted at all times. The jaw rarely sags. The head and shoulders can be held erect for hours without a sign of fatigue. This ability sometimes is referred to as muscle tone. Muscle tone also helps explain why we are able to maintain our posture and balance against the constant pull of gravity. Because humans walk erect, their muscles must defy gravity to a greater degree than those of animals that walk on all fours.

Besides the big muscles that permit us to walk and run erect, to lift weights, dance, or swat a baseball, there are a number of muscles that reveal our feelings. These are the muscles of expression. We use them to appear surprised or angry, when we sneer or wink, smile or frown. These muscles are small bundles of fibers located mainly around the eyes, mouth, and nose.

A sheet of muscles running over the forehead raises the eyebrows when we are surprised. Still another sheet of muscles, running from the lower jaw to the chest, makes the skin of the neck tense.

Where the tendons rub against each other or against bone or cartilage, they are enclosed in sheaths, or tunnels, which are lubricated. Groups of muscles are separated from other groups by membranes that help reduce the friction of movement. Within a muscle group, individual muscles are further separated by membranes. And within the individual muscles, groups of fibers are enclosed in sheaths. Finally, the muscle fibers are covered by individual membranes.

Sometimes a protective sheath is called a

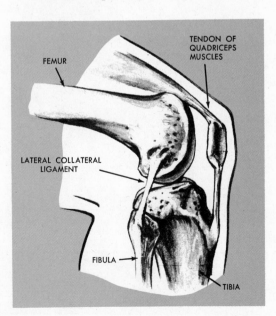

FEMUR

TENDON OF QUADRICEPS MUSCLES

LATERAL COLLATERAL LIGAMENT

FIBULA

TIBIA

bursa, which means "purse." The bursa is shaped like a sac rather than a tunnel and has a slippery fluid on its inner walls.

Sometimes a bursa becomes irritated and inflamed. This ailment is known as bursitis. Other ailments that may occur in the muscles and related body structures are strains and cramps. A cramp occurs when a muscle contracts and will not relax again. This happens frequently during vigorous exercise or when the limb is fatigued or subjected to cold. Muscle cramp may develop during swimming and cause even an expert swimmer to drown. The muscle usually can be relaxed by working the limb or by rubbing the muscle.

A strain is the result of continuous use of certain muscles for such activities as walking, bicycling, or gardening. The muscles and tendons ache but they recover after a period of relaxation.

Physical training can increase the size of the skeletal muscles and lack of exercise can result in muscles decreasing in size. Scientists report that muscle fibers actually grow larger because of exercise. Exercise, in moderation, also leads to changes in blood circulation and breathing habits that give the person with "trained" muscles the ability to perform athletic feats with greater ease. A bonus benefit of physical training is that of improved muscular coordination, which reduces effort in work or athletics.

While working or playing hard we sometimes need a "second wind." Strenuous effort burns the glycogen in the muscle tissue faster than the oxygen in the body can dispose of the waste products. During a sprint, the racer may need several times as much oxygen as his body can absorb during the race. But the muscles continue their work without the additional oxygen—for a limited period of time. During this period, we say the racer builds up an oxygen debt. After the race, the sprinter will breathe hard for several minutes, until the oxygen debt is repaid.

CHAPTER FOUR

THE CIRCULATORY SYSTEM

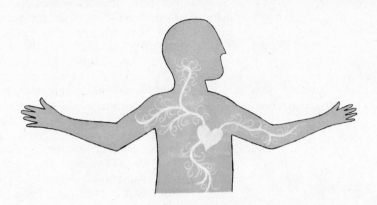

YOUR HEART is a bundle of muscles about the size of your fist. If you clench your fist, open it, and then clench it again, you can get a rough idea of the action of the heart. But if you open and close your fist, again and again, at a rate of a little more than once every second, your muscles will feel tired after a couple of minutes.

Your heart, meanwhile, is contracting and dilating at an average rate of 72 times a minute, which adds up to about 100,000 times a day or nearly 40,000,000 times a year. And the only rest the heart muscles get is the fraction of a second pause between beats.

The work done by your heart is about equal to the work you would perform if you lifted a 10-pound weight three feet off the ground and repeated this task twice every minute for your entire life.

The heart consists of several layers of muscles arranged in circles and spirals. When the muscles contract, the spirals and circles tighten and the blood is literally squeezed out of the chambers. The contraction that squeezes the blood from the heart is call systole and the subsequent relaxation of the heart muscles is called diastole.

A number of large arteries and veins runs into the top of the heart, carrying blood to and from other parts of the body. The walls on one side are thicker than the other, and the surface is covered with a number of small arteries and veins. The arteries on the surface of the heart are called the coronary arteries. They carry the blood which, in turn, carries the oxygen, food, and other necessary materials to the muscle fibers of the heart.

If we could see the inside of the heart we would find four chambers—two at the top called atria and two at the bottom called ventricles. Each atrium and ventricle on the right are separated from their counterparts on the left by a wall of muscle called a septum.

By tracing the paths of the blood through the heart, we see that this organ actually is a double pump. Blood flows from the right atrium into the right ventricle (the first pump), which squirts the blood into the lungs. The left ventricle, or second pump, squeezes the blood into the arteries that extend to all parts of the body. The septum prevents blood on the right side of the heart from mixing with blood on the left, and vice versa.

The thick ventricle walls do most of the blood pumping. The atria serve mainly as reservoirs, although they do give the blood a boost into the ventricles. A closer look at the pattern of flow shows that "used" blood from all parts of the body reaches the heart through big veins called the superior and inferior vena cava. The smaller veins from the head and arms drain into the superior vena cava. The inferior vena cava drains the blood from the lower parts of the body. The venae cavae open directly into the right atrium. The blood which has been used by the heart itself drains into the right atrium through a vessel known as the coronary sinus.

Valves in the Heart

The valve that separates the right atrium from the right ventricle prevents the dark or "used" blood from being pushed back into the atrium when the ventricle contracts. This valve is the tricuspid, so called because it has three cusps, or flaps, of tissue. The cusps are controlled by tiny papillary muscles. When the papillary muscles contract, they pull on cords attached to the cusps and thus pull open the heart valves.

With the tricuspid valve closed to prevent

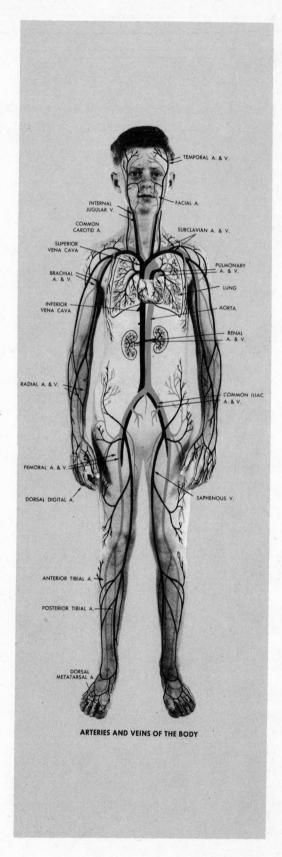

INTERNAL
JUGULAR V.

TEMPORAL A. & V.

FACIAL A.

COMMON
CAROTID A.

SUBCLAVIAN A. & V.

SUPERIOR
VENA CAVA

PULMONARY
A. & V.

BRACHIAL
A. & V.

LUNG

INFERIOR
VENA CAVA

AORTA

RENAL
A. & V.

RADIAL A. & V.

COMMON ILIAC
A. & V.

FEMORAL A. & V.

DORSAL DIGITAL A.

SAPHENOUS V.

ANTERIOR TIBIAL A.

POSTERIOR TIBIAL A.

DORSAL
METATARSAL A

ARTERIES AND VEINS OF THE BODY

backflow, the right ventricle squeezes the dark blood upward and into the pulmonary artery. The pulmonary artery has left and right branches extending into the lungs on either side of the body.

When the blood returns through the pulmonary veins it will enter the left atrium. From the left atrium it will be boosted through the mitral, or bicuspid, valve into the left ventricle. During the next contraction, the fresh blood will be squeezed into the aorta, the great artery from which branches run to all parts of the body. Again, by closing of the valve cusps, the blood is prevented from flowing back into the left atrium.

Valves to prevent backward flow of the blood also are located where the aorta and pulmonary arteries join the ventricles. Since the left ventricle must squeeze the blood throughout the body, its muscle is thicker than that of the right ventricle, which must only squeeze the blood into the air sacs of the lungs.

The approximately 72-beats-per-minute rhythm of the heart begins in a knot of tissue in the atria known as the sinoatrial, or S-A, node. The node contains nerve cells and fibers and muscle cells. It is called the "pacemaker" because it generates the "spark" or impulse that starts the wave of muscle contraction in the heart. The wave spreads over the muscles of the atria and apparently triggers an impulse in a similar node near the junction of the atria and ventricles.

The Pulse

The pulse is caused by the blood pressure impact on the arteries as the heart beats and can be felt by placing a finger on the radial artery, at the wrist. Doctors can tell much about the strength and regularity of the blood flow by feeling the pulse of a patient.

After vigorous exercise, your pulse may speed up from around 72 beats-per-minute to more than 120. But it should return to the original 72 beats within three minutes. Some deviation from these values may be normal for certain individuals; if there is any doubt, a medical opinion should be sought.

Blood Pressure

Blood pressure also permits doctors to study the health of the heart and circulatory system without actually viewing the organs. Each contraction of the ventricles (systole) causes the blood to spurt through the arteries and increases the pressure of blood flow. During the relaxation part of the rhythm (diastole), the pressure decreases.

From the heart, blood surges through the aorta to the arteries throughout the body. From the arteries, smaller vessels called arterioles branch out. From the arterioles, the blood flows to the smallest vessels, the capillaries. The capillaries carry the blood to the individual cells of the body where oxygen and other chemicals are delivered and waste products are collected. The capillaries then connect with venules, which run into veins which, in turn, flow into the venae cavae.

Except for the microscopic spaces between the cell walls of the capillaries, the blood flows through a sealed conduit of vessels that total some 70,000 miles in over-all length. The lin-

ing of the system is a membrane of cells called endothelium. The endothelium is so thin that even when magnified 1,000 times it appears no wider than a chalk mark. But it forms the smooth inner layer of the heart and all the blood vessels.

The arteries have layers of smooth muscle cells, elastic fibers, and connective tissue. One layer of muscle cells is circular and another layer of muscle fibers runs lengthwise. In the larger arteries with thick walls, smaller arteries run through their layers of muscle and fibrous tissue. Nerve fibers also accompany the muscle fibers that control the size of the opening in the arteries. The arterioles are barely visible without a microscope. They are constructed of a single layer of endothelial cells with an outer layer of muscle cells. The veins are built somewhat like arteries except their walls generally

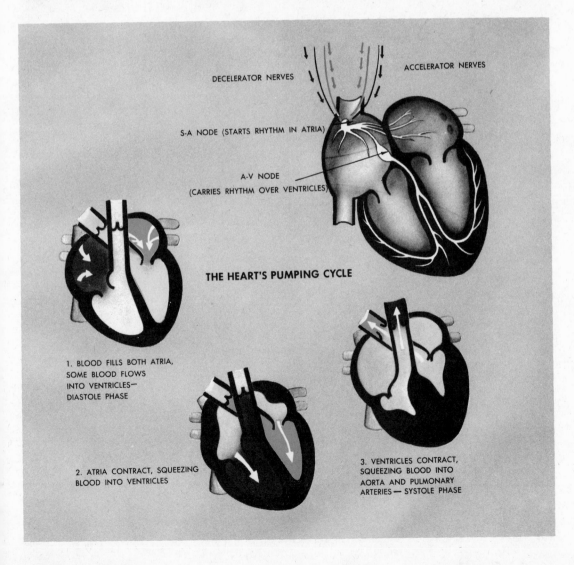

DECELERATOR NERVES

ACCELERATOR NERVES

S-A NODE (STARTS RHYTHM IN ATRIA)

A-V NODE
(CARRIES RHYTHM OVER VENTRICLES)

THE HEART'S PUMPING CYCLE

1. BLOOD FILLS BOTH ATRIA, SOME BLOOD FLOWS INTO VENTRICLES— DIASTOLE PHASE

2. ATRIA CONTRACT, SQUEEZING BLOOD INTO VENTRICLES

3. VENTRICLES CONTRACT, SQUEEZING BLOOD INTO AORTA AND PULMONARY ARTERIES — SYSTOLE PHASE

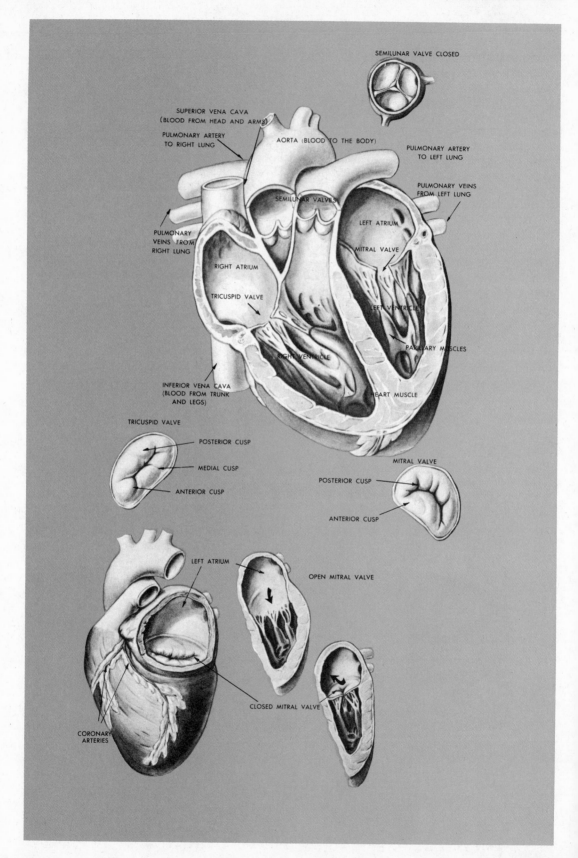

are thinner. A vein has an inner layer of endothelial cells, a layer of fibrous tissue, and a layer of muscle cells. The venule has an inner layer of endothelial cells and an outer layer of fibrous tissue.

The blood flow from the arteriole to the capillary is controlled by a circle of muscle fibers called a sphincter. The capillary system is so vast that if all of its vessels were opened at one time, they could swallow up the body's entire supply of blood. Yet the individual capillaries are so small that the red blood cells have to pass through them in single file. The red blood cells are, in turn, so small that a line of 3,000 of them would fall a little short of an inch in length.

Of the human body's total 70,000 miles of blood vessels, the largest percentage by far is capillaries. They could hold the body's entire blood supply (about five quarts). But only a part of the capillary system has blood flowing through it at any instant. The capillaries open and close first in one area, then in another. Tissues that use more blood, such as the arm and leg muscles, contain a greater share of capillaries than tissues that are not active.

The endothelial walls of a capillary are solid enough to keep the red cells from leaking out of the "closed circuit" of blood vessels. But white cells, chemicals, and small amounts of liquid can leave the blood stream by squeezing through tiny openings between the cells that make up the walls of the capillary. The blood flow is very slow at this point. It takes a minute for the blood to go through an inch of capillary tube. (Blood travels through the arteries at a speed of more than 40 miles an hour.) But during the slow trip through the capillaries, the food and oxygen needed by the body cells leave the tiny blood vessels and go into the tissues. A liquid called lymph, which bathes the tissue cells, also trickles through the capillary walls, as do the ingredients needed for repair and maintenance of the tissues.

At the same time, the carbon dioxide and other waste products from the tissue cells enter the capillary and are carried away. The lymph seeps into a special set of capillaries which return it eventually to the blood through a special vein near the heart.

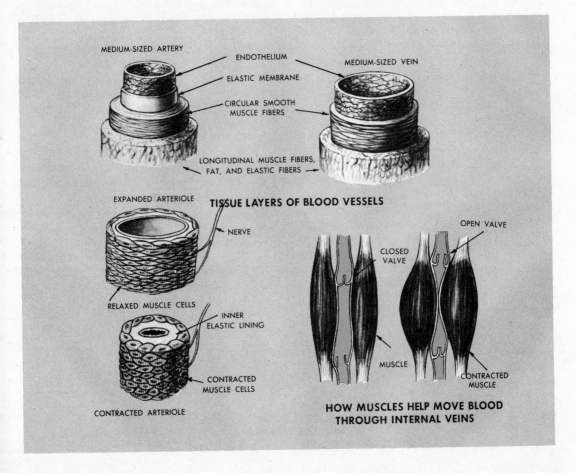

MEDIUM-SIZED ARTERY
ENDOTHELIUM
ELASTIC MEMBRANE
MEDIUM-SIZED VEIN
CIRCULAR SMOOTH MUSCLE FIBERS
LONGITUDINAL MUSCLE FIBERS, FAT, AND ELASTIC FIBERS

TISSUE LAYERS OF BLOOD VESSELS

EXPANDED ARTERIOLE
NERVE
RELAXED MUSCLE CELLS
INNER ELASTIC LINING
CONTRACTED MUSCLE CELLS
CONTRACTED ARTERIOLE

OPEN VALVE
CLOSED VALVE
MUSCLE
CONTRACTED MUSCLE

HOW MUSCLES HELP MOVE BLOOD THROUGH INTERNAL VEINS

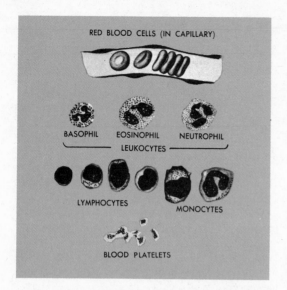

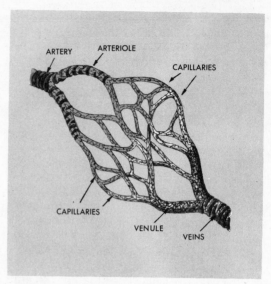

The dark, used blood in the upper part of the body can flow downhill from the capillaries to the heart. But what about the blood that has finished its trip through the capillaries in the hands and feet? Nature has provided for the need to push the used blood back up to the heart by two unique devices. One is the location of the veins between the skeletal muscles. The other is a system of valves which permit used blood to flow only toward the heart.

Good examples of these devices can be found in the legs. The veins in the legs are woven among the muscles so that when each muscle contracts, it squeezes a vein. Squeezing the vein pushes the blood closer to the heart. The valves in the vein prevent the blood from flowing backwards when the muscle relaxes.

If we spend too much time standing or sitting in one position, the used blood from the lower part of the body does not get the push it needs to return to the heart. That is why we may experience fatigue or sluggishness after standing still for a long time or after a long ride in a car or train. Varicose veins result from a failure of the used blood in the legs to return to the heart at the proper rate. The veins may lose some of their elasticity or the valves may fail to close properly. The used blood then accumulates and causes the veins to swell. Varicose veins occur frequently in the legs of people whose jobs require that they stand a great deal.

Blood

When blood is taken from the body and studied in a laboratory, it can be separated into two main parts. A little more than half of the blood is a watery fluid called plasma. The remainder is composed of red blood cells, white blood cells, and platelets.

The red cells give blood its color. They are tiny disks, so small that you could hide 40 or 50 of them beneath the period at the end of this sentence. They are thinner in the center than along the edge—which permits them to fold over when passing through an opening smaller than their own diameter. The human body contains nearly 25,000,000,000,000 red cells. Each lasts only four months. They simply wear out and break up in the blood. New red cells are produced by the bone marrow at the rate of around 1,000,000 a second and they wear out at the same rate.

Red cells are colorless when they are first produced. They acquire their color just before they are released into the bloodstream. The color comes from an iron pigment which is combined with a protein. The chemical combination is called hemoglobin. It is the hemoglobin that carries the oxygen from the lungs to the capillaries, where it is released to the individual tissue cells. The hemoglobin also attracts carbon dioxide and carries it in the red blood cells to the lungs, where it is exhaled.

Because of the ability of hemoglobin to hold large quantities of oxygen, animals can be smaller and more efficient than if the plasma itself had to carry the oxygen. For hemoglobin enables the blood to move up to 60 times as much oxygen as would be possible if the oxygen had to be dissolved in water or plasma. In other words, without hemoglobin, humans would need up to 300 quarts of blood instead of just 5. Even the muscles contain hemoglobin. It permits the muscles to build up a reserve of oxygen for the spurts of energy release we need when running, playing, or working hard.

The oxygen is held very loosely by the hemoglobin. In simple terms, the hemoglobin acquires a lot of oxygen when oxygen is abundant—as in the lungs after we inhale. And the hemoglobin gives up its oxygen when it reaches a region where oxygen is scarce—as in the areas where the capillaries branch among tissue cells.

Carbon dioxide similarly is picked up by the hemoglobin where carbon dioxide is plentiful and released in the lungs, where it is comparatively scarce. Unfortunately, hemoglobin also is strongly attracted to carbon monoxide, the poison gas that comes from automobile exhaust and faulty furnaces. The carbon monoxide crowds the oxygen out of the hemoglobin and the body tissues literally suffer from oxygen starvation.

When the number of red cells in the blood is too small or the red cells do not contain enough hemoglobin, the body is not able to get the proper amount of oxygen. The muscles and other tissues are not able to burn all of their supplies of fuel. The result is that the body cannot get the energy it needs. We call this condition anemia. If anemia is caused by a lack of hemoglobin, the shortage can be overcome by eating foods rich in iron, such as eggs and meat, particularly liver. Since hemoglobin is a protein, good quality protein foods are needed in the daily diet.

White cells are less common in the bloodstream, but they still number in the billions. The proportion is about 1 white blood cell for every 600 or 700 red blood cells. And there are several kinds of white cells. One kind, the granular leukocytes, develop in the bone marrow, along with the red blood cells. Another kind, the lymphocytes, develop in the lymph nodes, tonsils, and adenoids. The leukocytes play an important role in defending the body against the invasion of bacteria. These white cells can move around and literally chase down the bacteria.

As we mentioned earlier, the white cells can squeeze through even tiny openings in the walls of capillaries. When they corner bacteria, they engulf and digest them. One result of the battle is pus—a thick yellowish fluid composed of lymph, bacteria, and dead white cells.

Blood platelets are much smaller than red blood cells. They help blood to clot, or coagu-

late. When a blood vessel is cut, the platelets collect at the site of the injury. Many of the platelets break into smaller pieces and a complicated chemical process follows. Almost instantly, tiny threads appear from the platelets. The threads, called fibrin, form a tangled mass with the blood cells and platelets. This is the clot. The red blood cells give the clot its dark color.

The platelets do not perform the task of clotting by themselves. Chemicals in the injured tissue cells, the white cells, and the plasma are used by the body to form a clot.

The plasma is about 90 per cent water. The remainder is made up of minerals, such as sodium, calcium, potassium, and phosphorus, plus enzymes, antibodies, fats, sugars, and the plasma proteins. The plasma proteins include fibrinogen (one of the clotting chemicals), albumin, and serum globulins. Some oxygen and carbon dioxide are dissolved in the plasma.

When blood is lost through injury or disease, it can be replaced by transfusion. The blood is obtained from another person, but the blood of the donor must be compatible with that of the person receiving the transfusion. The main types of blood are classified as A, B, O, and AB. If the types are not compatible, the transfused blood cells may form clumps that can block the small vessels. It also is necessary to differentiate between Rh-positive and Rh-negative blood. Serious consequences may result if incompatible blood is given.

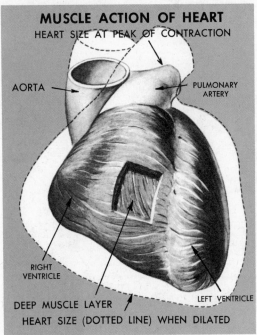

MUSCLE ACTION OF HEART
HEART SIZE AT PEAK OF CONTRACTION

AORTA

PULMONARY ARTERY

RIGHT VENTRICLE

DEEP MUSCLE LAYER

LEFT VENTRICLE

HEART SIZE (DOTTED LINE) WHEN DILATED

CHAPTER FIVE

THE RESPIRATORY SYSTEM

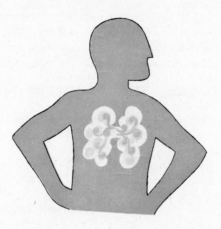

MAN CAN LIVE for weeks without food. He can live for days without water. But he can exist without air for only a few minutes. Without air, skeletal muscles will not contract, the brain cells will fail, the heart will not beat.

The smallest animals, like amoebae, get their oxygen directly from their environment, while insects may have millions of microscopic air pipes or tracheoles that deliver air from the outside directly to cells in the middle of the body.

Humans, like other larger and more complicated animals, have their oxygen delivered to the body cells indirectly—through the blood. The blood contains a chemical that is part protein and part iron pigment, called hemoglobin. The hemoglobin attracts oxygen when the blood flows through regions where oxygen is plentiful—as in the body cells. Similarly, the carbon dioxide produced when the body cells burn their fuel is attracted by the hemoglobin as it flows through the tissues where carbon dioxide is plentiful. And it is released in the lungs where carbon dioxide is comparatively scarce.

The act of respiration always is divided into two parts. The part of the process in which the body cells trade carbon dioxide for fresh oxygen is called internal respiration. The part involved in getting oxygen into the blood stream in the lungs and expelling carbon dioxide and water vapor is called external respiration.

External respiration begins and ends with the nose. The nose has many other duties besides detecting odors. It filters the air entering the breathing equipment, warms it, and moistens it. The nose also influences the sound of your voice—as you may have noticed the last time you had a head cold.

The Nose

The nose has been compared to an air-conditioning unit because it controls the tem-

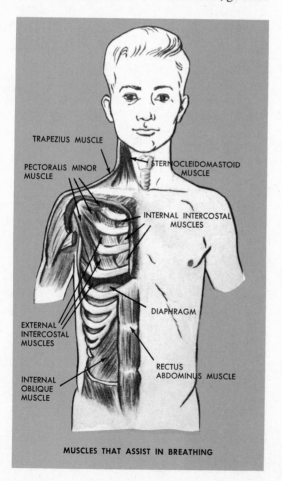

TRAPEZIUS MUSCLE

PECTORALIS MINOR MUSCLE

STERNOCLEIDOMASTOID MUSCLE

INTERNAL INTERCOSTAL MUSCLES

EXTERNAL INTERCOSTAL MUSCLES

DIAPHRAGM

INTERNAL OBLIQUE MUSCLE

RECTUS ABDOMINUS MUSCLE

MUSCLES THAT ASSIST IN BREATHING

perature and humidity of the air entering the lungs and filters foreign particles from the air. The interior of the nose is divided by a wall of cartilage and bone called the septum. Near the middle of the nasal cavity, and on both sides of the septum, are a series of scroll-like bones called the conchae, or turbinates. The purpose of the turbinates is to increase the amount of tissue surface within the nose so that incoming air will have a greater opportunity to be "conditioned" before it continues on its way to the lungs. The surfaces of the turbinates, like the rest of the interior walls of the nose, are covered with mucous membranes. These membranes secrete a fluid called mucus. The film of mucus is produced continuously and drains slowly into the throat. The mucus gives up heat and moisture to incoming air and serves as a trap for bacteria and dust in the air. It also helps dilute any irritating substances in the air.

In addition to the mucus, the membrane is coated with cilia, or hairlike filaments, that wave back and forth a dozen times per second.

The millions of cilia lining the nasal cavity help the mucus clean the incoming air. When we breathe through the mouth, we lose the protective benefits of the cilia and mucus.

A number of large nerve filaments extending into the nasal cavity from the base of the skull are part of the special sense organ that is associated with smell. The filaments relay information on odors to the olfactory nerve which leads to the brain.

The Sinuses

The nasal cavity has several small openings leading into the sinuses. There are eight sinuses, four on each side, with mucous membranes that are continuous with the lining of the nose. The sinuses help equalize the air pressure in the nasal cavity, and give resonance to the voice. Their air-filled spaces reduce the weight of the skull. The sinus cavities are the frontal, on each side of the forehead; the maxillary, in the cheekbones on each side; the

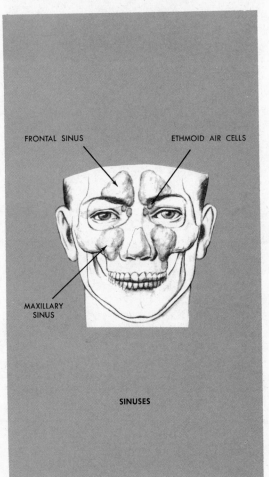

FRONTAL SINUS

ETHMOID AIR CELLS

MAXILLARY SINUS

SINUSES

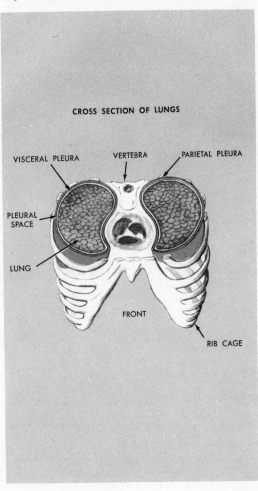

CROSS SECTION OF LUNGS

VISCERAL PLEURA

VERTEBRA

PARIETAL PLEURA

PLEURAL SPACE

LUNG

FRONT

RIB CAGE

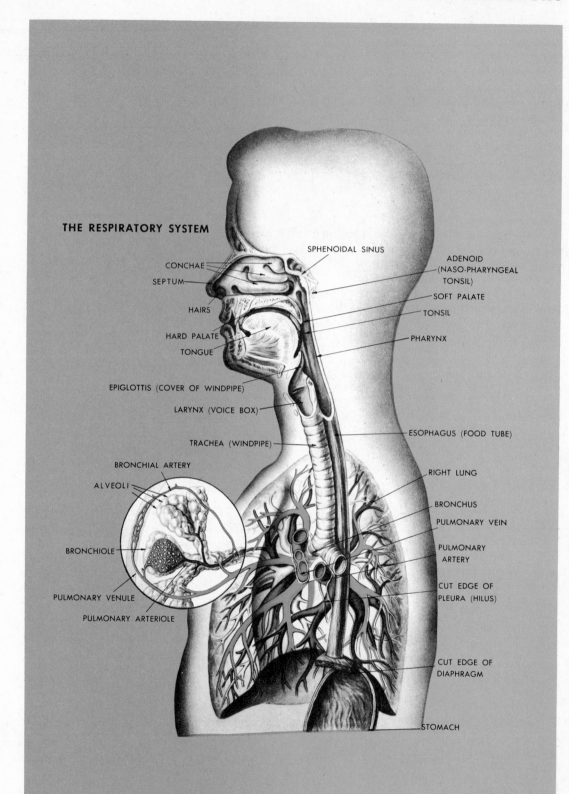

THE RESPIRATORY SYSTEM

SPHENOIDAL SINUS

ADENOID
(NASO-PHARYNGEAL
TONSIL)

CONCHAE

SEPTUM

SOFT PALATE

HAIRS

TONSIL

HARD PALATE

PHARYNX

TONGUE

EPIGLOTTIS (COVER OF WINDPIPE)

LARYNX (VOICE BOX)

ESOPHAGUS (FOOD TUBE)

TRACHEA (WINDPIPE)

BRONCHIAL ARTERY

RIGHT LUNG

ALVEOLI

BRONCHUS

PULMONARY VEIN

BRONCHIOLE

PULMONARY
ARTERY

CUT EDGE OF
PLEURA (HILUS)

PULMONARY VENULE

PULMONARY ARTERIOLE

CUT EDGE OF
DIAPHRAGM

STOMACH

ethmoidal, a honeycomb of bone in the walls between the nasal cavity and the eye sockets; and the sphenoidal, behind the nasal cavity.

Because they are linked to the nasal cavity, the sinuses are easily irritated by the spread of infection from the nose. Blowing the nose too hard can speed the spread of infection from the nasal cavity.

The Pharynx

The incoming air that has been filtered, warmed, and moistened in its trip through the nasal cavity next passes into the pharynx. The pharynx is one of the more complicated parts of the body since it serves as a passageway for both food and air. We all are aware that swallowing food and breathing cannot take place at the same time—without choking.

The incoming air travels through the nasal cavity, into the pharynx, and through the larynx, or voice box, by crossing over the path used by food on its way to the stomach. Similarly, food crosses over the route of air on its way from the nose to the larynx. But, when food is swallowed, a flap of cartilage called the epiglottis folds over the opening of the larynx. The base of the tongue pushes down the epiglottis as the food is moved back into the throat during the swallowing action.

On each side of the pharynx, behind the mouth cavity, are tonsils. Tonsil tissue also is located at the base of the tongue, and it may appear at the back and sides of the pharynx as adenoids. Tonsils usually are more prominent in children than adults. Their purpose is to guard the body against infections that may enter through the mouth or nose.

The Larynx

The larynx, also called the voice box, is at the top of the column that finally takes the air into the lungs, the trachea. However, it is the air expelled from the lungs, rather than incoming air, which is used to make voice sounds.

Two folds of membrane, the vocal cords, are attached to the front of the larynx wall and held by a pair of tiny cartilages. The cartilages are attached to muscles that contract and relax to move the vocal cords toward or away from the center of the larynx.

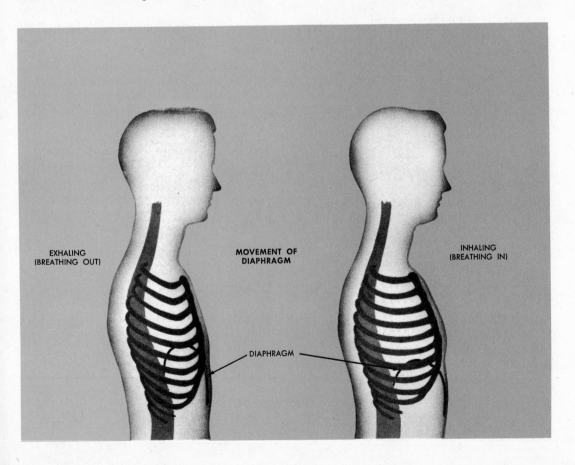

EXHALING
(BREATHING OUT)

MOVEMENT OF
DIAPHRAGM

INHALING
(BREATHING IN)

DIAPHRAGM

The Windpipe

Below the larynx, the trachea, also called the windpipe, continues down the neck and into the chest. A series of C-shaped rings of cartilage hold open the trachea. Lack of rigidity of the trachea permits us to bend the neck. The path of the esophagus, which carries food to the stomach, runs immediately behind that of the trachea. At the point behind the middle of the breastbone, where the aorta arches away from the heart, the trachea divides into two branches—the right and left bronchi. Each bronchus divides and subdivides many times into smaller cartilage-ringed branches that reach deep into the right and left lungs.

The Lungs

The tiniest bronchi, almost too small to be seen without a microscope, have cartilage rings in their walls. However, as the tubes become still smaller, they have little or no cartilage but instead have muscle cells in their walls. Bronchi of this size are called bronchioles. Finally, the bronchiole ends in a tiny air sac called an alveolus. The lungs contain nearly a billion of these microscopic, balloon-like alveoli. The alveoli, with their spaces air-filled, make the lungs appear somewhat like large sponges.

The respiratory nerve centers in the brain control our "living bellows," but what actually moves the bellows? The primary moving force is the diaphragm, a dome-shaped sheet of muscle fibers and tendons separating the organs in the chest from the organs in the abdomen. The diaphragm is attached to the breastbone on the front, to the spinal column at the back, and to the lower ribs on the sides. When the muscle fibers of the diaphragm contract, the sheet of tissue is drawn downward, creating a partial vacuum in the chest cavity. This causes air to flow into the trachea, the bronchi, and the alveoli. Expiration occurs when the diaphragm muscles relax, closing the "bellows" and forcing the air out again. The intercostal muscles, between the ribs, also participate in the breathing action. In forced breathing, abdominal muscles assist in expiration and the neck muscles assist in inspiration by pulling upward and outward on the first rib and the breastbone. This has a chain-reaction effect on the other ribs, increasing the capacity of the chest.

The rate of respiration is about 18 per minute for young adults. The rate is much higher for babies. It also is higher for adults engaged in active work or play. And in disease—or anything causing higher than normal temperature—the respiration rate is always increased.

A man carries two quarts of oxygen in his blood, lungs, and body tissues—enough to last about four minutes. Beyond that time there is damage to body tissues, beginning with the most sensitive cells in the brain. He also has about a quart of nitrogen dissolved in his blood and body tissues. The body makes no use of nitrogen and it eventually is breathed out again.

CHAPTER SIX

THE DIGESTIVE SYSTEM

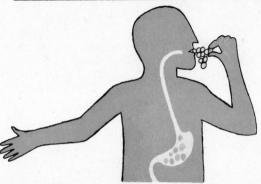

THE HUMAN BODY is sometimes described as a chemical engine that selects its own fuel. This generally is true. We are able to walk and talk and perform other tasks because of the energy we get from food. And, within the limits of the menu or the supermarket, we usually can choose from a wide variety of fuels for our bodies.

For much of the trip through the chemical refinery, or digestive system, food is either squeezed or pushed by muscles. It also is dissolved by a series of digestive juices. The digestive juices (or enzymes) serve as catalysts—they produce chemical changes in the food we eat without becoming part of the chemical produced.

In the mouth, the food is crushed and chopped by the teeth, which are brought together with the powerful forces of the jaw muscles.

The tongue itself is a bundle of muscles. The tongue muscles can change the shape of that organ, making its surface convex or concave. They also raise or lower the tongue and move it from side to side, as needed to assist in chewing food. On the surface of the tongue are sense organs called taste buds. The taste buds are scattered among the tiny papilla that give the tongue its rough, rasp-like surface. Taste buds can detect four taste sensations—sweet, sour, salty, and bitter.

Some of the sensations we call taste actually are smells detected by the olfactory organs in the nose.

The teeth have specialized jobs in preparing food for digestion. The incisors and canine teeth, at the front of the jaw, cut and tear food into smaller pieces. The molars, at the rear, grind the food.

The Saliva

While food is being pulverized into the pulpy mass called a bolus, the digestive juice of the salivary glands begins a breakdown of the carbohydrates. An enzyme in saliva splits the molecules of starch into smaller molecules of sugar. This enzyme can not break down starch grains that are still enclosed in their natural cellulose envelopes. For this reason, starches should be cooked before eating.

The fluid of the salivary glands serves several other purposes. It provides moisture needed by the taste buds. Saliva also has a cleansing action on the teeth. It washes away food particles that otherwise might provide a home for bacteria.

The salivary glands look like bunches of tiny grapes. The largest, the parotid, is located in front of the ear. Two salivary glands in the lower jaw are the sublingual, under the tip of the tongue, and the submandibular, under the edge of the lower jaw. There is a set of the three glands on each side of the mouth.

When the bolus of food has been thoroughly chewed, it is ready to be passed into the stomach—by swallowing. The muscles of the cheeks, the tongue, and the roof of the mouth form a chute. The tongue presses upward and backward against the hard palate.

The soft palate is raised as the food passes toward the back of the mouth, simultaneously closing the opening to the nasal cavities. At the same time, the epiglottis, a lid made of cartilage enclosed in the mucous membrane and located at the base of the tongue over the larynx at the top of the windpipe, closes. Also at the same time, the larynx moves upward against the lower surface of the epiglottis. This seals off the windpipe at the instant of swallowing.

After the food enters the esophagus it is moved along by muscle action called peristalsis, which is carried out by involuntary muscles. The digestive tube has two layers of involuntary muscles. The inner layer forms a series of circles about the tube. When any of these muscle fibers contract, the tube becomes

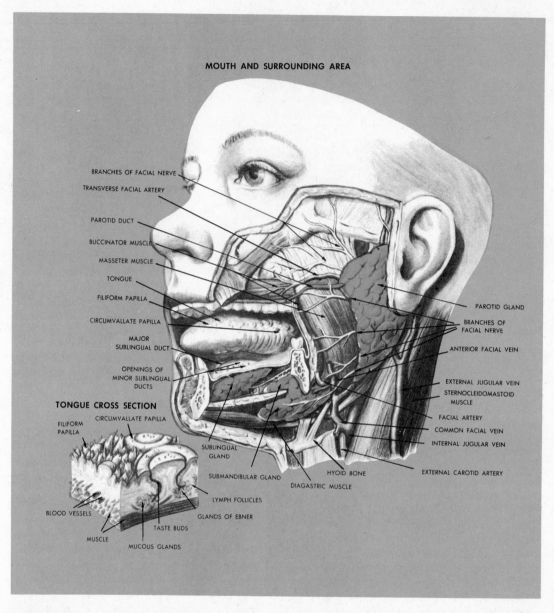

MOUTH AND SURROUNDING AREA

BRANCHES OF FACIAL NERVE
TRANSVERSE FACIAL ARTERY
PAROTID DUCT
BUCCINATOR MUSCLE
MASSETER MUSCLE
TONGUE
FILIFORM PAPILLA
CIRCUMVALLATE PAPILLA
MAJOR SUBLINGUAL DUCT
OPENINGS OF MINOR SUBLINGUAL DUCTS

PAROTID GLAND
BRANCHES OF FACIAL NERVE
ANTERIOR FACIAL VEIN
EXTERNAL JUGULAR VEIN
STERNOCLEIDOMASTOID MUSCLE
FACIAL ARTERY
COMMON FACIAL VEIN
INTERNAL JUGULAR VEIN
EXTERNAL CAROTID ARTERY

SUBLINGUAL GLAND
SUBMANDIBULAR GLAND
HYOID BONE
DIAGASTRIC MUSCLE

TONGUE CROSS SECTION

FILIFORM PAPILLA
CIRCUMVALLATE PAPILLA
BLOOD VESSELS
MUSCLE
TASTE BUDS
MUCOUS GLANDS
GLANDS OF EBNER
LYMPH FOLLICLES

smaller at that point. The outer muscle layer is longitudinal—its fibers run the length of the tube. The longitudinal muscles contract as the circular muscles relax. The alternate contraction and relaxation of the two sets of muscles pushes food along the digestive tube in peristaltic waves. Because of peristaltic action of the muscles in the esophagus, swallowing is possible in any body position.

The Stomach

The walls of the stomach are muscular. They contain not only the layers of circular and longitudinal muscle fibers, but a third layer of oblique muscle fibers. The muscles are particularly important for the stomach because it is the job of this organ to break up the food into tiny particles. Frequently, the stomach must grind up food which was not chewed thoroughly.

The mucous membrane that lines the entire digestive system is thick and velvety and has many folds. Like other mucous membranes, the lining contains mucous glands. But in the stomach, between the mucous glands are tiny gastric glands which secrete digestive juices. The lining of the stomach contains about 35,000,000 glands.

The stomach's gastric glands secrete hydro-

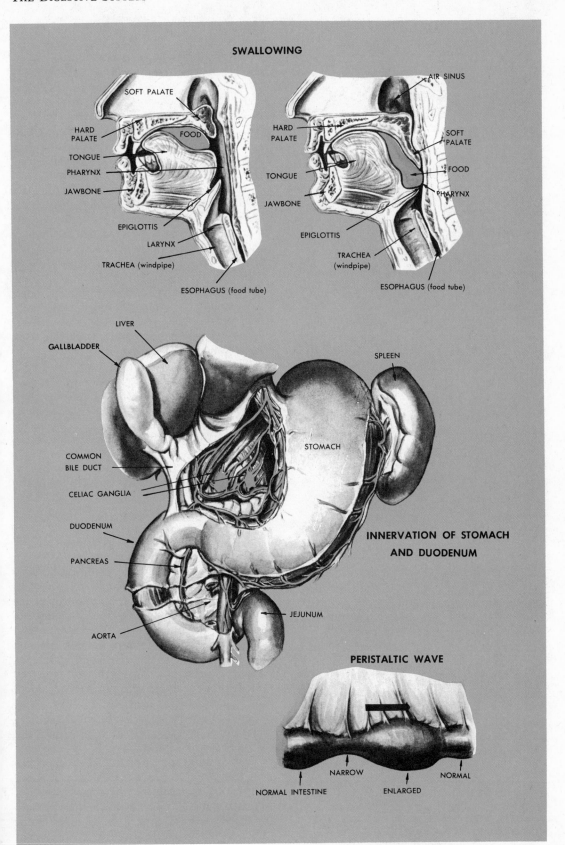

SWALLOWING

SOFT PALATE

HARD PALATE

FOOD

TONGUE

PHARYNX

JAWBONE

EPIGLOTTIS

LARYNX

TRACHEA (windpipe)

ESOPHAGUS (food tube)

AIR SINUS

HARD PALATE

SOFT PALATE

TONGUE

FOOD

JAWBONE

PHARYNX

EPIGLOTTIS

TRACHEA (windpipe)

ESOPHAGUS (food tube)

LIVER

GALLBLADDER

SPLEEN

STOMACH

COMMON BILE DUCT

CELIAC GANGLIA

DUODENUM

INNERVATION OF STOMACH AND DUODENUM

PANCREAS

JEJUNUM

AORTA

PERISTALTIC WAVE

NARROW

NORMAL

NORMAL INTESTINE

ENLARGED

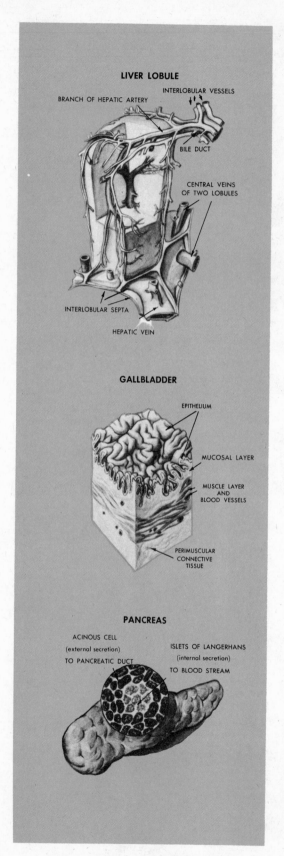

LIVER LOBULE

BRANCH OF HEPATIC ARTERY

INTERLOBULAR VESSELS

BILE DUCT

CENTRAL VEINS
OF TWO LOBULES

INTERLOBULAR SEPTA

HEPATIC VEIN

GALLBLADDER

EPITHELIUM

MUCOSAL LAYER

MUSCLE LAYER
AND
BLOOD VESSELS

PERIMUSCULAR
CONNECTIVE
TISSUE

PANCREAS

ACINOUS CELL
(external secretion)
TO PANCREATIC DUCT

ISLETS OF LANGERHANS
(internal secretion)
TO BLOOD STREAM

chloric acid and several enzymes. One enzyme, rennin, curdles milk. The same enzyme has been used for many years in the production of cheese. Another enzyme, lipase, splits certain fats, including those in cream and egg yolk. The hydrochloric acid combines with proteins to form a new chemical. A third enzyme, pepsin, splits the chemical formed by the proteins and hydrochloric acid into smaller units. The pepsin enzyme also digests the milk curds formed by the rennin.

The time taken for a meal to be changed by the stomach into a semifluid called chyme varies from about three to five hours. Fluids, as might be expected, pass through the stomach within minutes. Carbohydrates, among the solid foods, are handled most quickly by the action of the stomach's muscle contractions and the digestive juices. Proteins take a longer time, and fats require the most time. Some fats, in fact, slow down the digestive process for other foods in the stomach by slowing down the secretion of the gastric juices.

The pyloric sphincter at the lower end of the stomach controls the emptying of chyme into the next station along the digestive route, the small intestine. Like the cardiac sphincter between the esophagus and the stomach, the pyloric sphincter is a thickened band of circular muscles. Waves of peristalsis push the chyme through the opening formed by the pyloric sphincter and into the small intestines.

The Small Intestine

The small intestine is so named because of the diameter of its tube. It is about 20 feet long, or about four times as long as the large intestine. The first part of the small intestine is a short horseshoe-shaped section known as the duodenum. More digestive juices are added to the chyme entering the duodenum. Also added to the chyme are fluids from the pancreas and bile from the liver. The pancreatic fluid contains a number of enzymes that act upon all kinds of foods—proteins are broken down into amino acids, large sugar molecules are changed to simple sugars, and fats are reduced to fatty acids in preparation for absorption into the blood or lymph vessels.

Insulin also is secreted by the pancreas but it is absorbed directly into the blood. It is destroyed by exposure to the digestive juices, which explains why it cannot be taken by mouth by diabetics for control of blood sugar levels. The oral pills for diabetics have effects similar

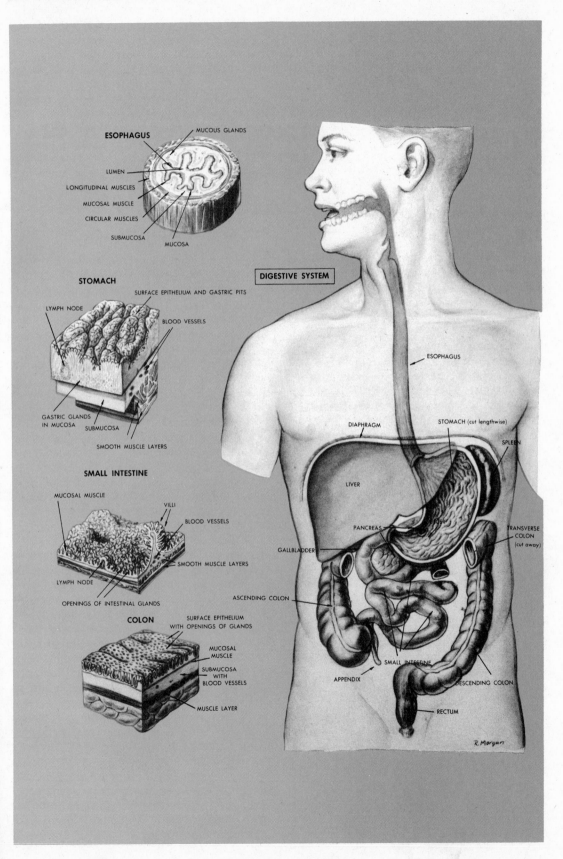

ESOPHAGUS

MUCOUS GLANDS
LUMEN
LONGITUDINAL MUSCLES
MUCOSAL MUSCLE
CIRCULAR MUSCLES
SUBMUCOSA
MUCOSA

STOMACH

SURFACE EPITHELIUM AND GASTRIC PITS
LYMPH NODE
BLOOD VESSELS
GASTRIC GLANDS
IN MUCOSA
SUBMUCOSA
SMOOTH MUSCLE LAYERS

SMALL INTESTINE

MUCOSAL MUSCLE
VILLI
BLOOD VESSELS
SMOOTH MUSCLE LAYERS
LYMPH NODE
OPENINGS OF INTESTINAL GLANDS

COLON

SURFACE EPITHELIUM
WITH OPENINGS OF GLANDS
MUCOSAL
MUSCLE
SUBMUCOSA
WITH
BLOOD VESSELS
MUSCLE LAYER

DIGESTIVE SYSTEM

ESOPHAGUS

DIAPHRAGM
STOMACH (cut lengthwise)
SPLEEN
LIVER
PANCREAS
TRANSVERSE
COLON
(cut away)
GALLBLADDER
ASCENDING COLON
SMALL INTESTINE
APPENDIX
DESCENDING COLON
RECTUM

R. Morgan

to insulin, but are not insulin. When the pancreas is unable to supply insulin to the body, diabetes results.

Bile, an orange-colored fluid, may enter the duodenum through a duct directly from the liver or from the gall bladder, where bile is stored. Bile is composed mostly of water, but it contains pigments from red blood cells that have been destroyed. The pigments undergo chemical changes in the intestine and eventually are excreted, giving the yellow-brown color to feces. The iron from these cells is reabsorbed, however. Bile also contributes to digestion by emulsifying fatty foods and making them easier to absorb. Bile also reduces the acidity of the chyme.

Beyond the duodenum, there are about 8 feet of small intestine called the jejunum and beyond that about 12 feet known as the ileum. The diameter of the small intestine gradually decreases along its length. At the junction of the small and large intestine, the bore is about half the diameter of the duodenum.

The interior of the small intestine is carpeted with microscopic finger-like projections called villi. The cells which cover the villi permit the absorption of water and the final products of digestion into the vessels that carry away the blood and lymph. Small amounts of products of digestion are absorbed through the walls of the stomach but most of the small molecules of sugars, amino acids, and fat products are absorbed through the millions of villi in the small intestine. The villi are in constant motion, swinging back and forth and changing in length. The motion of the villi keeps the chyme thoroughly mixed with the digestive juices while molecules of food pass through the cells on their surface. Fat products generally enter lymph vessels in the villi while sugars and amino acids enter blood capillaries.

The blood vessels carry the food products to the liver while the lymph vessels move their food units into a duct which empties into the subclavian vein, near the top of the rib case.

The Large Intestine

After traveling along the chemical refinery's conveyor belt to the end of the small intestine, about all that remains of a meal is water and waste products. These pass into the large intestine through a valve which prevents a backflow into the small intestine. The large intestine, about five feet long, has the general shape of a picture frame as it runs upward, across, and back down through the abdominal cavity. It has no villi and fewer folds than are observed in the small intestine.

Much of the water is absorbed through the walls of the large intestine. The waste products form the semisolid feces that are excreted through the rectum. Some waste products, including salts and proteins, are filtered from the blood, along with excess water, by a series of tubules in the kidneys. This waste is excreted as urine.

Food products carried by blood vessels from the walls of the digestive tube are delivered to the liver, the largest organ in the system and an important chemical plant. The reddish-brown liver manufactures proteins, processes carbohydrates, absorbs fat products, and makes them available as fuel, serves as a storehouse for vitamins and minerals, processes iron for the blood system, and renders harmless some of the poisons that enter the bloodstream. It also dispatches sugars to the tissues to burn as body fuel.

A thin membrane called the peritoneum lines the walls of the abdominal cavity and covers the organs within the cavity. A double layer of peritoneum connects some of the organs, helps hold them in place, and carries blood and lymph vessels. The membrane in some places may have quantities of fat which help the organs conserve body heat and protect them against injury.

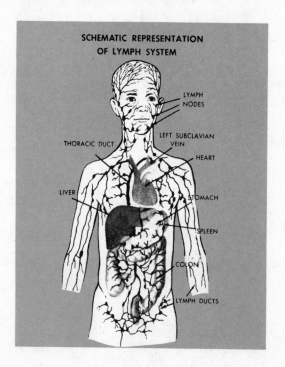

SCHEMATIC REPRESENTATION
OF LYMPH SYSTEM

LYMPH NODES

THORACIC DUCT

LEFT SUBCLAVIAN VEIN

HEART

LIVER

STOMACH

SPLEEN

COLON

LYMPH DUCTS

CHAPTER SEVEN

THE NERVOUS SYSTEM

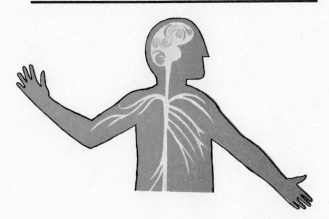

YOU MAY NOT have been aware of it, but all of your life you have been living in a continuous storm of stimuli, the small physical and chemical forces from the world around you. You have been bombarded hourly by impulses of light and sound. You have shivered in a cold wind, recoiled from pain, balanced yourself against gravity, and felt the sensation of pressure. You have found smells and tastes that were pleasant and unpleasant, and you have also jerked your hand away from a dish that was too hot.

If you stepped on a sharp object with your right foot, you quickly flexed the muscles of your right leg and extended your left leg so you could maintain your balance while avoiding the painful stimulus. And you reacted without stopping to think even a moment about what you should do about the situation. The various parts of your nervous system received and analyzed the message from your foot and decided automatically what should be done.

Sometimes you have participated directly in decisions of the nervous system, as while eating breakfast you decided whether the orange juice was sweet or the milk sour. And when you left the table, a feeling in your stomach helped you decide whether you were still hungry. As you started to leave your home, you remembered where you could find your hat and coat. And your eyes found the rectangle in the wall that was the door.

When you stepped outside, the muscles in the iris of each eye instantly and automatically adjusted the size of the pupil for the change in light. You were responding almost every second to impulses picked up by the millions of nerve receptors scattered over your body. Sometimes you made the decisions and sometimes your body decided for itself, but in each case messages were flashed back and forth through the nerve network that controls every action you take.

We can't see the nerve impulses as such, but if we could, the nervous system might appear like crowded highways radiating from a big city on a weekend. The body has millions of pain, pressure, and hearing receptors and each eye contains over 100,000,000 light receptors. Add to these the taste, smell, sound, and other radar-like receptors feeding impulses along the nerve paths to the brain, which alone contains over 12,000,000,000 nerve cells, and it is not difficult to think of the nervous system in terms of computers.

However, the human nervous system is in some ways more efficient than an electronic computer. It has been estimated that an electron-tube computer would have to be the size of a New York City skyscraper to contain the equipment having the same capabilities as the three pounds or so of human brain.

How a Nerve Works

To understand better how a nerve works, let's take a close look at a single nerve cell. Under a microscope, a nerve cell, or neuron, may appear as a tiny irregular or rounded blob with one or more threads extending from it. The threads are the nerve fibers and the blob is the cell body that serves as "local" headquarters for the nerve unit. There is one fiber longer than the others. Called the axon, it always carries nerve impulses away from the cell body. The shorter fibers are called dendrites. They carry nerve impulses toward the cell body. The fibers may be a fraction of an inch in length, or as much as three feet long in the case of some that extend to the feet.

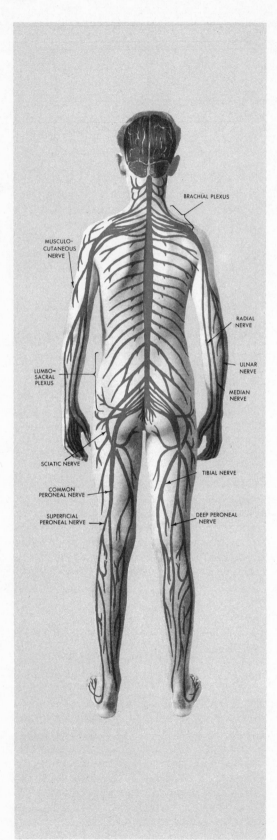

BRACHIAL PLEXUS

MUSCULO-
CUTANEOUS
NERVE

RADIAL
NERVE

ULNAR
NERVE

LUMBO-
SACRAL
PLEXUS

MEDIAN
NERVE

SCIATIC NERVE

TIBIAL NERVE

COMMON
PERONEAL NERVE

SUPERFICIAL
PERONEAL NERVE

DEEP PERONEAL
NERVE

When a nerve fiber is cut or crushed, the part of the fiber still connected to the cell body continues to transmit impulses, but the part on the other side of the injury gradually degenerates and finally disappears. However, if the nerve is protected by a sheath and the parts of the damaged fiber are not too far apart, the damaged nerve may be replaced. Surgeons sometimes sew the divided nerve parts together. This does not restore the usefulness of the fiber that is separated from its cell body, but it does provide a path for the new fiber to follow. Unfortunately, damaged fibers of the optic and auditory nerves as well as those within the central nervous system cannot be repaired by this method.

In moving through the network of nerve fibers, the impulse travels by a sort of chain reaction. One nerve cell triggers the next cell along the route. At the end of the fiber, the impulse jumps to the next by crossing a junction, called a synapse.

Certain chemicals secreted around the synapses help or retard the jump of the nerve impulse. One chemical acts as a conductor to speed the impulse on its way and the other acts as an insulator to slow up the impulse.

The exact nature of the nerve impulse is not known, but it apparently is a combination electrical-chemical action. Chemical changes are produced along nerve cells when an impulse is transmitted. And scientists have been able to trace electrical charges passing along a nerve fiber when an impulse is being transmitted. They have measured the voltage of a nerve. But they know the action is not entirely electrical because a dead nerve fiber is not a good conductor.

Central Nervous System

The central nervous system includes the brain and the spinal cord. Connected to the central nervous system is the peripheral nervous system, which includes the 12 cranial nerves running to sense organs, the heart, and other internal organs. The peripheral system also includes the 31 pairs of spinal nerves, both sensory and motor, that reach to skeletal muscles throughout the body.

Each of the spinal nerves joins the spinal cord by splitting into two roots. One root carries sensory-type fibers to the cord. A small bulge on the rear root called a ganglion, contains nerve cell bodies. The other root of the spinal nerve, the front root, enters the cord at

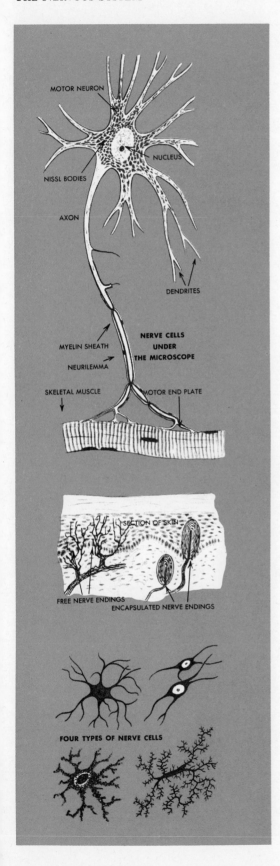

MOTOR NEURON

NUCLEUS

NISSL BODIES

AXON

DENDRITES

MYELIN SHEATH

NEURILEMMA

NERVE CELLS UNDER THE MICROSCOPE

SKELETAL MUSCLE

MOTOR END PLATE

SECTION OF SKIN

FREE NERVE ENDINGS

ENCAPSULATED NERVE ENDINGS

FOUR TYPES OF NERVE CELLS

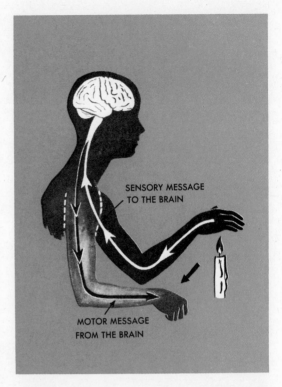

SENSORY MESSAGE TO THE BRAIN

MOTOR MESSAGE FROM THE BRAIN

the horn of the gray matter directly below the horn entered by the rear root. The front root carries motor-type nerve fibers. The cell bodies of the front root are inside the gray matter of the spinal cord.

In several parts of the body, nerve fibers branch out and connect with other nerve bundles. Such a group of branching and interconnecting nerves is called a plexus. One of the best known of these is the solar plexus located in the back of the stomach.

Autonomic Nervous System

There also is a network known as the autonomic nervous system that controls the smooth muscles of the internal organs.

The autonomic nervous system is separated into two sets, the sympathetic and the parasympathetic. One set of nerves causes activity among the smooth muscles of the body; the other reverses the action. The sympathetic nerves dilate the pupil of the eye; the parasympathetic constrict the pupil. The sympathetic nerves constrict the blood vessels and speed up the heartbeat; the parasympathetic nerves dilate the blood vessels and slow the heartbeat. These are automatic actions, involving the involuntary muscles, hence the name autonomic.

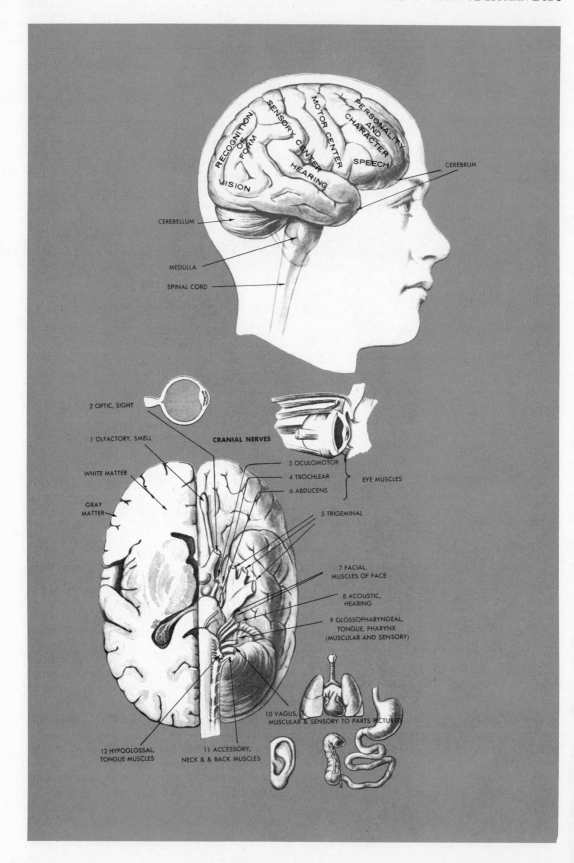

The Cranial Nerves

The cranial nerves are attached to the central nervous system through the base of the brain. Most of the dozen pairs of nerves in the system are both sensory and motor. The cell bodies of the cranial nerves' motor fibers are within the brain and, as with the spinal nerves, the sensory nerve cell bodies are located in ganglia outside the brain.

The cranial nerves include the olfactory which runs to receptors in the nasal cavity and provides us with our sense of smell, and the optic, which runs to the retina of the eye. Three other cranial nerves control the muscles that move the eyeballs. Still another, the acoustic, carries impulses from the sound receptors in the ear. Cranial nerves also include fibers running to taste buds in the tongue, muscles of the face, jaw, and neck, as well as the vagus, which reaches the heart, lungs, larynx, stomach, intestines, liver, pancreas, spleen, and kidneys.

The brain itself develops in the embryo as a ball at the end of a hollow tube that later becomes the spinal cord. As the ball expands, it divides into the cerebrum and the other major parts of the brain, the cerebellum, medulla, and the pons. The cerebrum, which eventually dominates the cranial cavity, grows much faster than the other parts of the brain. It folds back upon itself a number of times, producing the convolutions that give the human brain the appearance of a huge gray walnut. The convolutions almost conceal the medulla and the cerebellum, but enable the brain to carry an immense amount of surface area in a small space. The gray matter that gives the cerebrum its color is only a bark-like covering, about an eighth of an inch thick. Called the cortex, it contains nerve cells with axons that extend into

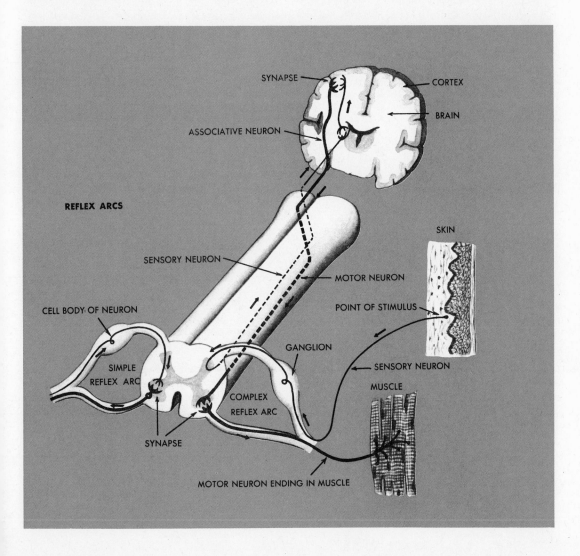

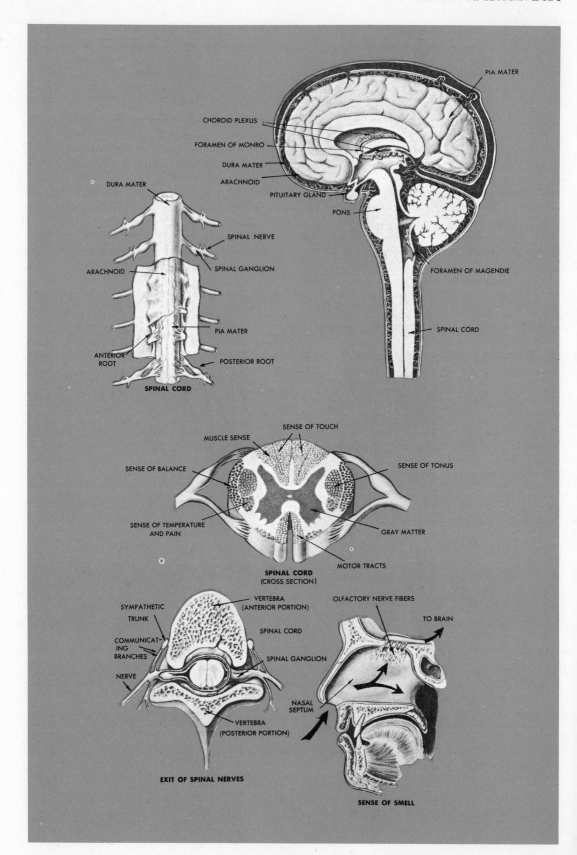

PIA MATER

CHOROID PLEXUS

FORAMEN OF MONRO

DURA MATER

ARACHNOID

PITUITARY GLAND

PONS

FORAMEN OF MAGENDIE

SPINAL CORD

DURA MATER

SPINAL NERVE

SPINAL GANGLION

ARACHNOID

PIA MATER

ANTERIOR ROOT

POSTERIOR ROOT

SPINAL CORD

SENSE OF TOUCH

MUSCLE SENSE

SENSE OF BALANCE

SENSE OF TONUS

SENSE OF TEMPERATURE AND PAIN

GRAY MATTER

MOTOR TRACTS

SPINAL CORD
(CROSS SECTION)

SYMPATHETIC TRUNK

VERTEBRA (ANTERIOR PORTION)

OLFACTORY NERVE FIBERS

TO BRAIN

SPINAL CORD

COMMUNICAT- ING BRANCHES

SPINAL GANGLION

NERVE

NASAL SEPTUM

VERTEBRA (POSTERIOR PORTION)

EXIT OF SPINAL NERVES

SENSE OF SMELL

a layer of white matter beneath.

The furrows and folds of the convolutions may seem haphazard, but they divide each half of the brain into distinct regions. One deep furrow starting near the middle of each hemisphere and running downward and forward is called the central sulcus. This is an important dividing line between sensory and motor nerve areas. The region behind the line contains nerves that bring stimuli from the hands, feet, face, tongue, and various other outer and inner parts of the body. In front of the central sulcus are nerves related to movement of the muscles in the hands, feet, face, tongue, and other areas.

In humans, machines have detected areas of the brain that react to lights, odors, and other stimuli. Knowledge of the sensory and motor areas of the brain helps locate the source of certain diseases involving the nervous system. For example, doctors for generations have known that nerve fibers from the right side of the body cross over in the brain stem to the left side of the brain. Similarly, nerve fibers from the left side of the body cross over to the right side of the brain. Thus, when a person becomes paralyzed on the right side, doctors can assume safely there has been damage to the motor area on the left side of the brain. Damage to the association areas of the cortex may be revealed when a person can see simple printed words but cannot recognize them. Or, if the motor association area is damaged, the person suddenly is unable to perform such a simple task as writing his name.

One region of the cerebrum that has defied mapping is the so-called silent area of the frontal lobes. This portion of the brain, behind the forehead, seems to be related to emotions and moral traits rather than simple sensory-motor functions. When fibers connecting the frontal lobes with the rest of the cerebrum are cut, the person may lose initiative, become careless, or even become unable to understand a joke. The frontal lobes may be cut surgically, however, to help mental patients who are extremely depressed or violent.

We mentioned earlier that electrical currents in nerve fibers could be measured and traced. The brain not only shows evidence of electrical activity, but it produces small current changes known as brain waves. The brain waves may appear at a frequency of about 10 per second, but they vary in frequency and size. Each person is said to have a brain wave pattern that is as distinctive as his handwriting.

The study of brain waves is a complicated field requiring expensive electronic equipment. But the information gained from the study of "brainprints" has been valuable in helping victims of epilepsy and other nerve disorders.

Because of their common origin the brain and spinal cord have the same set of protective membranes, although these vary slightly in different areas. The innermost of the three layers, the pia mater, fits over the convolutions of the brain like a tight, delicate glove. It carries many fine blood vessels that nourish the brain. Covering the pia mater is the middle membrane called the arachnoid. It resembles a filmy spider web. The outer layer, the dura mater, protects the central nervous system from being damaged by contact with bony surfaces of the skull and spine, and serves as a support for these.

The dura mater also forms partitions between the major divisions of the brain, giving them support and extra cushioning.

The Cerebellum

At the base of the cerebrum, where it joins the spinal cord, are three structures known as the pons, the medulla, and the cerebellum. The pons looks like a bridge made of coarse fibers. The fibers connect the medulla with the higher centers of the brain. The medulla, just below the pons, is an important switching center for nerve impulses going to and from the higher brain centers. It is also headquarters for many vital body functions. Body temperature, heart rate, breathing, swallowing, and the size of the openings in blood vessels are controlled by the medulla through the autonomic nervous system of the medulla.

The cerebellum, second largest of the brain divisions, is divided into ribbed hemispheres. And, like the cerebrum, much of the cerebellum areas have been mapped. The front and back areas control muscle tone. An area behind the back lobe is concerned with equilibrium. And the two main hemisphere areas control coordination of voluntary movements. Thus, the cerebellum is important for such activities as walking, dancing, playing ball, or even for such routine tasks as tying a shoelace or lifting a glass of water to the lips. If the cerebellum is damaged, many activities requiring coordination could be lost. Even talking distinctly would be difficult because the cerebellum helps coordinate the muscles of the vocal cords.

CHAPTER EIGHT

THE SENSE ORGANS

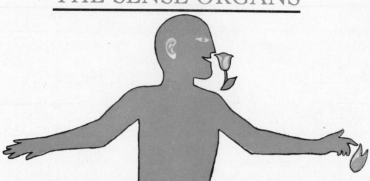

THE EYEBALL frequently is compared to a camera. The analogy is not entirely true, but we can learn a few things about the eye by thinking of it in terms of various parts of a camera. Both the eyeball and the camera are light-tight containers with dark inside walls. The camera is usually shaped like a box while the eyeball is spherical, of course. The walls of the camera usually are made of a rigid metal or plastic. The outside of the eyeball, the sclerotic coat, is made of tough fibrous tissue. The eyeball is further protected by its location in the bony orbit of the skull. The orbit is lined with a cushion of fatty tissue to protect the eye mechanism from shock damage.

The eyeball has a layer just inside the sclerotic coat, the choroid, which is filled with blood vessels to nourish the living tissues of the eye.

The Lens

Both the camera and the eye have a lens to focus the image on a light-sensitive surface. The light-sensitive surface in the camera is the roll or plate of film. In the eye it is a layer of light-sensitive nerve cells called the retina. In the camera, the distance between the lens and the film usually can be changed to keep the image in focus for objects both near and far away. In the eye, the shape of the lens is changed automatically, by small muscles, so that we can see clearly objects at various distances.

A further similarity between the eye and the camera is that of the iris, the curtain at the front of the eye that can be opened or closed to permit various amounts of light to pass through the lens. In the camera, the iris may be controlled by energy from a photoelectric cell or it may be adjusted by hand. The iris of the eye adjusts automatically to changes in light intensity, again by the action of tiny muscles it contains. The opening in the iris of the eye is called the pupil.

In the cases of both the eye and the camera, simple lenses do not produce clear images without some "correction." The outer edges of the lenses bend rays of light at different angles than do the center parts of the lenses. Camera lenses are corrected by making them from combinations of different kinds of glass. The human eye is partly corrected by nature's design of the cornea, a transparent extension of the sclerotic coat in front of the pupil. The curvature of the cornea varies slightly to compensate for visual errors produced by edges of the lens. In some people, however, the surface of the cornea becomes irregular and vision is blurred. This condition is called astigmatism.

The front of the eyeball is protected by a smooth, transparent layer of tissue called the conjunctiva. A similar membrane covers the inner surfaces of the eyelids. The eyelids also contain dozens of tiny tarsal glands that secrete an oil to lubricate the surfaces of the eyeball and eyelids. Still further protection is provided by the lacrimal gland, located at the outer edge of the eye socket. It secretes tears to clean the protective membrane and keep it moist.

The region between the cornea and the lens is filled with a salty, clear fluid known as the aqueous humor. The eyeball behind the lens is filled with a jelly-like substance called the vitreous humor.

The Retina

The innermost layer of the eyeball, the retina, is itself made up of eight layers of nerve tissue. Most of the layers contain nerve fibers or nerve nuclei. But the layer most directly involved in vision contains specialized nerve cells called rods and cones. They get their names from the rod and cone-like shapes seen when the layer is viewed under a microscope. The rods are more sensitive to light than the cones. The cones, on the other hand, are sensitive to colors. When we are trying to see an object at

SCHEMATIC DRAWING OF THE EYE SHOWING ANATOMIC LAYERS AND VASCULAR PATTERN

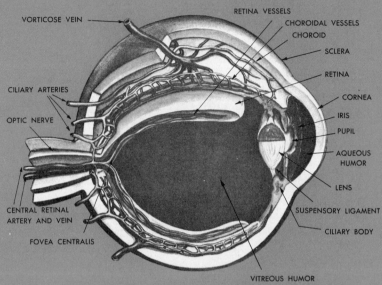

VORTICOSE VEIN

RETINA VESSELS

CHOROIDAL VESSELS

CHOROID

SCLERA

RETINA

CILIARY ARTERIES

CORNEA

IRIS

OPTIC NERVE

PUPIL

AQUEOUS HUMOR

LENS

CENTRAL RETINAL ARTERY AND VEIN

SUSPENSORY LIGAMENT

CILIARY BODY

FOVEA CENTRALIS

VITREOUS HUMOR

MUSCLES OF EYE

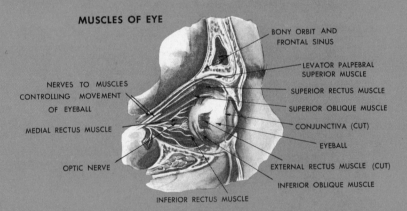

BONY ORBIT AND FRONTAL SINUS

LEVATOR PALPEBRAL SUPERIOR MUSCLE

NERVES TO MUSCLES CONTROLLING MOVEMENT OF EYEBALL

SUPERIOR RECTUS MUSCLE

SUPERIOR OBLIQUE MUSCLE

CONJUNCTIVA (CUT)

MEDIAL RECTUS MUSCLE

EYEBALL

OPTIC NERVE

EXTERNAL RECTUS MUSCLE (CUT)

INFERIOR OBLIQUE MUSCLE

INFERIOR RECTUS MUSCLE

TEARS

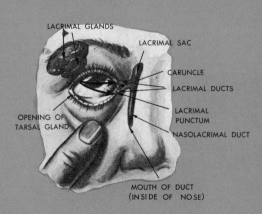

LACRIMAL GLANDS

LACRIMAL SAC

CARUNCLE

LACRIMAL DUCTS

LACRIMAL PUNCTUM

OPENING OF TARSAL GLAND

NASOLACRIMAL DUCT

MOUTH OF DUCT (INSIDE OF NOSE)

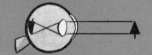

A NORMAL EYE FOCUSES IMAGE ON RETINA

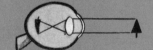

A NEARSIGHTED EYE (MYOPIA) FOCUSES IMAGE IN FRONT OF RETINA

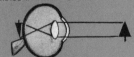

A FARSIGHTED EYE (HYPEROPIA) FOCUSES IMAGE BEHIND RETINA

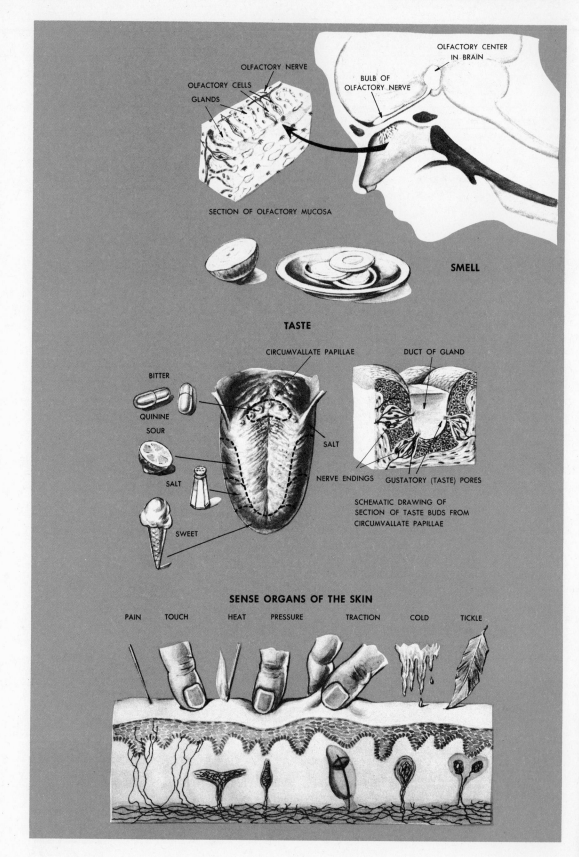

OLFACTORY NERVE

OLFACTORY CELLS

GLANDS

OLFACTORY CENTER IN BRAIN

BULB OF OLFACTORY NERVE

SECTION OF OLFACTORY MUCOSA

SMELL

TASTE

CIRCUMVALLATE PAPILLAE

DUCT OF GLAND

BITTER

QUININE

SOUR

SALT

SALT

SWEET

NERVE ENDINGS

GUSTATORY (TASTE) PORES

SCHEMATIC DRAWING OF SECTION OF TASTE BUDS FROM CIRCUMVALLATE PAPILLAE

SENSE ORGANS OF THE SKIN

PAIN   TOUCH   HEAT   PRESSURE   TRACTION   COLD   TICKLE

night, perhaps by moonlight, we depend upon the rods. The faint amounts of light passing through the lens fall upon the retina and stimulate the rods which transmit, through the optic nerve, the messages that produce the visual image in the brain.

As the intensity in light increases, cones begin to dominate the action of image formation in the brain. The rods might continue firing messages to the brain in bright light, but they apparently contribute very little to the image in such cases. Animals such as rats and owls, which sleep during the day and forage for food at night, have only rods in the retinas of their eyes.

Eye Defects

Visual acuity may be affected by several types of eye defects. Astigmatism, mentioned earlier, is one abnormal condition. Other common defects are myopia (nearsightedness) and hyperopia (farsightedness). Myopia occurs when the rays of light entering through the lens are focused in the vitrous humor, in front of the retina. Hyperopia results when the image is focused, theoretically, behind the eyeball. Both near and farsightedness may result from abnormal curvature of the lens or cornea or from abnormal shape of the eyeball.

Taste and Smell

There are four basic taste sensations, sweet, sour, salty, and bitter. The receptors for taste are located mostly on the tongue, although there are a few taste buds, as they are called, on the soft palate and epiglottis. The taste buds on the tongue are found at the tip, on the sides, and at the back. Taste buds are more plentiful in babies than in old people.

Although taste buds look alike under a microscope, those at the back of the tongue transmit the bitter sensation. Taste buds at the tip generally produce the sensation of sweetness. Those along the sides at two points, near the tip and again near the back of the tongue, are related to the taste sensation of saltiness. And buds along the sides but toward the back of the tongue transmit sour sensations.

If your mouth were completely dry, you would not be able to taste anything. Taste sensations occur only when the substance in the mouth has been moistened. The moisture usually is supplied in sufficient quantities by your salivary glands.

The organ of smell helps to detect substances at a distance or things not visible, and may act as a warning of danger. It is apparently much more important in lower animals than in humans.

Our sense of smell is contained in the olfactory organ located in the top of the nasal cavity. A long bulb of nerve tissue extends along a ledge of skull bone separating the nasal cavity from the brain. There is a series of tiny holes through the bony ledge, and through the holes nerve fibers pass to a layer of hair cells in the nasal mucous membrane. The size of the membrane area containing the odor receptors is only about $1/4$ of a square inch in humans, but the olfactory receptor area in a dog is about 40 times as large—indicating the relative importance of the sense of smell between the two species.

The olfactory smell receptors are a type of chemical detector. To be "smelled," an odor first must be dissolved in the mucous secreted by the nasal mucous membrane. Scientists have found that only substances that can pass a certain set of "smellability" requirements will be detected by the nose.

The olfactory organ is a sensitive and complicated chemical plant capable of sifting through many sizes and shapes of molecules, giving you a computer-quick decision on which odoriferous substances are close to you. The receptors are sensitive enough to detect a substance diluted to as much as one part in 30,000,000,000.

Ears

Have you ever tried to carry on a conversation near the center of a big city during the rush hour? If so, you can remember the continuous din of elevated trains, police whistles, taxi horns, shouts of newsboys, and the clacking of shoes on sidewalks.

Most people can hear sounds between about 40 cyles, or vibrations, per second and 20,000 per second.

How do sounds that begin as air vibrations reach the part of the brain that identifies and catalogs them? The vibrations travel down the tube leading from the outer ear to the eardrum. The tube is called the external auditory canal. It is lined with hair and glands that secrete ear wax. The tube is funnel-shaped to help collect sound waves and guide them to the eardrum, or tympanic membrane.

On the inner side of the tympanic membrane

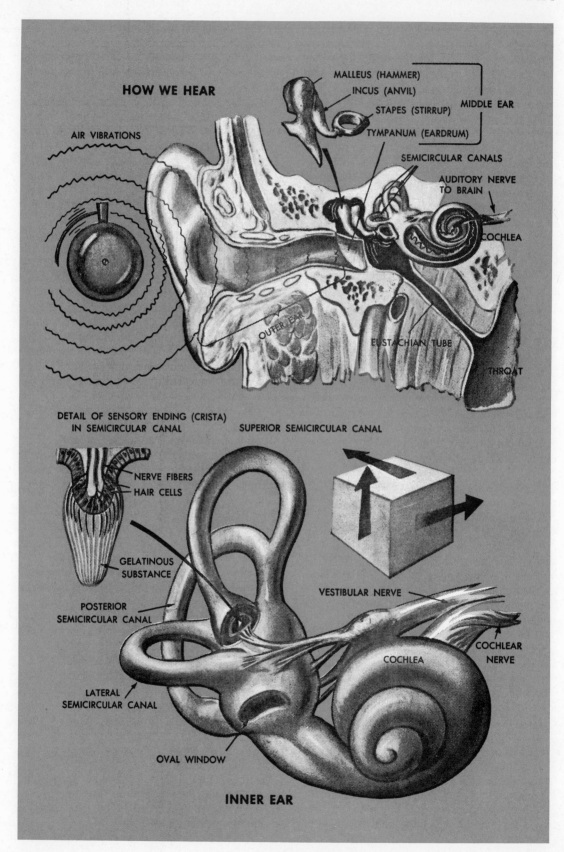

HOW WE HEAR

MALLEUS (HAMMER)
INCUS (ANVIL)
STAPES (STIRRUP)   MIDDLE EAR
TYMPANUM (EARDRUM)

AIR VIBRATIONS

SEMICIRCULAR CANALS

AUDITORY NERVE
TO BRAIN

COCHLEA

OUTER EAR

EUSTACHIAN TUBE

THROAT

DETAIL OF SENSORY ENDING (CRISTA)
IN SEMICIRCULAR CANAL   SUPERIOR SEMICIRCULAR CANAL

NERVE FIBERS
HAIR CELLS

GELATINOUS
SUBSTANCE

VESTIBULAR NERVE

POSTERIOR
SEMICIRCULAR CANAL

COCHLEAR
NERVE

COCHLEA

LATERAL
SEMICIRCULAR CANAL

OVAL WINDOW

INNER EAR

is the middle ear, which as we have said earlier, contains three tiny bones, or ossicles. The bones, called the hammer, anvil, and stirrup, are stretched across the cavity of the middle ear to relay the vibrations from the eardrum to the fluid-filled cavity of the inner ear. Sound waves vibrate the eardrum and the hammer attached to it. The hammer pushes the anvil which, in turn, moves the stirrup.

The stirrup acts as a piston on the membrane of the oval window as it pushes against the fluid in the inner ear. The inner ear contains the cochlea, a snail-shaped spiral tunnel in which the organ of Corti—the true organ of hearing—is located. The inner ear also contains the semicircular canals which help give us our sense of balance.

The Hearing Organ

The organ of Corti consists of specialized nerve cells that follow the spiral of the cochlea. The cells rest on the basilar membrane, which is made up of connective-tissue fibers. The nerve cells have hair-like projections and the tips of the hairs are in contact with a membrane above, the tectorial membrane. The spongy bone that forms the core of the cochlea has many tiny tunnels through which the nerves carry impulses to the brain.

Each middle ear is connected with the throat in back of the mouth by a passageway called the auditory, or Eustachian, tube. The job of this tube is to equalize air pressure in the middle ear with the atmospheric pressure.

The Organ of Balance

The organ of equilibrium, or balance, has two kinds of nerve receptors. They are located in three membrane-like tubes, called semicircular canals, and two small sacs in the inner ear next to the cochlea. The semicircular canals are set at right angles to each other—like the top and adjacent sides of the corner of a box. The nerve receptors in the semicircular canals are hair cells with the tips of the hair embedded in a plume of gelatin-like material. When the head is moved, the fluid flows against the plumes, called cristae. This pressure triggers the receptors which transmit to the brain the message that the head is changing position.

The second kind of receptor is located in the two small sacs. It also uses hair cells with the hairs embedded in a gelatin-like material. But the surface of the gelatinous mass in the two sacs is coated with a layer of tiny grains of limestone. Movement of the head causes the grains, called otoliths, to shift. This causes the hair cells to send out nerve impulses.

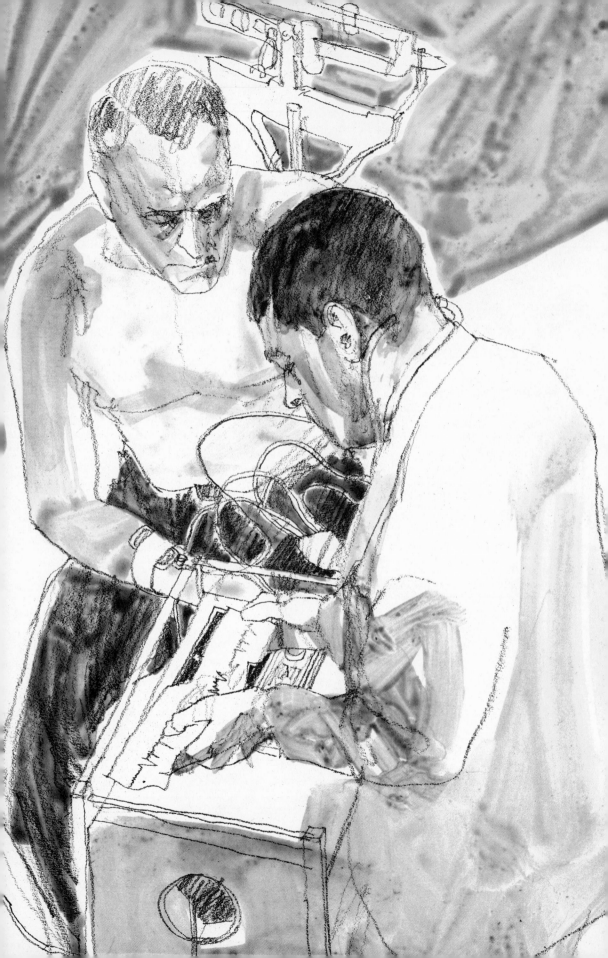

PART IV

Safeguarding Your Health

CHAPTER ONE

THE PERIODIC HEALTH EXAMINATION

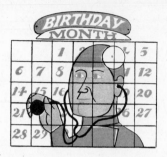

EVERY CHILD born in the United States today will enjoy an average life expectancy of at least three-score and ten years and a freedom from communicable disease unequalled in history. This fortunate state has been made possible largely by the public health worker and the medical scientist. Throughout the era of health improvement, little effort has been required of the average citizen to obtain these important benefits.

The future will be different. Immunization, better sanitation, and superior nutrition have already made probably their most useful contributions to our well-being. However, many diseases still cannot be prevented by these means; for these, early detection and correction are necessary. Further advances can be expected only when each individual assumes responsibility for his own health and fitness. Longevity will depend more and more upon our active participation in programs for health betterment—this must be a "do-it-yourself" project.

The chronic diseases, with their quiet approaches, make "undercover" progress to depress our vigor and shorten our active years. Diabetes, cancer, and high blood pressure seldom cause symptoms in their earlier stages, yet treatment is more effective, less extended, less painful, and less expensive when it is begun at the onset of a disease. Thus, the best hope for control of these dread diseases lies in their early detection.

The regular health examination is the only practical method we have at present for detecting disease in its earlier stages. The practice of examining infants and young children at frequent intervals has given us the healthiest children and the lowest death rates for these age groups ever achieved in the history of our country. Mortality from disease is unbelievably low among infants and, until maturity, accidents cause more deaths than disease. As adults, we should adopt this effective type of

disease control and share in the benefits our children enjoy. Why wait until pain or other symptoms appear to motivate us? If industry has found the regular inspection of expensive machines a source of profits, it is even more logical that we should examine the human machine for which spare parts are not yet an actuality. With reasonable attention the body astounds us with its capacity for self-regulation and repair.

Your family doctor, who is acquainted with your background and personal problems, is the person best equipped to give the health examination. He is interested in you, and you have faith in his competence—this sympathetic bond is very necessary for mutual understanding and cooperation in the maintenance of health.

How Often Should You Be Examined?

While experience has established the annual examination as practical for the normal, healthy adult, the interval is not fixed. For those under the age of 40 and free from symptoms, an examination every second year may provide sufficient protection. When symptoms appear, prompt re-examination should be sought to ward off serious disease.

Time passes rapidly and it may be advisable to link the annual checkup to an anniversary date. Many persons select birthdays. Whatever the date chosen, regularity of examination counts most.

The health examination can be completed within an hour, although some additional time may be needed for analyzing x-ray and laboratory tests. Part of this period is spent with the physician, the rest with the nurse or technician.

The Examination Procedure

Your doctor will first ask you some questions about your living habits. He will want to know about your work, your daily diet, and hours of

Sample of Patient's History Form approved by the
American Medical Association

Form A   **PATIENT'S HISTORY FORM**
NOTE—Answer "yes" or "no" wherever possible. Give date, number, or other information where requested.

Name_____ Birth date_____Birthplace _____

Address_____ Single____ Married____ Widow____ Widower____ Divorced____

Work experience: Present occupation_____When started_____Previous work_____

Is your work

Regular____   Hazardous____   Smelly____   Hot____   Seated____   Hours per week____

Satisfying____   Fatiguing____   Noisy____   Cold____   Standing____   Days vacation____

Monotonous____   Indoors____ Out____   Crowded____   Damp____   Walking____   Do you like your work____

In your work are you subjected to

Skin irritation____ Dust____ Fumes____ (If "yes," describe)_____

Have you ever changed work for health reasons ____ (If "yes," describe)_____

Other work problems____ (If "yes," describe)_____

Living conditions

Live with own family____   Alone____   Congenial____   Quiet____   Room to yourself____

Live with another family____   Number in household____   Depressing____   Irritating____   Time to yourself ____

Additional comments about home conditions_____

Personal habits

Is your sleep: Restful____   Disturbed____   Sleep alone____   Average hours of sleep____

How many servings of the following foods do you eat daily:

Fruit____   Meat____   Bread____   Leafy vegetables____   Other vegetables (specify)____

Eggs____   Fish____   Cereal____   Cheese____   Other milk products (specify)_____

How much do you drink daily of: Water____ Milk____ Tea____ Coffee____ Soft drinks____ Alcoholic drinks____

Are your bowel movements: Regular____   Without physics or cathartics____

Do you smoke: Cigarettes____ Cigars____ Pipe____ How many____ For how long_____

What medicines do you use regularly: Aspirin____ Sleeping pills____ Allergy drugs____ Others (specify)____

What exercise do you take in addition to your work_____ Frequency_____

What sports do you pursue_____ Frequency_____

Sex life: Are there problems you wish to discuss_____

Form A   **PATIENT'S HISTORY FORM**

NOTE—Answer "yes" or "no" wherever possible. Give date, number, or other information where requested.

Illnesses, injuries, and immunizations

If you have had any illness, indicate by the approximate age at which you had it

Chicken Pox___	Hepatitis___	Syphilis___	Bronchitis___	Others (specify)
Measles___	Encephalitis___	Migraine___	Pneumonia___	_____
German Measles___	Poliomyelitis___	Rheumatic Fever___	Asthma___	_____
Whooping Cough___	Meningitis___	Tuberculosis___	Allergy___	_____
Diphtheria___	Gonorrhea___	Pleurisy___	Nervous Conditions___	_____

Do you ever have

Loss of appetite___	Abdominal cramps___	Numbness___	Chronic cough___	Discharges___
Nausea or vomiting___	Muscle cramps___	Tingling___	Chest pain___	Convulsions___
Headaches___	Palpitation___	Wheezing___	Trouble with urination___	_____
Dizziness___	Shortness of breath___	Swelling of feet___	Bleeding___	_____

Injuries or broken bones (specify)_____

Surgical operations (specify)_____

Immunizations (Enter date of last booster dose)

Smallpox___ Tetanus___ Diphtheria___ Polio___ Whooping Cough___ Others (specify)_____

Dental health: Date of last visit to dentist_____How often do you visit dentist_____

Family health history	Father	Mother	Brother or sister	Wife or husband	Children
Any deceased	___	___	_____	_____	___
Cause of death	___	___	_____	_____	___
Any now ill	___	___	_____	_____	___
Nature of illness	___	___	_____	_____	___

Menstrual history

Monthly periods: Regular___ Last how many days___ Does flow seem excessive___

Pregnancies: Number___ Any problems during pregnancy (discuss with doctor)_____

Do you consider yourself to be in good health ___ If not, what is your complaint_____

What additional information should the doctor have about you_____

_____

_____

_____

_____

_____

_____

_____

sleep; in particular, he will seek information about habits which affect health; such as smoking, drinking, and exercise. If your parents are no longer living, he may wish to know their ages at death and the causes, for diseases often run through the family. Even minor symptoms will be listed in your history, such as slight changes in digestion or elimination. Have you been disturbed over an emotional problem? Apprehension and anxiety can cause physical symptoms, even interfere with the functions of vital organs. Give your doctor frank answers.

For the examination your doctor may ask you to disrobe in part, so that he may check your posture and balance, and make other necessary observations. In beginning his head-to-toe scrutiny, he examines your eyes, ears, nose, and throat. Any enlargement of the thyroid gland or lymph nodes in the neck will be noted. He will listen to your heart and lung action, check your pulse rate, take your blood pressure, and examine your abdomen. He will note the condition of your arteries and the nerve reflexes.

While a chest x-ray is now a routine procedure, other x-ray investigations are a matter for his medical judgment.

The Laboratory Tests

When a sample of blood has been collected from an arm vein, a white blood count and hemoglobin determination are usually made. If your doctor has not previously ordered a test for syphilis, he may do so. A urine specimen is collected and other tests will be arranged when your doctor believes they are indicated for you.

Because you may have questions to ask, the discussion with the doctor which follows the examination may be the most valuable portion of the whole procedure. When your health is good and disease is not present, the doctor may wish to make some recommendations in regard to your living habits or he may suggest that certain immunizations be repeated. When defects are located, he stands ready to give information and guidance toward their correction. His advice is far more reliable than that given in lay journals or by your friends. Follow it. Never become the victim of fads and quackery.

Keeping the Record

Most physicians have their own system for keeping records. The American Medical Association has devised a pattern form for health records, a sample of which is reproduced here. This will give you a general idea of what information the doctor will ask you for, and of what the examination consists, as already described. The doctor may modify the examination procedure as circumstances warrant, but the general outline will usually be followed.

Everyone, young and old, needs a regular periodic physical checkup. Many reasons can be found for having it, few excuses for omitting it. Serious disease is only occasionally found, but many persons will carry the "seeds" of chronic ailments which may become disabilities later in life. We all have some habits which may be keeping us from enjoying vigorous, positive health. Finally, regular examination provides a continuous record of your physical state—a baseline for judging changes in your health as they occur. So, for more robust health, and a longer and more active life, have the annual health inventory, ask your physician's advice, and follow it closely.

Chapter Two

THE HEALTH OF WORKERS

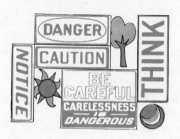

AMERICA'S GREATEST ASSET is its nearly 80,000,000 productive workers, in business, industry, and agriculture. Upon their good health depend the prosperity and productivity of our economic system. The worker who is absent from his job because of illness or injury stops producing, and both his family and society suffer through loss of his earnings and services. The complex nature of modern industrial techniques exposes workers to many new physical and chemical hazards which would increase accidents, occupational diseases, and loss of time from work if precautions were not taken to protect the safety and health of these workers.

Recognizing the importance of preserving the health and safety of workers, many industries have organized safety programs and preventive industrial health programs. Physicians and safety experts are often employed by industry to supervise these programs. Industrial hygienists study the job hazards and set up standards for safe operation to protect the worker from accident-causing procedures. Safety equipment is provided for machines, and protective equipment for workers.

Physicians examine job applicants to assure that their vision, their hearing, and their physical condition are well adapted to the safe performance of their particular jobs. In case of sudden illness or injury, doctors are available for prompt medical care to prevent further harm to the worker and to restore him quickly to full employment. Physicians give the worker appropriate inoculations against diseases to which the job may expose him. Industrial nurses work under the physician's direction to teach the worker safety and health and to advise him about his health problems.

Industrial management usually provides these health programs as a part of the employer's responsibility to maintain a safe workplace. Workmen's compensation laws require that management do so, as well as to furnish medi-cal care for job-related injuries of illnesses. Some unions also provide such health maintenance services. They are equally in the self-interest of the worker and the employer.

The Worker's Responsibility

The worker himself can greatly assist in supporting such health maintenance efforts. In order for such programs to be successful, he should carefully observe the safety rules prescribed by the safety team in his shop. He should regularly use such protective equipment as safety glasses, safety shoes, gloves, masks, and hard hats as necessary. He should handle carefully those dangerous materials which his job involves and not take "short-cut" chances that make accidents more likely.

He should get prompt dressings from the nurse for minor abrasions and scratches that could become infected and disable him. He should take advantage of the voluntary physical examinations, immunizations, and other services recommended by the medical department. And he should avoid needless exposure to gases, fumes, solvents, dusts, cleaning agents, and other irritating chemicals through careless handling. His careful cooperation with the safety team is in his own interest even more than in his employer's. To become disabled is of no advantage to anyone—especially to the worker's family.

Every employee should have a personal physician, whether or not there is an industrial physician at his place of employment. If there is no industrial physician, the family physician may fulfill this function anyway. In addition, many illnesses and injuries which are not related to his work can just as effectively deprive him of his job as can an accident at work. Prompt medical treatment of a minor illness may prevent a major, disabling one. Periodic check-ups by the family physician are therefore a part of good health maintenance to preserve good earning capacity, especially as the worker grows older. Early diagnosis of heart disease, diabetes, cancer, or emotional troubles—with consequent treatment and cure—may save years of productive employment and avoid forced invalidism or retirement.

Many illnesses which happen to employed persons are not directly related to their jobs. Acute conditions like colds, digestive disturbances, headaches, or hangovers may happen to anyone, and are related to the job only conditionally if at all. Chronic illnesses such as allergies, heart diseases, arthritis, high blood pressure, diabetes, vision and hearing disturbances are not, as a rule, due to the job, although in some instances they may be made worse, or improved, by a change in employment. These illnesses reside in the person, and not in the job. They are therefore the responsibility of the worker, not of the company.

Some employers choose to provide assistance to the worker and his doctor through

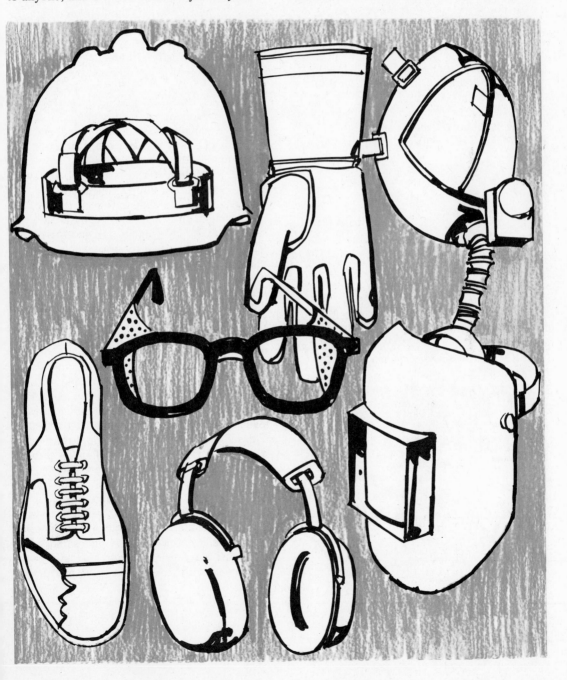

making available the more expensive laboratory tests at nominal cost or even for free. The treatment of the patient remains the function of the physician chosen by the individual, and the responsibility rests between doctor and patient, involving the company only incidentally as a voluntary and helpful factor. One type of such helpfulness is the adaptation of work load and type of work by personnel officials of the company for workers with handicaps which can be overcome—temporarily or permanently —by modification of working conditions.

Common Job Hazards

Among the commonest job hazards that produce temporary or permanent disability to workers are the following:

- burns, either from acid or caustic chemicals, or from hot objects or steam;
- fractures, especially of the hands or feet,

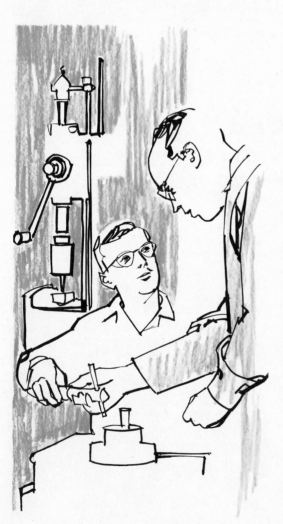

from improper handling of machines and other heavy objects;

- skin rashes from irritating chemicals or solvents;
- chemicals or foreign bodies in the eye, from splashes, dusts, or abrasives;
- back injuries, often sustained by improper lifting techniques;
- poisonings, from unprotected exposure to chemicals or gases;
- lacerations and bruises, usually resulting from impulsiveness in handling materials or machines.

In addition, continuously appearing new processes in industry, shipping, and agriculture require never-ceasing vigilance in adaptation of safety procedures to new hazards, as in such fields as radiation, air pollution, and plastics. Only by continual conscientious ingenuity can the work environment be improved and the safety and health of the worker protected in these rapidly advancing fields.

The promotion of the health and safety of workers is a team effort, which involves the understanding and cooperation of the worker and his industrial and family physicians, the safety director, the nurse, the industrial hygienist, his union, and the management at his plant or office. Effective health maintenance works best when all these people work together for safeguarding the workplace, the home, and the worker. Industrial physicians should not provide care for home injuries or ordinary illnesses, but by cooperation with the family physician, they may help in maintaining the worker's general health. Similarly, the safety director or employer may not be able to force compliance with all desirable health and safety standards, but the worker can greatly assist the team by a helpful attitude toward the health and safety of the group of employees with whom he works, for the good of all concerned. The whole philosophy of safety and health maintenance depends on friendly cooperation in a community of all the people involved. To this end, all can make a contribution toward lowering accident rates, helping to maintain a productive economy, and at the same time, protecting the wage earner and his family from avoidable disaster.

CHAPTER THREE

FOODS AND NUTRITION

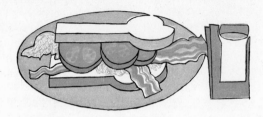

GOOD NUTRITION is vital to our physical and emotional well-being. It gives us the vigor and stamina we need both to carry on and to enjoy our daily activities. Because most of us eat our most important meals at home, what comes from our kitchen to our dining tables largely determines the quality of our nourishment.

Food contains the nutrients such as protein, carbohydrates, fats, vitamins, and minerals that we need for growth, maintenance, and repair of body tissues and energy production. All of the nutrients that man requires are found in ordinary "everyday" foods readily available in all parts of the country the year around. We normally have no need for dietary supplements of vitamins and minerals when our diet is properly varied. To be certain that she is giving her family all of the needed food values, the homemaker must make careful food selections in the market place and then prepare her food attractively while conserving its nutrients.

It is not necessary to memorize the details of the nutrient composition of foods in order to achieve a nutritionally adequate diet. Simply choose foods from the four basic groups: milk, meat, vegetable-fruit, and bread and cereals. These foods offer us a wide variety and assure us the basis of a healthful diet.

Milk Group

The consumption of an adequate amount of milk or other dairy foods is particularly important during growth, pregnancy, and while nursing a baby. The milk group includes not only whole, skim, and evaporated milk and buttermilk, but also butter, cheese, and ice cream. Milk and its products can improve the value of almost any meal.

The dairy foods, with the exception of cream and butter, are interchangeable so far as their contribution of calcium to the diet is concerned. Thus, a one-inch cube of cheddar cheese can change places at mealtime with 2/3 cup of milk; 1/2 cup cottage cheese can be used for 1/3 cup of milk, and 1/2 cup of ice cream is interchangeable with 1/4 cup of milk if a treat is desired.

Milk or some milk product is recommended every day for everyone in these minimum quantities:

Eight-ounce cups of fluid whole milk

Children . . . . .3 to 4 cups
Teen-agers . . . . .4 or more
Adults of all ages . . . . .2 or more
Pregnant women . . . . .4 or more
Nursing mothers . . . . .6 or more

Milk is our richest food source of calcium and is a valuable source of protein and riboflavin. Milk is counted on to supply adults with an important vitamin, vitamin D; so be certain that the brand you buy has this vitamin added.

Meat Group

In addition to meat, fish, and poultry, eggs, dry beans and peas, and nuts are included in the meat group because they contribute similar important food benefits—protein, B vitamins, iron, and other nutrients for the family meal.

Choose two or more servings from the meat group every day. A minimum adult serving of meat is two to three ounces of lean, cooked meat, poultry, or fish without bone. Larger servings may be needed for growing and active persons; smaller servings will do for children. It is recommended that some meat, poultry, fish, or eggs be eaten at each meal. Eggs (two for a serving), dry beans, dry peas and lentils (1 cup, cooked, per serving), peanut butter (4 tablespoons), and nuts can be used in place of one serving of meat when menu variety is desired. A thick peanut butter sandwich does not look much like roast beef, but it can accomplish about the same thing in the body.

Do not be hasty in condemning luncheon meats, hamburgers, and frankfurters; they are rightful members of the meat group and may provide a tantalizing attraction for the "meal skipper." Do not overlook the less expensive cuts of meat either. Use of a little time, imagination, and possibly a meat tenderizer can turn inexpensive meat cuts into gourmet delights just as nourishing as the more expensive cuts. The decision to broil, roast, boil, or fry the foods in this group, of course, depends on your preference and tolerance for fat. Roasting and broiling reduce the fat content of these meats somewhat.

Vegetable-Fruit Group

Vegetables and fruits are the foods most frequently neglected by children and young people. This is unfortunate because vegetables and fruits provide important nutrients.

Your diet should include four or more servings from vegetable-fruit group every day. There should be one good source of vitamin C or two servings of a fair source.

There should be also one serving, at least every other day, of a good source of vitamin A. If the food chosen for vitamin C is also a good source of vitamin A, the additional serving of vitamin A food may be omitted. The remaining one to three or more servings may be of any vegetable or fruit, including those that are valuable for vitamin C and vitamin A.

A serving for an adult, for example, is 1/2 cup of vegetable or fruit, or one medium-sized whole fruit or potato, or half of a medium-sized grapefruit or melon.

The following are sources of vitamin C: *Good*—grapefruit or grapefruit juice, orange or orange juice, cantaloupe, guava, mango, papaya, raw (fresh) strawberries, broccoli, green pepper, and sweet red pepper. *Fair, but also important*—honeydew melon, tangerine or tangerine juice, watermelon, asparagus tips, Brussels sprouts, raw cabbage, collards, garden cress, kale, kohlrabi, mustard greens, potatoes and sweet potatoes cooked in their jackets, spinach, tomato or tomato juice, and turnip greens.

Vitamin A is stored by the body so that a daily source is not needed; two or three servings a week are sufficient. Foods that provide vitamin A are: dark-green and deep-yellow vegetables and a few fruits, namely apricots, broccoli, cantaloupe, carrots, chard, collards, cress, kale, mango, persimmon, pumpkin, spinach, sweet potatoes, turnip greens, winter squash, and other dark-green leaves.

Bread-Cereal Group

This group includes all breads and cereals that are whole grained, enriched, or restored.

Cereals seem to be the forgotten food group, just as fruits and vegetables are often the neglected foods. The drift away from the use of cereal foods occurring in recent times is a reflection of our affluent way of life. It is lamentable, since cereals at relatively low cost add both variety to our diet and worthwhile amounts of important nutrients.

A serving is one slice of bread; one ounce of ready-to-eat cereal; 1/2 to 3/4 cup of cooked cereal, cornmeal, grits, or macaroni products. Four or more servings daily from this group are recommended; for example, three slices of bread and one serving of cereal. If no cereals as such are chosen, you should have an extra serving of bread or baked goods. Choose from breads, cooked and ready-to-eat cereals, cornmeal, crackers, grits, rice, rolled oats, macaroni, spaghetti, noodles, and baked goods made with whole grain or enriched flour.

Other Foods

The foods suggested above provide the minimum foundation for an adequate diet. Other foods will be needed to complete or round out the diet. Additional or extra-large servings of foods listed in the daily plan can be used as well as such foods as fats, oils, sugars, and unenriched refined cereal foods which are not emphasized because they contribute mainly calories. The amount of food each person eats each day (the size, the number of servings) will be determined primarily by his energy needs. The minimum servings recommended in the daily food guide will provide from 1250 to 1450 calories. Most people will need from a third to a half more calories than the basic plan provides for. Strict adherence to the basic plan would turn it into a weight reduction regimen. The bathroom scale is a good guide as to whether one is getting enough calories or too many.

There are several important concepts to keep in mind when following this nutrition guide:

●No single food will provide all of the nutrients needed. Variety in the diet is the surest way to be certain of proper nourishment. Excessive dependence on even such a good food as milk can interfere with achieving an adequate diet. Learn enough about foods to be able to make wise substitutions for tiresome or unliked foods so that health needs will be met.

●Be certain that your children are exposed to a variety of vegetables and fruits while they

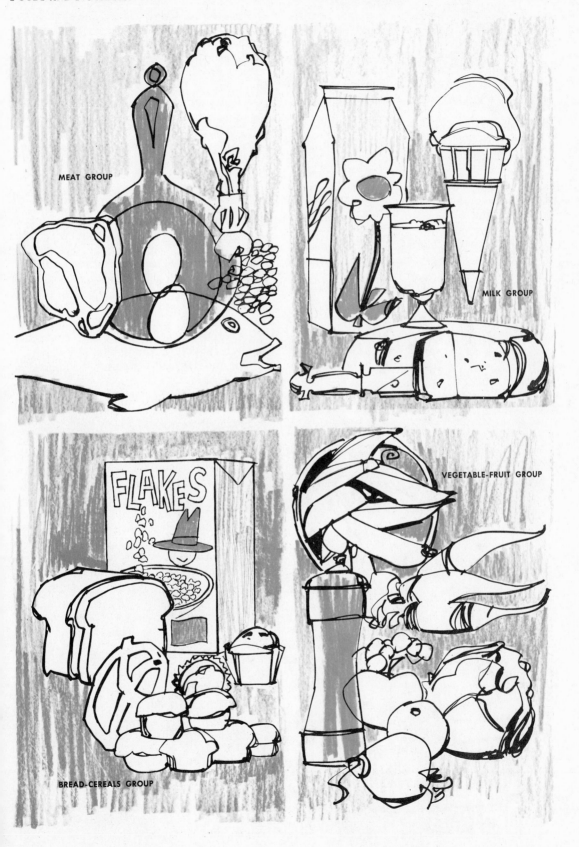

are young so that their interest in these essential foods is stimulated. Also cook them in appetizingly different ways. Frequent repetition of the same vegetable prepared in the same old way is sure to destroy its popularity.

●The less food one consumes, as in caloric restriction for weight reduction, the more important it becomes to choose food wisely. The preferred way to reduce weight is to cut down on the amount of food consumed. One should cut *down,* however, not cut *out.* Many people have the mistaken notion that some foods are fattening and should be avoided; this is not so. No one food can be considered fattening because each food contributes a certain percentage of the day's calories. The true cause of overweight is the total amount of food calories one consumes per day.

●Each meal is important, one no less than

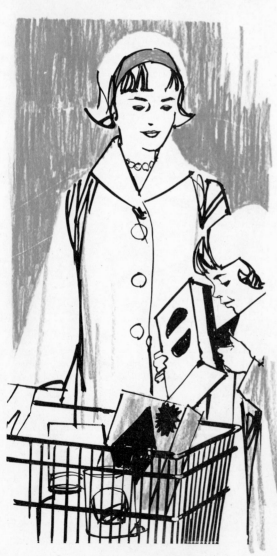

the other. If breakfast is a neglected meal at your house, the reason why should be sought and corrected. Trying different foods and methods of preparation may keep the family from being bored. There is nothing sacred about the conventional American breakfast of toast, eggs, cereal, or pancakes. Simple sandwiches may be a welcome change, or a small steak or chop. Perhaps a slight modification of the kinds of foods served, the frequency of their use, or the size of servings will bring the family's appetites back to the table and their meals up to acceptable standards.

●Although we may prefer fresh foods in season, there is so little loss of nutritive value by the modern methods of preservation that canned and frozen foods can be used with confidence. It is fashionable today to criticize processed foods as being so highly refined as to be devoid of nutrients. Such criticism is usually made either by those who have something else to sell or by zealots who do not understand modern methods of processing.

Our food industry prevents contamination and deterioration of foods by processing and makes available the most nutritious and attractive food products known. Processing techniques now utilized give us canned, frozen, and dehydrated foods with nutritive values comparable to those in the foods grandmother prepared fresh from her farm. Some heat sensitive vitamins (vitamin C, the B vitamins, and ascorbic acid) are lost in the canning process and in blanching prior to freezing, but these losses are insignificant when the total diet is considered. Dehydration, a fairly new process on the consumer market, results in only slight losses of the B vitamins. Cured and fermented products have nutritive values similar to foods preserved by other methods. Foods preserved in these various ways differ in physical characteristics from the fresh food, but they have the advantage of safe storage for long periods of time. Refined cereals which lose nutrients in the milling process are restored to at least the nutritive level of the whole grain product; vitamin D is added to milk, and iodine added to salt.

●Selection and final preparation is the homemaker's role in food production. She should look for the enriched products when purchasing foods that can be enriched. The cooking process she employs will affect the heat-sensitive and the water-soluble vitamins. The homemaker can conserve these vitamins by cooking most foods in as short a time and with

DAILY FOOD GUIDE

	CHILD	PRETEEN & TEEN	ADULT	AGING ADULT
milk or milk products (in cups)	3-4	4 or more	1-2	1-2
meat, fish, poultry, eggs (in servings)	1-2	3 or more	1 large	1 large
green & yellow vegetables (in servings)	1-2	2	2	at least 1
citrus fruits & tomatoes (in servings)	1	1-2	1	1-2
potatoes, other fruits & vegetables (in servings)	1	1	1	0-1
bread, flour, & cereal (in servings)	3-4	4 or more	3-4	2-3
butter or margarine (in tablespoons)	2	2-4	2-3	1-2

1. The need for the nutrients in 1 or 2 cups of milk daily can be satisfied by cheeses or ice cream. (1 cup of milk is approximately equivalent to 1½ cups of cottage cheese or 2-3 large scoops of ice cream.)

2. The recommended daily serving of meat, fish, and poultry (3 oz.) may be alternated with eggs or cheese, dried peas, beans, or lentils.

3. It is important to drink enough fluid. The equivalent of 3-5 cups daily is recommended.

as little water as possible. Many nutrients are carelessly discarded in unnecessary trimming and unused left-overs.

Between-Meal Snacks

Should snacking or between-meal eating be allowed? The rapidly growing child and teen-ager generally need more food than they can eat in three meals. Evidence is accumulating that shows that several smaller meals per day may be more desirable. Children and teenagers often get hungry or "run out of gas" long before a meal. Tiredness and upset appetites result. Snacking is acceptable, when necessary, but usually needs some supervision by parents who understand that snacks should be nutritious—not simply a sweet treat. Consider them as "junior" meals. Each person must be the judge of the time and amount of the snack. If weight is a problem, let the snack be such foods as celery or carrots. The adult, so long as he eats adequate meals, should have little need for any food between meals.

Soft drinks and candy can become a problem if they are consumed out of proportion to other foods in the diet. Be sure they do not replace other foods which offer more adequate nutritive quality to the diet. Drinks and foods in which sugar is replaced by nonnutritive sweeteners are becoming popular. Be sensible in the use of less valuable foods and drinks; young people require a considerable amount of food energy and nutrients which such drinks do not provide.

Food habits change with age. This is neither surprising nor a cause for alarm. Old age does not necessitate a greater intake of calories, vitamins, minerals, and protein. Except for total calories, people 60 years of age and over have the same nutrient requirements as people in middle age. Caloric requirements decrease with age largely because of a reduction in the metabolic rate and a gradual reduction in physical activity. This means less food need be consumed, but greater care must be exercised in the selection of that food so as to satisfy all nutritional needs. Adherence to the principles of good nutrition enumerated in this chapter will assure an adequate diet.

Food habits of older people are influenced directly by such factors as income, social status, isolation, marital status, presence of disease, earlier training, and psychological and physiological conditions. Loneliness, boredom, a feeling of rejection, or perhaps of guilt because of imposing on loved ones can act to destroy appetite. In some cases, these factors may have quite the opposite effect.

Foods are now available that can facilitate the feeding of elderly people with chewing problems, impared gastrointestinal functions, or with almost any dietetic problem. In rather extreme cases, one can resort to liquid formulae, chopped and pureed foods, as well as a whole host of foods for special dietary uses. Consult your physician for ideas.

Special Diets

If it becomes necessary to prepare special diets, the first step is to be certain to understand perfectly what is expected. The physician should answer all questions; the patient should not leave his office until he understands what the doctor recommends. Fortunately, most special diets are now designed to be modifications of the normal diet. If one understands the basic facts about normal nutrition, it should be possible to prepare attractive meals built around special diets. Creative menu planning and food preparation are a "must" for the homemaker in this situation. In addition to avoiding foods forbidden by the special diet, perhaps the next most important thing is to learn to read food labels. Many foods for special dietary use are now on the market. These include diabetic packs, low or restricted sodium foods, and foods with modified fats.

Eating out has often been frustrating for those faced with dietary restrictions. Limiting food choices from an elegant restaurant menu or shunning the tempting delicacies offered in a friend's home present definite problems for dieters who either enjoy eating out or must do so often. Since most diets are only a variation of the so-called average American diet, the solution may be easier than it appears. Check first with the physician to determine just how flexible the diet is. Possibly a regular meal can be eaten or other substitutions can be made now and then. If one eats out often, a restaurant with a sympathetic management should be selected. Some restaurants prefer to be called ahead of time when special meals are required; others advertise special menu items such as the "low-calorie" meal for the dieter. Choose those places which, although they may have an exotic menu, also have a simple a la carte menu, for this gives more variety of selection. Such restaurants often also are ready to prepare something the dieter knows he can have. When

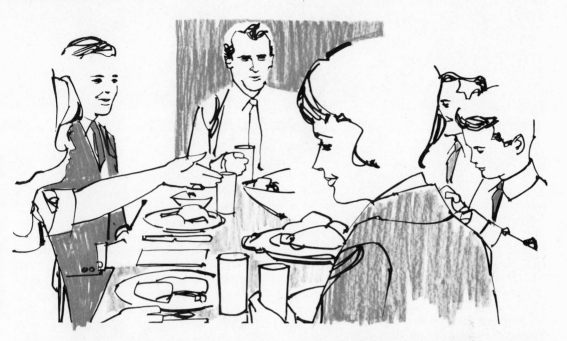

visiting a friend's home for a meal, a brief explanation of the dietary limitations to the host will usually suffice. Eating out is a fun time. So enjoy the company, forget what cannot be eaten, and *enjoy what can!*

The Homemaker's Role

The homemaker with a family to feed is a key member of the health team. Her job is to plan and prepare the most attractive, appetizing, and nutritious meals possible—and, also, to see that these meals are consumed by the family. Mention has already been made of the need for variety in meals, in methods of preparation, and of serving. The gradual development of good food habits is an important feature of an emerging personal health program. Food habits usually become established before the onset of the teens. If children have not learned by this age to demand and accept a wide variety of foods, they probably never will. What is accomplished prior to adolescence will, in large measure, determine how well nourished the children will be during adolescence. The feeling of independence and often of rebellion so common in teenagers can play havoc with food habits that are not well established. Parents and older children must set a good example for all other members of the family. Everybody should eat something of everything served. Somehow convince Dad that he must act like a pacemaker and avoid making unfavorable comments about the choice of foods or how they are cooked. Such differences should be discussed privately. The family meal is a time for congenial family fun and warmth. Food eaten in an atmosphere of love and understanding will certainly be accepted and digested more readily.

Chapter Four

OBESITY

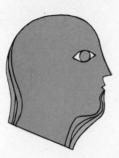

Most physicians consider obesity to be an important factor in personal health for three reasons:

1. It is common.
2. It is associated with increased sickness and death rates, notably in respect to heart, circulatory, kidney, and metabolic disorders as well as surgical and obstetrical complications.
3. It can be treated with success as one practical way to help control associated medical conditions.

The assumption that illness can be reduced and death delayed through the correction of obesity depends on whether two things are true: that weight reduction can and does lower the risk of disability and death and, that weight reduction can be achieved and maintained.

Medical experience strongly suggests greater risks for overweight persons in respect to most of the major disorders besetting our population. Statistical reports, notably from life insurance sources, provide the principal support indicating increased hazards associated with overweight. Although overweight and obesity are not the same, most overweight persons are obese; that is, they have an excess of body fat that amounts to more than 15 per cent over the average weight for their height and sex. A cause and effect relationship between overweight and increased danger to health has not been established, and available information does not supply positive proof of beneficial effects directly due to weight reduction. On the other hand, the evidence for generally adverse effects from obesity seems too massive and too consistent to be ignored. Unless and until definite evidence is forthcoming to the contary, it appears reasonable to advise apparently well and afflicted individuals alike to avoid overweight, and, if overweight, to reduce and then stay reduced.

Taking fewer calories than are needed seems within the theoretical capability of almost every person. Yet reported results suggest that this frequently attempted experience is difficult and is seldom achieved. Irrespective of source and of circumstances, reliable, unbiased, and sufficient long-term observations indicate poor over-all success for most "dieters."

Obesity is not always readily subject to treatment, and correction of obesity does not always insure elimination of the added risks associated with this condition. Yet it must be acknowledged that efforts toward its control seem justified by the relative health advantages currently identified with normal weight status.

The practical management of obesity may be divided into four interdependent and overlapping aspects: psychological, pharmaceutical, physical, and dietary. General management of obesity is directed toward establishing an energy balance in an individual with the right kind as well as the right amount of body weight. Proper management requires a correct diagnosis as well as an attempt to assess the "specific" causes of obesity in each instance.

Psychological Considerations

Psychological (emotional) factors are operative in every person whether he is obese or not. There does not appear to be a single psychological problem peculiar to the obese state, nor one common to all obese persons. However, psychological factors may cause overweight, or help to maintain it through their influence on dietary habits.

The role of psychic and emotional factors must be assessed especially when anxiety is a conspicuous feature and the person eats more calories than proper hunger calls for. Attempts at weight reduction may have adverse effects in some individuals with more serious psychological problems. The doctor may avoid or at least postpone treatment in those few situations where it may actually be harmful.

Psychiatric consultation or treatment is required for only a small portion of obese patients. The general practitioner, the internist, or (for children) the pediatrician usually can provide suitable guidance and support as part of total patient management. The indispensable will to lose weight is most readily induced by that physician with the most complete knowledge of the patient, his family, and his unique environment, especially if he assumes responsibility for the patient's over-all care above and beyond the reducing regimen. Rather than concentrating on the management of obesity, the aim of treatment now is more appropriately thought of as the guidance of the patient who is obese—of the whole person.

Pharmaceutical Preparations

It is not our purpose to list the many and varied products available to further weight reduction. They may be classified into broad groups, notably: drugs that reduce appetite; drugs that promote a feeling of well-being; tranquilizers and sedatives; stimulants to metabolism (body chemistry); bulky foods to satisfy hunger; cathartics; and drugs to eliminate excess fluids.

Agents that reduce food intake sometimes are prescribed at the outset or, in stubborn cases, as short-term aids to dietary treatment providing they do not interfere with taking necessary foods. Beyond their specific actions, these drugs admittedly meet the frequent need for a "gimmick," the element of magic for which the wavering will power inevitably reaches out. However, they also serve as a crutch, detracting and diverting from the essential emphasis on dietary regulation. At best, they appear to afford only initial temporary help. They merely postpone the day when facts must be faced.

Physical Factors

Among the current—though scarcely new—developments in the management of obesity is the revised emphasis on the role of exercise. Once regarded as a major factor in the treatment of overweight, physical activity was later accorded less importance in the wake of revelations that considerable effort was required to shed even one pound of adipose tissue. The small amounts of energy expended during a 36-mile walk or a 6-hour swim discouraged a majority of would-be reducers who were too readily convinced that they lacked the resources to work off even a small part of their

DESIRABLE WEIGHTS FOR MEN OF AGES 25 AND OVER

Weight in Pounds According to Frame (In Indoor Clothing)

HEIGHT (with shoes on) 1-inch heels Feet Inches		SMALL FRAME	MEDIUM FRAME	LARGE FRAME
5	2	112–120	118–129	126–141
5	3	115–123	121–133	129–144
5	4	118–126	124–136	132–148
5	5	121–129	127–139	135–152
5	6	124–133	130–143	138–156
5	7	128–137	134–147	142–161
5	8	132–141	138–152	147–166
5	9	136–145	142–156	151–170
5	10	140–150	146–160	155–174
5	11	144–154	150–165	159–179
6	0	148–158	154–170	164–184
6	1	152–162	158–175	168–189
6	2	156–167	162–180	173–194
6	3	160–171	167–185	178–199
6	4	164–175	172–190	182–204

DESIRABLE WEIGHTS FOR WOMEN OF AGES 25 AND OVER

Weight in Pounds According to Frame (In Indoor Clothing)

HEIGHT (with shoes on) 2-inch heels Feet Inches		SMALL FRAME	MEDIUM FRAME	LARGE FRAME
4	10	92– 98	96–107	104–119
4	11	94–101	98–110	106–122
5	0	96–104	101–113	109–125
5	1	99–107	104–116	112–128
5	2	102–110	107–119	115–131
5	3	105–113	110–122	118–134
5	4	108–116	113–126	121–138
5	5	111–119	116–130	125–142
5	6	114–123	120–135	129–146
5	7	118–127	124–139	133–150
5	8	122–131	128–143	137–154
5	9	126–135	132–147	141–158
5	10	130–140	136–151	145–163
5	11	134–144	140–155	149–168
6	0	138–148	144–159	153–173

For girls between 18 and 25, subtract 1 pound for each year under 25.

Source: Metropolitan Life Insurance Co.

surplus. Moreover, they found spiritual as well as bodily comfort in some expert opinion that calories expended through exercise would be immediately replaced as a result of an automatic increase in appetite. The only exercise that mattered, they were persuaded, was the thrice daily practice of pushing themselves away from the table "soon enough and far enough."

At present, fortunately for fitness as well as for fatness, exercise has been restored to grace

36-mile hike within the span of hours, a walk of just 1 extra mile per day for 36 days is a simple, even pleasant device for shedding an extra pound of fat. The total loss of 10 pounds thus achieved in a period of a single year represents a rate of loss which, with few exceptions, is greatly in excess of that at which corpulence is normally acquired. The average obese individual typically accumulates his 10 to 30 per cent surplus over a span of approximately as many years.

Sport	Cal/min.
Canoeing (2.5 mph)	3.0
Horseback riding (walking gait)	3.0
Volleyball	3.5
Walking (2.5 mph)	3.6
Bowling	4.5
Cycling (5.5 mph)	4.5
Golfing	5.0
Swimming (20 yd/min)	5.0
Rowing (2.5 mph)	5.0
Walking (3.75 mph)	5.6
Skating	6.0
Table Tennis	6.0
Tennis	7.1
Water Skiing	8.0
Horseback riding (trotting gait)	8.0
Skiing	9.9
Squash	10.2
Cycling (13 mph)	11.0
Rowing (race speed)	14.0
Running (10 mph)	15.0

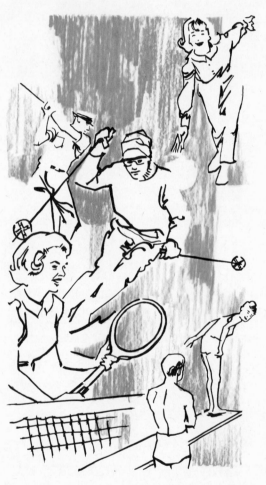

and enjoys respectability. Exercise is advocated for weight control for at least three reasons:

1. It helps expend calories.

2. Within the usual range of activity, exercise need not stimulate a corresponding increase in appetite to offset the energy deficit.

3. The energy output required to offset a pound of fat is approximately 3,500 calories, but the weight need not be lost in a given time period.

Instead of the exhausting, often impossible

Exercise also furthers physical, mental, psychological, and social fitness. It provides an outlet for emotional tensions, promotes self-confidence, wholesome social activity, and good sportsmanship, and enhances the real, albeit intangible, sense of general well-being that provides the will power to confront and master personal challenges—including a reducing regimen.

Present evidence indicates that physical activity does not modify the distribution of fatty tissue in various undesired localities. This is determined by factors governing body build.

Dietary Aspects

It is generally agreed that given adequate determination, weight can be lost on virtually any dietary plan, good or bad, that insures a calorie intake less than what is required by the energy used. It is equally apparent that many diets are only temporarily effective and do not promote the fundamental purpose of permanent loss, not to mention good eating habits.

The principles of the good reducing diet continue to be essentially these:

●The diet should be individualized in harmony with income, national origins, religious principals, and personal circumstances. It should literally be a personalized prescription.

●The diet should be practical, consistent with work patterns and other everyday obligations and responsibilities. It should keep the individual functioning at his usual job and should not encourage invalidism, real or imagined. Inappropriate or excessive devotion to diet above and beyond actual need can be still another form of disability.

●The diet should be flexible, and should allow for a variety of foods so that the patient can exchange one of which he has tired for another that furnishes the same food values, not merely the same calorie count. The diet should be elastic, but the dieting should within reason be rigid. Any departures from the prescribed diet should be intentional and planned, not accidental or due to carelessness. The reducing

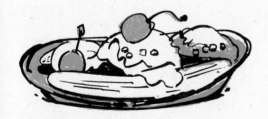

diet may include an item such as ice cream, a commonly forbidden treat, prescribed not just permitted, once or twice weekly.

●The diet should utilize readily available commonly preferred foods which all members of the family can be encouraged to enjoy, as distinct from unusual or "dietetic" foods.

●The diet should be consistent with accepted health practices and compatible with any medical conditions, such as liver, kidney, and heart disorders, which may exist.

●The diet should be balanced and complete in conformity with the Recommended Dietary Allowance of the National Research Council (see preceding chapter). Only the attending physician can assure the dieter on this point.

●The diet, basically, should be a pattern for life not only for the period of weight reduction, but also for the long-term maintenance of "normal" weight and optimum health.

Adjusting Caloric Levels

The total caloric prescription depends upon the weight level and the desired rate of loss. Excessive rates of loss not only fail to provide an adequate period for adjustment to a revised living pattern but, particularly in the case of greatly overweight adults, appear to increase the risks of serious circulatory mishap. The usual goal of one or two pounds' loss per week is achieved by a daily intake of 500 to 1,000 calories less than the estimated caloric intake needed to maintain the weight at which reducing was begun.

Prescriptions for diet range widely and are commonly set at some arbitrary level between 1,000 calories and the energy level sufficient to maintain the estimated desirable body weight. Satisfactory working estimates may be computed readily through such simple formulas as 15 calories per pound of desired weight with no reckoning for physical activity, plus an additional 25 to 50 per cent, depending on physical activity. This factor is often crucial.

Obviously the calorie level can and should be adjusted in accordance with response. There is no substitute for trial and error. It is also currently emphasized that 1,000 calories represent the smallest practical energy vehicle that can provide the recommended daily allowances of essential minerals and vitamins through usual food sources. For children, notably during puberty and adolescence, the minimum figure for a satisfactory diet on which to lose weight is close to 1,600 calories, with 1,800 often recommended to insure a margin of safety as well as to encourage adherence.

The protein component of the diet usually is calculated at one gram per two pounds of ideal body weight, of which at least two-thirds should be of animal origin, that is, of high nutritional value. Although this represents 12 to 20 per cent of the total calories, higher proportions still are advocated by some, more in the interest of lowered fat and carbohydrate content than of protein supply.

RECOMMENDED DAILY DIETARY ALLOWANCES, REVISED 1963

Designed for the Maintenance of Good Nutrition of Practically All Healthy Persons in the U.S.A.

(Allowances are intended for persons normally active in a temperate climate)

	Age[2] Years from—to	Weight kg.(lbs.)	Height cm. (in.)	Calories	Protein gm.	Calcium gm.	Iron mg.	Vitamin A Value, I.U.	Thiamine mg.	Riboflavin mg.	Niacin Equiv.[4], mg.	Ascorbic Acid, mg.	Vitamin D I.U.
Men	18-35	70 (154)	175 (69)	2,900	70	0.8	10	5,000[3]	1.2	1.7	19	70	
	35-55	70 (154)	175 (69)	2,600	70	0.8	10	5,000	1.0	1.6	17	70	
	55-75	70 (154)	175 (69)	2,200	70	0.8	10	5,000	0.9	1.3	15	70	
Women	18-35	58 (128)	163 (64)	2,100	58	0.8	15	5,000	0.8	1.3	14	70	
	35-55	58 (128)	163 (64)	1,900	58	0.8	15	5,000	0.8	1.2	13	70	
	55-75	58 (128)	163 (64)	1,600	58	0.8	10	5,000	0.8	1.2	13	70	
Pregnant (2nd and 3rd trimester)				+200	+20	+0.5	+5	+1,000	+0.2	+0.3	+3	+30	400
Lactating				+1,000	+40	+0.5	+5	+3,000	+0.4	+0.6	+7	+30	400
Infants[5]	0- 1	8 (18)		kg.x115 ±15	kg.x2.5 ±0.5	0.7	kg.x1.0	1,500	0.4	0.6	6	30	400
Children	1- 3	13 (29)	87 (34)	1,300	32	0.8	8	2,000	0.5	0.8	9	40	400
	3- 6	18 (40)	107 (42)	1,600	40	0.8	10	2,500	0.6	1.0	11	50	400
	6- 9	24 (53)	124 (49)	2,100	52	0.8	12	3,500	0.8	1.3	14	60	400
Boys	9-12	33 (72)	140 (55)	2,400	60	1.1	15	4,500	1.0	1.4	16	70	400
	12-15	45 (98)	156 (61)	3,000	75	1.4	15	5,000	1.2	1.8	20	80	400
	15-18	61 (134)	172 (68)	3,400	85	1.4	15	5,000	1.4	2.0	22	80	400
Girls	9-12	33 (72)	140 (55)	2,200	55	1.1	15	4,500	0.9	1.3	15	80	400
	12-15	47 (103)	158 (62)	2,500	62	1.3	15	5,000	1.0	1.5	17	80	400
	15-18	53 (117)	163 (64)	2,300	58	1.3	15	5,000	0.9	1.3	15	70	400

[1]Food and Nutrition Board, National Academy of Sciences.—National Research Council: Recommended Dietary Allowances, sixth edition, 1964, Publication 1146.

[2]Entries on lines for age range 18-35 years represent the 25-year age. All other entries represent allowances for the midpoint of the specified age periods, i.e., line for children 1-3 is for age 2 years (24 months); 3-6 is for age 4½ years (54 months), etc.

[3]1,000 I.U. from preformed Vitamin A and 4,000 I.U. from beta-carotene.

[4]Niacin equivalents include dietary sources of the preformed vitamin and the precursor, tryptophan. 60 mg. tryptophan represents 1 mg. niacin.

[5]The calorie and protein allowances per kg for infants are considered to decrease progressively from birth. Allowances for calcium, thiamine, riboflavin, and niacin increase proportionately with calories to the maximum values shown.

Fat should contribute 25 to 30 per cent of the total energy supply; however, 45 to 50 grams seem a minimum for practical purposes considering the appetite-satisfying and energy values of fats.

The carbohydrate remainder, some 40 to 60 per cent of the total calories, should also provide suitable bulk with sufficient fiber content (roughage) for normal bowel function and to sustain useful intestinal bacteria.

These figures represent tentative, average, and admittedly arbitrary proportions of the principal food sources. Enthusiasm for more extreme prescriptions—for example high fat or high carbohydrate diets—are revived periodically by experimental and clinical observations, and occasionally by those more interested in making a fast dollar than reducing fat. These programs commonly are without adequate scientific foundation. They apply to only a relatively small proportion of obese people, and are inconsistent with good long-term dietary practices.

Salt intake, although ordinarily in excess of needs, should not be restricted in reducing diets except when directed by the physician. In all likelihood, prohibiting the use of salt has contributed to weight reduction as much by decreasing the appeal of food as well as by causing water loss.

Fluids should be consumed as desired, preferably in sufficient quantities to permit a daily urine output of at least one quart. They combat the tendency to constipation that sometimes troubles patients in the initial stages of a re-

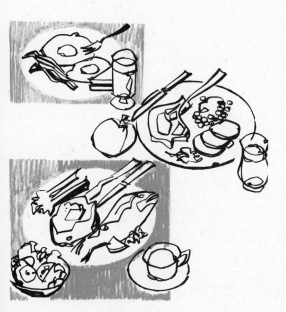

ducing program. There is at present insufficient information to recommend routine limitation of fluid intake as a means of caloric control.

Liquid formula diets unquestionably have helped many persons to lose weight. Although some of these preparations combine the merits of economy, acceptability, and nutritional balance, these too lend themselves chiefly to short-term intensive weight loss, postponing the day of reckoning when practical considerations inevitably oblige the patient to return to more usual and probably more complete foodstuffs. Without developing proper eating habits, the prospects for effective maintenance of desired weight seem poor.

Dietary Objectives

For some dieters the total day's prescription may perhaps be distributed among three meals with calories represented equally. For others, it may follow a two-fifths, one-fifth, two-fifths pattern—40 per cent breakfast, 20 per cent lunch, 40 per cent dinner. Each meal should contain all the food components, especially complete proteins and essential nutrients in suitable proportions. When this ideal is too difficult, a balance over the day should be sought.

Recent reports indicate that smaller, more frequent feedings may be more conducive to weight loss than the more usual three-meal regimen and may also be more protective against nutritional disease. Somewhat in contrast, short periods of complete fasting are advocated by other competent physicians whose patients have achieved impressive weight losses. After fasting there has been good acceptance of regimens involving periodic complete abstinence without apparent adverse effects. Hospitalization is sometimes recommended, at least initially, in these and other cases where close supervision is essential.

Obviously, a fasting or starving person will lose weight, but the publicity given to huge losses may tempt the observer to try to do this on his own initiative. Such drastic methods are strictly for selected cases under medical care, and usually in the hospital. As a do-it-yourself procedure they are extremely dangerous.

Timing of Meals

Of great importance, but commonly ignored, is the timing of meals. These, whatever their number, should be consumed at regular, though not necessarily equal, intervals. Meal schedules should be set and followed consistently seven days a week. Only in this manner can the rhythmic pattern be developed that is essential for long-term adherence to a reducing and especially a maintenance regimen. Meals should be leisurely, stress-free, preferably family occasions where quarreling and other upsetting emotional elements are not allowed to interfere with eating. Here too, the sound general nutrition practices embodied in the reducing regimen hopefully will be emulated by other members of the family circle, especially the youngsters. In the event of disagreement, it is the others in the family rather than the patient who must be urged to conform.

Results unquestionably depend upon how often the patient sees his doctor, notably in the early stages of the regimen when weekly visits are all but essential. The desired permanent weight is commonly achieved in practical stages through a succession of short-term goals. Although planned interruptions reportedly are desirable in some instances, weight loss seems generally best accomplished by a steady downward progress.

Weight objectives may be set for periods of 4 to 12 weeks. Regardless of the criteria adopted, the patient should be given family as well as medical support throughout the period of weight loss. This support should continue to the point where his maintenance program hopefully will become an established way of life. He should become free from the thrice or more daily decisions about what and how much to eat that jeopardize adherence to his permanent program of weight control. Weight reduction is never an objective in itself. It is part of the total program for helping the obese person become generally well-nourished and adjusted.

Good nutritional therapy directed to an obese person may favorably influence the eating pattern of other members of the family, primarily the mother who plans, purchases, and prepares the meals for her spouse and children. The resulting general improvement in dietary habits should help to prevent all types of malnutrition including overeating.

Since there is nothing really new in the management of obesity, emphasis must be on this and other preventive aspects—especially in the younger age groups where many are otherwise destined to join the hard core of obese adults. The serious, sustained cooperation of parents unquestionably is essential, but a coordinated school program is equally important. Emphasis should be on the positive, dynamic ("thou shalt" rather than "thou shalt not") approach to weight control as an integral part of physical and total fitness. Example must be provided as well as encouragement. The educational potential of the school lunch program surely can be exploited to great advantage and school athletic facilities can be utilized more fully.

CHAPTER FIVE

MOUTH AND TEETH CARE

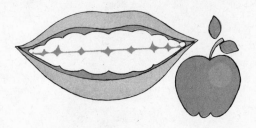

THE MOUTH is the most versatile of human organs. The food needed by the body for the life processes enters it. The first stages of digestion are accomplished in it by the teeth, the taste buds, and the salivary glands. Man's main means of communication—speech—comes from it. Its size and shape, especially the contour of its lips, strongly affect one's personal appearance. Thus it is clear that the mouth and its principal components—the teeth, the tongue, and the gums—should receive the best of care. Good dental health care is neither intricate, difficult, or expensive. All that is required is that good dental health habits be established early and be consistently maintained. Such a regime will prevent most serious dental disorders and maintain the mouth in a condition of good health throughout life.

Children

The child's first set of 20 teeth begins to form before he is born. Because these teeth, like all other parts of the unborn baby's body, are formed from the food the expectant mother eats, her diet during the prenatal period must be adequate and well balanced. She need follow no special diet to build good teeth. The wholesome diet prescribed by her physician for her general health and for the growth and development of the child is adequate.

Good nutritional habits should be instilled

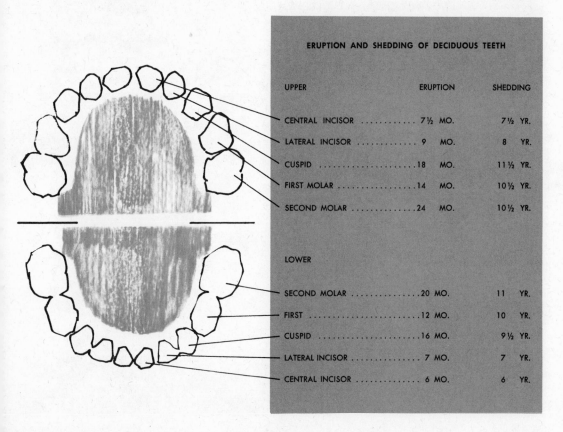

ERUPTION AND SHEDDING OF DECIDUOUS TEETH		
UPPER	ERUPTION	SHEDDING
CENTRAL INCISOR	7½ MO.	7½ YR.
LATERAL INCISOR	9 MO.	8 YR.
CUSPID	18 MO.	11½ YR.
FIRST MOLAR	14 MO.	10½ YR.
SECOND MOLAR	24 MO.	10½ YR.
LOWER		
SECOND MOLAR	20 MO.	11 YR.
FIRST	12 MO.	10 YR.
CUSPID	16 MO.	9½ YR.
LATERAL INCISOR	7 MO.	7 YR.
CENTRAL INCISOR	6 MO.	6 YR.

PLACE THE BRISTLES OF THE BRUSH POINTING TOWARD THE ROOTS OF THE TEETH. ROTATE THE BRUSH SO THAT THE BRISTLES SWEEP DOWN OVER THE GUMS AND TEETH IN THE DIRECTION OF THE BITING OR GRINDING SURFACE.

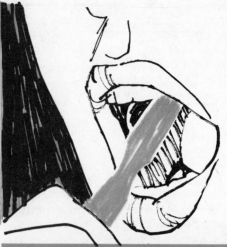

BRUSH THE CHEWING SURFACES OF THE UPPER AND LOWER TEETH.

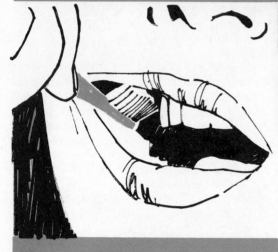

BRUSH THE OUTSIDE SURFACES OF THE UPPER AND LOWER BACK TEETH.

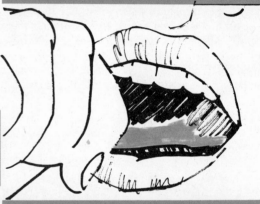

BRUSH THE INSIDE SURFACES OF THE UPPER AND LOWER BACK TEETH.

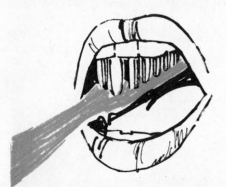

BRUSH THE INSIDE SURFACES OF THE UPPER AND LOWER FRONT TEETH.

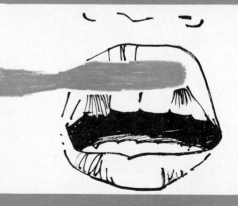

BRUSH THE OUTSIDE SURFACE OF THE UPPER AND LOWER FRONT TEETH.

in the child early in his life and maintained throughout the tooth-forming period, that is, until the child reaches young adulthood. Good nutritional habits established in those years are likely to be followed throughout life.

The same wholesome diet prescribed by the family physician for the well being of the growing child is also adequate for the well being of his teeth. Of primary importance from the dental health standpoint is the limiting of the intake of all forms of sweets because acids produced by the fermentation of sugars cling to the teeth and cause dental decay.

Usually by the age of two or two-and-one-half years the child's complete set of 20 deciduous or "baby teeth" will have erupted. Sometimes these newly erupted teeth are slightly defective. Therefore it is essential that the child be taken to the dentist at an early age so that he can correct any defects that may be present. The dentist will also clean the child's teeth and provide both the parent and child with proper mouth hygiene instruction. Visits to the dental office should be repeated as often as the dentist advises in order to keep the baby teeth healthy until they are replaced by their permanent successors.

Good daily home care also is essential to maintain the child's teeth in a healthy condition. The teeth should be brushed after each meal and, if possible, after each snack. During the child's early years some older person will have to do the brushing. Later, when the child becomes more adept he will be able to do the brushing himself, but the brushing should be supervised by the older person. The advice of the child's dentist should be followed concerning the type of brush and dentifrice to use and the most effective method of brushing.

Although many extravagant claims have been made for many dentifrices for many years, it was not until about 1960 that researchers developed a dentifrice that will do more than help the brush clean the teeth.

Research chemists developed certain dentifrice formulas which apparently help prevent dental decay. The claims for several such dentifrices have been accepted as sound by the American Dental Association. Other dentifrice manufacturers are working to develop similar products.

For many years, different toothbrush manufacturers have made claims for their particular product. Of late, the dental profession has generally recognized that a small, straight-handled brush with even tufts of bristles is the most satisfactory for both children and adults. Recently a number of different types of electric toothbrushes have been placed on the market. They are still very much in the trial stage and, while some of them appear to be satisfactory for adults, their value for use for children has not, as yet, been demonstrated.

Fluoridated Water

Children who live in communities that have fluoridated water are more fortunate than those who do not. It has been thoroughly proved that the addition of minute amounts of fluorine to the public water supply reduces the incidence of dental decay among children by at least 60 per cent.

Families who do not live in water-fluoridated communities may help safeguard their children's dental health by having their dentist apply a fluoride solution to their youngster's teeth at regular intervals.

Malocclusion

A growing number of American children appears to be affected by malocclusion or irregular teeth. It is impossible to attribute this condition to any one cause. In some instances it is inherited, in others acquired, and in still others it is due to a combination of both.

If a child inherits small bones from one ancestor and large teeth from another, various types of malocclusion may result. Prolonged sucking, biting, or sleeping habits may exert undue pressures that result in facial deformity. The too early loss of one or more deciduous teeth may cause others to shift, thus reducing the space intended for the succeeding permanent teeth. If the prematurely lost tooth is a molar, the dentist frequently recommends that the space be maintained by a device called a "space maintainer." Sometimes one or more deciduous teeth are retained too long. In such instances the dentist, aided by x-ray pictures, will determine the presence and state of development of the permanent tooth that is to replace it.

When the family visits the dentist regularly, he can detect the first signs of serious malocclusion in the child's teeth. He will advise the parents as to what orthodontic treatment is required and when it should be started. The condition may be such that the child's dentist may be able to correct it, or the services of an orthodontic specialist may be required.

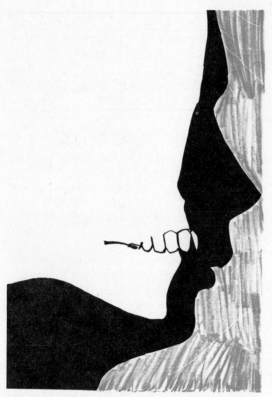

Teeth that do not meet (occlude) properly, cannot do their job. Teeth, bone, jaw joints will be damaged.

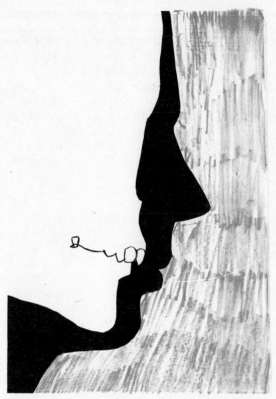

After orthodontic treatment, teeth occlude properly and work well with no harm to bone or jaw joint.

In many instances, serious disfiguring malocclusion can be avoided if preventive measures are begun early. Sometimes, however, even though preventive orthodontic measures are applied early, tooth irregularity may persist or grow worse, in which case orthodontic treatment should be instituted. Only a person trained in facial development can decide when such treatment should be started. Parents should rely on the dentist's judgment in instances of this kind—not on their own or that of well meaning relatives and friends.

The correction of most cases of pronounced malocclusion requires much time, patience, and skill on the part of the dentist and much cooperation on the part of the child and the parents. The cost will vary according to the seriousness and complexity of the condition, the number of visits required, and the amount of time required to obtain satisfactory results. In most instances, however, the satisfaction derived by the family and the child from good orthodontic treatment more than compensates for the time, effort, and money spent.

The increasing participation by American youth in contact sports has brought about a corresponding increase in accidents to the teeth and jaws. The National Alliance Football Rules Committee has ruled that boys playing in high school or college football games must wear a face guard to protect their teeth and jaws from injury.

If, through accident, a youth's permanent tooth has been completely dislodged from the mouth, it may be reinserted and anchored in its socket by the dentist where sometimes it may become firmly reattached. Although the conditions for a successful reimplantation must be ideal—which they usually are not—the chances of success are worth the effort. They can be increased if the displaced tooth is immediately immersed in water and the patient rushed to the dentist for prompt attention.

Four Dental Health Rules

Fortunate is the family that observes the four basic dental health rules:

1. Follow an adequate, well-rounded diet, one in which sweets are kept at a minimum.

2. Have early and frequent examinations and care by your dentist.

3. Cleanse the mouth thoroughly immediately after eating.

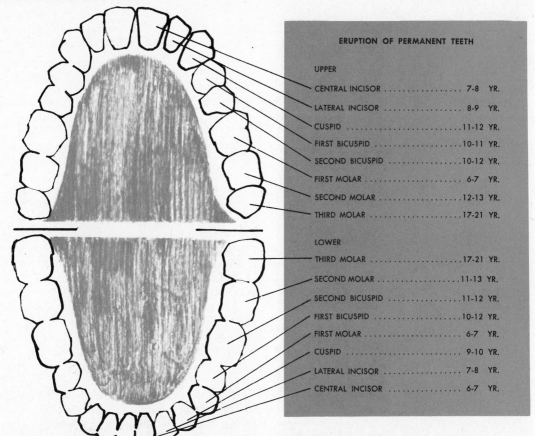

ERUPTION OF PERMANENT TEETH	
UPPER	
CENTRAL INCISOR	7-8 YR.
LATERAL INCISOR	8-9 YR.
CUSPID	11-12 YR.
FIRST BICUSPID	10-11 YR.
SECOND BICUSPID	10-12 YR.
FIRST MOLAR	6-7 YR.
SECOND MOLAR	12-13 YR.
THIRD MOLAR	17-21 YR.
LOWER	
THIRD MOLAR	17-21 YR.
SECOND MOLAR	11-13 YR.
SECOND BICUSPID	11-12 YR.
FIRST BICUSPID	10-12 YR.
FIRST MOLAR	6-7 YR.
CUSPID	9-10 YR.
LATERAL INCISOR	7-8 YR.
CENTRAL INCISOR	6-7 YR.

4. Drink fluoridated water or have fluoride solution applied by the dentist directly to the children's teeth.

Strict observance of these rules will help to maintain the 20 deciduous teeth in a healthy, serviceable condition until the permanent set of 32 replaces them. Furthermore, adherence to these rules will help maintain the permanent teeth and their supporting structures in a healthy condition throughout life.

Adults

The person who reaches adulthood with a complete set of 32 vital, healthy, and serviceable teeth supported by healthy bone and gum tissue is less likely to experience serious dental disorders later than if he neglected his teeth during youth.

Children lose teeth primarily because of dental decay; the majority of adult losses of teeth are because of disorders of the supporting bone and gum tissues. The most common diseases of this kind are gingivitis or inflammation of the gums, peridontitis, and periodontosis. The two latter conditions are commonly called pyorrhea.

In gingivitis the gums are red, swollen, and tender and they bleed easily. The cause is usually careless mouth hygiene habits which permit calculus (tartar) and food particles to accumulate on the teeth and irritate the surrounding soft tissues. Correction of this condition consists of the thorough removal of the deposits by the dentist or dental hygienist supplemented by thorough brushing of the teeth and gums after each meal.

If gingivitis is not corrected, it may develop into periodontitis. In this condition the gums become badly inflamed and tender. They draw away from the necks of the teeth forming pockets which become inflamed. As the condition becomes worse, the bone supporting the teeth is destroyed and the teeth become loose. Unless this condition is treated and checked by the dentist, the teeth eventually become so loose that they must be removed.

Adults sometimes are affected by another type of periodontal disease called periodontosis. In this condition, even though the mouth is kept clean, the bone supporting the teeth slowly wastes away. This disorder appears to be associated with a nutritional imbalance. Regular visits to the dentist, good home care

Progress of peridontal disease: (1) Irritations cause gums to withdraw from teeth.

(2) Further destruction.

(3) Most of the tissues have been destroyed.

(4) One tooth is lost—the other weakened.

of the mouth, and the observance of good dietary habits are the best measures for preventing periodontal disorders.

Vincent's Infection (trench mouth) is a not uncommon disorder that attacks the gums and other soft tissue of the mouth and throat. Many patients who contract this disease neglect to have it treated because in its early stages it resembles gingivitis. Such negligence is regrettable because the disease spreads with alarming rapidity and serious results. Unhygienic mouth conditions and lowered resistance of the mouth tissues are contributing causes of this disorder. In its acute stage the disease is recognized by its characteristic foul odor, pain, inflammation, and ulceration of the gums accompanied by an increased flow of saliva. The dentist should be consulted immediately when these symptoms occur because the longer the disease remains untreated, the greater the destruction to the periodontal tissues and the longer the time required to effect control and cure. Sometimes, months after all symptoms have disappeared, they may suddenly recur.

The soft tissues of the mouth are subject to many other disorders of less frequent occurrence. These include thrush, aphthous stomatitis (canker sores), pemphigus, actinomycosis, leukoplakia (smoker's patches), and burning tongue. The mouth tissues are also subject to lesions associated with systemic disturbances each of which presents characteristic symptoms. Although many of these conditions are of a minor character, some may be major and, if neglected, may have serious if not fatal results—precancerous lesions, for example.

Cancer of the Mouth

According to the American Cancer Society, approximately 36,000 Americans—mostly elder citizens—are stricken by cancer of the mouth each year. Of these, some 6,000 succumb to the disease. Although the specific cause or causes of cancer are not known, one or more of the following conditions are found in a cancerous mouth: chronic infections, smoker's spots, imperfectly fitting dental appliances, or broken, jagged teeth. Thus corrections of such conditions when they exist would seem to be a good way to prevent mouth cancer.

Cancer of the lip has been associated with sunburn, pipe smoking, and the habitual holding of nails, pins or other hard objects in the mouth. Cancerous growths vary so much in appearance that they are often difficult to recognize in their early stages. Cancer of the mouth can be eliminated if it is given early attention. The ever-present possibility that a pre-cancerous lesion may be attacking the mouth is an argument in itself for careful semi-annual dental checkups.

The person who observes the four basic mouth health rules—particularly the rule concerning regular dental examinations—is the least likely to experience serious disorders of the soft tissues of the mouth.

Toothache usually is, though not always, the result of dental neglect. In the majority of cases toothache is the reaction of irritated nerve endings within the tooth occurring because of decay or accident. In this type of ache the patient can usually locate the tooth because it hurts when a particle of food or hot or cold water enters the cavity. When the pain is caused by inflammation at the root end of the tooth, the offending tooth is more difficult to locate.

If the pulp—or so-called nerve—of a tooth dies and is not treated properly by the dentist, an abcess may form at the root end. Sometimes, particularly in children, the infection burrows through the jawbone and gum and drains into the mouth causing what is commonly called a gumboil. The dentist will probably recommend the removal of such infected teeth although in some instances he may treat and save them.

Because of the complex nature of the nervous system in the jaws and surrounding parts, it is frequently difficult for a person to determine which tooth is the offender. If the suspected tooth is obviously decayed, the pain may be alleviated temporarily by slightly dampening a small pledget of cotton with oil of cloves and inserting it into the cavity. Adults may also somewhat lessen the pain by swallowing one or two aspirin tablets. Children should be given a smaller dose. Never place an aspirin tablet on the gum tissue surrounding the offending tooth; that will seriously irritate the gum and will not relieve the pain. Hot or cold cloths applied to the cheek will sometimes give some slight relief. Which is the most helpful depends on the cause of the pain. Obviously the most effective treatment will be administered by your dentist. See him as soon as possible.

Unfortunately, some people who have always observed good dental health rules and—

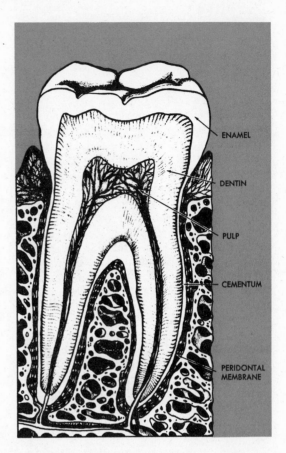

ENAMEL

DENTIN

PULP

CEMENTUM

PERIDONTAL MEMBRANE

understandably—many who have always neglected these rules may eventually lose one or more teeth. In most instances such teeth should be replaced with artificial substitutes in order to prevent the loss of more teeth and to restore chewing efficiency.

Even the loss of one tooth weakens the dental arch by causing the adjacent teeth and the opposing teeth to shift out of normal position. Such shifting causes undue pressure on the remaining teeth, injuring the supporting bone and soft tissue which surrounds the tooth root. The shifting of the teeth—however slight—permits food particles to lodge in the crevices between the teeth which irritate the soft tissues and frequently result in periodontal disease. Lost back teeth should be replaced promptly to prevent further destruction of the dental arch and to maintain masticating efficiency. Lost front teeth should be replaced to improve personal appearance as well as to improve health and chewing efficiency. Your dentist will advise you whether the lost teeth should be replaced by a fixed or removable appliance. The prompt replacement of one or several teeth by means of some type of dental appliance will restore the mouth to a serviceable condition and prevent or greatly postpone the need for further artificial dentures.

Dentures

Frequent and adequate dental care and close adherence to the rules of nutrition and mouth hygiene do not guarantee against the loss of teeth. In time the teeth, like other organs of the body, become impaired through use and abuse, in which case they may need to be replaced by artificial dentures. Efficient as they are, artificial dentures cannot be expected to function as well as a full complement of healthy natural teeth. In most instances the new wearers of dentures must learn how to use them for both eating and speaking. Lower dentures are particularly difficult to keep in place, but in most instances practice and determination will overcome the difficulty.

Artificial dentures, like natural teeth, must be cleaned daily—after each meal if possible—to preserve the health of the mouth. The dentist can advise the best materials and the best methods to use for this purpose. Additionally, the patient should have the dentures examined and cleaned by the dentist as often as the dentist advises.

Most denture wearers learn that, in time, the bony ridges of their jaws recede or shrink so that their dentures become loose. When this occurs the patient should obtain new dentures or, if possible, have the loose dentures rebuilt to fit the altered shape of the mouth. People should never try to reline their own dentures, as they may do irreparable harm to the soft tissues and ridges of their mouths. Relining must be done by the dentist. It is unwise to wear loose, ill-fitting dentures because the irritation which results can be a predisposing cause of mouth cancer. Inasmuch as artificial dentures are somewhat fragile and subject to breakage, the prudent denture wearer will own a second, emergency set.

Bad Breath

Unpleasant breath (halitosis) may be caused by disease in the mouth, such as has been described previously, or simply by neglecting ordinary mouth cleanliness. It may also come from infections in the nose, throat, and lungs, and sometimes even may originate in the stomach.

If the mouth is clean and healthy and the teeth are in good condition and bad breath still exists, a physician should be consulted. Indigestion, lung cancer and lung infections, diabetes, and other conditions may cause unpleasant breath. Only a physician can manage these ailments.

Mouthwashes can do nothing more than camouflage an unpleasant breath for a limited time. The only sure cure is to find and remove the cause. It is apparent that if the cause is elsewhere than in the mouth, no mouthwash can be expected to do any good. The American Dental Association states: "The usual commercial mouthwash has no medicinal value. Clear drinking water is just as effective for rinsing the mouth to clear it of loose food particles or soluble substances. There are times, however, when your dentist will prescribe a special mouthwash for certain conditions of the gums or other tissues of the mouth."

CHAPTER SIX

EAR CARE

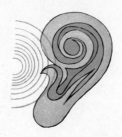

THE OUTER EAR, because of its prominence and its thin tight skin, is especially subject to sunburn and frostbite. Thus, it often needs to be protected from the elements. The ear canal leading to the middle ear is normally kept healthy by wax which protects it from drying and scaling or from damage by water while you are swimming or bathing. The wax, however, may accumulate to such an extent as to obstruct the canal and interfere with hearing. It will then need to be removed by your doctor. Foreign objects accidentally lodged in the ear can be dangerous and should also be removed only by a physician. A live insect in the ear canal can be very annoying or painful. If professional help is unavailable, light mineral oil can be dropped into the canal, suffocating the insect and quieting it until it can be removed.

Picking the ear canal with tooth picks, hair pins, or similar objects can be dangerous. Doing so may cause an infection in the canal or puncture the ear drum. Even frequent wiping of the canal with cotton applicators may cause irritation and a local infection. The normal healthy ear needs little attention other than to be washed with a washcloth covering the end of your finger. After a shower and after swimming the ear should be dried by draining it on a dry towel on the finger.

The Middle Ear

The middle ear is a closed air space separated from the outside by a membrane tightly stretched across the deep end of the ear canal. This membrane is called the ear drum. In a healthy ear the air pressure inside is kept equally balanced with the outside pressure through the eustachian tube. The eustachian tube connects the middle ear with the nose and opens and closes when we swallow or yawn. When we change altitude rapidly, we notice this exchange of air in the form of "popping" of the ears.

Any condition or disease that interferes with the normal opening of the eustachian tube will result in an imbalance of air. This in turn will interfere with hearing and favor development of disease in the middle ear. Large or infected adenoids and tonsils, colds, allergies, and sinus infections are some conditions which may be responsible for an imbalance. Under these circumstances the middle ear may develop an excess of moisture and fill with fluid or mucus. If it becomes infected, an abscess of the middle ear will form. A feeling of fullness or of heaviness or muffling of sound is noticed first. Then comes an earache which at first is a dull throb rather than severe pain. A small child or baby, because he cannot report the early symptoms, may respond to the inflammation only by crying and a high fever. The ear infection may be discovered only by an examination or if the child pulls at the ear, turns his head frequently, or becomes especially fussy.

Varying degrees of inflammation and fluid accumulation sometimes occur without pain. The only symptom then is hearing loss. A test for hearing, an examination of the ear, nose, and throat by a doctor, and proper treatment is the only way that complications can be prevented. The medical treatment will include nose drops and ear drops and the application of heat to the ear. The doctor may prescribe antibiotics. It is often necessary to incise or lance the ear drum to allow the pus to drain, as this is preferable to letting the drum burst.

Frequently the inflammation may subside but leave the middle ear filled with fluid or mucus. This condition may also require incision or drainage and possibly the insertion of a plastic tube for a few weeks to keep the ear open and draining. Inadequate care or delayed care of an earache can result in a mastoid infection which may have other serious complications. Permanent loss of hearing is possible and can be guarded against only by proper care at the proper time.

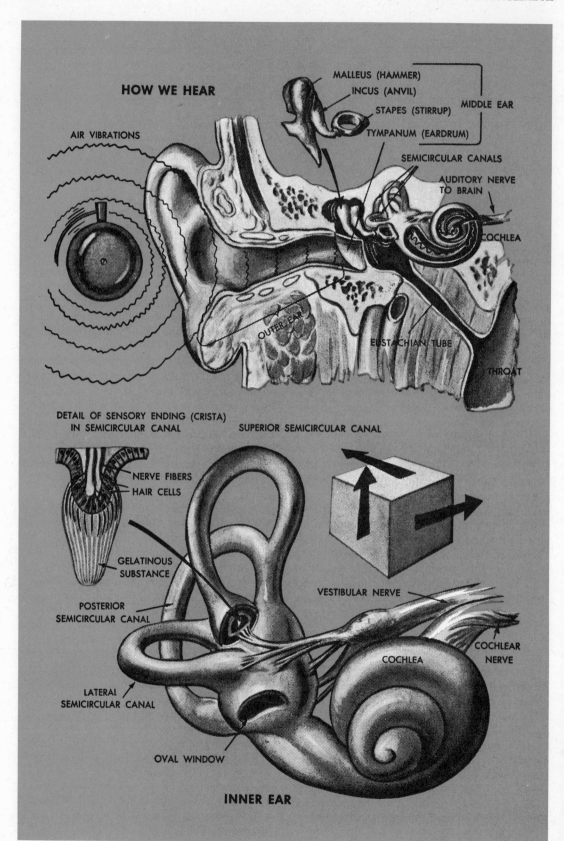

HOW WE HEAR

AIR VIBRATIONS

MALLEUS (HAMMER)
INCUS (ANVIL)
STAPES (STIRRUP)
TYMPANUM (EARDRUM)
MIDDLE EAR

SEMICIRCULAR CANALS

AUDITORY NERVE
TO BRAIN

COCHLEA

OUTER EAR

EUSTACHIAN TUBE

THROAT

DETAIL OF SENSORY ENDING (CRISTA)
IN SEMICIRCULAR CANAL

SUPERIOR SEMICIRCULAR CANAL

NERVE FIBERS
HAIR CELLS

GELATINOUS
SUBSTANCE

POSTERIOR
SEMICIRCULAR CANAL

VESTIBULAR NERVE

COCHLEA

COCHLEAR
NERVE

LATERAL
SEMICIRCULAR CANAL

OVAL WINDOW

INNER EAR

Proper care of acute colds and respiratory infections, is also important in caring for your ears. Vigorous nose blowing is always dangerous, and is especially so if the nose is obstructed tightly or if pus or nasal secretions fill the nose and nasal passages. Blowing may force these secretions into the middle ear through the eustachian tube.

The Inner Ear

The inner ear has two functions. The fluid that fills it carries sound vibrations to the nerve cells in the fluid and on to the brain. The same fluid also supports the semicircular canals with nerve cells which respond to movement such as turning, bending over, and lying down. This mechanism helps us keep our balance.

One quite common condition called Meniere's disease results from an imbalance of the fluid pressures in the inner ear. Because the same fluid contains nerves having to do with both balance and hearing, Meniere's disease affects both functions and causes impaired hearing, abnormal noise sensations (tinnitus), and a sense of turning or vertigo. The vertigo, or dizziness, may be so severe as to produce nausea, vomiting, weakness, perspiration, and a feeling of helplessness. Feelings of fullness, roaring, muffling of sounds, or loss of hearing may occur without the vertigo. The cause of Meniere's disease is not entirely known, but it may be related to emotional stresses. It usually tends to be slowly progressive and comes in attacks of varying degree and frequency. Medical treatment includes drugs, a special diet, limited fluid intake, and proper regulation of habits. In most cases this treatment will decrease the attacks and control its progress. Several types of surgery are available for severe cases which do not respond to medical treatment. A recently developed operation achieves a proper balance of fluid pressure by opening a connection between the fluids in the ear and those surrounding the brain.

Deafness

Mild hearing loss may pass unnoticed. When loss of hearing is sufficient to cause difficulty in communicating, the victim is said to be "hard of hearing." When one has lost so much hearing that he cannot understand a loud voice or a voice amplified by a hearing aid, he is spoken of as being deaf.

The outer ear and middle ear carry sound waves to the fluid of the inner ear. The waves stimulate the nerve cells of the inner ear so that they carry the sound to the brain by electrical impulses. The outer and middle ear handle the "mechanics" of carrying sound waves, while the inner ear deals with the "electronics." Surgery can restore hearing loss in a high percentage of patients who have trouble with the "mechanics" (conductive deafness) but surgery does not offer much hope at present for trouble with the inner ear (nerve deafness).

Corrective Surgery

When congenital deformity, inflammation, or injury closes the outer ear canal, a plastic reconstruction of the canal can restore hearing if the middle and inner ears are sufficiently well developed.

An ear drum may be partially destroyed as a result of infection, but may later be repaired by plastic surgery to the drum. If the middle ear bones (ossicles) or their ligaments are damaged or scarred by infection, in some cases these can be restored by corrective surgery.

Otosclerosis, a common form of deafness which comes on without any known cause but tends to occur in families, usually begins in young adults. It affects the stapes, one of the small ear bones, which vibrates in the oval window between the middle and inner ears. Bone grows around this window and eventually prevents vibration. An operation called fenestration can successfully restore hearing by cutting a new "window" in the horizontal semicircular canal and covering it with a skin flap. Since this operation was first developed, it has been found that fenestration is not necessary when the stapes can be mobilized. An operation to do this is now generally used in place of fenestration except in unusual cases. It has had much success in restoring hearing to people who would otherwise need hearing aids.

Such ear operations have been made possible by the perfection of the otologic microscope, which magnifies the tiny operative field of the middle and inner ear. With it a skillful and experienced ear surgeon can offer improved hearing to most hard-of-hearing patients with conductive deafness.

Hearing Aids

Proper hearing evaluation is the only way hard-of-hearing persons can determine whether they are suited for surgery or for a hearing aid. The ear specialist can make this judgment only after a complete ear, nose, and throat examination. Only then can it be known whether a hearing loss is the result of a correctable disease, a dangerous disease such as mastoid complication, an abscess or tumor, or other cause. The degree and type of hearing loss must also be established. Until all this is known, a hearing aid should not be bought.

Many good hearing aids are now available. Some persons can use any one of several makes, while others cannot profitably wear any type of hearing aid. Ethical hearing aid dealers will cooperate with the physician and audiologist to provide the most effective hearing aid. To this end, the medical profession has established various hearing centers. These have special equipment and are staffed by qualified audiologists to assist the ear specialist with difficult diagnostic hearing problems and to assist in choosing the proper hearing aids. An audiologist is a professionally trained person, usually with a doctorate degree, whose profession is the diagnosis of the types and degrees of deafness and the re-education and rehabilitation of the deaf and hard-of-hearing.

Early Detection Vital

It is important that hearing loss or deafness should be detected as early in life as possible. It may be suspected in newborn babies and infants who do not exhibit either the eye-blinking reflex or the surprise reflex (a sudden drawing up of the legs and bringing forth the arms as for an embrace) in response to a sudden loud noise. After the first few months of life, the child with normal hearing will respond to sounds by stopping whatever movements he is making and holding still for a moment. He will also begin to turn his head in the direction of a sound. If this response is not present by eight months, one should suspect hearing problems. From one year on, awareness of noises increases in the average child along with efforts to imitate language.

By two years the average child will be expanding his words to short phrases. If his speech does not develop, he may not be hearing properly. Early evaluation by your doctor and the beginning of an educational program are necessary when this problem is discovered. Early examination by audiometry is now practiced in many schools. Suspected hearing losses reported by these tests should be followed up by further evaluation and examination by your

doctor. Children who are hard-of-hearing need special care and placement for educational progress.

Here are some helpful suggestions for parents of both preschool deaf and hard-of-hearing children:

Some Do's

1. Do let him know that you have confidence and pride in him.

2. Do let him see that his whole family loves and needs him.

3. Do treat him as if you expected him to speak, and know he understands you when it is obvious that he does.

4. Do make a game of playing with him and let him watch your face when you talk.

5. Do make a game out of playing in front of a mirror so that he can enjoy watching you in imitating facial movements.

6. Do give him a chance to grow up and take some responsibilities.

7. Do read to him and show him pictures.

8. Do talk to him and ask others to do so, more and more, not less and less.

9. Do give him a chance to develop his special abilities and interests.

10. Do talk to him in a normal voice and in full sentences.

11. Do expect from him what is socially within his age and mental level.

12. Let him do alone the things he can do. This gives him self-confidence.

13. Do help him when you are teaching him to help himself.

14. Do use encouraging, positive, and specific direction to elicit desirable conduct.

15. Do stress success.

16. Do cooperate with the doctor, the health examiner, the educational specialist, the teacher, and the principal of the school.

17. Do teach him obedience.

18. Do have patience and time and effort.

19. Do explain painstakingly the most vital occurrences of everyday life in the home.

20. No matter how small the residuum, do make use of the remaining hearing which he may possess. It is invaluable in learning language, acquiring speech elements, and in regulating the pitch and placement of the voice.

21. Do begin immediately to train his eyes to substitute for his ears, or at least to complement his remnant of hearing.

22. Do face the light always when you are talking to him. Light on your back throws

shadows on your face and makes lipreading more difficult.

23. Do teach him what is his and what belongs to others.

24. Do keep a daily record of his principal activities as an index to his general progress.

25. Do talk into his ear to store up auditory impressions which will some day aid the mastery of speech by oral methods.

26. Do let him know you think he is a fine and important person.

Some Don'ts

1. Don't listen to the neighbors and relatives when they say thoughtless things about your child.

2. Don't feel you must apologize for him or be ashamed of him.

3. Don't keep him away from other children because he has no speech and doesn't hear as well as they do. They may be some of his best teachers.

4. Don't let his handicap worry you too much. He will sense your anxiety, and it will cause him worry too.

5. Don't forget that Father, as well as Mother, is an important person in the child's life.

6. Don't compare him with his brothers and sisters or with the neighbor's children.

7. Don't blame yourself for his handicap, but start now to try to help him.

8. Don't let any member of the family "baby" him. Don't wait on him hand and foot.

9. Don't be afraid to let him grow up and develop in other ways like any child.

10. Don't talk in single words. He probably understands more than you give him credit for.

11. Don't shout at him.

12. Don't exaggerate your lip movements. This makes speech harder to understand.

13. Don't correct every word he uses; accept and encourage his speech.

14. Don't expect his development to be spasmodic; development is continuous.

15. Don't be his greatest handicap.

16. Don't dream of miracle "treatments" and "cures."

17. Don't threaten him.

18. Don't be negatavistic; try to build on the things he achieves.

19. Don't display a "dead pan" expression when you talk to him. Make him think you are more interested in talking to him than anything else you could do.

Different age groups have different hearing problems. A hearing aid or an operation is not always the solution. Elderly people, for example, find it especially difficult to accept a hearing aid and often their deafness is a type that cannot be helped. In such instances, the earlier the patient learns to read lips, the better he will adapt to his progressive deafness.

CHAPTER SEVEN

EYE CARE

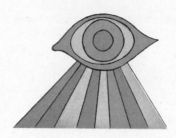

THE EYE, in common with the heart and other organs of the body, has great endurance and can withstand enormous use without damage. However, there is a difference between use and abuse, and it is important that we use our eyes properly and recognize the danger signals that indicate the need for immediate examination by a skilled eye physician.

Before discussing eye problems, perhaps a few definitions are necessary. The words *ophthalmologist* and *oculist* refer to the medical eye doctor who has had a complete medical training, followed by an internship and an additional three years of specialization in the study of eye diseases. Almost every medical doctor of this type has passed examining boards known as the American Board, qualifying him as an expert in his field.

The word *optometrist* refers to a person who has had college training plus one or two additional years of study in methods of examining the eyes and prescribing eyeglasses. The optometrist is not trained in any aspect of the field of medicine and therefore is not qualified to substitute for the medical eye specialist. He cannot use drops or prescribe medications.

The word *optician* refers to a person who manufacturers eyeglasses on the request of a medical eye physician or optometrist. Most states license opticians only after a certain period of training and require them to follow certain standards for the measurement of frames and grinding of lenses for eyeglasses. In addition, some opticians also fit contact lenses on the prescription of the medical eye physician or optometrist.

The Infant's Eyes

The eyes of the newborn infant have most of the components necessary for seeing. Some portions continue their development until about six months after birth. The newborn, however, can see form and movement. Several months after birth, he focuses on persons or objects. An infant should be able to fix his eyes on an object by the third to sixth month after its birth. Wandering movements of the eyes, however, will be present until 12 to 18 months of age.

Abnormal positions of one eye in relation to the other also occur during this period, so that this lack of coordination of the eyes should not be cause for worry unless it occurs constantly in one eye. The parents should watch the eyes, especially the pupils, because growths of various types and other lesions can be detected very early by careful observation. Ordinarily if something is wrong the defect appears as a whitish or yellowish reflex in the pupil.

Any infant who develops a constant crossed or wall eye should be examined immediately by a physician. Ordinarily this can be done with special magnifying instruments after the pupils are dilated with drops. Only medical eye specialists are allowed to dilate the pupils for such examinations.

Most newborn infants have some slight discharge from the eyes during the first four to five days after birth. Ordinarily this is small in amount and quite often is related to the drops used in the eyes at the time of birth to prevent the development of infection. Occasionally, however, a newborn baby develops an acute infection in both eyes, with discharge, and with redness and swelling. If this occurs after discharge from the hospital, your physician should be consulted at once.

Another condition to watch for is a lump under the skin at the inner corner of one or both eyes. Pressure on this lump causes a discharge of mucus into the eye socket. The cause of this is blockage of the tear draining apparatus and a resultant infection of the tear sac. This type of blockage can be cured in almost every instance by giving the child a light anesthetic and passing a small silver probe down

SCHEMATIC DRAWING OF THE EYE SHOWING
ANATOMIC LAYERS AND VASCULAR PATTERN

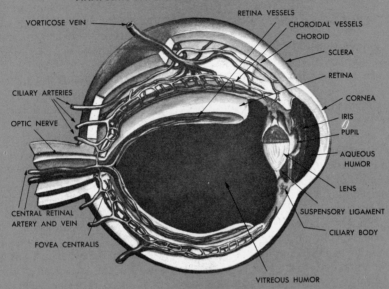

VORTICOSE VEIN

RETINA VESSELS

CHOROIDAL VESSELS

CHOROID

SCLERA

RETINA

CORNEA

CILIARY ARTERIES

IRIS

PUPIL

OPTIC NERVE

AQUEOUS HUMOR

LENS

CENTRAL RETINAL ARTERY AND VEIN

SUSPENSORY LIGAMENT

CILIARY BODY

FOVEA CENTRALIS

VITREOUS HUMOR

MUSCLES OF EYE

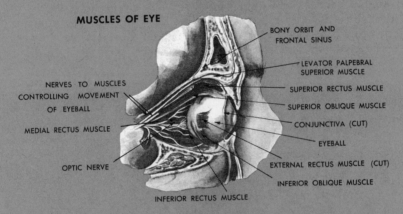

BONY ORBIT AND FRONTAL SINUS

LEVATOR PALPEBRAL SUPERIOR MUSCLE

NERVES TO MUSCLES CONTROLLING MOVEMENT OF EYEBALL

SUPERIOR RECTUS MUSCLE

SUPERIOR OBLIQUE MUSCLE

MEDIAL RECTUS MUSCLE

CONJUNCTIVA (CUT)

EYEBALL

OPTIC NERVE

EXTERNAL RECTUS MUSCLE (CUT)

INFERIOR OBLIQUE MUSCLE

INFERIOR RECTUS MUSCLE

TEARS

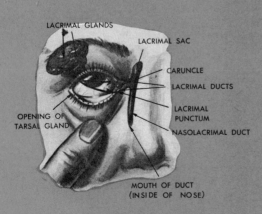

LACRIMAL GLANDS

LACRIMAL SAC

CARUNCLE

LACRIMAL DUCTS

LACRIMAL PUNCTUM

OPENING OF TARSAL GLAND

NASOLACRIMAL DUCT

MOUTH OF DUCT (INSIDE OF NOSE)

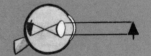

A NORMAL EYE FOCUSES IMAGE ON RETINA

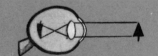

A NEARSIGHTED EYE (MYOPIA) FOCUSES IMAGE IN FRONT OF RETINA

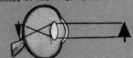

A FARSIGHTED EYE (HYPEROPIA) FOCUSES IMAGE BEHIND RETINA

the tear ducts to the nose to relieve the obstruction.

The Child's Eyes

The two or three-year-old child has almost complete development of vision. Most three-year-olds will be found to have at least 20/30 vision in each eye. For this reason it is important for the ophthalmologist to check the vision of every three-year-old child. If the vision is found to be poor in one or both eyes, the proper remedies can be instituted and most often the vision can be restored to normal. If, however, diagnosis and treatment are deferred beyond age seven, it is too late to correct the sight in the affected eye.

Strabismus, known as crossed-eye or squint, is extremely common. In most cases the turning of the eye is due to a defect in the coordination of the brain and eye. At times it is due to an infection of the nerves running to the muscles or of the muscles themselves. Less common but more serious cases of strabismus are caused by poor vision in an eye resulting from a tumor or an infection. In cases of this type

the eye turns out of place because of the poor vision. Any child who develops a persistent inward or outward turning of an eye should be examined immediately.

Some types of strabismus can be controlled with glasses. It is necessary to test the eye for glasses with the pupils widely dilated with special drops. Ordinarily it takes two or three days to dilate the pupils properly. The ophthalmologist can carry out refractions in this way even in very small infants.

If the child is found to be quite farsighted, glasses can be ordered to correct the turning of the eyes. Quite often this is all that is needed. If the child also is found to have poor vision in one eye, glasses are ordered, and the good eye is patched with tape. This forces the child to use the eye with poor vision. Ordinarily within one to three months the vision will improve markedly in the eye which has been turning. If glasses do not correct all of the crossing, surgery is often necessary. This type of surgery usually is very successful.

If a child with strabismus is allowed to go without treatment, he almost always develops extremely poor vision in the eye which turns

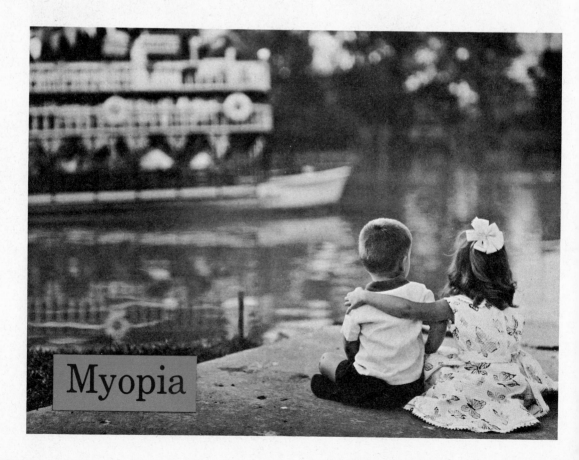

Myopia

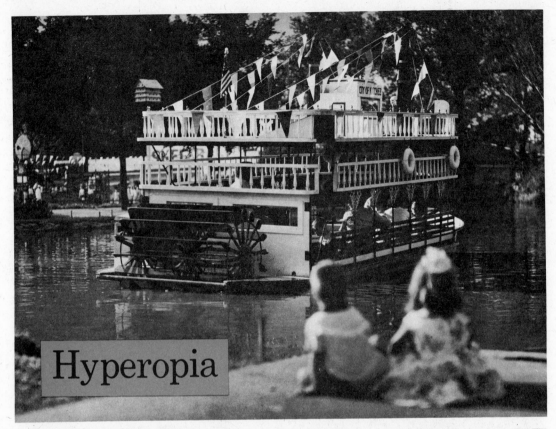

Hyperopia

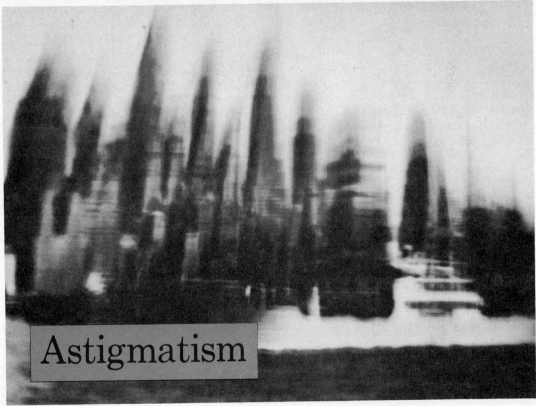

Astigmatism

because he fails to use this eye. For this reason it is extremely important to carry out early treatment.

All children should have their eyes examined—both with and without drops—to determine whether glasses are needed. The extremely farsighted or nearsighted child needs glasses for constant use, otherwise he may fail to read or use his eyes properly. This is especially true during the school years when the child must study. Because of their physical activity, it is best for children and teenagers to wear lenses that are specially hardened or "shatterproof." Lenses of ordinary glass may shatter and lacerate the eyeball.

It is perfectly safe for the child or teenager to use his eyes extensively, provided they are used under proper conditions. Studying should be done at a properly lighted desk. Ordinarily the light from a 100 watt bulb on a table or floor stand coming from the left side above the desk provides fairly ideal illuminations. Reading in bed should be prohibited unless a backrest allows an almost vertical position, and proper lighting is present at the bedside. Nearsighted children should always wear their glasses for close work and should be prohibited from reading in bed under any circumstances.

Television has no harmful effect on the eyes, but to prevent fatigue, the room should be moderately lighted.

Eye Infections

Eye infections have become less common in recent years because pneumonia and other infections are less common. However, infections quite often occur in association with such diseases as measles, influenza, streptococcal diseases of the throat, and ordinary acute upper respiratory infections. The infection can be detected because the eye becomes scratchy, hot and red, and there is considerable discharge. Occasionally the infection spreads to the cornea, the clear window in front of the pupil. In this case a painful and dangerous ulcer forms which should have prompt treatment. This type of inflammation of the eye was formerly known as pink-eye, but this name is now used to describe quite a large number of types of infections of the external eye.

Children and teenagers often injure their eyes themselves or are injured by one of their playmates. Self-injuries most often result from a sharp instrument, such as a knife, fork, kitchen utensil, or a toy with a sharpened point.

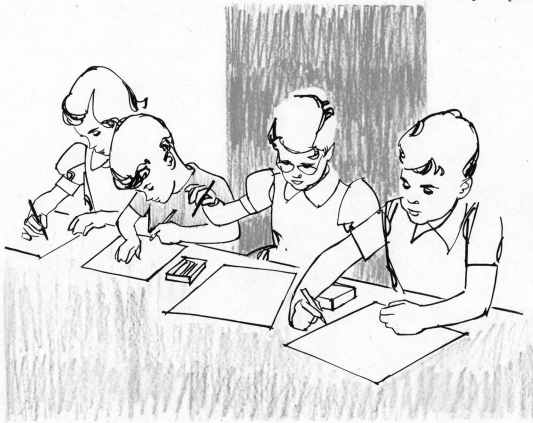

One of the most common types of injury is due to the B-B gun. It is wise to select toys for infants and small children which are not likely to cause injury. They should be composed of a flexible material and be of such size that they cannot enter the eye. They should also not have projections or sharp points which could injure the eye.

Another type of serious injury in older children can result from looking at eclipses of the sun. Many parents and even some teachers are not aware of this danger and a large number of eyes are damaged because of a failure to observe proper viewing precautions.

To view an eclipse properly, the sun should be made to shine through an opening in one piece of cardboard onto another piece, where it will produce an image. By this indirect method, the eclipse can be observed with complete safety.

Many children get foreign bodies in their eyes while playing. Most often these are small specks of dust, but quite often larger particles —such as small stones from passing cars and blades of grass or barbs from growing grain— may enter the eye. An injury of this type may occur and then be quickly forgotten. A few hours later there is sensitiveness to light, a tendency to hold the eyelids closed, and a beginning redness. A foreign body should be suspected even though the child fails to remember an injury. There is no particular point in trying to remove foreign bodies of this type by washing the eyes because quite often they are trapped in small folds and the washing fluid does not get into the proper place. It is better to pull the lower lid down and to have the child look upward. This tends to open up most of the folds in the lower portion of the eye. Quite often the foreign body will be revealed.

Foreign bodies that get trapped under the upper lid are more difficult to find. To reveal them, the child should look downward and the parent inverts the upper lid by holding the lashes and turning the lid inside out over the index finger of the opposite hand. In this way the inside of the lid can be seen very clearly and the presence of a foreign body detected.

Foreign bodies sometimes lodge on the cornea of the eye. These are more difficult to see. In cases where there is obvious irritation but a foreign body cannot be found, it is always best to take the child to a physician for immediate attention.

Many children sustain lacerated injuries or cuts of the eyeball without remembering the

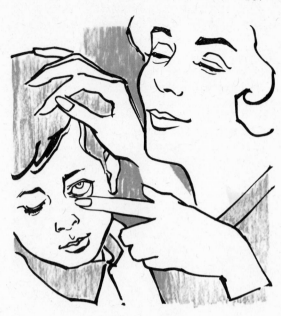

injury. Quite often injuries of this type are not detected until 24 or more hours after they occur. In such cases serious damage may be done to the eye. If the child tends to keep an eye closed, if the lids are swollen, or if there is redness the parents should seek immediate medical advice.

Cataracts

A cataract is a clouding of the lens, which lies behind the pupil. Children may be born with cataracts but they might not be detected until somewhat later in childhood. If the cataract is large and causes a considerable amount of whiteness in the pupil, it is easily seen by the physician and the parents. But if it is small, it may go unobserved.

If both eyes are affected the child very often has reduced vision, and the poor vision then creates the need for medical care. If the cataracts are extensive enough so that vision is affected, surgery is indicated. At times a blow or a tiny puncture wound will cause a cataract in any eye. Because of the injury the eye becomes inflamed and a white opacity develops in the pupil which indicates the presence of a cataract. Other cataracts develop because of low-grade chronic inflammation on the inside of the eye. Quite often inflammations of this type are so quiet that no one realizes the eye is diseased. It is only when vision is found to be defective, or when the parents notice the presence of a cataract, that the cause of the poor vision is discovered.

Surgery for cataracts in children and teen-agers is extremely successful. Removal of the cataractous lens, however, leaves the child without ability to focus the eye properly. For this reason, it is then necessary for the child to wear glasses if the cataracts affect both eyes, or a contact lens on the operated eye in order to restore proper focus.

Eyelid inflammation in which there are scales and crusts on the edges of the lids and around the eyelashes is called granulated eye-lids. In it, a brownish discharge forms on the eyelid margins and the inner corners, especially in the morning on awakening. The redness of the lids eventually causes some thickening. Most often granulated lids are due to a skin disease known as seborrhea. In these cases the seborrheic condition becomes infected with an organism known as staphylococcus. The com-bination of these two diseases causes the red-ness, scaling, and discharge. This condition can be controlled by proper treatment of the in-fection as well as the basic skin disease.

Sight-Saving

Children who have poor vision as a result of cataracts, astigmatism, strong nearsightedness and farsightedness, or poor development of the retina require special care in the pre-school and school periods. Help should be obtained, through the physician, from local agencies devoted to the assistance of children with re-duced vision.

Standard children's books with large print can be obtained. Magnifying lenses of a special type may assist materially in reading slightly smaller print. When the child reaches school age, he may, if necessary, be placed in a class arranged particularly to help the child with reduced vision. Special books and teaching equipment are available in almost every com-munity to help such children. Teachers are trained especially in the methods of handling children with problems of this type.

Generally it is better for children with sub-normal vision to be in a regular school with ordinary classmates than placed in a school for the blind or in a special school where other children with reduced vision are taught. The child with poor vision can develop a better per-spective on life if he has contact with active people.

One type of glaucoma which affects infants and newborns, and also appears in childhood, is a condition known as congenital glaucoma.

This may occur in either an acute or a chronic form. In this disease the ability of the eyes to remove fluids which accumulate is impaired as a result of faulty development of the drainage apparatus of the eye. The fluid which accumu-lates raises the pressure and causes what is known as glaucoma.

If the pressure persists over a long period of time, it interferes with the nourishment of the retina or seeing layers. As a result they are destroyed and vision is lost. Almost all chil-dren who have congenital or childhood glau-coma require surgery. Quite often this is extremely successful.

The disease can be detected by the parents because the eyes appear larger than normal. Also the corneas or the transparent window in the front of the eye are less clear than they should be. Treatment of glaucoma is an emer-gency and no time should be lost in contacting a physician for proper surgical care.

Adult Eyes

Young adults in high school or college may use their eyes for almost any amount of time, provided they do so under proper lighting conditions and with frequent rest. It is best to stop about every fifteen minutes and look into the distance or look out a window at distant objects in order to give the eyes a rest.

Excessive use of the eyes for close work over a period of six to eight hours often causes head-aches, especially on mornings after the eyes have been used a great deal the previous night. This has no serious significance and does not mean that the eyes are defective or that any-thing has gone wrong because of use of the eyes. It simply means that your eyes are tired just as leg or arm muscles may be sore after too much exercise on a preceding day.

Refractive errors in vision should be cor-rected if the person is doing a considerable amount of close work. The need for correction is determined by the use of eye drops followed by examination to ascertain the degree of far-sightedness, nearsightedness, or astigmatism. Glasses may be required, but quite often only for close work or in long distance viewing. Older adults have lost considerable amount of their focusing power and therefore examination of their eyes can be done without the use of eye drops. However, the pupils still should be di-lated to rule out the possibility of some serious disease inside the eye which can be seen only after the pupils are well dilated.

The older person who is beginning to lose his focusing power for near vision may require glasses just for close work. In case the distant vision also has diminished, it may be necessary for him to have two pairs of glasses or to have one pair of glasses called bifocals which correct both distant and near vision. Bifocal glasses still may need to be worn only at the time the person is doing near work, in case he does not like to wear glasses all the time.

Glaucoma

Glaucoma is an increasingly serious disease which occurs most frequently in persons over the age of 30 and affects at least two per cent of people over 40. One type of glaucoma, called chronic glaucoma, causes no symptoms until severe damage has been done. It can be detected only by the medical eye physician who uses an instrument to measure the degree of pressure in the eye and another instrument to measure the size of the visual field, or side vision. Every adult over 40 should have a test for eye pressure as well as a test for visual fields when he goes for an eyeglass check.

The second type of glaucoma which affects people over 40 is called acute glaucoma. In this ailment the pressure suddenly rises to a very high level and the attack is accompanied by severe pain, redness, and markedly blurred vision. Most often the patient must be placed in a hospital immediately and undergo surgery to relieve the pressure. This is successful in almost every patient, but prompt treatment is very necessary.

Cataracts

Cataracts may occur in any adult from the age of 35 on. They are more common after the age of 50. The cataracts affect only the lens of the eye, which lies just behind the pupil. When a cataract develops, the lens simply becomes milky and cloudy. Because of this cloudiness, light cannot get through to the seeing portions of the inside eye.

When vision is reduced, cataract surgery becomes necessary. It is not necessary to wait until the cataract becomes "ripe" as was formerly the practice. New surgical techniques permit the cataract to be removed at almost any time. It is necessary for the person who has had a cataract removed, however, to wear either contact lenses or bifocal glasses after the operation.

Adults, like children may develop various types of conjunctivitis, or inflammation of the mucous membrane beneath the eyelids. In such cases the eye becomes scratchy and red and has discharge. Most often the cause is bacteria entering the eye. Another fairly common type of infection in adults is cold sores on the anterior surface of the eyeball. This can lead to blurred vision, scarring, and permanent damage to vision. It may affect one or both eyes and quite often recurs because of exposure to the sun, wind, and dust. Early treatment is necessary to prevent damage to the cornea and it is therefore wise to consult the physician as quickly as possible.

Inflammations of the interior eye are common in adults. One of the most common is of the uveal tract, which is the middle coat of the eye. This middle coat contains most of the blood vessels and nerves that supply the eye. Inflammation of this type damages the retina, the lens, and the cornea. Uveal inflammations are quite often associated with such other diseases as joint, lung, or diseases of the intestinal tract. A search must be made for the disease elsewhere in the body which might cause the eye problem, and then the primary cause should be treated. The eye should also be treated to prevent damage to vision.

Some individuals are sensitive to tobacco, developing an impairment of vision known as amblyopia. This is not the result of external smoke irritation, but is due to absorption of toxic substances such as grain or wood alcohol, tobacco, or drugs which affect the nerves in the retina. The condition improves and the patient may recover completely when the cause is removed. Persons susceptible to amblyopia should not smoke at all, since the condition is often due to excessive smoking.

Degenerative Diseases

Because the number of elderly people in the population is increasing, a larger number of degenerative diseases due to poor circulation is being seen. One of the most common types affects the back part of the eye (retina). In it, hemorrhage and swelling in the most vital part of the visual system almost always lead to scarring and to permanent damage to vision. Quite often if treatment is started promptly, further damage can be prevented. Delay leads to repeated hemorrhage and extensive scarring with severe loss of vision.

Another type of degenerative disease is

retinitis pigmentosa. This most often is an inherited defect of the eye which commences in early childhood, in the teenage period, or even in early adult life. One of the first symptoms is night blindness characterized by difficulty seeing at night. The cause of this disease is not known and, even if it is discovered early, there is no specific treatment. If the disease is discovered in a child or young adult, proper sight saving methods may be employed so that the patient will be able to carry out a profession which requires only limited vision.

Another type of degenerative disease is due to closure of the main blood vessels which supply the brain and the eye. Just like water pipes, the blood vessels of the body can become corroded over a period of years. If the main vessels that lead from the heart to the brain develop this type of corrosion, there may be blockage of circulation to the brain and the eye. Sometimes only the smaller vessels which lead from the main vessels are affected. In this case the circulation of the eye may be cut off suddenly and all vision lost. Prompt treatment in some instances will prevent further damage to the other eye. If the blockage of the vessel is in the proper place, the affected eye may be successfully treated within the first three to four hours.

Contact Lenses

Contact lenses have become increasingly popular in recent years and their types have also increased. The physician is becoming more skilled in their use, and more and more people seem to be able to wear such lenses for longer periods of time. There is no danger in wearing contact lenses—providing they are properly fitted and are comfortable to use. If the lenses are properly fitted and checked by the physician with a special microscope and if no damage is found after wearing the glasses six to eight hours, there is very little likelihood they will do any permanent damage to the eye. The lenses, however, should probably not be worn for more than 10 to 12 hours a day. The habit that some teenagers have of pushing the contact lenses off the cornea beneath the upper lid while sleeping at night should be condemned because the eyeball may be seriously scratched.

Eye Surgery

Modern methods of surgery have completely revolutionized the treatment of many eye diseases. A large number of conditions now can be successfully operated on that formerly would have been allowed to go without treatment. The development of new instruments, very fine needles, and special threads for stitching have made it possible to carry out the most delicate eye operations.

One disease which seems to be increasing in frequency in adults is retinal detachment. This condition is discovered when it produces symptoms of flashing lights in front of one eye, followed by the development of a curtainlike loss of vision. It formerly was fairly hopeless, but now can be cured in 80 to 90 per cent of cases if the patient consults a physician promptly.

CHAPTER EIGHT

SKIN CARE

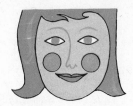

MOST PEOPLE become especially concerned about skin and hair problems because disorders of the dermis (which includes both hair and skin) are extremely apparent, both to the victim and to those about him. Such conditions are seldom fatal or even disabling, but they may well produce psychological problems which in turn may contribute to physical illness. For example, the girl or boy with acne may become depressed, begin overeating, gain weight, and aggravate the acne. Thus even a simple type of skin problem may start a chain reaction that damages the body.

Proper care of the skin and hair is an investment which will pay dividends in better health. Prompt treatment of even minor skin disorders is important. An entire field of medicine—dermatology—concentrates on studying the structure and functions of the dermis. These studies have resulted in many improved treatments for skin and hair problems.

Hair and Scalp

Many people have difficulties with their hair and scalp. Unlike the skin from which it grows, hair serves no indispensable function—many bald people live to a healthy old age. But the appearance of the hair is psychologically important. Attractive, well-groomed hair helps a person feel poised and confident; and this feeling has indirect physical effects. Also, proper care of the hair—especially cleanliness—may help control skin problems.

The quality and amount of hair on any body area are inherited characteristics, just like eye color or skin texture. This can be observed by comparing the amount of facial hair, tendency to baldness, hair texture, and color in the members of any given family or nationality. Not all members of the group will be alike, but definite patterns will be seen in successive generations.

Baldness

Hair growth is affected by sex hormones. Because many more men than women become bald, the male hormones are probably involved in this. The influence of sex is also shown in the parts of the body involved. In "male pattern baldness," all the scalp hair except a rim may be lost, while a luxuriant beard remains. In women, hair loss is more likely to be diffuse, but occasionally a pattern baldness occurs also in women. This usually occurs after menopause when a woman's hormone balance changes.

Hair loss can not always be explained by hormone-heredity patterns. Baldness in younger women has become more of a problem recently. Among the many possible causes, no one knows yet which is the true cause. On the other hand, hair loss due to the breaking off of hair above the scalp surface is probably increased by too frequent permanents and dye treatments, curlers which pull at the scalp, and rough teasing or ratting of the hair. Loss of hair in both men and women sometimes results from factors in their physical health or environment. These can often be corrected.

Many of the theories put forth explaining baldness are completely unscientific. You can disregard such "explanations" as lack of nourishment to the hair roots, excess tightness of the scalp, lack of nerve endings, or lack of circulation. Bald men's scalps do not lack blood supply, nutrients, or nerves, and any treatment aimed at these supposed causes—such as massage, vibration, and "electric" treatments—will naturally fail.

Dandruff

Another hair and scalp problem is dandruff. While a mild accumulation of castoff cells, oil, bacteria, and dirt is normal, and can be controlled by regular shampooing with thorough rinsing, some cases require more involved treatment. One should see a dermatologist if dandruff is very heavy or if it is accompanied by itching and redness; these may be symptoms of a more serious disorder, such as a disturbance of the oil glands (seborrhea). There are many medicated shampoos and drugs available which your doctor can recommend to treat these conditions.

In hair disorders, an ounce of prevention is worth a pound of cure. Women should fasten hair rollers so that they will not tug at the scalp. Any other prolonged pulling of the hair root, such as the ponytail hairdo of a few years ago, should also be avoided. Hair may be dyed, curled, and straightened, but such treatments should not be harsh or repeated frequently. Brushing will clear scalp of debris and will make the hair neat and glossy, but it will not forestall baldness.

Hair Removal

While not much can be done for hereditary baldness, there are various effective ways to remove or conceal superfluous hair. Shaving is an effective and inexpensive, but temporary, way of removing leg hair. So far as women are concerned, it is unsatisfactory for removing facial hair because a stubble shows after a day or two. However, hairs on the face and arms can be bleached with peroxide so that they are hardly noticeable. Manual epilation (hair removal) is tedious and impractical except for the eyebrows, where it is desirable to remove some hairs and leave others.

Epilation on a large scale can be accomplished by the use of hot wax, which is spread on the skin and allowed to harden, then removed rapidly, taking the hair with it. While this method gives longer lasting results than shaving, it still has to be repeated every few weeks, and is uncomfortable. Chemical depilatories give similar results. All these procedures can cause irritation.

Shaving and epilation are often blamed for coarsening of hair. Actually, a woman who needs these treatments probably already has hair which is getting darker and coarser. It occurs in spite of, not because of, hair removal.

Electrolysis is a permanent way of removing hair. This process involves the insertion of a small needle into the hair follicle and the application of a burning current to the hair root so that it is completely destroyed. It is the best available method for hair removal in small areas.

When a woman has excess facial hair, she should consult a dermatologist who will establish whether this is due to a disease, the use of certain drugs, or is the result of natural physiological processes. If he thinks electrolysis is the best way to treat the patient, he can usually refer her to a number of qualified electrologists. When the process is performed by a well-trained technician, it is safe, only minimally uncomfortable, and can yield very good permanent results. However, even the best technicians will miss one out of every five or six hair roots so that they will regrow. Also, downy hair may become larger and have to be removed eventually. Electrolysis can be irksome, slightly painful, time-consuming, and moderately expensive.

X-rays are effective—but extremely dangerous—hair removers. The dangers of hair removal by x-ray include skin cancers developing after a number of years. When any commercial hair removal system is under consideration, the potential user should be absolutely certain that it is not based on x-ray. Even physicians do not employ x-ray for removing hair. Certain chemical hair removers based on thallium have also been found to be toxic and have been removed from the market.

Skin Care

Regular cleansing of the skin is desirable for both health and cosmetic reasons. Cleansing removes sebum (oily secretion), sweat, dead skin, dirt, cosmetics, and some bacteria. This process can be carried out most quickly and effectively with water and a mild soap or detergent.

Many factors influence the degree of dryness of the skin: geographical location, time of year, relative humidity in living and working conditions, and excessive use of soaps and detergents. Some people may find that regular use of a cleansing cream or lotion with occasional soap and water cleansing is more comfortable than washing regularly with soap and water followed by the application of a moisturizing cream.

It is believed that oily skin is influenced by heredity, emotions, activity, and climate. Washing with a moderately drying soap two or three times a day and using a nongreasy cleanser should decrease excessive oiliness of the face. If it persists, an astringent may be used two or three times daily on such oily areas as the nose, forehead, and chin. But if any unusual redness or irritation develops, the use of these preparations should be discontinued.

Four major processes account for the difference between the old and the young face. One, the skeletal framework of the face thins and requires less space. Two, natural lines of

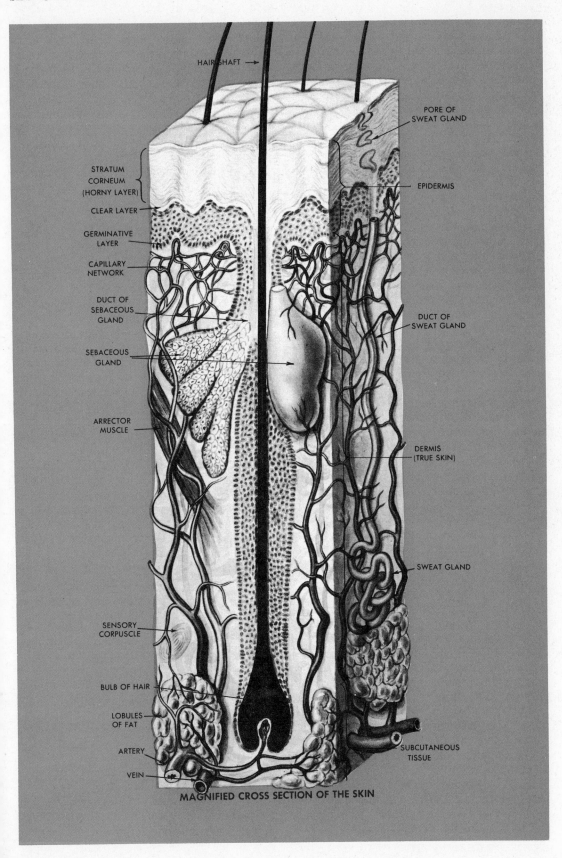

MAGNIFIED CROSS SECTION OF THE SKIN

expression and action of the face and neck deepen and become obvious. Three, the skin becomes lax and sags into characteristic folds and pouches. And four, skin color changes.

At present there is no preparation or method that will permanently rid an individual of these four characteristics, but certain preventive measures can slow the aging process. Because sunlight is a primary factor in aging, one should avoid overexposure to the sun's rays. Facial lines are more noticeable when the skin is dry; thus such areas should be lubricated. Plastic surgery can temporarily alter the contours of the aging face, but usually such surgery has to be repeated at varying intervals in order to maintain the improved appearance.

The enlarged pore represents the opening of a special type of hair follicle, the sebaceous follicle, which has a very fine, almost invisible hair. The term sebaceous comes from the fact that this hair follicle has larger sebaceous (oil) glands than most. It is questionable whether significant shrinking of the pore will occur from the use of any product. A cover-up type of cosmetic can be used to camouflage enlarged pores. Excessive use of these preparations, however, will aggravate the condition.

The cause of brittle nails is not definitely known. Contrary to popular legend, brittle nails do not result from a deficiency in protein, vitamins, calcium, or any other known nutrient. Brittle nails are probably due to external stresses such as detergents, solvents, or manicure preparations. Brittleness also increases with age.

The nails are very plastic when moist, brittle and rigid when dehydrated. Probably the constant use of polish removers, which contain solvents, leads to a loss of waterholding capacity. While some studies indicate that gelatin taken daily in large doses may be beneficial, the present consensus among dermatologists is that significant improvement does not result from treatment with gelatin. Some cases of brittleness are due to systemic disorders, such as circulatory disturbances and impaired thyroid function.

If brittleness occurs without known external cause and is persistent and severe, consult your doctor. Some cases can be helped by proper administration of vitamin A, thyroid extracts, or other drugs.

Dark circles under the eyes usually have no relation to physical disease. The condition is dependent on several anatomic factors and may reflect a family trait. The skin of the eye-lids is thin and contains little fatty tissue. The blood which passes through the large veins close to the surface shows through to the surface of the skin. This produces a bluish-black tint in the skin. When one is fatigued and pale, the color is accentuated. Darkening of the circles may also be accentuated during menstruation and the latter part of pregnancy. When aging, the discoloration may become more obvious and permanent.

Cosmetics are often effective in camouflaging dark circles. A lighter make-up can be used around the eyes, with darker make-up used elsewhere.

A wart is a viral infection of the outer layer of the skin. It is now believed that there is only one kind of wart; however, the warts are classified according to their location; for example, plantar warts on the soles of the feet. Ordinary warts are always benign (not liable to become cancerous) and always remain so.

Treatment for warts varies from removal by freezing or by electric sparks to suggestion. If the patient has faith in a certain treatment—no matter how ridiculous or unscientific—that treatment often appears to him responsible for the coincidental disappearance of his warts.

Other skin blemishes which mar the appearance or create minor annoyance, depending on their location, include the following:

Wens are plugged sebaceous (oil) glands in which the secretion hardens. They may grow to a considerable size, and if they are located where they interfere with clothing, or where they are unsightly, they should be removed. This is accomplished by a minor surgical operation.

Fatty tumors consist of growths filled with fat. They may be numerous and very disfiguring. Usually they are best left alone, since their number renders surgery impractical.

Fibromas are small hard growths of scar or connective tissue which are usually harmless and best left alone unless they become troublesome.

Neurofibromas are tumors connected with the nerves; they are not susceptible to any known successful treatment.

Skin tags are small superficial growths which can easily be removed by a physician if conditions warrant.

None of the preceding conditions is of a cancerous nature, nor likely to become so.

Moles are of several varieties, most of which are harmless. They should either be left alone, or if they are annoying in any way, they should

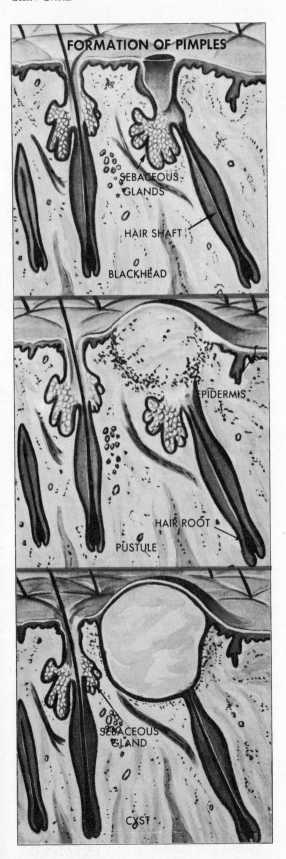

FORMATION OF PIMPLES

SEBACEOUS GLANDS

HAIR SHAFT

BLACKHEAD

EPIDERMIS

HAIR ROOT

PUSTULE

SEBACEOUS GLAND

CYST

be called to the attention of a physician. If any mole changes color, bleeds, grows, or shows any other sign of change, it requires prompt attention to forestall a rapidly growing and spreading tumor known as melanoma, which is dangerous to life.

Birthmarks are of serveral varieties, and their handling depends on their type. One kind which is common and very disfiguring is the port-wine mark, named for its dark red wine-like color. Occurring on visible parts of the skin, it is an embarassment, though it is harmless medically. It cannot be removed, but it can be covered with a preparation available at most well-stocked cosmetic counters. This is an application which is not like either ordinary makeup or stage makeup, but is waterproof and practically undetectable when its color is skillfully matched to the individual's own complexion. The matching is done by the cosmetic technician in much the same way as face powders are blended.

Other varieties of birthmarks, especially those called spider nevi and those including hair growth, require medical attention.

Body Odor and Deodorants

Body odor is commonly related to perspiration. Perspiration itself is essentially odorless; the odor develops as the result of the action of bacteria on the secretions from the skin's glands. This indicates that bathing is a primary method for the control of body odor.

Deodorants are products which are formulated to mask or diminish body odor. Various chemicals may be incorporated into the preparations to perform this function. Deodorants, however, do not in any way affect the flow of perspiration.

Antiperspirants, as the name indicates, incorporate chemicals which are intended to reduce the amount of perspiration which reaches the skin's surface. Effectiveness will vary, depending on such factors as the individual's amount of normal perspiration and activities, climate, and ingredients used in the product. Antiperspirants usually also have a deodorant effect.

Acne

A common problem in dermatology is acne. In this disorder, which afflicts almost all teenagers and some adults, blackheads, pimples, and red inflamed swellings appear on the face, chest, and back. The severity of the acne varies enormously: it may occur in the form of only a few blackheads or bumps, or it may become manifest as many blackheads, pustules, and cysts (inflamed sacs deep in the skin), which last for several years and leave permanent scars. In the normal course of events, acne continues from puberty to the early 20's, but in some it occurs through adulthood.

We do not know the cause of acne. As in baldness, both hormones and heredity appear to play a role in its appearance. During sexual maturation, there are hormonal changes which trigger the onset of acne in persons who have inherited a tendency toward it. Since the specific cause is not understood, we can only treat the symptoms. Also, we can avoid foods and irritants which aggravate the condition.

The first visible disturbance in acne occurs in the hair follicles and oil glands of the skin, which share common openings onto the skin surface. When acne is active, the oil (called sebum) hardens and forms plugs in these apertures. The hardened plugs are what we call blackheads; they are dark because of oxidation of the light-colored oil and other products on exposure to air. If one of the follicles becomes inflamed and fills with pus, it is called a pustule (or, more commonly, a pimple). A pustule may remain sterile or may become secondarily infected.

Effects of acne can be unfortunate, both temporarily and permanently. Teenagers are acutely aware of the facial disfigurement, even when it is mild, since they are at a very self-conscious age. This makes it likely that they will squeeze the lesions, increasing the danger of permanent scarring. If the pimples are infected, squeezing them may force the bacteria into the bloodstream.

Proper home care may help greatly to prevent acne or to keep it from getting worse. Cleanliness appears to be one important preventive measure. Good personal hygiene, especially frequent handwashing, is just as important as washing the face. Clean hair and scalp can be achieved by shampooing and brushing the hair often, keeping brushes and combs clean, and having the hair kept short. Most persons with acne should scrub their faces thoroughly three times a day with a rough washcloth. Besides cleansing the skin, washing with soap or detergent dries it and causes its surface to peel. This helps keep the follicles open so that plugging does not occur. Also, cleansers break down protein, emulsify oils,

remove debris, and may have an antibacterial effect. A slightly drying soap is the most effective. Many mild cases of acne can be managed by correct washing alone.

Skin problems may reflect the person's general health. Acne can be improved, at least to some degree, by getting enough sleep, exercising moderately, and having regular eating and elimination habits. Emotional upsets and tension may add to the problem. Irritants, such as permanents and heavy cosmetics, should be avoided during active flare-ups of acne. Because heavy makeup clogs the pores, it should be left on only for limited periods of time and removed as soon as possible. Medicated, drying make-ups are available without a prescription, and some of them are helpful. Some exposure to sunshine may be beneficial, but intensive exposure may make acne worse. A boy whose skin is irritated by an electric razor may be helped by wet shaving, and vice versa.

No one can be healthy unless he is well nourished. The acne victim should include foods from each of the four basic food groups (fruit-vegetable, milk-cheese, meat, and bread-cereal) every day. On the other hand, some foods may make acne worse and should be avoided. Among these might be chocolate, and foods containing chocolate; nuts, including peanut butter; seafood and shellfish, including tuna fish; large amounts of dairy products, dark-colored carbonated beverages; foods containing tomatoes; fried foods; sweets; spicy foods.

If acne persists in spite of these simple measures—cleanliness, good health, avoiding irritants, and good nutrition—a dermatologist should be consulted. Not only can he help control acne, but he can make sure that it is not some other disorder masquerading as acne.

The doctor will work out an individualized program of control. This is important because each person's problem is individual and because, even in the same patient, a drug may have different effects at different times.

Various prescription drugs are available for acne. Antibotics are often helpful, and other drugs, with different modes of action, are being tested for their effects on this disorder. Much work is being done on the correction of acne symptoms and on the causes which have been theorized for it.

For some patients, other procedures may help. The dermatologist decides which methods to use after making a careful diagnosis of the individual problem. Since there is no simple, "one-shot" cure for acne, he may try various approaches, and the treatment may last for several years or until the patient outgrows the condition.

The scarring which may follow severe acne can be treated with some success. Skin planing, called dermabrasion since it involves scraping or smoothing the skin, improves some acne scars. Results depend upon the shape and depth of the scars and upon the skill of the operator. Scars on the cheeks and, to a lesser degree, on the forehead and temples respond to dermabrasion. But scars on the chest, back, shoulders, and neck respond poorly. Scars of recent origin respond better than do old scars. Complications, such as changes in skin color, sometimes occur. A physician who is experienced and competent in this area can determine whether dermabrasion is likely to be helpful.

Problems of skin and hair disorders often become magnified in the sufferer's mind, seeming more important than they really are. While they must have proper medical care and follow prescribed programs for as long as necessary, the patient should also avoid dwelling on his condition. If he becomes absorbed in the things and people around him, he will see the problem in its proper perspective. This will help counteract the psychological effects which may accompany the physical disorder.

Skin problems as skin cancers, moles and fungus infections should be handled only by a physician.

Cosmetics

It is generally difficult to measure scientifically a significant difference between brands of cosmetics. Thus, the best guide for cosmetic selection becomes personal preference and experience. Price is not always the best guide to quality in cosmetics. Several low-priced cosmetic products have proved, through years of satisfactory use, to compare favorably with some similar more expensive products.

Each cosmetic product should be evaluated on an individual basis. Many women may prefer to try a new product of a brand name familiar to them. While, in general, a manufacturer tries to maintain a certain level of quality, the goal is not always reached. This does not mean that new cosmetic products and brands should not be used, but rather that their use should be accompanied by healthy skepticism until they prove themselves satisfactory.

Since the passage and enforcement of the Federal Food, Drug, and Cosmetic Act of 1938, the incidence of cosmetic quackery has been significantly reduced. Claims for cosmetics which are obviously without scientific basis and mislead the public are subject to action by Federal authorities. Although outright exploitation by cosmetic manufacturers is far less frequent than previously, it still exists.

The majority of cosmetics on the market today are satisfactory for the purposes for which they are advertised. Though in some cases their actual effect on the skin may not be spectacular, the psychological effects for an individual may well justify the expenditure.

As with foods and drugs, the ultimate test of safety of cosmetics remains in the consumer's hands. If an individual's experience seems to indicate a personal sensitivity to a given product, prudence would suggest its avoidance.

Creams

Cold cream belongs to the broad category of cleansing agents. The average cold cream is a water-in-oil type of emulsion whose cleansing action may depend on a combination of two effects. First, the mineral oil portion dissolves the fatty skin secretion (sebum) and loosens the particles of grime. Second, the suspending effect of the formula facilitates the removal of dirt with a soft towel or tissue.

A non-emulsified variant is the so-called liquefying cleansing cream. A typical formula might contain mineral oil which, instead of being emulsified, is solidified by the addition of paraffin or petrolatum to a consistency which makes it melt when in contact with the warm skin. This oily film is intended to dissolve sebum and loosen grime for removal with a tissue or towel.

Cold creams and other types of cleansers are intended to remain on the skin for only a short time, since the cleansing operation calls for removal of the cream together with the impurities picked up from the skin.

All lubricating, conditioning, moisturizing, and night creams can be placed in the same category. They are intended to remain in contact with the skin longer (overnight) than cold creams or cleansing creams. Their purpose is to promote skin smoothness by relieving drying and roughness. They do this by furnishing lubricant, emollient (softening), or humectant (moisture attracting or retaining) action— and preferably a combination of any two of these three effects. The film of cream on the skin shuts out the air, and the water in the cosmetic contributes a moisturizing effect, which may be assisted by humectant ingredients such as glycerine or sorbitol.

Foundation creams (of which vanishing creams are the best example) are a variant of the lubricating preparations, since they incorporate similar moisturizing ingredients. Foundation creams, as the name implies, are applied prior to make-up to provide a fine residual film that serves as a base for powder and rouge and furnishes some protection against soot and grime.

Many manufacturers advertise claims for cosmetics with mysterious ingredients such as royal jelly, orchid pollen, mink oil, turtle oil, "formula X9," placenta extract or "milk serum," and with vitamins and hormones, which state that women over 35 years of age can obtain a more youthful appearance by using these products. Such claims are based on flimsily conducted experiments reported under the guise of scientific articles.

Since the amount of the special ingredient is limited and the cosmetic base is basically good, these products can be used safely. The purchaser, however, is getting nothing more than a good cold cream at an exorbitant price.

Most of the commercial so-called bleach or freckle creams contain ammoniated mercury as their principal ingredient. This chemical is a keratolytic (peeling) agent. It hastens the normal process of sloughing or flaking of the epidermis (outer layer of the skin). This rids the skin of pigment cells near the surface, temporarily making the skin look lighter. It is questionable whether freckles are lightened by these preparations, even temporarily.

To avoid absorption into the system, a bleaching cream should not have a concentration of mercury exceeding 5 per cent. It should not be applied to irritated or damaged skin or to large areas of the body. No children under 12 should use such preparations. If any type of skin irritation develops, use of bleaching compounds should be immediately discontinued. Since mercury compounds cause severe reactions in some people, it would, therefore, be wise to make a patch test to determine sensitivity before using one of these preparations.

Hair Treatments

Static charges, which make hair fly, usually develop after it has been shampooed. Hair tangles easily and may break in combing.

Also, shampooing decreases the oily film and gives it a dry and dull appearance. Creme rinses are intended to help control these problems. They make the hair more manageable and give a feeling of softness to the hair. Since a creme rinse is applied after the hair has been rinsed with water, it leaves a light film on the hair which may improve its gloss.

Protein rinses, such as egg shampoos, have been suggested as beneficial to damaged hair, but there is no scientific evidence to substantiate this claim. Many scientists feel that there is little if any evidence that protein from such shampoos or rinses can penetrate the hair to give any reconstructive effects. Hair shafts are lifeless structures. These shampoos may influence the physical behavior of the hair, much as creme rinses do, by coating the outer surface. This, of course, would make the hair more manageable.

A weak acid such as vinegar or lemon juice reverses the chemical action between ordinary tap water and soap, which forms "scum" (insoluble precipitate) on the hair.

Hair Dyes

Permanent dyes are often referred to as tints rather than dyes, although the terms are synonymous. Generally, a tint is a hair coloring preparation containing aniline derivatives and utilizing an oxidizing agent, such as peroxide, to develop hair color. A tint penetrates the hair shaft into the second layer of the hair (cortex) to produce a permanent effect. Tints will lighten the hair, but unless the hair is prebleached, the degree of lightening is usually limited to no more than two shades.

Usually each brand states on the package in a clear, concise manner what results can be expected. The directions will indicate that if your hair is color "X" it can go to no lighter than color "Z."

A tint always requires a developer (oxidizing agent). The use of the developer helps the consumer identify the product as a permanent tint.

The package directions will also say that a color test should be performed on a lock of hair. This test will indicate just what color to expect from your hair in its present condition. It is important to carry out this test, for unexpected color reactions can result.

The oxidation dyes are more commonly used professionally, in beauty parlors, but a number of brands are available for home use.

They may be used satisfactorily at home if the hair is in good condition. When the hair is in poor condition as a result of overdyeing, over-bleaching, or poor permanent waving, the result may be breakage and splitting of hair and irregular coloring.

If a person desires to lighten the hair by more than two shades, pre-bleaching is required. In pre-bleaching, hydrogen peroxide mixed with a hair lightener is applied to the hair to bleach out much or all of the color. The purpose is usually to increase the porosity of the hair fibers or to achieve extreme lightening prior to blonde toning. Ordinarily, after pre-bleaching, a toner (which is a highly diluted tint) is applied; this gives just a small amount of color. Because bleaching increases the porosity and brittleness of hair, it may be more damaging to the hair than simple tinting.

There should be an interval of about four weeks between tintings. More frequent tinting may result in overlapping of colors and streaking. One should not try to change the color of one's hair too frequently or too radically—say from blonde to brown to red. One may get green hair instead, or the hair may break off close to the scalp. One of the large cosmetic firms indicates that the greatest number of complaints are received from people who have tried to change the color of their hair drastically in relatively short intervals. Drastic color changes require professional techniques—and even then damage to the hair cannot always be prevented.

Semi-permanent preparations are fully-formed hair dyes which do not require mixing. They also contain aniline derivatives and, according to brand, may be applied as a shampoo or following shampooing. These products achieve a semi-permanent effect by penetrating into the cuticle, the outer layer of the hair (tints penetrate into the cortex). The color produced by semi-permanent preparations is claimed to last through several shampoos.

There are two classes of semi-permanent preparations. The dyes in the first class do not utilize an oxidizing agent but do alter the color of the hair. They give highlights rather than producing drastic changes; they will brighten "mousy" hair and will cover gray hair to a limited extent.

Dyes of the second class use air as the oxidizing agent. It takes about 15 minutes for oxidation to occur. Results are generally comparable to those of the first class, with the added advantage that better coverage of gray hair is claimed. There is no satisfactory way for the consumer to differentiate between the two classes.

Temporary preparations in the form of rinses, shampoos, or color sticks can be used to touch up roots which begin to show the hair's natural color. These preparations are water-soluble and can be removed by shampooing. Their labels will state this information and serve as a means of identification.

Metallic salt dyes usually contain a lead or bismuth compound. The salts undergo a chemical change to deposit a colored film along the hair shaft without penetration. These preparations have several disadvantages from a cosmetic point of view. Since the coloring substance is deposited on the outside of the hair like a plating, the natural luster is obscured. Also, several applications of the metallic salt dye may be required to produce an appreciable change in hair coloring. Years ago, enterprising manufacturers exploited this deficiency by calling these products "hair color restorers" to imply that color gradually would return to gray hair. This term was banned as misleading.

Another disadvantage is the limited number of available shades. These dyes tend to produce dark and intense colors rather than muted lighter shades. In addition, the metallic salt dyes may interfere with permanent waving.

On the other hand, these dyes have the advantage that they are very easy to use at home. Self-conscious persons, particularly men, use these dyes in the belief that their associates may not realize the fact, since the change in color is produced very gradually and the transition is more likely to pass without notice.

Finally, these dyes are probably safe when properly used. There is little if any evidence that persons become allergically sensitized to the metallic salts as they do to the organic dyes. Most metallic salt dyes carry warning statements as "for external use only" or "contains ingredients which may cause skin irritation," although there is no legal requirement for special labeling to identify ingredients and possible toxic effects.

Evidence is strong that metallic salts are not absorbed through intact skin. However, care should be exercised to prevent their contact with mucous membranes or skin lesions and to avoid accidental swallowing.

Although the use of metallic salt dyes is limited today, a number of different brands are available. The fact that they promise permanent effects distinguishes them from the temporary preparations. The absence of caution statements and directions for patch testing on the labeling will generally distinguish them from the permanent or semi-permanent organic dyes.

All of the aniline products, permanent or semi-permanent, are required by law to carry a caution statement on their labels and include directions for patch testing. This helps to distinguish them from metallic dyes, but it also serves a more important purpose. The label should be read carefully and the directions should be followed. The caution label will read: "Caution—this product contains ingredients which may cause skin irritation in certain individuals, and a preliminary test according to accompanying directions should first be made. This product may not be used for dyeing eyelashes or eyebrows—to do so may cause blindness."

The patch test involves the application of a small amount of dye, mixed as for actual use, to the skin behind the ear or on the inside of the elbow. This test area should remain uncovered and untouched by eyeglasses, combs, or other objects for 24 to 48 hours. If redness, burning, itching, blisters, or eruptions appear at this site during that time, the reaction is positive and under no circumstances should the dye be used.

A negative reaction simply indicates that a person is not sensitive at that particular time and under those conditions. It indicates a low degree of risk to use of the specific dye at that particular time. One cannot predict which persons will become sensitive at a later date, particularly if the brand or color of the dye is changed. Thus the skin test must be performed before each application of the dye.

The relative tendency of the oxidation and semi-permanent dyes to produce allergic reactions is about the same. Although the incidence of reaction is low (about 5.5 per 1,000,-000 is reported by one company), the products are still considered to be potential sensitizers. For this reason, the caution statement and directions for use should be read and followed very carefully.

The person who has developed a sensitivity to one of the oxidation or semi-permanent dyes may be able to use a metallic salt dye safely, although the cosmetic results are less satisfactory.

Frosting, tipping, and streaking are all processes that involve bleaching portions of the hair. In frosting, a plastic cap is put on the head and some strands of hair are pulled through small holes in the cap. These hairs are then treated with bleach for various time intervals. The process gives the hair a salt-and-pepper appearance. Frosting has two advantages: the bleaching solutions do not reach the scalp, and all of the hair is not involved. The effect on the fibers that have been treated is the same as in the bleaching process. Frosting or bleaching aids in the manageability of fine hair because these processes do give the hair some body.

Once the hair has been colored there is really no satisfactory way to remove the dye. New undyed hair must be allowed to grow out. There are preparations known as color removers available for removing dyes from the hair, but these products should only be applied professionally. Even then, damage may result, particularly if the hair is already harmed by overbleaching, overdyeing, or overprocessing from permanents.

Soaps and Detergents

The chief difference between soaps and detergents is that synthetic detergents, most of which are made of petroleum derivatives, do not deposit "hard water scum" on the skin, bathtubs, or fabrics. Soaps—nonsynthetic detergents made of animal and vegetable fats—combine with the minerals that make water hard (chiefly calcium and magnesium salts) to form an unattractive and insoluble scum.

The chemical composition of synthetic detergents varies greatly. Most range from extremely mild to moderate; some are severly irrating to the skin. Most of them on the market today, however, are said to be equivalent in mildness to the soap products used for the same purpose. But individual sensitivity varies.

Since both soaps and synthetic detergents dissolve fatty materials, washing with them removes some of the skin's natural oily coating, along with the grimy and oily soils, bacteria, and skin debris. Actually, water alone, especially if hot, will remove significant quantities of the skin oils.

The consumer must rely on label information to make the distinction between soaps and detergents. However, there is no standard statement that is consistent from product to product that would unequivocally indicate the nature of the contents. Most soap products carry the word "soap" prominently, and most synthetic detergents carry reference to "no soap scum" or a similar distinction.

CHAPTER NINE

NOSE AND THROAT CARE

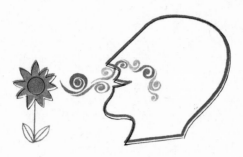

THE NOSE has two chief functions. In it are the nerve ends by which we perceive and distinguish smells. Second, and most important, the nose acts as a vent or channel through which the air we breathe is prepared or conditioned for passage into our trachea or wind pipe to our lungs. In the lungs the oxygen in the air is absorbed into the blood stream and is exchanged for carbon dioxide.

Pressure changes which occur during breathing assist in the exchange of gases in the lungs. As we breathe in, the resistance produced by the nose and air passages reduces pressure in the lungs; as we breathe out, the pressure in the lungs is increased because the air is slowed down by the nasal passages. This fluctuation in pressure helps the lungs exchange fresh oxygen for the poisonous carbon dioxide in our blood.

The nose is really two noses (nostrils) divided by a partition called the septum. On the side walls inside the nose are baffles with curved surfaces, called turbinates, around which air circulates and is made moist and warm. These turbinates have blood spaces which fill and empty automatically as we breathe, normally in a regularly balanced fashion. This process allows the turbinates to swell and obstruct the nose at times and to contract and open the nose wide at other times. Cold weather, irritants, cold feet, and other body disturbances may throw the balancing mechanism off. The result may be either an obstructed nose or a wide opened nose which tends to get uncomfortably dry.

The nose is normally wet or moist inside, being kept moist by mucus and a thin watery secretion given off by small glands in the lining of the membranes. Both flowing and drying goes on continuously with excess fluids and mucus being swept backward to the throat. This accounts for the normal amount of mucus

in the throat called postnasal drip. While some people have more than others, it usually represents a normal healthy process. If this drip becomes excessive or heavy and colored, it may indicate some disease and merits professional investigation.

The sinuses are air spaces closely connected to the nose; each sinus has an opening into the nose for the free exchange of air and mucus. The sinuses are located in the cheeks below the eyes (maxillary sinuses), between the eyes (ethmoid sinuses), in the forehead (frontal sinuses), and in the center of the head behind the nasal spaces (sphenoid sinuses).

An abnormal shape of either the external nose, the septum, or the turbinates may cause an obstruction of the nose which can be corrected only by appropriate surgery, such as a reconstruction operation on the nose or septum done by an ear, nose, and throat surgeon. Occasional obstruction or stuffiness may be caused by such conditions as acute colds, hayfever, nasal growths, variations in circulation, and emotional episodes. Any prolonged or habitual obstruction should be investigated by a physician.

When the nose is blocked, people often tend to get panicky and to feel that something must be done to keep the nose open. They may resort to frequent use of nose drops or constant nose blowing, sniffing, and snorting. This is not necessary and may be harmful.

As far as breathing is concerned, the mouth is a good safety valve for free breathing when necessary. If the nose is completely blocked, any amount of nose blowing is not likely to open it. Forceful blowing may force infection into the ears through the tube that connects them with the throat, or the sinuses, or may cause nosebleed or increased irritation. Blowing your nose is safe only when air can pass through it with reasonable ease. While blowing

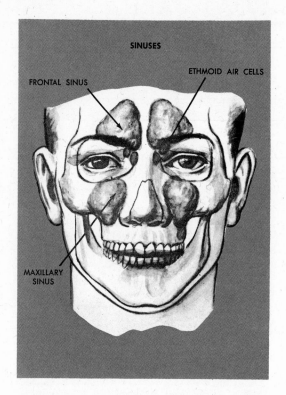

SINUSES

FRONTAL SINUS

ETHMOID AIR CELLS

MAXILLARY
SINUS

your nose, you should hold your handkerchief loosely in front of your nose and not pinch your nose shut tightly.

Nasal obstruction, however, may be dangerous in the very young infant before he has learned how to get air through his mouth. Use of nose drops gives only temporary relief and is often followed by a greater congestion. Frequent and habitual use of drops results in a vicious cycle with more and more obstruction developing the longer you use the drops. Oily nose drops are particularly dangerous for infants and young children because their use often leads to pneumonia.

The common habit of "picking" the nose or pulling out hairs may also introduce infection or start bleeding. Infection in the area of the nose is particularly dangerous because of the direct drainage between the nose and the brain along the path of the nerve of smell.

Colds and Sinus Infections

During an acute cold or other infection, one or more sinuses may become inflamed. The opening from the sinus into the nose may swell shut. This results first in a feeling of fullness and pressure and finally in pain as secretions and pus form in the sinus. A large majority of simple acute colds and sinus infections clear up spontaneously as the pus or secretions drain into the nose and the throat.

Use of nose drops once or twice a day during this time favors drainage, but their use should not be continuous. Active pain and obstruction usually require the help of a physician. Medical treatments include drugs, local suction treatments, and possible sinus drainage by catherization (inserting a tube) after careful anesthetization of the nose.

Simple home management will be adequate for most less severe cases. The important points in home care are: Get more rest in bed than usual. Avoid late hours and all types of dissipation such as overeating, drinking, smoking, and exposure to cold. Do not sit around in chilly rooms or with cold feet. Take a hot shower or bath on going to bed to help decongest the respiratory passages. Take a simple hot foot bath and breathe plain steam for added relief. This remedy can be repeated frequently.

The diet should be light and nutritious and fluids should be taken freely. The judicious use of aspirin and nasal decongestants as prescribed by a physician often decrease the severity of some of the symptoms. Traveling or flying at high altitudes except in properly pressurized cabins is inadvisable without instructions from a physician.

All headaches are not due to sinusitis. Chronic sinusitis does not typically produce headache. You should tell your physician about recurring headaches so that he can check to rule out endocrine and other medical causes—tension, tumors, or the like.

Nosebleeds

Nosebleeds (epistaxis) occur at any age and are especially common in children. The most common form comes from a small varicose vein near the front of the septum. Bleeding from this area can often be stopped by pressing the soft parts of the nostrils together tightly, close to the face, and holding them closed for several minutes. Nosebleeds from farther back are more difficult to stop. They frequently require the aid of a physician and may require hospitalization and nasal packing.

During active nosebleed, one should not lie on one's back, particularly a child who may strangle in his own blood. The proper position is to lie down on one's side, with the face looking downward into a basin or a towel to catch the blood. Pinching the nose tightly between the fingers or plugging the nose snugly with cotton is the most practical procedure while waiting for the doctor or while on the way to the doctor's office or hospital.

A relatively minor injury may fracture the nasal bones, or displace or fracture the cartilages, or cause a blood clot or hematoma in the soft tissues of the nose. Such injuries in children may result in permanent deformities if they go untreated. This makes it advisable to have a careful examination after any nose injury. Proper surgical drainage and reduction of fractures and splinting by the physician are often required, especially in small children.

The Throat

Several structures in the throat act as "lines of defense" against infection. These include the tonsils, adenoids, lingual tonsils, and the lymphoid tissue of the eustachian tube area. Any or all of these tissues may become infected. Repeated or severe infections may overwhelm their protective function and they then become a health hazard. They may need to be removed surgically.

Excessive smoking, or in some individuals even moderate use of tobacco, may produce irritation in the throat and the larynx, giving rise to a hacking cough known as "cigarette cough" or "smoker's throat." This can be relieved only by exercising greater moderation or in some instances, discontinuing the use of tobacco.

The adenoids are masses of sponge tissue resembling the tonsils. They lie in the nasophar-ynx high in the throat above and behind the soft palate. This is in the line of the air passages from the nose and closely associated with the openings of the eustachian tubes.

Adenoids tend to get small and disappear as we get older, but in childhood they may become infected and very much enlarged. In such a state, they interfere with both the nose and the ears and often cause sinus and ear infections. It is then necessary to remove the adenoids. They may also occasionally become enlarged in adult life and have to be removed.

Around the eustachian tubes are lymphoid tissues in smaller patches, which may become inflamed and infected and cause ear troubles. These may enlarge with the adenoids or even after the adenoids have been removed. In such a case a second operation in the adenoid area becomes necessary.

Examination of the nasopharynx is often very difficult, especially in children. Satisfactory examination may require a general anesthetic. In cooperative adults and children, it may be examined with a small mirror, similar to that used by dentists, or with a special electrically lighted instrument called the nasopharyngoscope.

The tonsils are visible on each side of the throat between the arches of the palate. It is believed that they have no function after about five years of age. Reasons for removal of the tonsils include: very large tonsils, repeated acute infections with sore throats, large lymph nodes in the side of the neck, or illnesses that

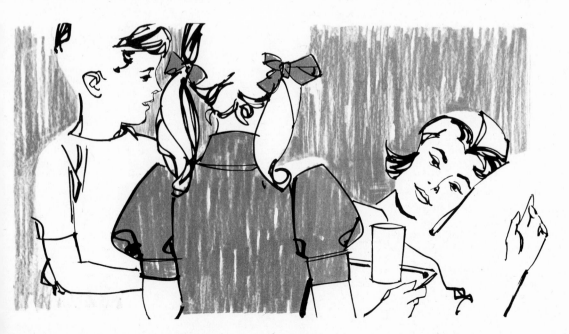

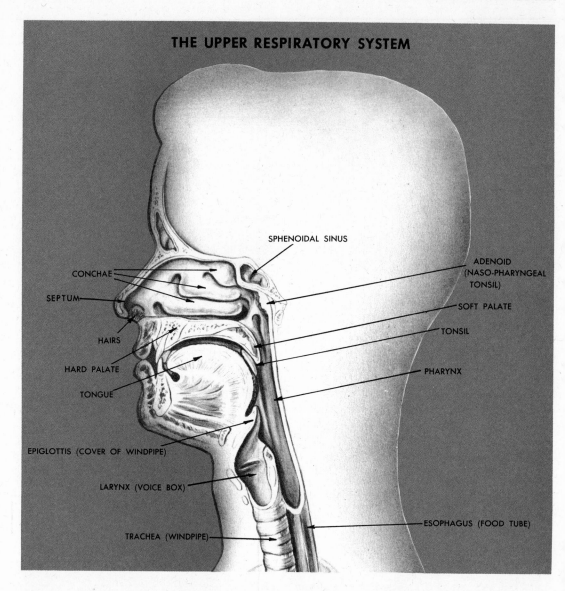

THE UPPER RESPIRATORY SYSTEM

(Labels: SPHENOIDAL SINUS, CONCHAE, SEPTUM, HAIRS, HARD PALATE, TONGUE, EPIGLOTTIS (COVER OF WINDPIPE), LARYNX (VOICE BOX), TRACHEA (WINDPIPE), ADENOID (NASO-PHARYNGEAL TONSIL), SOFT PALATE, TONSIL, PHARYNX, ESOPHAGUS (FOOD TUBE))

suggest a chronic focus of infection. Tonsils generally should not be removed in cases of acute infection, acute illness of any type, and severe blood disease that might interfere with proper clotting and healing such as hemophilia. Tonsils can be removed at any age.

The lingual tonsils are separate from the throat tonsils. The linguals are out of sight on the back of the tongue in the lower throat. They become enlarged and may suffer the same diseases as the throat tonsils. In such cases they may need surgical or medical treatment.

Inflammation or infection of any structures in the throat may produce a "sore throat." This can occur even after removal of the tonsils and adenoids. Many different germs and diseases may be responsible. In all cases of persistent or

recurring sore throat, or in seriously ill patients, a careful history and examination by a physician is necessary. Blood counts and bacterial tests may reveal unsuspected diseases. Tests which indicate that specific antibacterial drugs should be used may save more than the cost of the test by avoiding the use of wrong and costly medications.

Strep throat is a term commonly applied to a very severe sore throat associated with fever and toxicity. It is often followed by rheumatic fever. Unless a laboratory test for bacteria is made, not even a physician can truly diagnose a strep throat.

Diphtheria, though now rare, is still a serious type of throat infection. It produces poisonous substances that may damage the heart and certain parts of the nervous system. An active case of diphtheria may affect the larynx and trachea to such an extent as to cause obstruction and suffocation unless an opening is made in the windpipe below the voice box (tracheotomy). The only reason diphtheria is now rare is because of the widespread practice of immunizing children with diphtheria toxoid early in life.

Acute infectious mononucleosis is a fairly common contagious disease in young adults, It does not respond to antibiotics but is associated with a very sore throat, large glands, large spleen, and usually severe toxicity. Recovery may take several weeks.

The Larynx

The larynx or voice box is the organ that produces the voice. It also protects the air passages, or trachea, by closing tight during swallowing. This prevents food or liquids from entering the trachea.

Inflammations, infections, tumors, foreign bodies, injuries, or anything else that causes the vocal cords to swell may interfere with breathing. This obstruction may require immediate care or an emergency tracheotomy, which consists of making an opening in the neck directly to the windpipe.

Hoarseness is a common effect of any type of disease in the larynx. In all cases of hoarseness lasting longer than two weeks, a medical examination should be made.

The huskiness and hoarseness associated with colds ordinarily clear up with recovery from the cold. Moist atmosphere, steam, abundant fluid intake, and voice rest are the most important things for relief of symptoms.

In small children the inflammation may cause swelling and result in croup. Steam may help this condition, but if breathing becomes difficult, a physician should be called.

Other diseases associated with sore throats include leukemia, bacterial allergy, rheumatic fever, tumors, and virus infections.

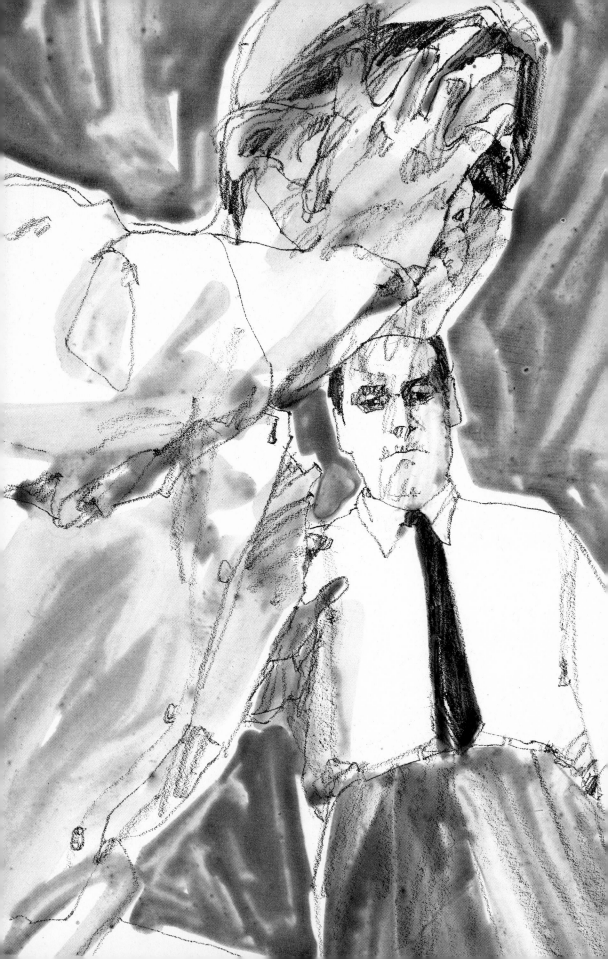

PART V

Mental and Emotional Health

CHAPTER ONE

THE MANY FACES OF MENTAL ILLNESS

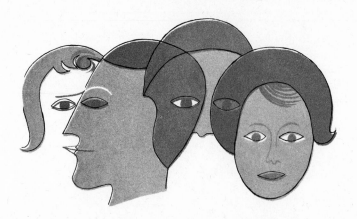

MENTAL ILLNESS is regarded by many as the most important health problem in the United States. The American Hospital Association reports that one of every two hospital beds in the country is occupied by a person who is mentally ill. One out of every four Americans will at some time in his or her life suffer such serious mental illness as to require hospitalization or intensive clinic or office treatment. Case studies in both rural and urban areas disclose that 8 out of 10 of us will some time in our lives be disturbed enough to need psychiatric help or to have benefited from it if it could have been obtained.

It is estimated that 50 to 70 per cent of the patients going to a family doctor suffer from illness of an emotional rather than a physical nature. In addition to the enormous amount of disability caused by this foremost of all crippling diseases, mental illness is also a leading cause of death. Suicide, an obvious result of mental disease, is now stated to be the eighth cause of death in America. The figure would be higher if automobile fatalities were included, for traffic authorities are convinced that about 20 per cent of fatal accidents are actually successful suicides. These, then, are the simple but startling dimensions of the problem of mental illness.

The problem is complicated by other factors. First of all, since the human body can react in only a limited number of ways, mental illness often mimics the symptoms of physical illness. Differentiation between the two is impossible for the medically-untrained person, and it is often difficult for the physician.

Second, it is now an accepted fact that certain kinds of emotional upset can actually bring about physical changes in the body, either in its function or in its anatomical structure. Ex-

amples of such physical illnesses deriving from psychological causes are high blood pressure, peptic (stomach or duodenal) ulcers, migraine headache, some types of colitis, asthma, and hives. There are many other illnesses, thought in the past to be purely physical, in which an emotional cause is suspected but not yet proved beyond doubt.

Third, there is some confusion in the use of terms. Some would use the phrase "emotional illness" to refer to those illnesses of a mild nature, caused by purely emotional factors, and the diagnosis "mental illness" to refer to major disease, especially that produced by some physical or chemical change in the brain.

However, at the present time, the term "mental illness" is generally accepted as the over-all designation of all these forms of disease. It includes all illnesses whose manifestations are primarily behavioral disturbances, whether the primary cause be physical or psychological, and also those diseases, often called "psychosomatic," in which there is a mixture of emotional cause and physical effect.

Mental Health

Doctors are often asked what constitutes good mental health. This is a difficult question. Physicians know much more about mental illness than they do about mental health. However, it can be said that sound mental health means that a person is assuming the responsibilities that a person of his or her age and intellectual and physical capacity should assume and is carrying them out.

Mental health includes emotional stability and maturity of character as well as the strength to withstand the stresses of living without undue or persistent symptoms, physical or psychological. Mental health implies the ability to judge reality accurately and to see things in terms of long-term rather than short-term values. It implies the ability to love, to be able to sustain affectionate relationships with other persons. It means the ability to work in one's chosen field both pleasurably and productively. It demands the presence of an effective conscience, realistic and independent, and at the same time a practical code by which to live. Finally, it entails the gratification of certain basic needs—such as hunger, thirst, self-assertiveness, and sex—in such a way as to not hurt other people or one's self.

To achieve this ideal of mental health we need more than the services of physicians and other persons who treat the mentally ill. We need the kind of society and the kind of family life that will develop such attitudes and responses. It is not enough for professionals to treat those who have become ill. The responsibility for prevention lies not with the physician. It lies with those who shape the social, political, and economic structure of our country. It lies, therefore, in a democracy and with every citizen of it.

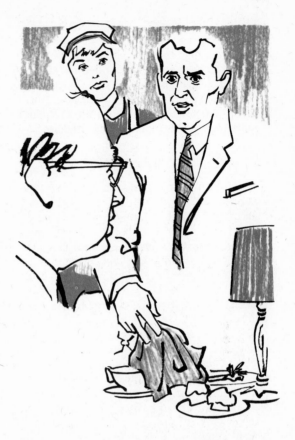

Mental Diseases

There are five major conditions affecting the human mind. The first of these is mental retardation. Some persons are born without the mental capacity to cope with the world. This may be due to unfortunate accidents in heredity or congenital defects. It may also be due to illness of the mother affecting the unborn child.

There are about 5,500,000 such unfortunates in the United States. For them our only present answer is training and education within their limits. As for the future, our major hope is to cure mental deficiency by its prevention through research into its causes.

A second category of mental illness, known medically as dementia, is the loss of mental and emotional capacity through physical changes in the brain. Such changes can occur after severe brain injury, with the destruction of the brain areas by accident, a cancer, or an infection. They occur most commonly, however, as a result of hardening of the arteries in the brain, or by its degeneration with age, usually called senile degeneration.

Such illness obviously becomes more common as medicine conquers more and more causes of death and a greater number of people live into old age. It can be said that all of us—if we survive long enough—will finally develop brain degeneration and thus end up mentally ill, in the sense that we shall have lost our former faculties to a greater or lesser degree.

The third kind of mental disease is that which most people think of when they picture the mentally ill. This is psychosis, or, to use the ordinary word, insanity. This type of illness may manifest itself by profound changes in mood so that the sufferer is deeply depressed and discouraged and thinks himself worthless, a disease commonly known as depression, and probably the foremost cause of self-destruction. It may show itself by an opposite change in mood, with abnormal cheerfulness, out of keeping with reality, usually accompanied by difficulty in maintaining a consecutive conversation and inability to follow through on plans, with consequent unproductiveness.

More usually, this form of major mental illness may show such symptoms as the holding of ideas which are contrary to fact (delusions), hearing voices which are not present or seeing things which are not present (hallucinations), or notions that someone is after the patient, persecuting him, spying on him, reading his mind (paranoid ideas). Such persons have lost touch with reality, live in a world of their own, do not see things as most people see them.

Here has been simply described the disease known as schizophrenia, or split personality, or, in an older term, dementia praecox. These are the unfortunates who constitute the major population of our mental state hospitals.

Psychoneurosis

The fourth mental illness is the most common one and that from which, to some extent, all of us at one time or another suffer. To most of us, it is just nervousness, a sense of being fearful and anxious and depressed about the problems we face in living. Only if it continues or develops into other symptoms can it truly be called an illness—something which impairs our capacity to carry on our personal business of living.

Most often this illness is seen as a state of anxiety or tension, an undefined sense of worry and apprehension, often accompanied by such physical signs as trembling, sleeplessness, headache, and upset stomach. In some degree every one of us has known such symptoms. It is only when they persist into a regular and unbroken pattern that a diagnosis of an "anxiety state" can fairly be made.

Since anxiety is the most intolerable of all sensations, some mentally ill persons develop physical impairments in its place. Such persons are said to suffer from hysteria. This means a loss or change in physical function without any physical explanation. Such hysterical disease may present itself as a paralysis or loss of feeling in an arm or leg, a sudden loss of consciousness or awareness of one's surroundings, a loss of one of the special senses, such as sight or hearing, feeling, or smell. When the doctor speaks of "conversion hysteria," he means that the patient has found his fears unbearable and has converted them into a physical disability.

Another kind of ordinary mental reaction is depression. Almost everyone has experienced the normal kind of depression that grief produces. But when it becomes a prolonged sense of the lack of any worth in living, it is designated by the diagnostic term "depressive reaction." Another variety is a sense of chronic fatigue and weakness, of not being quite up to the demands of daily life. An older term called this "neurasthenia." We now call it "asthenic reaction."

There are also persons in whom minor mental illness takes the form of specific obsessive fears (phobias), such as fears of closed spaces, high places, crossing the street, certain animals, and crowds. Or they may develop certain special habits that they persist in—such as the child avoiding stepping on the cracks in the sidewalk, or the man who must go back several times into his house before he leaves it to be sure the stove has been turned off, or the woman who is excessively tidy in her housekeeping. These are called compulsions.

This group of the mentally ill is usually diagnosed as suffering from what is known as an "obsessive-compulsive" sickness. All of these individuals—the anxious, the hysterical, the depressed, the tired, the obsessive—fall into the category of neurosis, or, as the physician will ordinarily call it, psychoneurosis.

We all are, or have been, or will be at some time and to some extent neurotic. Basically, all the forms of neurosis are ways of handling the problem of anxiety, of fear, or worry. Often we unwittingly fall back on the solutions we used in earlier life for the problems of stress and its consequent fear. Others, equally unknowingly, recognize what we are doing and hence use such criticisms as, "Act your age." or "When are you going to grow up?" or "Stop being childish." The understanding of anxiety is the root of treatment for all the neuroses.

Character Disorders

The forms of mental illness that most people find it most difficult to accept as illness belong to the group called "character disorders." These occur in individuals who persistently show abnormal personality disturbances. They include those who seem merely inadequate and ineffectual, those who are abnormally angry and aggressive, those who deviate from normal sexual patterns, those who are unsocial, those who use alcohol excessively or become addicted to drugs, and those who commit crimes.

Such people in general are characterized by a repetitive sort of self-defeating behavior, by an inability to learn from experience, and by being incapable of conforming to the ordinary rules of society. We find it hard to accept them as ill because we see them as lacking in will-power, moral judgment, and strength of character.

They are, however, ill, unable to live in such a way as to let them get along with their fellow human beings. Their psychological problems have shaped their ways of doing things, their characters, their personalities. Therefore we call their symptoms "character disorders," "personality disturbances," "character neuroses." You will also hear such persons called by an older term, "psychopathic personality." It must be remembered that these people are sick.

It should be noted, finally, that some experts believe that there is no hard and fast dividing line between the psychoses, neuroses, and character disorders. Rather they feel that many people facing stresses of living that cause anxiety to develop, retreat into some kind of behavior that solves their problems, however inadequate the particular solution may appear to the outsider. Each of these persons has developed a certain kind of defense against the impact of the strains of the world. What kind of defense this is spells out the special illness from which he suffers. Thus the anxious man, the psychopath, the schizophrenic may turn to the solutions of alcohol or narcotics.

Much of modern psychiatry is devoted to understanding the nature and purpose of these defenses. Most of all, it must be understood that these mental illnesses are not willful, not rationally chosen, not deliberate falsifications. Rather they are the result of forces that are truly unconscious, forces the patient is not aware of or able to control until he has had treatment.

Mental illness is the result of unconscious—*not* conscious—motivations within the patient. The simulation of disease, the faking of illness, known technically as malingering, is rare. When it does occur, it is itself a sign of mental illness.

The Signs of Mental Illness

The suspicion of the onset of any illness always arises either in the patient or in some person who is living with him or is close to him. This is as true of mental as of physical disease. Therefore the original indication of mental illness will usually be observed in the home or at a person's place of employment. The symptoms of mental disturbance are so many as to be beyond counting. They run the gamut from temper tantrums to hallucinations, from mild melancholy to juvenile delinquency, from headache to alcoholism, from a fear of cats to blindness.

A certain amount of anxiety, discouragement, or uncertainty lies within the limits of normal behavior. Concern is justified, however, when such reactions are out of keeping with the severity of the circumstances that seem to trigger them, or when they persist long past the immediate impact of stress.

Concern is justified when the symptoms are obviously out of keeping with reality, as are hallucinations, abnormal suspiciousness, or delusions. Concern is justified when a person's behavior is clearly self-defeating, as in someone who is drinking excessively, or using drugs

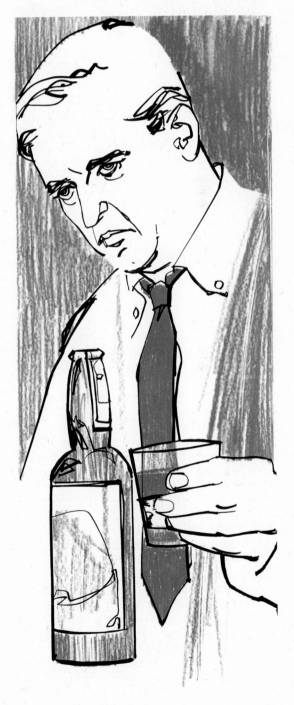

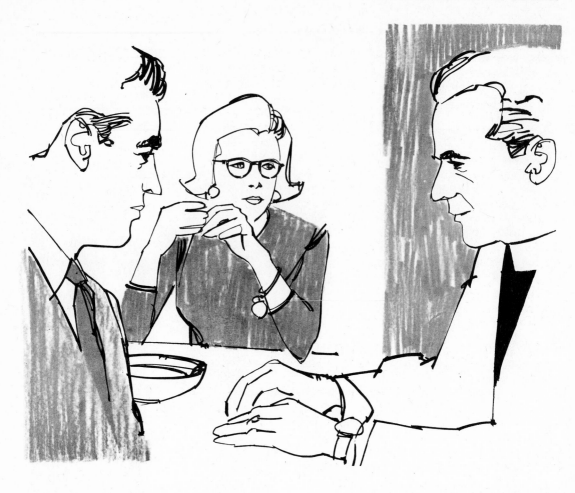

without a physician's prescription, or engaged in activities that run counter to the broad dictates of society.

Concern, finally, is justified when there is a change, slow or abrupt, in an individual's behavior or personality, and when that change persists. If such symptoms are not recognized by the patient himself so that he seeks help, it may be necessary for a friend or relative to take the first steps toward solution.

As people begin to recognize how common mental illness is, and to realize what the physician and psychiatrist can do to treat it, fewer persons resist the idea that they or their relatives may have a mental illness. Yet this reluctance still persists to some extent. So do certain misconceptions. For example, contrary to popular prejudice, mentally ill persons are rarely violent. There is no need to fear them, as a rule. There are, of course, some who in their sickness manifest a wish to hurt other people, and they must be restrained so as to save them and others from their impulses. But

on the whole, in the home, there is little reason to fear the mentally ill member of the family.

There is no point in arguing with a mentally ill person. His thoughts are real to him. It is better simply to state that you know how he feels but perhaps he will feel differently when he feels better. With a mentally ill person it is imperative to be reassuring and encouraging, not critical and scoffing.

Above all, no one should ever tell the mentally ill person that his troubles are just imaginary or that he should pull himself together and snap out of it. Often, particularly with depressed persons, such well-meant admonitions will merely increase their anxiety and guilt and make the illness worse. Mental illness is genuine illness; it will be no more cured by sarcastic advice than would a broken leg or pneumonia.

Threats of suicide should always be taken seriously. There is a tragic misconception that people who say they are going to kill themselves never do. Quite the contrary is true;

most people who commit suicide have warned others before of their intention. A threat of suicide is always a reason for taking immediate preventive action.

The Treatment of Mental Illness

Once a person sees in himself the signs of mental illness or once such signs are observed by his relatives or friends, the question arises as to the proper place to go for help. In the rare cases of violent action toward others or an actual suicidal attempt, it may be necessary immediately to call on the police or emergency rescue squads to prevent an urgent threat to life. Few cases of mental illness require such drastic management.

In most instances the patient should go himself or be quietly urged to go to his family doctor. The family physician is in 99 per cent of all cases of mental illness the first source of help. Sometimes, in the case of persons who resist medical advice, it may be helpful to enlist an influential friend or the family minister, priest, or rabbi. Some members of the clergy have come to know much about mental illness and can be very helpful to the family in steering a stubborn mentally ill person to proper professional help. They would be the first to acknowledge that final treatment must be placed in the hands of physicians and their professional associates.

In the vast majority of cases the family doctor will be able to care for the mentally ill person without referral to anyone else. This is true especially of the neurotic and psychosomatic illnesses which constitute most of the mass of mental disease. In more severe cases the general practitioner may refer the patient to a specialist in the field of mental disease—the psychiatrist. The latter may treat the patient himself or may in turn use the services, under his supervision, of specially trained persons such as marriage counsellors, psychiatric social workers, or clinical psychologists.

There is still confusion in the minds of many persons as to the distinction between a psychiatrist and a psychologist. A psychiatrist is a doctor of medicine who has had special training in the diagnosis and treatment of mental illness.

A clinical psychologist is not a physician, but rather a person who has been trained in the study of human behavior and psychology, and who with further special preparation can undertake the treatment of some forms of mental illness. The clinical psychologist is also trained in psychological testing, the laboratory procedures of the field of mental diseases. Such tests help in the diagnosis of mental disease and often in indicating the line of treatment that should be undertaken. Psychological tests are as important to the family physician and the psychiatrist in dealing with mental disease as are x-rays of the chest in the diagnosis of tuberculosis or an electrocardiogram in the diagnosis of heart trouble.

The psychiatric social worker may, under adequate supervision and with special training, treat some cases of mental illness. More usually, however, he will be concerned with collecting information, helping the family adjust to the circumstances brought about by the mental illness of one of its members, and keeping relatives abreast of developments as the patient is treated.

Psychotherapy

The prime method of treating mental illness is known as psychotherapy. This may take several forms, but in essence it is an attempt on the part of the doctor to change the abnormal behavior that brought the patient to his office by getting him to understand the causes of that behavior so that he can then change it. The doctor's role is more one of listening and suggesting than one of offering advice. We all know how helpful it is at times just to get our troubles off our chests.

In mild cases of mental illness, psychotherapy may be just letting the patient talk his troubles out, reassuring and encouraging him and helping him to create a mentally healthier way of living. This is particularly true in cases of acute anxiety or depression. With more deeply seated difficulties, psychotherapy may require a prolonged exposure of the unconscious problems that have led to the illness. Sometimes group therapy is used, in which a group of patients meets regularly with a psychiatrist, or perhaps a psychologist or psychiatric social workers, so that each patient begins to understand his own problems as he sees those of the others in the group.

The most prolonged and most probing type of psychotherapy is that known as psychoanalysis, in which the effort is made to explore all of the recesses of the personality in order to root out the mental illness. There is widespread confusion about psychoanalysis, and very often psychiatrist and psychoanalyst are used as synonymous terms. Accurately, psychoanalysis is a specialty of the field of psychiatry. Psycho-analysis is both a theory of human psychology and a method of treatment.

The method of treatment is one in which the patient is allowed, at his own pace and by his own association of ideas, to come to an understanding of his problems. This is best done when the patient is relaxed and free from distraction; therefore he often lies on a couch during the therapy.

All forms of psychotherapy have one aim—getting the patient to talk about himself in meaningful terms, so that he understands his motivations, the causes of his symptoms, and can reconstruct his life in a more mentally healthy fashion. This is what is called "insight." In gaining it, the patient must do the major work. In the last analysis, he knows more about himself than anyone else does.

The role of the physician, the psychiatrist, the psychoanalyst is one of helping the patient to express his ideas, challenging those that may be premature, helping to interpret to the patient the meaning of what he is saying. It is rarely one of outright advice, and still more rarely one of dogmatic instruction.

Medical and Other Treatments

Measures other than psychotherapy do enter into the treatment of mental illness. Certain drugs can be used to alleviate the very genuine physical symptoms that may be present. Sedative drugs are used to promote sleep. The tranquilizing drugs are used to lower the level of anxiety. Mood-elevating drugs are used to lift a patient out of depression. All these are powerful agents and should be used only on the advice and prescription of a physician.

Some of them have very real dangers. Even the mildest tranquilizers may cause the patient to become addicted. The sedative drugs, especially the barbiturates, have the same risk and furthermore, if taken in overdosages, can cause death. The use of sleeping pills is the most common way of committing suicide in this country.

An ultimate aim in all treatment of mental illness is the elimination of such drugs—even though they may have been needed along the way as crutches—so that the patient can get along in his world the way it is, without the need for escape into the unreal world of drugs.

Other treatment techniques should be mentioned. Electric shock therapy is used on some severe mental illnesses, primarily those with a predominant depressive coloring. In this treatment an electric current of low voltage passed through the brain causes unconsciousness. In ways not completely understood, this is often the quickest way to end a serious depression. Another form of shock treatment produced by giving the patient insulin is sometimes used in schizophrenia.

A third form of physical treatment is lobotomy, in which pathways in the brain are surgically destroyed. This is little used in this country now, and only in desperately ill and essentially unmanageable patients. All these forms of therapy are being used less as knowledge of psychotherapy increases and as drugs are found which control acute symptoms.

Hypnosis

Hypnosis deserves a special word. Hypnosis is the production, by suggestion, of a state of suspended consciousness and dependence on the hypnotist. Except perhaps for its use in anesthesia when ordinary anesthetics are unsafe for one or another reason, hypnosis should never be used by anyone who is not trained in psychotherapy. It is merely a psychotherapeutic tool. It is not difficult to learn how to hypnotize, but the tool is a double-edge one, and hypnosis can do great harm if used improperly by untrained persons. The use of hypnosis as entertainment should be forbidden without reservation.

Hospitalization

Serious cases of mental illness require hospitalization. This may be in a local community hospital, in a private mental hospital, or in a state or federal mental hospital. Preferably admission to any of these hospitals should be voluntary. However, in some instances patients are so ill as not to be able to recognize their need for care and must be legally committed. In most states this process is provided for by laws that try to guarantee an easy and non-embarrassing admission as well as more adequate safeguards for the patient's rights.

As a rule two physicians must testify before a judge, though in some states admission is allowed on the word of a single doctor in emergency situations. The likelihood of anyone's being "railroaded" into a mental hospital is so remote as to be virtually nonexistent. Stories of normal individuals having been forced into mental hospitals and then kept there against their wills are almost totally fictitious. This sort of thing just does not happen.

If a friend or relative is admitted to a private psychiatric hospital, one can be assured that he will in all probability obtain excellent care. If he is admitted to a state hospital the care may be less exhaustive, and there may well be fewer niceties. On the whole, nonetheless, the family of a mentally ill person sent to a state hospital can rest easy in the knowledge that adequate and prompt care will be given. Some of the country's state hospitals are centers of research and education in mental illness; in them the patient will receive care unrivaled anywhere in the world.

The admission of a mentally ill individual to any hospital involves many problems and difficulties which may be particularly harrowing to relatives. A whole book could be written on the arrangements for getting a patient admitted, for taking him to the hospital, how to leave him there, how relatives should behave during visiting periods, on the hospital atmosphere and its activities, on when to write the patient and what to write him. In fact, such a book has been written.

Every family should own it. It is *Mental Illness: A Guide for the Family* by Edith M. Stern, and it can be obtained from the National Association for Mental Health, or from any local mental health society. It contains specific answers to all these questions.

When a mentally ill patient is discharged from the hospital as being sufficiently improved to live in the outside world, both he and his family and friends face problems in adjustment. So far as the patient is concerned, this is a time for neither pampering nor pushing. The family at this time particularly needs the advice of whatever physician is superintending this part of the patient's recovery. In some states such supervision is carried out by the hospital itself, in others by local mental health clinics, in still others by private physicians.

The sooner the patient can get back to the care of his own family physician, the better. It may be necessary for the patient to continue on medication for some time after discharge from the hospital. This must be given under a physician's direction, and under no circumstances should any other medications be given by relatives who sense the patient's discomfort and think they can thereby relieve it. After-care will usually be necessary for a time; it will be administered by a physician or one of his professional associates and final decisions must be left in his hands.

Unfortunately, local facilities for the hospital care of mentally ill persons are still far from satisfactory. Any citizen interested in mental health can do no greater service to his community and his friends than to work toward their development. He should support the establishment of mental health clinics, child guidance centers, and particularly, psychiatric facilities in the local general hospital.

Mental illness of all sorts, including alcoholism, is just as much the business of every community hospital as physical illness. The ultimate aim in any community should be the possession of such facilities as will take care of that community's mentally sick. Eventually the state hospital should be only for the incurable, who require long-term custodial care. The individual citizen can assist in this aim by joining the efforts of his local mental health association and by contributing to and supporting in every way his already existent mental health facilities. He can also lend his voice to the demand that health insurance cover mental illness as it covers physical illness, so that mentally ill persons can be cared for in local private and community hospitals.

As with all illness, some cases of mental illness are incurable. This fact is as difficult to face as incurable cancer or a fatal heart attack. The old, whose brains are suffering a degeneration that cannot be reversed, are not going to recover. But proper hospital care can make their final days more comfortable.

There is now greater hope for the young people who have schizophrenia and were formerly thought incurable. More of them are being discharged from the hospital than ever, thanks to new psychotherapeutic understanding and the use of new drugs. Medicine has reached the point where one never gives up hope for the apparently most hopeless psychotic patient.

The feeble-minded may have to remain hospitalized for life, but modern institutions give them a world of their own where they do not have to face the stresses of ordinary society and in which they can live happily and often productively.

Brain Disease

It has already been noted that physical and mental illness may be difficult to differentiate. This is particularly true in cases of disease of the brain. Because the brain is the organ of behavior, disease of the brain may produce disorders of behavior as well as symptoms of disturbance in motion, sensation, and strength.

As with any part of the body, the brain may be attacked by various disease processes. In mentioning them here, the point is that small symptoms are to be taken seriously; they may be the initial signs of either physical disease of the brain or mental illness of psychological origin. It takes a doctor to tell the difference.

Infections of the brain or its coverings will be accompanied by the acute signs of infection, such as fever, pain, and toxic feeling. There may be simultaneously disturbances in behavior. In the same way the brain may be invaded by tumors or cancers, with a combination of physical and emotional symptoms. Injury to the brain may have the same double effect, and so may disturbances of the blood supply.

Strokes are the result of either broken blood vessels producing bleeding in the substance of the brain, or blocking of the vessels producing temporary or permanent loss of function of the part of the brain supplied by the vessel. Particularly in the case of so-called "small strokes," the changes in personality may overshadow such physical symptoms as paralysis or loss of speech.

The brain can be poisoned, as other organs can be. This is especially true with alcohol, and sedative drugs, such as the barbiturates. These characteristically produce alterations in behavior, and mental as well as physical symptoms. (See Part X, Chapter Seven.)

The brain has some diseases peculiar to itself. Among these are the so-called "degenerative" diseases such as amyotrophic lateral sclerosis, or the diseases in which the insulating material of nerve cells is lost, such as multiple sclerosis. The early symptoms of these diseases may be difficult to understand and may seem psychological when they are actually physical.

Another such disease is Parkinson's disease—paralysis agitans, known to our elders as the "shaking palsy"—characterized by stiffness of the joints, tremor of the hands, change in facial expression, and difficulties in walking. (See Part X, Chapter Five.)

Another disease peculiar to the brain is epilepsy. This may be likened to an explosion in the normal electrical activity of the brain. Depending on the part of the brain in which the abnormal electrical discharge takes place, various symptoms can result. The patient may have brief twitching or loss of contact (petit mal epilepsy) or may have behavioral disturbances of an extreme sort (psychomotor epilepsy). Most commonly he may have an epileptic seizure (grand mal epilepsy), with a warning cry, unconsciousness, and some of the following symptoms—stiffness, jerking, tongue-biting, loss of control of bowel and bladder, and, afterwards prolonged sleepiness.

Fortunately, very, very few epileptic attacks result in death; the patient usually recovers spontaneously. The occurrence of such an attack, however, demands medical attention. It may point to a growing brain cancer, or in an older person to a stroke, as well as to the disease of epilepsy itself.

This brief mention of diseases of the brain, diseases often called neurological, underlines the need of the family to depend on its personal physician and its right to do so. Only he, together with his fellow specialists and associated professionals, can unravel the web of mystery that an illness of the brain, psychological or physical, may present. Do not hesitate to call him. It is better to be wrong than to be too late.

CHAPTER TWO

DAY-BY-DAY LIVING

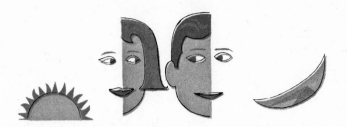

MENTAL AND EMOTIONAL health is not just the concern of those who suffer from severe mental illness. Keeping mentally fit is as much of interest to everyone as is keeping physically fit. To prove this point, take a look at these questions:

Are you always tired?

Do you sleep poorly?

Do you have vague pains?

Are you worried about your job?

Are you getting along badly with your wife? Or husband?

Are you in trouble with your boss?

Are you in financial difficulties?

Have you lost a close relative, perhaps your husband, your wife, a son or daughter?

Are you facing disease, disability, or impending death yourself?

Are you sure that your good breaks can't possibly last?

Are you vaguely uneasy and don't quite know why?

Do you think people tend to "have it in for you?"

There are few of us who now or at some time in our lives would not have to answer "yes" to one or more of these questions. The list represents only some of the common fears, anxieties, frustrations, and problems which beset people in a confused and threatening age. Almost all of us could add to this list. Behind, above, and through our lives hang the recurring fears of disaster. It is no wonder that we live in an era of tranquilizers, pep pills, and sleep potions, and that about half of the patients in doctors' offices are suffering from ailments based on emotions.

A few centuries ago man's great problem was keeping alive. Today, thanks to medical progress, economic advances, and the availability of labor-saving devices, conveniences, and comforts, man's difficulty lies mainly in coming to terms with life.

When people make jokes about psychiatrists and psychiatry, there can be little doubt that the problem of how to live with life is the overshadowing challenge which faces everyone, beginning in childhood and extending beyond into sixth and seventh decades—those dividend years the advances of medical science have given us.

All this has little to do with severe mental illness. One need not be a schizophrenic, a paranoic, a manic-depressive, or a senile dementia patient to have mental or emotional problems. These problems are the lot of almost everyone at some time, and there is no shame in having them. Nor is there any shame in asking for help from professional sources, just as one would do if he had a broken leg, acute appendicitis, or any other disabling illness.

Most persons with such health problems, however, do not seek professional help. As a matter of fact, if all in need were to seek it, there would be a severe shortage of professional persons in psychiatry, psychology, and even in general medicine.

The question then arises: What can people in such situations do for themselves or with the aid of existing resources? The answer is that there are many things that every person can do, some of them quite simple.

To begin with, anyone with mental or emotional problems should realize that he is not alone in this. His dilemma is not unique. Thousands of others have similar difficulties. Is it fear of death or bereavement? Is it financial concern? Is it striving for success or worrying about failure? Whatever your dilemma, you may be sure that it is shared by millions of others. Understanding this fact, knowing that you are not unique or queer, can in itself be a comfort.

A missionary's wife, often separated from her husband or uprooted from her home to travel with him—perhaps into danger—has modeled her life around faith in the God whom they serve plus a philosophy which she applies to every adverse circumstance. She says, "This, too, will pass." There is great comfort in knowing that time is a potent healer. If you can accept this fact, you will often reduce your problem to a manageable dimension.

Another comfort is found in the philosophy of a lady in her nineties. Her life had been good, but not without its troubles. Widowed relatively early, she worked to support herself. She had a severe attack of crippling arthritis in her sixties, and in her seventies survived five major operations for cancer in less than one year. Her philosophy has always been that it is not what happens to you that matters, but how you rise to the occasion.

Living Day by Day

There are three ways to meet a situation: One may face, fight, and conquer. One may face and examine, then observing that nothing can be done, adjust oneself. Or, one may run away and hide from reality behind illness or other psychological retreat. Obviously the first two solutions are sound.

Alcoholics Anonymous has expressed the proper approach in the prayer "God grant me the serenity to accept the things I cannot change, courage to change the things I can, and wisdom to know the difference." Members of Alcoholics Anonymous make one other impor-

tant point about living with one's difficulties. They endeavor to live day by day. They take no long-term pledge. They face each day as it comes. As each day passes, crowned with success, strength grows with the experience.

This approach is applicable to many of life's crosses. A loved one dies. You face a long and dreary future of loneliness. Financial disaster strikes after a life of prosperity. A friendship is broken by misunderstandings. A chronic physical disability is suffered. A marriage is wrecked. A trust is betrayed. You look despairingly down the desolate years ahead. But you can face today, and triumph. Today is the tomorrow you worried about yesterday. Tomorrow may never come. Life is lived from day to day.

Talking It Out

Sharing the burden comforts the troubled person. Although no one advises the perplexed individual to be a bore by prating incessantly of his problems, there are times when it is essential to talk things out with an understanding and sympathetic friend. Every doctor has listened to patients tell about their difficulties and, before he has had the opportunity to do anything, has had the patient suddenly smile and say, "Doctor, I feel better already. Just telling you about it seems to help."

An understanding but not unduly sympa-

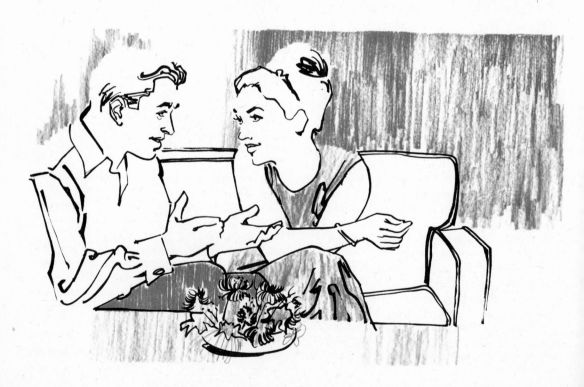

thetic confidant can help you put problems into perspective and afford you the relief of talking about the matter. Our language contains such expressions as "opening the heart" or "getting it off the chest." These are literal descriptions of the relief gained from sharing troubles, considering alternatives, considering or accepting advice, and making a new start.

The benefit of these experiences comes from the knowledge that there are sympathetic persons with whom one can share and that frustrations are common. The discussion helps to identify and define the problem. Thus, we face it more effectively. A child with trouble instinctively runs to a parent. Young people, especially, often find it helpful to talk with older and more experienced persons. Older persons too may receive help in their moments of anxiety or frustrations by talking things over with someone they love and trust, a brother, a sister, or a friend. A most natural sharing is between husband and wife.

The greatest mistake is to attempt to fight a problem alone when there is help as near at hand, as a loving relative. The endless "hashing over" of trifling problems is not encouraged, but in genuine emergencies two heads are better than one and two hearts are even better than two heads.

But here a word of warning is in order. Mental and emotional problems are not a proper subject for amateur treatment, except the immediate help of friendly and sympathetic understanding. Persons who receive the compliment of being accepted as confidants should not presume to give advice which can come properly only from qualified professional people. If sharing the burden does not give adequate immediate aid to a troubled mind, professional help should be sought.

There are many professional sources to which an individual can turn if he needs more than the opportunity to talk things over. Many clergymen are not only sympathetic and helpful, but also experienced in dealing with emotional problems. One should not expect the clergyman to replace the psychiatrist, but a firm religious faith is one of the best sources for tranquility and inner peace, and the clergyman can often be a source of help. (See also Part II, Chapter Eight.)

Another source is the family doctor. He, like the clergyman, usually understands people and is familiar with their problems. The good family doctor is patient, understanding, competent, and sympathetic. In most instances he can give adequate professional help without referral to a psychiatrist. If he advises consultation with a psychiatrist, you should show no hesitation in accepting this advice. A psychiatrist is a doctor of medicine and there is no stigma attached to consulting one. It is as sensible to seek help for an illness of the emotions as it is for an illness of the body. Indeed, an emotional illness often appears as an illness of the body.

Working It Out

Of the three ways there are to meet a situation, the most constructive is to face, understand, and conquer it. The stimulus of activity is better medicine than the deadening opiate of actionless worry. Working at a solution immediately results in whittling the problem down. It may not be completely eradicated, but it can be cut down to a manageable size. Constructive activity is in itself a partial solution and a help.

The second attack is to accept problems when they cannot be overcome. This does not necessarily mean inactive acceptance. One may look at the situation and decide that it cannot be changed. Purposeful activity often will take away the distress of unsolved problems. You cannot avoid the fact of the impending death or serious illness of a relative. But you will be much happier and more useful if you devote your time and energy to comfort the sick or dying person and his family or assist in other constructive ways.

A wise proverb from the Orient says "I complained because I had no shoes until I met a man who had no feet." Filled as our world is with people who have no shoes, there are still too many who have no feet who may need help even from those who themselves need help and who can help themselves most by helping others.

Among the more constructive approaches to problem solving is one being stressed by physicians and others who work with the handicapped. Until recently a man who lost a foot was a cripple. If he even used crutches, he was an exception. Such a catastrophe often reduced a man to a wheelchair and a life of bitter futility. Today, such people are walking unnoticed with ingeniously devised artificial limbs and playing a full part in life's battles.

Along with this progress goes an attitude which is applicable to every problem, great or small. In considering a handicapped person, rehabilitation experts now emphasize his remaining abilities rather than his disability. They build on these. In like manner, the individual who has troubles in one area gains perspective by looking at the more favorable areas of his life. This also applies to situations when all the bad news seems to pile in at one time.

The author Max Wylie, writing of his reactions to the brutal murder of his daughter, said that the most help to him in his grief came from the introductory words of the minister at his daughter's funeral: "We are gathered here to give thanks for the life of Janice Wylie."

After many happy, prosperous and fortunate years, a family suddenly had what seemed to be an exceptional concentration of illness and misfortune. One member developed serious arterial disease and required extensive surgery with the possibility of losing a limb. A grandchild, ill with unusual blood changes, raised the specter of leukemia in the minds of apprehensive relatives. Another member required gall bladder surgery while an elder in the family developed what might well prove to be a fatal illness. All these blows struck in a very short space of time, yet the family attitude was "We will not complain. We have had many good years, and we must expect to have our share of bitter along with the sweet."

Tension

Physical symptoms due to emotional causes have been frequently misdiagnosed. They have been called "nervous breakdowns" and often the individual was brushed off with the statement that he was "enjoying poor health." Emotional ailments have been mistaken for physical illnesses and treated medically or surgically with poor results. It is now well realized that the emotions can produce or aggravate physical symptoms.

This realization does not mean that all disease is due to our emotions. It does not support any vague theory of "mind over matter," nor does it confirm the theory that disease is due merely to some form of mental or emotional malfunction. The emotional basis for physical symptoms is largely the state which physicians call "tension."

Tension is a state of physical being in which nervous impulses secondary to anxiety cause changes in the function of certain body organs. Tension is often associated with peptic ulcers and many bowel complaints. In other cases, tenseness affects the circulatory system and

may cause high blood pressure, which in turn may result in heart disease. These symptoms can often be improved or removed by relief of the underlying tensions.

One of the more common manifestations of tenseness is the tension headache. The victim suffers periodically from severe headaches more or less coincident with a let-down from an extended period of tension.

Prolonged and repeated tensions may alter the functions of the glands of internal secretion. This influence upon the tissues of the various organ systems may result in chronic disease, notably arteriosclerosis, heart disease, peptic ulcer, and spastic colon. The more firmly these physical symptoms become entrenched, the less likely it is that they will be improved by the removal of the underlying tensions.

Tensions result in part from outside stresses. They are also determined by the capacity of the individual to receive and to react to stresses. It is important to remember that individuals differ in this regard. We speak of some persons as excitable, others as nervous, others as flighty, others as calm, and still others as lethargic. These are external observations and may be deceptive. The person with a calm exterior may be boiling inside and the individual who overreacts to minor stimuli may meet severe stresses with unexpected poise.

Meeting Stress

We live in a world of stress. It is possible that we have so exaggerated the stresses that we have created a new stress, namely the fear of stress. It is true that we are threatened with possible nuclear warfare and that we are pressured on all sides to earn more, to meet increased demands in our social, economic, or personal lives. The worship of status has created severe tensions in the effort not only to keep up with the Joneses, but to surpass them. It is significant that the greatest incidence of heart disease from stress in industry seems to be neither among senior executives nor the ordinary workers, but rather among the young junior executives who struggle fiercely to outdo their fellow workers.

And yet the world was never without its stresses. Primitive man had to combat the elements and wild beasts. Medieval man had his crusades, his tournaments, his fear of disease, pestilence and witchcraft, and his eternal wars. The pioneer conquered the wilderness with an axe in one hand and a rifle in the other.

Man has never been without stress and it is not conceivable that he ever will be. The question then arises, not how one can avoid stress, but how can one meet stress successfully. Everyone must learn to deal with it, for no one can consistently avoid stress if he faces his responsibilities.

It therefore becomes important in establishing a pattern for living that troubles and difficulties be confined to a proper place in the scheme of things and not be allowed to dominate life. Here are some basic pieces of advice which, if they can be followed, will tend to minimize one's frustrations and difficulties, or at least prevent them from gaining the upper hand:

- Learn to understand and accept yourself as you are. Recognize not only your capacities and your strengths, but also your weaknesses.
- Set realistic goals and ambitions for your life, those which offer you both a challenge and a reasonable chance of success.
- Measure your success by your whole life, not merely by the negative or positive aspects of small areas of interest or brief spans of time.
- Don't try to push people around and don't let anybody push you around; don't try to progress by pushing others down.
- Credit other people with the same good motives that you possess, and keep the chip off your shoulder.
- Remembering the corrosive power of hates, keep yourself free from resentments and "slow burns."
- Try at least to like and understand your neighbor if you cannot always love him.
- Be as cheerful as you can under the circumstances.
- When you are annoyed with someone, have it out in a frank and friendly manner.
- Bear in mind that you are neither alone in trouble nor even in your own particular brand of trouble.
- Give the other fellow the benefit of the doubt as you would like him to give you.
- Keep as constructively busy as you can.
- Allow time for fun and recreation.

- Laugh often, especially when you really want to cry.
- Be ready to help those who need help more than you do.

There are no panaceas. There is no simple and easy recipe for achieving good mental health. There just isn't any magic formula for successful living. There are books that will help you, but there is no book that will change your life without an effort on your part. There are sources of good advice, but no one can live your life for you. Help and strength and encouragement can be had from friends and relatives, from clergy and physicians, and from special counselors in mental health, but there is no one who can look life in the eye for you, except you yourself.

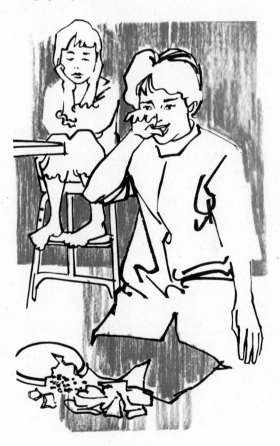

CHAPTER THREE

GOOD GRIEF

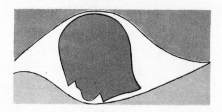

WHEN WE THINK of grief, we often think only of death, but other losses bring on almost identical reactions. People going through a divorce experience grief; so do people who have lost their health. Grief is also common to the aging person. A man in his middle sixties facing mandatory retirement may show grief reactions. People who have lost a child through marriage and now find the house empty may experience grief.

Ten Stages of Grief

Ten stages of grief are commonly seen by doctors, ministers, and others who deal with the problem. Everyone goes through some or all of these stages whenever he loses anything or anyone very important to him. In other words, what we are really talking about is *good* grief, normal grief, not abnormal grief. This healthy kind of grief, if not carried to extremes, can help a person move through an important loss with minimum harm to himself, either physical or mental.

The first stage of grief is shock. The person is in a sense temporarily anesthetized against the overwhelming experience he is facing. This state of shock is helpful to him because he does not have to comprehend all at once the magnitude of his loss.

The second stage of grief is emotional release. This comes about the time it begins to dawn on the person how dreadful his loss is. In this stage clergymen are often faced with a particular kind of problem. Many people appear to have the impression that a person who has a mature religious faith should not grieve. When people are asked about this, they say, "Well the Bible says 'sorrow not.' " They forget that the verse goes on to say, "sorrow not, even as others who have no hope." This is quite a different thing. They have confused a stoic attitude toward life with religious faith. The clergyman has to encourage his people to realize that emotional release is normal and natural—that there are times when we must all give vent to our feelings.

The third stage is the stage of utter depression, loneliness, and a sense of isolation. The person feels that there is no help for him. He is down in the depths of despair; nothing could be so awful as his depression. This too is a normal kind of experience. Many people like to consider themselves being attuned to another's needs. This stage of grief is a time when they should show their concern. We have not begun to use the many volunteers within our churches who would be willing to visit with grieving people.

The fourth stage of grief brings physical symptoms of distress. The percentage of people who come to doctors' offices because of symptoms closely related to a great loss is very high. For example, a man of 45 had been working for 15 years for a small company, expecting to take it over when the owner retired. He had worked diligently, including evenings, Sundays, and holidays at no extra pay, to be ready for this new responsibility. But when the elderly owner retired, his nephew was brought in to take over the job. The disappointed man soon entered a hospital as a patient with physical evidences of illness. Many people are in the hospital because of some loss so great that they have not been able to face it. People can be helped through this stage most effectively by being helped to understand the grief process.

The fifth stage of grief begins when people become panicky. They become convinced that there is something wrong with them as persons. They begin to feel that because they can concentrate on nothing except their loss, they must be losing their minds. For this reason it has been suggested that clergymen ought to preach a sermon about once a year on the handling of grief, so that people may know in advance that such panic is normal, natural—that this is *good grief*. They must know that they can expect this to happen to them whenever they lose anything or anyone who is important to them. Then, when they begin to think that this is unique, they can recall what their pastor said and their panic need not be so great.

At the sixth stage the person begins to feel

guilty about everything related to his loss. We have heard much about neurotic guilt in recent years. Now we are hearing more about real guilt. Some clergymen have been guilty of glossing over guilt. They have been tempted to encourage their people, to reassure them, and to say "though your sins be as scarlet, they shall be as white as snow." But no clergyman should say this before he gives the person a chance to admit his sorrow and his repentance for his guilt. When guilt is real, it must be dealt with.

It is often helpful to seek the advice of a clergyman, and to lay all the facts before him. Some churches do this through a formal confessional; virtually all encourage the idea on a voluntary basis. Not until he has unburdened himself of his guilt, is it possible to give the individual the aid he needs.

Grief's seventh stage is one of hostility. Now the person is beginning to feel a little better. He is beginning to come out of his depression and to express himself. He is hostile toward people he thinks may have contributed to the problem he now faces. This may include his doctor or his nurses, as well as people he feels responsible for his loss. Hostility is normal, too. While we should not encourage a person to be as hostile as he can, we must recognize that it is the nature of man. What the hostile man is really saying is, "They can't do this to me. Why did this have to happen to me? What have I done, more than others, to deserve this?" This is a natural hostility and has to be dealt with.

At stage eight the person seems unable to return to his usual activities. No matter how much he tries to get back to normal, he cannot quite do it—something seems to stop him. One of the causes of this may be related somewhat to our American culture and the way in which we handle grief. We make it difficult for people to grieve openly in America. Formerly, people wore black veils or a black armband, and everyone knew they were in mourning. We took this into account in the way we dealt with them. Today we offer our sympathy once after the funeral or after a great loss, and then we say, "Let's get back to business as usual." So the person has to carry his grief all by himself.

For example, a husband and wife were out riding with a widow of a year's duration and happened to go by a golf course where the man recalled a funny incident that happened in relation to the widow's husband. He was about to tell the story but thought, "No, I don't want to open this wound because Martha has been getting over it so well. I won't bring it up." We all tend to make this mistake.

How much better it would have been if he had spontaneously told the funny story and Martha would have laughed with him and enjoyed it very much. Had he said, "I'm sorry. I really shouldn't have told that," her reply in all probability would have been, "Shouldn't have told it? You don't know what a wonderful lift it gives me to know you still remember George. Nobody ever mentions him anymore!" In America we tend to make our friends suffer in silence, to carry their burdens by themselves. It is essential that we seek to minister to the aging person who carries a sense of loneliness and isolation all by himself.

In stage nine we gradually begin to overcome our grief. One cannot predict when this is going to happen. It may come in a few months, or not for a year or two. But little by little, if the person is sustained and encouraged by those around him, proper emotional balance returns.

At the last stage, we readjust our lives to reality. The last stage is not "we are our old selves again." We are never our old selves after we have had a great grief experience. We are different from what we were before. But we believe that we can be stronger people and deeper people, and better able to help others because of what we have experienced.

Among people who go through earthshaking experiences of grief, those whose religious faith was mature and healthy to begin with have come through the experience better able to help others who face similar tragedies.

On the other hand, those who have an immature or childish faith tend to face loss in an unhealthy way. They usually never work through their grief, and so months, even years, later are still fighting battles within themselves which the spiritually mature person has been able to wrestle with effectively.

Obviously, people of mature faith do not just suddenly acquire it when they need it. Like athletes who must stay in training, maturely religious people are always in training for whatever may come at anytime, When grief assails them, they are ready for it. It is just one of the many problems they have learned to wrestle with creatively.

CHAPTER FOUR

UNDERSTANDING YOUR CHILDREN

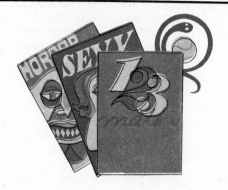

PARENTS have been rearing children for so long that it would seem there could not possibly be any more problems in child management. It would seem that grandparents, teachers, doctors, psychologists, and others would know exactly what to tell parents to do with their children to help them grow up to be perfectly behaved, hard working, happy adults who obey the laws and get along with their fellow men.

Somehow the job isn't quite that simple. As most parents know, while plenty of advice is available to them about child rearing, too often this advice is confusing and conflicting. One grandparent says "be strict" and another says "let the child have his way." And, to make matters worse, a newspaper or magazine article advocates a third course of action.

It is no wonder that many parents are confused and lack confidence in their qualifications and ability to rear their youngsters successfully. Too often parents feel that there is only one right way to raise their child. They are likely to feel that bringing up a child is like building a house or working a jigsaw puzzle. Accordingly, they may look diligently for the correct set of plans or strive to make each piece fit into a proper place. When the plans or pieces cannot be found, such parents become anxious and discouraged. This state of mind often interferes with the enjoyment of their children, and, consequently, keeps child-rearing from being the rewarding task it can be.

The purpose of this chapter is not to furnish easy answers for such everyday questions as "What can I do to make my child mind?" or "How can I teach Susie good manners?" or "How can I make two-year-old Johnny share his toys with his friends and neighbors?" or "What makes my child so fidgety?" Rather, the purpose is to help parents overcome some of their uncertainties and worries and to give them—in general terms—information about child rearing and management.

Parents should be reassured by the fact that no single mistake is fatal. On the other hand, they must recognize that continued disregard of proper principles can cause serious later problems. The most important single principle is that everything must be done for the child in a spirit and an atmosphere of love, acceptance, and understanding. The emphasis on proper child management is not on naughty children, but on good children who sometimes do naughty things.

What to Expect

Happy is the parent who knows what to expect of his child for he shall less often be annoyed, puzzled, and disappointed. Understandably, parents become confused, anxious, defeated or worn out by their 18-month-old who is wetting his pants, their 2-year-old who is saying "no" to everything, their 2½-year old who can't make up his mind, their 4-year-old who hits and bites, or their 13-year-old who is moody and goes to his room and locks his door. But they can tolerate, if not enjoy, such behavior if they realize that it is normal for the child at his particular age.

Parents feel better when they realize that the child's journey from helpless infancy to one of responsible adulthood takes 18 to 21 years. It takes a long time for his muscles and coordination to mature sufficiently for him to walk or write his name. It takes a longer time for him to get control of the necessary parts of his nervous system so that he can take disappointment without crying, learn to respect the rights of others, or concentrate on what the teacher is saying to him in school.

No parent needs to carry in his hand a reference book on child development which will tell him what to expect of a particular child at a particular age in a particular situation. Nevertheless, it does help parents if they know something about the child they are dealing with. The mother with her first child and with little previous knowledge of child development and child rearing can hardly be expected to know how children grow. But this knowledge is not difficult to acquire, especially when taken gradually in small doses from one's family physician or pediatrician or from one of several readily available and readable books.

Parents may be helped when considering any typical behavior problem by realizing that all children behave that way some of the time, but none do all the time. However, parents should not assume that the unpleasant characteristics appearing at various ages are necessarily approved of or that nothing should be done about them.

Children learn by patient, repetitious guidance and discipline. Parents must learn to handle unacceptable behavior until children can grow up sufficiently to behave the way their parents would like them to.

Behavior Patterns

The following paragraphs outline briefly the age periods and the general character of childhood behavior in each. It should be remembered at all times that these behavior patterns

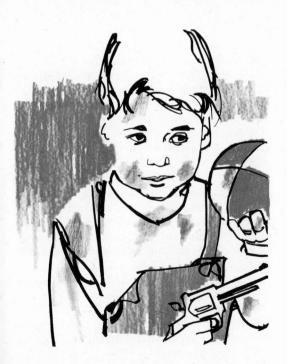

do not appear according to a hard and fast schedule, and that one phase merges into another gradually. Perhaps most important of all is the constant realization that children differ, and that each child must be considered in the framework of his own personality and his own growth pattern.

The first three months of a baby's life, especially the first one, are seldom smooth. Behavior difficulties during this time include excessive crying, spitting up, getting day and night mixed up, waking up at all hours of the night for feedings, and crying even when there doesn't seem to be anything to cry about.

From 9 to 12 months some parents are disturbed, but need not be, when the baby's appetite falls off, when he becomes afraid of grandmother and other strangers, and when he is messy and throws everything out of the high chair or bed onto the floor.

Between 18 and 30 months the child often still wets. He can't be reasoned with; he says "no" to almost everything. He often eats poorly. He may be a perfectionist and want everything just so. He may have a tantrum when he doesn't get his way.

At two-and-a-half years he is apt to say "yes" and then "no." This can be one of the most difficult and exasperating ages. But understanding his characteristics, abilities, and limitations helps to make him more interesting and enjoyable. The "no" stage gives way to a stage of uncertainty and indecision on the part of the child. He wants to have his cake and eat it too. He simply can't make up his mind. You may have a struggle getting him into the bathtub and then you have an equally hard struggle getting him out again. He wants to put on his coat and go outdoors, but as soon as you get him bundled up, he decides he wants to stay in the house. By the time you get his clothes off again, he may simply sit down on the floor and cry, saying, "I don't want to do anything."

Parents can often work around him and avoid head-on clashes. Directions should be simplified and he shouldn't be asked for a decision. Instead, invitational words should be used such as "Let's eat lunch now" or "How about a walk?" or questions such as "Where did it go?" or "How can we do this?"

The two-and-a-half-year old may stutter. Do not call attention to it or you may make it worse. (See Chapter Five of this Part.) The mind of this age child can work faster than his tongue. Don't worry, the mind and mouth will usually get together eventually and he should learn to speak as well as you—but no better, if your own speech is careless. In managing a two-and-a-half year old, parental patience is essential. It is true your patience will wear thin, but you can be encouraged by the fact that as he approaches three he will become a much more pleasant child to live with and manage.

At three he may be eager to please and better able to do so. He will be more able to profit by experience, to share, take turns, and make some decisions.

The four-year-old may present some difficult behavior patterns, characterized by hitting, biting, throwing rocks or breaking toys, and running away. He is apt to be angry one minute and laugh the next. He may pick up words and take delight in using them. He may threaten his mother with such statements as "I hate you" or "I'm going to get a cannon gun and shoot you." Because he is out of bounds in all directions, the management of the four-year-old is dependent upon firm discipline. Limits must be set; lines drawn and adhered to.

Five seems to be a much better age, as parents observe with a sigh—but it doesn't last. The six-year-old child has to make the sometimes difficult adjustment of starting to school. Often he seems to be in constant emotional conflict with himself. At that age he seems to "have to be right" and he seems to "have to win." Parents are often distressed but should not be surprised if he sometimes tells lies, cheats, or steals. Explain desirable behavior. Be patient. He needs your approval very much, your understanding, praise, and encouragement. If you or the school push too hard or expect too much, he may become tense and nervous and develop such physical symptoms as stomachache, headache, and fatigue.

The eight-year-old tends to be exuberant, expansive, and cocky. He is apt to be sloppy, to lose things, to have bad table manners. He may tackle things with great eagerness but fail to finish them—and he may be upset over his failure. At this age most children are eager and friendly. They are more able to accept moderate responsibilities and they want to do well. However, much praise and encouragement from adults are needed, as are reasonable explanations. The child at this age doesn't want you to talk down to him. It is particularly important for you to protect him from undertaking overly difficult tasks and to avoid excessive criticism when he fails at something.

Ten years is a more comfortable age, though some children may develop emotional prob-

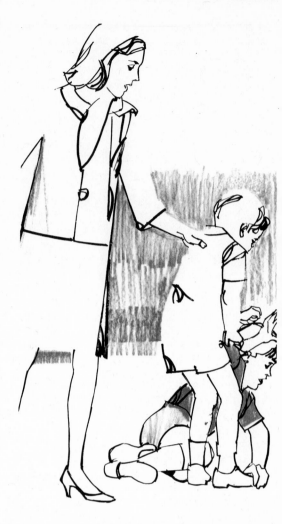

lems at this time. Parents of a 10-year-old are often able to feel relaxed and successful because they have such a "nice child." Children at this age actually try to be good. The parents are still law, but the child is flexible and doesn't take things too seriously. Perhaps never again will parents be so completely accepted. It is particularly important for parents—especially busy fathers—to do things with their children at this age rather than to wait until the child is "more interesting and a little older." It is not going to be very long before the child has interest and concern only for those of his own age, with little time for his parents and less interest in what they are doing or in doing things with them.

The 11-year-old is apt to be rude, argumentative, and overanxious. He may sulk around the house and complain that he doesn't have anything to do. He may quarrel more with his brothers and sisters and get "fed up" with his chores around the house. This age has been called the pre-adolescent period. Children at this time begin to "spread out" and girls begin to mature physically in preparation for menstruation—in fact, some will menstruate at eleven or even younger. Children may worry because they are taller, skinnier, fatter, or shorter than some of their classmates.

Since children do not usually like to be different, it is important for pre-adolescent youngsters to have some knowledge of growth and development and, more specifically, a great deal of information about sex. (See Part II, Chapter Six)

The 13-year-old may at times be withdrawn and moody. A girl nearly always wants a room to herself. And don't be alarmed if she goes there and locks the door. At this age children may worry about popularity, school, money, and the future. Advice on dealing with children at this age cannot be given simply and in a few words. Parents should be available if their children want to talk things over, but they should not pry. Give praise when you can and, when you have to correct, don't overdo it and try to pay some compliment at the same time.

The 14-year-old who seems to be more friendly and joyous and straightforward, may become sullen, restless, and exasperating by 15. At this age young people seem to be furthest away from their parents and may even separate themselves from the family circle. They may enter the house and go directly to their rooms without a greeting, or may sit in the same room with parents without noticing them at all. Attracting the other sex is particularly on their minds at this age. Parents need to show trust and confidence in their youngsters, but at the same time they should know where they are and with whom they are going out. "Going all the way" in sex relationships may take place if supervision is completely absent. Pregnancy in high school girls is increasingly common.

At 16 many youngsters are apt to be happy, friendly, good tempered, and self-assured. They are more likely to take parents into their confidence, sometimes even discussing their friends of the opposite sex, their plans for the future, and so on. They show more pride in their parents and admiration of mother's good looks, dad's hard work, and other accomplishments. Although youngsters themselves may occasionally show "thorny behavior," usually such behavior is short-lasting and handled in a more mature way. Some 16-year-olds, however, are difficult to handle and insist on privileges for which they are insufficiently mature.

It cannot be overemphasized that parents should remember that the stages of development are not cut-and-dried. Stages may appear either earlier or later than in the typical patterns presented. Most children will display a mixture of patterns, at times shifting temporarily to a behavior typical of the preceding or later period.

Persistent abnormal behavior at any age, whether it is severe colic in infancy, unusually hostile behavior in a four-year-old, or extremely withdrawn behavior or moodiness dur-

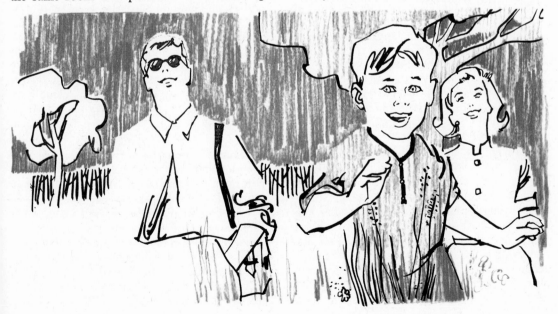

ing adolescence, may signal the need for help from your family physician. Don't be afraid to get professional advice and counsel when your common sense tells you it is needed.

Children Are Different

As already indicated, even though parents can learn a great deal about what to expect of children at a particular age, they still need to remember that their own particular child is different from every other child who was ever born. Each child is unique. What he is at a given moment depends on many, many things including the traits he has inherited from his parents and his grandparents, his greatgrandparents and their grandparents before them. Some children are born to be tall and slender, others to be short and stocky. Some are born to be placid and sedate, others to be active and "into things." Each child is born with a different type of intellectual endowment. The son of a famous author and writer may be a slow reader and the son of a mathematical genius may not have a head for figures. The 200-pound fullback's son may "take after" a great uncle who is small and weighs only 130 pounds, soaking wet.

Children's general physical make-up differs from child to child. One child may have a slight defect in his vision and another may have a mild hearing problem. Some children inherit a tendency to allergy and have more colds and infections than others. Whether or not a child has been sick and has to go to the doctor frequently for injections or other treatments may influence his reactions to strangers. Some children who do not feel well may "misbehave." This may get them into trouble sometimes, especially if the cause has not been detected. Any child who is presenting behavior problems of any type should have a careful medical examination to make sure he is not physically ill or has an unnoticed physical defect.

The child's situation in the family has a considerable influence on his life and his behavior. Often we expect more of our first child than we do of later children. As other youngsters come along many parents realize that often thay have been too tense with their first ones. Jealousy of a baby brother or sister may profoundly upset some youngsters. Younger children, on the other hand, may have difficulty keeping up with an older child in the family, especially if the latter has been outstanding in

studies, athletics, or popularity. Family crises, including death, divorce, sickness of parents, financial problems, moving, all require adaptations and adjustments by the child, and all of these things influence the child's behavior.

Emotional Crises of Childhood

Every child faces certain stresses, crises, or threats. They are the lot of every child by virtue of the fact that he is a human being living among other human beings, and in a society that generates dangers and threats of dangers. How the child meets these threats or stresses in large part determines how the child's personality develops and how he solves the problems that he will face at various stages of his growth.

It is extremely important in the development of the child's personality at what age these crises or stresses impinge upon him. If they occur before the age of 5, their effect is much greater and differs in quality than if they occur at the age of 5 or 6, or at 9 or 10. Needless to say however, at whatever age they occur they will have a tremendous effect upon all the child's later attempts at learning.

The most important stress or threat to the child that can arise in his early childhood is that of abandonment, desertion, or isolation. This—as with the other stresses that follow—can be either a real threat or it can be a fantasy conceived by the child as a result of circumstances in his family group or the attitudes of people toward one another or toward him.

A very important threat in early childhood and extending into the school-age period is the threat of mutilation. The child may fear disfigurement by disease, injury, operation—or even the removal of organs.

At numerous times during childhood, up to and through adolescence, most children are troubled by death. The child fears his own death or that of his parents or others essential to his security and well-being. Sometimes his death fears concern others, especially brothers or sisters, who constitute rivals to him for the attention and affection of his parents.

A recurrent threat to the child is the threat of deprivation. This does not necessarily mean that he fears total loss of everything he and his family own. It does not mean either that the threat of deprivation is real, for it may be entirely a fantasy built by the child upon some misinterpretation of the attitudes of persons in his world. The sense of deprivation most probably will be a comparative one. The child will feel he is not given the same amount of love and attention as his brothers or sisters, or that he is not given the same amount of food or clothing as they or other children. Or he may feel deprived in respect to the toys other children around him receive.

By the time the child is in the middle of the school-age period he is acutely aware of the effects of disease and the possibility that he may become a victim of disease. He notes the occurrence of acute and chronic diseases and their effect on children in his own group. With these observations he realizes that such disasters may be visited upon him. Similar to this fear is that of physical or mental disability. This threat develops as the child begins to compare his own capabilities and talents with those of other children about him. He soon learns that children of his own age have a wide range of physical abilities and physical powers. In school he learns that there is also a wide divergence of intellectual powers and attainments among children of the same group. Such comparisons many times lead the child to develop anxieties about his own physical or mental capabilities.

During the school-age period and thereafter, the child faces the ever present threat of defeat or loss of prestige. This again involves an estimate of himself, or a comparison between his own and the accomplishments and acts of others in his age group. Finally, the child always faces the possibility of disgrace. He is acutely aware of this possibility as he struggles to overcome impulses that may result in his breaking his group's or society's moral code.

The above paragraphs summarize in brief form some of the important crises in child development. Many of these stresses occur from time to time in spite of the parents' best attempts to see that they do not. Knowing that they do and probably will occur, parents may then be on the alert for their possible emergence and do their best to modify their effects. Parents can accomplish this best by endeavoring to present the child with a renewed sense of security and trust in them, and by placing renewed emphasis on the worth and basic goodness of the child himself.

Personality Growth

Each school-age child must face and solve certain milestones in personality growth. The child will meet them between the time he is about 5 years old to the beginning of adolescence at 12.

First in order—and of extreme importance —is the child's ability to withstand a separation from the parents (particularly from

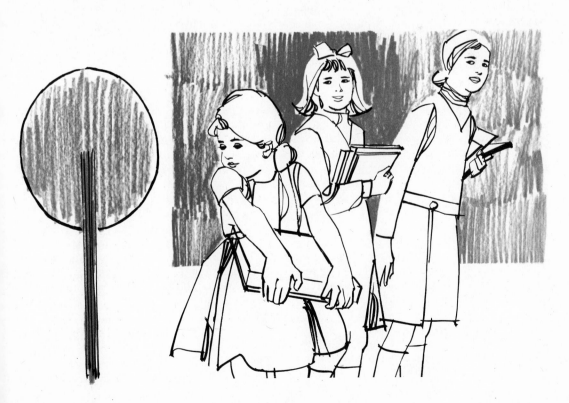

mother). It is to be expected that children meet this problem in graduated steps from early preschool years onward. At first they are usually left with relatives and for short periods of time. Also they usually remain at home and are in familiar surroundings.

A further step in this growth process is being left with persons who are not family members and for longer periods of time, but still remaining in the home. Most children can take these increased lengths of separation without feeling anxiety or distress if they are with persons they know and trust. The important point for parents to emphasize is that they will return at a stated time, such as before supper, before bed time, or while he is asleep. The parents should be faithful in carrying out their promises.

The real test as to whether the child can be satisfactorily separated from his parents comes when he starts school. Here the child leaves both his mother and his home. Also he has to accept both a new authority and forced association with children who are strangers to him. Fortunately for the child, his parents and his preschool playmates have almost certainly made him aware that this experience is coming, that it has been faced without harm by other children before him, and that he has little to fear. He should certainly be told how he will enjoy school experiences, how much he will learn, and how proud his parents will be when he goes to school.

There is one possible aspect of separation fear of which many parents are unaware. Most parents go to great lengths to allay any fears that the child may have relative to what may happen to him in school. But they fail to assure the child that everything and everybody will be all right *at home* while he is in school. Some children with mild or severe anxieties may worry most as to what possible dangers might beset mother or younger brothers or sisters at home. Parents can alleviate this anxiety by quiet, sincere, but definite reassurance as to their own safety (and lack of loneliness) when the child leaves them.

A major task of the school-age child is to learn to control and sublimate his aggressive drives. Generally, control of the child's aggressive drives develops by steps or stages whereby he gradually impersonalizes these drives. These drives were initially person-directed—that is, toward frustrating individuals or even toward himself—but now they must slowly but definitely be modified in both aim and object. Soon they are directed toward things and objects,

and eventually toward ideas and ideologies which are a justifiable target for the child's hostility. Finally these drives have as their end the child's desire for mastery of both himself and his environment.

Closely allied to the control of aggressive and destructive impulses is the child's task of socialization. This refers to the ability of the child to get along with other children of his own age, to enjoy their presence, and to gain satisfaction from cooperating or competing with them in the usual childhood games and activities. The child must acquire certain personality characteristics to make this socialization effective—or to make it possible at all.

In the first place he must develop the willingness to share—share enjoyments with others and share playthings and toys. Much of this ability to share is established in the child at home with his brothers and sisters. That is, it is established if parental guidance and insistence have made this type of behavior the only type that is acceptable to them.

Secondly, the socialization of the child can really begin—or be expanded and enriched—only after the child has learned that in the long run his greatest satisfactions in play will come if he understands the need to follow rules. He must learn that alteration of rules for his own benefit will only result in spoiling his fun.

Both the home and the community can help in teaching socialization by providing group activities. Clubs, recreation areas, cub scouts, and the like—should be supervised so as to ensure a child's acceptance, his desired and deserved participation, and his protection.

The fourth major task that confronts the school-age child is to develop the drive and the essential habits for learning. The motivation to learn, the joy in the satisfaction of curiosity, competence in learning—plus the freedom to achieve in competition with other children of his own age level—constitute a very complex bit of behavior. These complexities still baffle experts in education and child psychology.

However, we do know that parental attitudes both toward learning and toward education itself—and parental attitudes toward their own child as one who is able to learn—are very important in establishing the child's attitude toward schoolwork. They establish within the child a feeling of competence and an assurance of his ability to learn. Expressed negative attitudes toward learning or the child's learning ability will hinder the child's attempts to develop habits that are so necessary in learning.

CHAPTER FIVE

BAD HABITS IN GOOD CHILDREN

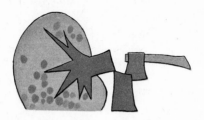

PARENTS WILL MAKE few mistakes if they realize that children are almost never either "good" or "bad." Any child may at times be fidgety, nervous, disorderly, hostile, mean, bullying, inattentive, daydreaming, or excessively timid. Although there is rarely a single cause which can explain anything so complex as a child's behavior, anyone dealing with children must be willing to seek and understand the reasons behind it.

Parents have every reason to be somewhat confused about discipline since so many "experts" in the past generation have proffered different or conflicting advice. One group who held sway for a while preached the old philosophy of "spare the rod and spoil the child." Then along came another group who seemed to say the opposite. These experts would have parents feel that they should be very "permissive" and should rarely keep children from doing anything that they want to do.

More recently, experts in child care have tended to follow a more sensible, middle-of-the-road approach which encourages love and affection and, at the same time, maintains reasonable discipline and respect for authority. It is this philosophy that governs the following advice on meeting certain common problems of child behavior

Feeding and Bowel Problems

When Bobby was a month old his mother complained that he was constipated. His bowels moved only once daily, and at times he would even miss his daily evacuation but for the help furnished by the mother. As a rule the baby was given a suppository, and if this did not produce results, a laxative of some sort was used.

Her physician advised that there was little harm in letting an infant miss one or even two days since the baby ate only liquids and there might not be enough stool to afford the stim-

ulus necessary to produce an evacuation. The mother, however, had read books and pamphlets on infant care, and she insisted that her boy's bowels must move twice—or at least once —every day. If this did not occur voluntarily, she would use force.

Eventually, the mother was prevailed on to offer the boy a chance for intestinal independence. The agreement was based on physiologic principles which, the young mother readily admitted, sounded plausible.

Most babies go through a period of what is often taken for constipation. The stool represents the residue of undigested food and a certain portion of intestinal secretion. By a series of muscle contractions in the walls of the intestines, this mass of unused material is moved slowly down to the rectum. In this area the bulk ultimately sets up a stimulus to the muscles guarding the opening of the rectum, the anal sphincter, and by the aid of contraction of the abdominal muscles the stool is finally propelled outward. It becomes clear therefore that bowel evacuation is a complex physiologic mechanism involving the presence of residue, the contraction of muscles, and the production and transmission of nerve stimuli.

The young infant's diet consists mainly of milk—an almost completely digestible food with little residue. The intestinal secretions are small in amount and the intestinal muscles are thin and comparatively feeble in their contractions. The nerve endings are not fully mature and are therefore slow in transmitting impulses. Thus it is illogical to assume that when an infant does not have a bowel movement every day he is constipated. Constipation in older babies does exist and is usually the result of indiscriminate use of laxatives, suppositories, or enemas in early infancy when there is little justification and practically no need for forcing.

Bobby, at the age of six months, appeared to enjoy the tumult produced by his constipation, and so he cultivated it to the point where he would rather suffer than give it up. It took a complete change of attitude from obsession to indifference on the part of his mother to correct this pernicious habit of "holding back" the stool in order to command sympathy and attention. By means of a sound feeding regimen and discontinuation of cathartics and other uncalled-for procedures, the problem was solved. At the age of eight months, Bobby had his "natural movement."

His mothers's satisfaction, alas, was of short duration. Those who deal with the vagaries of childhood are often impressed with the tendency of one undesirable habit to follow another.

At nine months, Bobby's mother began to complain, "He eats like a bird; I don't know what he lives on." Up to this time Bobby's record had shown no complaints about his eating habits, with the exception of one remark when he was seven months old that he did not relish string beans and refused mashed carrots.

In the healthy baby, refusal to eat can almost invariably be accounted for on the basis of a dislike for one particular food. Mothers fail to realize that in forcing a child to take this objectionable item they show stubbornness far less justified than that of which they accuse the infant. The baby in his turn is shown an excellent example of inconsiderateness on the part of his attendant, and at the same time he seizes the opportunity of making himself important by not eating. He soon learns to associate eating with fighting, and it affords him no small degree of success in matching his wits against those whom he can so easily defeat emotionally.

However, few children extend their fast to the point of appreciable loss in weight. A child who loses weight through not eating demands careful investigation; it is not merely a bad eating habit. Persistent refusal of food accompanied by a loss in weight indicates a departure from health.

It does not take much for a child to vomit. Practically every infant goes through a stage when spitting up or regurgitation occurs with great frequency. The recumbent position of the child, the nearness of the stomach to the mouth, and the shape of the stomach itself offer a condition which makes vomiting easy. At times, particularly when the stomach is overfull, the excess simply runs out. By the time the baby is several months old he has had ample experience in giving back food. It is therefore not uncommon to find youngsters who utilize vomiting as a weapon wherewith to muster all the attention available.

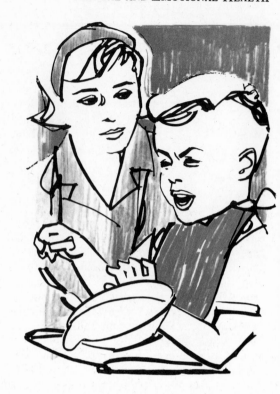

Furthermore, the nervous system of the young child is rather immature, and it needs but a small stimulus to induce expulsion of the stomach's contents. Every mother is acquainted with the frequency of vomiting as the initial symptom of almost any acute disease of childhood. Thus it is that vomiting usually commands a high premium for the child who is inclined to take advantage of the process; and to the baby it does not appear as an unpleasant indulgence. So far as is known, babies do not experience the nausea and sick feeling that precede vomiting among grown-ups.

An exception is repeated forceful vomiting with loss of weight, often accompanied by visible waves of muscular contraction in the abdomen. This may indicate an obstruction in the stomach; it requires immediate medical attention.

Rumination

Among the serious habits occasionally encountered in babies is rumination. The habit usually starts around the fourth month of infancy and may accompany or follow a period of vomiting due to some abnormal condition of the stomach. It occurs most often in poorly nourished, unhappy babies, although it may be seen in a thriving infant.

Ruminating begins within a few minutes after feeding, when the baby proceeds to suck his fingers. The suction pressure thus produced brings the liquid food up to the throat, and gargle-like sounds result from the back and forth movements of the tongue splashing against the contents of the throat. The food soon oozes out of the mouth, and the finger sucking is repeated until the entire feeding is thus spilled. Prolonged indulgence in this habit often leads to severe malnutrition and unless vigorous control is exercised, serious consequences may follow.

Rumination should not be confused with regurgitation. Most young babies regurgitate or spit up a small part of their feeding. Regurgitation is a harmless condition and is due to an overfilling of the infant's small stomach. It is simply the excess of food which runs out. It is not retained in the throat or in the mouth. In rumination, on the other hand, the food is purposely sucked up into the throat and is utilized as an unhealthy form of play.

While early in the course of this condition the habit may be corrected with comparative ease, later corrective methods become extremely difficult, involving not only careful medical supervision but also complicated appliances for restraint. Needless to say, an infant who shows a tendency to rumination calls for action and vigilance at the time the habit first appears. He should never be given the opportunity of becoming an expert at the task.

Since the bringing up of the food involves fist or finger sucking as the first prerequisite to the mechanism, it becomes evident that any attempt to stop rumination must include restraint of the hands. In the infant this is not difficult. A stiff cardboard splinted at the elbow is usually all that is necessary to prevent sucking of fingers. In the early stages of rumination this is all that is required. Obviously, strict attention must be paid to eliminate every possible underlying factor, particularly conditions producing irritation to the stomach.

Dirt Eating

Dirt eating, or pica, is another bad habit sometimes encountered in good babies. The word "pica" comes from the Latin and refers to a bird that eats everything unfit for food—a magpie.

Among young children the habit of putting everything in the mouth is well known. The reason for this is that in infancy the mouth is the main organ of tactile (touch) sensing. As the child grows and learns to rely on other means of mental communication, the hand-to-mouth method of judgment diminishes, and by the time the first year is ended the mouth is largely abandoned as a tactile organ. In some mild degree, however, the habit of placing things in the mouth persists among many children and even some adults.

Dirt eating among children is a different matter. It is not only a bad habit, but a habit which at times may lead to serious consequences. There are many cases on record of children being poisoned through this indulgence. Pica involves more than mere ingestion of earthy matter. It implies the swallowing of all things unfit to eat. Aside from being repulsive, the repeated swallowing of hair and other indigestible objects not infrequently causes actual obstruction of the stomach or the intestines. Reports have been made of numerous cases of lead poisoning in children who ate paint chips off household furniture and woodwork. An example of pica is a three-year-old girl with intestinal obstruction caused by eating mud pies.

While many little dirt eaters are not particular about the nature of the dirt they may imbibe, others are quite exacting in their taste. Thus one baby nibbles at each object within reach, whereas another limits his attack to the geranium pot and will not touch the dirt in the adjacent fernery.

Although swallowing of all sorts of bizarre objects is commonly seen among the insane, young children afflicted with this bad habit are not necessarily mentally unbalanced. Indeed some authorities state that in the majority of instances these children are unusually bright. In any case, the mental status of the child has little bearing on this unesthetic indulgence.

Physicians are agreed on the type of child susceptible to pica. Generally speaking, the condition is found in physically and emotionally inferior children. Many have rickets of active or latent degree. Many show marked evidence of malnutrition. Practically all of them have poor color and present other indications of anemia in mild or severe form. Many present a history of stomach or bowel disturbances. They are practically always an oversensitive, unhappy lot.

It was once thought, and with some justification, that dirt eating was brought about by mineral deficiencies in the child's diet. While there are undoubtedly many children who suf-

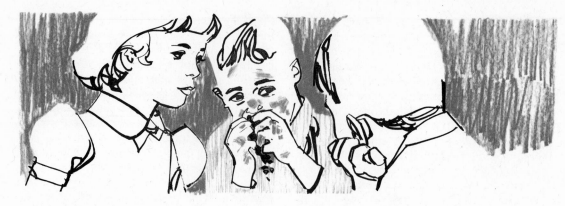

fer from shortage of certain essential elements, dirt eating is now generally recognized as a bad habit based on a perversion of the normal appetite.

As in all undesirable childhood behavior, prevention is the best cure. Any tendency on the part of the infant to indulge in pica is best stopped early by using effective disciplinary measures. Most babies who eat everything that is not food simply do not know any better. Time and experience will teach them food discrimination.

Obviously any child who is given to indulging in pica needs a thorough physical examination. Whether malnutrition is the cause or the result of this perversion of appetite is merely of academic interest. Practically all reports indicate that improvement in the nutritional state of the child is invariably accompanied by corresponding reduction in the practice.

Crying

During the early days of a baby's life, his wants are limited to basic needs: food, water, a comfortable bed, dry clothing, and other factors that contribute to his ease. If he is unsatisfied with his status, crying usually brings a change for the better. As he grows, life becomes more complex, and his desires begin to branch out. Gradually he becomes conscious of things about him. He is no longer satisfied with mere physical comforts. He begins to demand attention. But he cannot say just what is on his mind—he has neither the words nor even the image of his desires. He simply cries on the chance that someone may understand his social needs in the same way they did his physical requirements.

The mother who can recognize a legitimate cry seldom has to contend with crying as a problem. The normal infant quickly senses the limitations of crying as a means of ruling those about him. In contrast to this type of mother is the one who rushes to the crib alarmed and wondering what can be the cause of the tears. She suspects hunger in spite of a steady gain in weight. She suspects colic even though there are no gastrointestinal upsets. She suspects every illness it is possible for a child to have, in spite of the fact that a sick baby seldom cries loudly and practically never cries long.

She picks the baby up. He has won a victory and stops crying. He is put back in his crib, and the crying starts again and keeps up until the whole household—including baby—is exhausted. He falls asleep, but is too tired to rest for any length of time. Crying is soon resumed, only more vigorously after the rest.

Why do some babies cry all night and comparatively little during the day? The answer is simple. During the day the baby receives all the attention he wants and probably a good deal more than he needs. He feels that those who treasure him are close to him, are conscious of him in their waking hours. He knows that he receives ample attention even though he is asleep.

Normally, a baby does not cry when he has all that he wants. But at night, when his parents are asleep, he feels less sure of his status. So he utilizes the technique he acquired early in infancy—crying—and it usually brings results.

Psychologists have learned that in babies the making of sounds is associated with the movement of arms, hands, legs, and feet. During the crying spell a baby will throw his arms in all directions and kick his feet. Is it not strange then, that as the child reaches the age when crying is considered "baby-like" or "sissy-like," that the crying habit simply changes to bullying, pugnacity, or destructiveness. The original habit pattern for commanding attention is merely taking on a new form.

Parents faced with the crying habit must come to understand its underlying principles. Realizing that a continuous loud cry in a healthy baby is a demand for oversolicitude, they must quietly and tactfully—yet with determination—adopt the attitude that their child must simply learn to respect the comforts of the other members of the household. It takes but a few nights of judicious indifference to let the baby know you're on to him.

Thumb Sucking

Practically every baby is a potential thumb sucker. Indeed one seldom sees a young infant who at one time or another does not put his thumb in his mouth. Until the age of six weeks or two months the infant is not aware of his thumb. He does not recognize it as a part of his own body.

Gradually, after much gazing at the fingers on his hand, he ventures to find out something of the nature of these objects by sticking them in his mouth. Anatomically, in early infancy the four fingers of the hand move as a unit; the thumb is the only independent member of the hand. It is naturally easier to put the thumb in a small mouth than it is to insert the whole fist. Some babies, however, do even that.

Psychologically as well as physiologically, the mouth is a highly important part of the body. The importance lies in the fact that the mouth affords pleasure from the moment life begins. Through the mouth the infant takes food to appease his hunger and water to quench his thirst. As he grows, he is gratified to hear his own cooing or crying or babbling sounds. What is of particular significance is a mucous membrane on the lips which possesses highly specialized and sensitive nerve endings, stimulation of which produces pleasurable sensations.

In the adult, this zone is associated with sexual feeling and some parents relate the innocent pleasure of thumb sucking to unnatural sexual activity. The gravity with which such parents view thumb sucking usually makes them overanxious and their overanxiety gives their child an effective method for attaining attention.

Not infrequently, vigorous restraints on thumb sucking bring about lip sucking. The baby simply uses his upper or lower lip to exert suction pressure with his cheeks. Interestingly, we often encounter mothers who though shocked at the thumb sucking habit, do not hesitate to give the baby a pacifier or a teething ring which serves the same purpose.

In the opinion of most pediatricians, the deforming results accruing from thumb sucking have been unduly exaggerated except in extreme cases. It is true that when the habit is persistent and of long duration, an outward displacement of the teeth and a pushing out of the upper lip may take place. However, in the majority of cases if the parents approach the problem sensibly, the habit is soon abandoned. Simple diversion of the child's interest through suitable toys or play will usually accomplish more in the way of prevention than any restraining method in existence.

During the child's early infancy the mother is at times justified in tying a cardboard cuff around his elbows if the thumb sucking is too annoying. Generally, however, few babies would be afflicted with this habit if mothers and fathers had a saner attitude toward the normal expressions of the normal infant. The child who is physically healthy, mentally alert, and emotionally happy is seldom a trouble maker. Bad habits are often forced on a young child through misguided solicitude.

Undesirable acts become habits only when parents or other attendants place a premium on these acts. Thus most older babies and young children resort to thumb sucking only when they are tired or unhappy. Repeated exhortations and warnings and punishments for this diversion serve only to stress the power that the youngster possesses over those about him. He would be abnormal if at this early, unreasoning age he did not take advantage of such power.

Head Rolling

While crying and thumb sucking are natural phenomena and represent necessary steps in physical and mental development, head rolling and other unsightly head movements usually start from some irritative cause. Rickets, a common disorder of infancy, is probably the most frequent underlying factor in the production of the head rolling habit. At times, and this is particularly true of rickets in mild form, the disease is not even suspected because the symptoms may be so indefinite that the mother often attributes them to teething, hunger, or some other vague condition.

One of the early manifestations of rickets is sweating about the forehead. It is readily conceivable that the baby, dissatisfied with the perspiration, will turn his head from side to side in an effort to wipe the moisture on the pillow or the sheet. This procedure brings relief, and the child learns quickly to repeat the process when his forehead becomes moist. Also his restlessness brings attention from those who are not particularly pleased with this activity. He has found a new way of commanding attention, and he will hold to it as long as it remains effective.

Head rolling may also start as a result of faulty focusing of the eye muscles. In such cases the baby attempts to fix the eye on some object of interest to him, and tries to follow it by shifting his head from side to side. Placing a bright toy in front of the baby, as mothers often do to occupy his interest, not infrequently results in this habit.

Shyness and Stubbornness

Shyness in a grown-up person is an undesirable trait, always difficult and sometimes impossible to overcome. In the young child it is merely a bad habit, rather easily corrected, once the underlying cause is discovered and removed. It is important, however, to distinguish between shyness and indifference in the child; but this is not always a simple matter.

A four-year-old boy did not care to play with other children. According to his mother he was a "model boy" and had never caused any trouble from the day he was born. He was a bit slow to be sure, but he took after his father, the

mother hastened to explain. This child had a mild deficiency of the thyroid gland.

Appropriate treatment administered daily brought about an almost immediate cure for his "shyness." He is now eight years old and is doing fair work in the third grade in school. He is still taking the treatment. With the large majority of children, however, shyness is usually traceable to lack of understanding of the sensibilities of the growing child.

Some parents, unconsciously more concerned about their own personal importance than about their child's social progress, still cling to the Victorian dictum, "A child should be seen, not heard," and do not permit the youngster to enter into family discussions. The child no sooner opens his mouth than he is warned, "Daddy is talking." Constant reproval brings about an attitude of "What's the use?" Some parents make a fetish of obedience in protest against the "fad of the new freedom." Others are fearful of allowing their children to roam at large lest they may mix with undesirable elements in the neighborhood.

It should not be assumed that the child be reared without any sense of discipline. It is indeed well to implant the idea that the children in the household must learn to conform to the ideals and comforts of the entire family. One must remember however that neither conformity nor respect can be taught by exhortation or by squelching the youngster's desire for self-expression. The child should be encouraged to

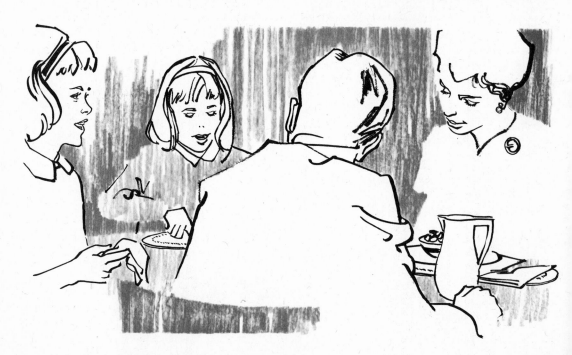

enter family discussions. His remarks, regardless of immaturity of judgment or misuse of words, should never be ridiculed. He must feel that he is a part of the family circle.

His inexperience in etiquette may make him a mild nuisance on occasion; but as he grows, he will acquire the finesse of conversation in accordance with the custom of his elders. The child learns by imitation. People who are anxious about the behavior of their offspring must recognize that the philosophy of the child is that of simplicity and frankness. Only in that light must his conduct be judged.

One occasionally meets the other extreme—the parents enthusiastic about the "new psychology." They allude to the three-year-old as the "little man" and give him as much freedom of action as if he were physically and mentally able to take care of himself. These pathetic little men go about with an exaggerated idea of their importance, lording it over their "inferiors" with scorn and derision. At times one jolt is sufficient to cause these premature adults to shrink back into their shell, taking with them their grievances and grudges. They often become the daydreamers in the classroom.

To sensitive parents every child, at one time or another, is a problem. Mothers and fathers with an inclination to make mountains out of molehills appear to be constantly at sea, worrying over methods and procedures to direct their child in the paths acceptable to society. They make sacrifices of every description to afford their offspring everything within—and too often above—their means, often with disheartening results. Their anxieties make their children anxious.

The child's attitude toward strangers must be interpreted broadmindedly. There is little justification for expecting a child to go into ecstasy over the approach of some one whom he neither knows nor probably cares to know. At times a child may be indeed terror-stricken by an overexuberant stranger who thinks it his duty to administer "a big hug."

Most children show a certain degree of diffidence or perhaps bashfulness toward strangers. This attitude is not due to lack of sociability on the part of the child, but rather to a lack of interest or mutual understanding. Shyness develops slowly. It builds as the result of exaggeration on the part of the parents and others.

If the trait is drilled into him over a period of time—with the great amount of attention usually connected with undesirable behavior—the child will cultivate it, and it truly becomes a characteristic. He is known as shy and afraid of strangers. At first he is looked on as a sensitive or nervous child. Gradually he becomes a problem in personality.

While shyness evokes parental sympathy as a rule, stubbornness usually produces frank displeasure and not infrequently even open hostility. Indeed, of all bad habits to which the child may be addicted, none is so intolerable to parents as stubbornness. That a child should challenge adult authority is a direct insult not easily overlooked and practically never condoned. Yet, stubbornness is nearly always provoked by the parents themselves.

A child is born neither shy nor stubborn. These undesirable qualities are generally forced on him by grown-ups. Shyness often develops when parents endeavor to inculcate excessive sociability, and stubborness when they attempt to teach obedience. Both traits are maintained by the youngster for the purpose of commanding attention and power—shyness by the sympathy which it invokes, stubbornness by the enduring contest in an uneven match.

Some children are by nature quiet, perhaps in the same way that some are thin and others stocky. To push a quiet child into boisterousness is as illogical as to overfeed a thin baby in an attempt to make him stocky. The latter procedure works havoc with the digestive system; the former is productive of emotional upsets, usually resulting in shyness.

A 15-year-old boy ran away from home in an effort to avoid constant nagging about his "shyness." He was a quiet, studious youngster, with a philosophic turn of mind.

Everything went smoothly until his mother decided to round out his interests. From then on the boy had no peace. He had to join the "Y" and learn to box. He would come home black and blue from bruises on his body. He had to go to school dances, though he hated girls and felt clumsy on the floor. His mother spent hours studying child psychology; and the longer she studied, the graver the problem loomed. All her son was interested in was writing poetry and reading the classics. What was to become of him?

One afternoon, instead of going to his boxing class, he hailed a west-bound motorist—and was finally returned under police escort from a neighboring city. The boy is now instructor in English literature in one of the state universities. He is still a poor boxer and, his wife asserts, a clumsy dancer.

But most children who have shyness drilled into them do not end up so fortunately, probably because they do not have an enhanced intellectual capacity to compensate for their shortcomings. As a rule, the longer we talk about the youngster's shyness, the better he likes it.

As for stubbornness, parents who complain about their youngsters are reminiscent of a cartoon of a man pulling at the halter on a mule, urging the animal onward in no uncertain terms. The mule, in stance befitting his species, carried the cartoonist's philosophic inscription, "My, what a stubborn man!"

Bladder Control

"The child wets the bed." The only complaint that is heard with greater frequency is, "He won't eat." Often, indeed, these two bad habits occur together. Like all unnatural behavior, enuresis is a product of civilization. It will undoubtedly remain a problem as long as our social culture continues to regulate the natural functions of man.

Before discussing bedwetting as a habit, however, it must be stated that from 12 to 15 per cent of the problem children present organic reasons for their enuresis. Many have structural defects of the genito-urinary system which easily account for the inability of the youngster to control his output; a few have diabetes of one form or another. Every child with enuresis is entitled to a thorough examination with the aid of all modern methods to determine that his bedwetting is a bad habit and not a symptom of disease.

Many children wet their beds from physical exhaustion. This is particularly true of the thin, underweight boys and girls who play too hard and too long, taking little time off to eat and practically none to rest. They remain at play from early morning until late at night. When their tired muscles finally relax, the bladder opening also relaxes and the urine flows out. This type of enuresis is easily cured, once the child's activities are restricted to his optimum capacity by an afternoon rest period and early retiring. This should be supplemented by better eating habits and encouragement. Mild sedatives are often necessary during the initial period of treatment.

Among untold thousands of healthy young children enuresis is a carry-over from infancy and represents an unreadiness of the child to control bladder evacuation. No training can be expected to hasten the maturity of this physiological mechanism. The fact is that overzealous parental attempts to secure a dry bed do more to delay than accelerate control. However, there is no objection to putting the child on the toilet seat three times daily to familiarize him with the use of the toilet.

The average two-year-old child empties his bladder 7 times in 24 hours. It is wise to make liberal allowances for individual variations and express no concern if the child wets the bed occasionally until he is three and one-half or four years old. At this age, five emptyings a day constitute an average.

If bedwetting continues beyond this age, it is well to study the elimination habits of the youngster and have him examined physically, including the analysis of his urine. Nagging the child about his bedwetting or shaming him is never advisable. In fact, it leads to the establishment of enuresis as a habit because of the attention that it brings. It is well at this early time to consider dispassionately the emotional status of the child and to do all that is reasonable in order to afford the youngster a maximum of happiness.

It is generally accepted that enuresis seldom develops in children who are happy. This is the case in spite of the fact that most youngsters thus approached deny any disagreeable feature in their environment. As a rule the child himself is unaware, consciously at least, of the situation or situations which bring about and maintain the annoying habit. Every youngster who wets the bed considers himself most unfortunate, and there is nothing that he would not do to overcome it. Many boys and girls remain in bed late in the morning in the vain hope of drying the traces with their little bodies.

Whether enuresis is a means of drawing attention or a defense reaction or a reversion to infantile pleasure, whether one or a number of such psychological phenomena are involved, experience has shown that the habitual bedwetter has ample cause for discontent in his surroundings.

Many cases of enuresis may be traced to parental bickerings. Some are quite apparent, even if mothers and fathers refuse to recognize them as such. One of the prominent causes common to all behavior disorders is a feeling of insecurity. Another is jealousy, especially by a child of a new brother or sister. Parental overanxiety often brings on the habit.

Of all the types of enuresis, none is so resistant to treatment as that in which there is an alleged hereditary tendency to the condition. In spite of evidence to the contrary, there are still many thousands of people who believe that bedwetting is handed down from one generation to the next. Recently a 14-year-old girl was troubled with a skin ailment. Her mother objected to the physician's questions about the child's bladder habits. Bedwetting, she insisted, "runs in the family." She herself had enuresis until she was married. Her sister, now 20 years old, has never dared to sleep away from home and missed going to college because of this handicap. A brother, a senior in high school, wets the bed practically every night. "It can't be a bad habit with all of us. It is simply a family curse." The mother cannot comprehend that faulty training may be the common factor underlying this curse. Her attitude remains: "You cannot fool nature."

Then there is the child who starts on his career of wetting the bed during an acute illness. It is not unusual to find that mothers in those cases build a veritable complex centering around the child's "weak kidneys." Jerry Fowler was trained to the nursery chair when he was less than a year old. He had not wet the bed for over five years. At six years of age, Jerry had measles. Complications set in, necessitating bed care for over two months. He had excellent nursing care but could never become reconciled to the use of the bed pan. The nurse was obliged to carry him to the toilet in order to make elimination possible. During the fever stage of the disease he would wet the bed only on rare occasions. Convalescence was slow. Bedwetting became frequent. The boy was ashamed and unhappy at first. So were the parents. To allay his worries his mother would say, "It isn't your fault; you are weak and run down."

At the age of eight years, Jerry was a bright, well-developed lad in excellent physical condition. All kidney function tests were normal. Asked whether he was happy, he mumbled, "I guess so, but I have weak kidneys."

From here on, Mrs. Fowler took up the discussion, and a sadder story is seldom heard. Her son had always been neat and clean and self reliant until this trouble set in. Even now he is a model boy, studious, obedient, considerate of his parents. "But the questions the child asks are maddening: Mother, why do I have to be sick? Mother, do you think I'll ever get well? Mother, what if I should....." The last sentence was too horrifying to complete.

It was obvious that mother and son were playing an exquisite drama with reciprocal torture as the central theme. Mrs. Fowler appeared unbelievably blissful in her despair. Jerry enjoyed complete happiness in his kidney weakness. Fortunately the heroine was finally convinced that the infirmity responsible for the theatrical reaction was no more real than the stage on which the performance was being enacted.

A sensible attitude brought about early but slow improvement. Several months later, Mrs. Fowler reported that Jerry had not wet the bed for over two weeks, "And if I understand my boy, he won't wet for a long time." Smiling with confidence she said. "Because my 'leading man' hates to wash and dry bed sheets, especially on cold winter mornings."

Sleep Disturbances

Until he is a month old, the average infant sleeps a total of 22 out of 24 hours. Premature infants, for several weeks after birth, are awake only during the time when they are fed. These long hours of sleep are necessary so that the nervous system may gain the opportunity to adapt itself to independent functioning. At birth the nerve sheaths are incompletely formed and some of these structures are poorly "insulated."

The "insulation process" takes several months. For this reason practically all infants for the first few months of life jump or startle at the slightest sound. All babies are extremely sensitive to vibration. This is a normal phenomenon, and not, as many people erroneously believe, a manifestation of nervousness. To be sure, nervous infants, like their adult counterparts, are jumpy, and at times excessively so, but the startle itself, early in life, is a sign of a normal nervous system.

As the infant grows and its nerve coverings increase in quality and amount, the periods of sleep decrease. At two months a baby usually sleeps about 20 hours out of 24. At four months he may be expected to sleep 16 to 18 hours a day, and at one year, 14 to 16 hours. There are wide variations, of course. If a child sleeps less but is happy during his waking hours, one need not be concerned. If he sleeps more, but shows normal mental reactions when awake, this, too, can be passed without worry. Babies, like adults, differ widely in the amount of sleep they require.

Young children are light sleepers. Not until they reach the stage of strenuous play do they begin to sleep soundly. Regardless of parental inability to keep up with what seems almost perpetual motion on the part of their young offspring, apparently few of these living dynamos suffer from physical or mental tiredness. Deep sleep as a rule does not develop until the age of four or five years.

Restless sleep and insomnia are not common among healthy children. There are many babies who at one year or thereabouts make it a practice to awaken in the middle of the night, crying without apparent reason. Many parents erroneously attribute this to teething. Why the teething pains abate promptly when the baby is taken into the parents' bed, they apparently do not stop to consider. The fact is that the awakening on the part of the child is merely an effort to obtain a little extra attention to which he is not at all entitled.

The only way in which this bad habit may be stopped is never to give it an opportunity to develop. The child must be made to realize from the beginning that he has not only privileges which he may enjoy, but also duties which he must fulfill. One of these duties is to respect the comfort of others.

A good practice to follow when the baby first awakens during the night is to investigate the cause. If he is thirsty, he should be given water. When he is through he should be tucked in without comment, and left alone. No child is entitled to a night feeding after the third month, except on specific advice of the physician. A baby knows the limitations of crying. He stops when he learns that it does not bring results.

Night Terror

Simple crying to obtain attention should not be confused with night terrors. These are quite common among children and occur most frequently between the ages of two to five years. The general pattern is that the child awakens suddenly after a period of sleep, varying from one to two hours, screaming and trembling with terror. He is confused and clutches at the person closest to him, though he recognizes no one. Often he breaks out in a profuse sweat. Consoling seems to have no effect on his confusion or his trembling.

The attack may last from several minutes to an hour or even longer, until the child relaxes and falls asleep again. The attack may occur once or several times during the same night. In the morning the child has no remembrance of the episode.

There are many explanations and theories regarding the cause of night terror, none of which is acceptable in its entirety. Nervousness and worms are the most popular as well as the most untenable explanations. Among physicians one theory proposes that night terrors are due to overeating preceeding bedtime. Another attributes them to a disturbance in carbohydrate metabolism.

According to a third theory the trouble is caused by partial asphyxia, resulting from large tonsils and overgrown adenoid tissue. Although the last two theories seem unrelated, functionally they bear the same significance in that carbohydrates play an important part in tissue oxidation. Some of these children respond favorably after a light evening meal, while others obtain relief from carbohydrate feeding before bedtime, and others show improvement with the removal of tonsils and adenoids.

It should be remembered, however, that many children suffering from night terrors appear to be in good physical and mental health. It is conceivable, of course, that if they lose sleep as a result of prolonged periods of night terrors, their health may ultimately suffer. Generally, however, that does not happen frequently.

A good rule to follow is to have the child examined by a physician during the beginning of the attacks, rather than wait until the child has lost weight, or until he has cultivated a fear of going to sleep in anticipation of night terrors. Some children learn before long that night terrors can be turned into an effective weapon against unsuspecting parents. Early examination and the reassurance parents receive can nip such a development in the bud.

CHAPTER SIX

SPEECH PROBLEMS

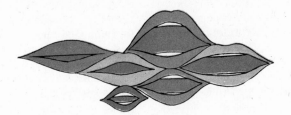

A CHILD BEGINS to acquire the skills in speech as soon as he is born. Your child is learning to talk as he sucks and swallows, belches and smiles, for the coordination he uses in these activities are also used in speech.

During the first six months the sounds your baby will make will consist mostly of crying, babbling, and vocal play. These occur as a response to pain, hunger, cold, or pleasure. A good deal of vocal play occurs when the child is alone, and this activity is important in the learning of speech. During the next six months your child will begin to understand a few words and will try to imitate them.

Between 12 and 18 months the normal child will begin to say his first meaningful words. These may sound far from perfect according to adult standards. For example, the baby may say "bah" consistently to refer in one way or another to his bottle. His saying "bah" may in some cases be a demand for food, simple recognition of his bottle, or some other meaning. He will use variations in facial expression, vocal inflection, gestures, and loudness of tone as a way of trying to communicate exactly what he means.

During his second year, the child's vocabulary grows at first slowly, and then with increasing rapidity. At 21 to 24 months of age the average infant uses combinations of words and simple sentences. By the age of three and one-half the average child is able to speak intelligibly—that is, he can be understood by persons unacquainted with him. If by this time your child does not use meaningful speech patterns you should consult with your physician.

All children experience some difficulties in learning to speak. With every child there will be occasional stammerings and other types of awkward speech. You should avoid setting too high a speech standard during the years your child is learning to talk.

Here are some ways parents can guide the speech development of normal children:

- Read stories aloud to him.
- Encourage him to talk a great deal.
- Have the child describe and interpret pictures for you.
- Take your child with you on your usual trips to the grocery store, post office, cleaner, etc. Explain in simple terms what you do there.
- Encourage the child to learn nursery rhymes, short poems and songs, especially those in which a certain sound is repeated many times.

The above suggestions, however helpful, do not guarantee that your child will not have difficulty with speech. Each child is different, and what is helpful to one may not be helpful to another. If your child appears to have difficulty

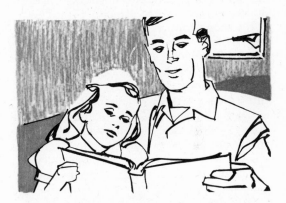

in speech although you have carried out the above suggestions for several months, consult a speech therapist or speech clinic in your area or ask your school about other sources of help for your child.

The Problem Called Stuttering

If you feel that your child stutters, you are concerned. This is perfectly natural. After all, you are a conscientious parent and you are faced with what you consider a baffling problem which deeply involves your young child. What has happened? Only a few days ago he was speaking normally and now you feel that he is stuttering. Can anything be done about it?

Fortunately, research and clinical experience in speech problems during the past 30 years have uncovered many reassuring facts. These have special meaning for you because, as you will see, you are a very important person in all this. You are a listener. And stuttering involves a listener.

Children who are considered to be stutterers are not generally abnormal or inferior. In fact, except for their speech behavior and the way they feel about it, they are so much like other children that nobody has found any way to sort them out. They are just normal, everyday, wonderful children.

Scientists have found it difficult in most cases, sometimes impossible, to see any difference between the speech of children who are *newly classified* as stutterers and the speech of other children. Just why this should be was explained by a recent study in which it was discovered that two, three, and four-year-old children repeat their words about 50 times in every 1,000 words of normal speech. No child was found who didn't repeat a little; some repeated as much as 100 times in 1,000 words. This is part of learning how to talk; as a matter of fact, adults repeat too. Just listen to yourself.

The speech of most young children who are taken by their parents to be stutterers is for the most part not unusual; it becomes unusual in some way *after* the parents begin to think of them as stutterers. In case after case, stuttering —as a serious problem—developed only after someone had decided that the child was stuttering. This judgment, or "diagnosis," in and of itself, is one of the chief causes of the stuttering problem. The judgment is made by the listener, who more often than not, is a parent, usually the mother.

Once she has attached the stuttering label to something the child does, she begins to hear all repetitions and hesitations as the thing which she has labeled them, that is, stuttering. She reacts with facial expression, tone of voice, body attitude. She disapproves because she disapproves of the label she herself has given it. The child catches her attitude; he begins to have feelings of uneasiness, of being disapproved of. He tries to do something about it. What he does, interferes with his speech even more. And the problem called stuttering begins to bloom.

It is suggested, therefore, that if a speech problem seems to be developing, first check with your family doctor to be sure that the child is in good health. Then, if he is healthy and alert, take your cue from the research find-

ings previously mentioned and try to follow these suggestions:

● Do nothing to call attention to the interruptions in speech; if your child has begun to notice them, let him know they are quite normal under the circumstances and so, of course, acceptable. You can make him self-conscious about his speech even by praising it, if you praise it too much. But err, if you must, by approving it more than is justified.

● If he hesitates in his speech more than most children do, and especially if he hesitates with strain or tension, look about him and at yourself, the rest of the family, and his playmates to find the conditions which are to blame; then do what you can to improve them. Look for situations of stress between people.

● In order to understand the problem better, try to notice the conditions under which he hesitates and repeats, the times he speaks smoothly and easily, the many ways in which he is a "regular boy," and the way other youngsters his age hesitate and repeat just as he does. There are certain conditions under which prac-

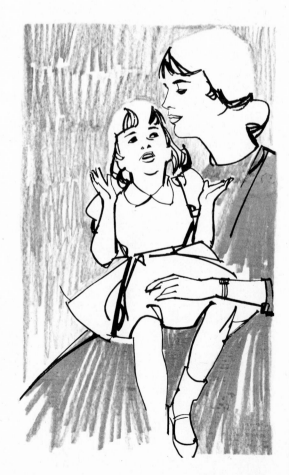

tically any child tends to speak smoothly and other conditions under which they tend to speak hesitatingly.

- Never, in talking to or about him, label him a stutterer or call his speech stuttering.
- Try to be the kind of listener a child likes to talk to; let him know that you enjoy hearing him talk; have fun talking with him and reading to him. Read to him whenever you can but never in a tense, impatient, or loud voice. Let him know that you love him.
- Try to cut down on scolding and use praise as often as you can. Try to keep things relaxed and pleasant in the home so that there isn't too much teasing or bossing around.
- Never ask him to "speak pieces" or show off his speech for anyone. That means family as well as neighbors or company.
- Finally, however drastic this may sound, try to be as friendly and considerate toward him as you would be toward a house guest.

Unless the speech problem that you and your child are in together is in some way unusual, these suggestions should prove helpful. Give them an honest trial. If, at the end of six months or so, you feel he is not talking as smoothly and as easily as he should, it is best to consult a speech clinician—preferably of course, one who is certified by the American Speech and Hearing Association, the recognized professional organization of speech pathologists and audiologists in the United States.

Your family doctor can tell you where to find one. There may be such an expert in your public school system.

Adult Stuttering

If you are an adult stutterer, you have no doubt seen yourself somewhere in the preceding paragraphs. What's more, you are to be congratulated for doing one of the most important things you can do about your problem: you have been reading, trying to get more information about it. You might also find it useful to follow the following suggestions:

- Seek out an accredited speech clinic and take advantage of the services if offers.
- Sort out your thinking about stuttering and take responsibility for it, because your stuttering is something *you do* because of your thinking about speaking and about stuttering and about yourself.
- Pay more attention to your normal speech than to what you think of as your stuttering.
- Pay enough attention to the things you do that you call stuttering to understand that they interfere with your otherwise good speech. Moreover, they are unnecessary and you can change or eliminate them.
- Do more, not less, talking.
- Work at being a "normal" speaker. Do more of the things you would be doing if you were talking "all right."

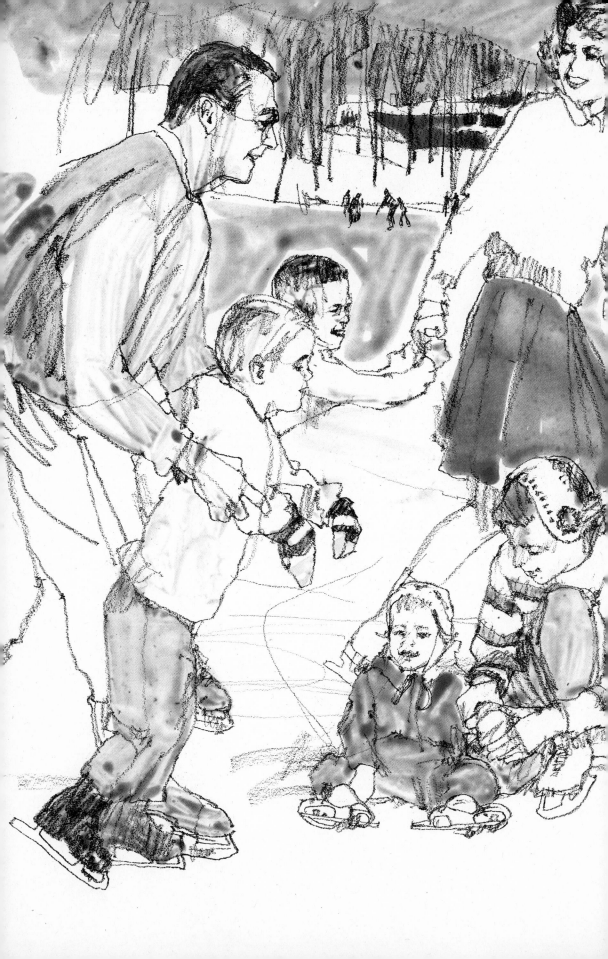

PART VI

Recreation
and Relaxation

CHAPTER ONE

PLAY AND RELAXATION

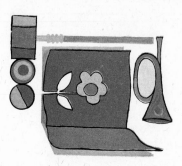

EVERY PARENT knows how important play is to the young child. Through play, he gains physical strength, develops physical skills, and establishes relationships with his parents, brothers and sisters, and friends. It has often been said that the child who does not want to play is sick and that the child who does not have a chance to play cannot grow physically and socially. But the values of play and recreation are not restricted to the young. All ages need relief from boredom, relaxation from tensions, and the self-fulfillment found in recreation. Through play, many of our most pleasant associations with other people take place. The change of pace from work and responsibility which we find in play may be as important to our health as rest.

Wholesome physical play can contribute to physical, mental, and emotional health. Recreation is not only physical activity, however. Recreation may range from active physical pursuits to quiet activities, such as reading. It may bring excitement or relaxation. It includes both solitary activities and those with groups. It may consist of long-span avocational interests or momentary pleasures, and may range from worthwhile cultural and educational pursuits to trivialities.

Satisfactions from recreation are personal. What may be satisfying to one person may seem like work to another; and what may appeal to a person at one age may bore him at another. Recreation is more a state of mind than a particular activity.

Home as a Play Center

Many agencies--governmental, voluntary, and religious—offer recreation programs. Yet the home remains the most important center, not only for recreation itself, but also for developing lifelong recreation interests, skills,

and tastes. Patterns set in the home for the use of leisure influence lifelong choices of forms of recreation. The parents' responsibility for establishing good patterns, then, is very great.

Formerly, when a large part of the population lived on farms, families were held together largely through economic necessity. Children were needed to milk the cows, care for the crops, or perform household chores. Today's city families have few home chores, and family relationships are more often cemented through play than work. Children—and parents as well—tend to drift away from homes in which they cannot play.

Homes differ tremendously in the provisions which they can make for recreation. A family with no financial worries can provide many facilities. Yards can offer gardens, children's play apparatus, game courts, swimming pools, patios, and barbecue pits. Inside the houses there can be recreation rooms, workshops, dark rooms for photography, music and television rooms, sewing rooms, and libraries. Most budgets can provide some of the above for the family's enjoyment.

Where space for recreation is lacking in the home and where money for books, supplies, and equipment is limited, there are still many opportunities for recreation. Never before have libraries, community centers, parks, voluntary agencies, schools, and religious groups made possible so many free or low-cost opportunities for families to participate in good recreation experiences.

Although schools and other community agencies teach recreation interests and skills, parents can be particularly helpful in developing desirable interests and encouraging participation in worthy leisure pursuits. Many forms of recreation can be enjoyed only if skills are developed and knowledge attained.

There is reason to believe that personality is

developed to an important extent in leisure. Young people who exhibit undesirable social behavior are often the ones who have never had the opportunity to learn how to use their leisure constructively.

Parents should observe some precautions in relation to family recreation. Recreation is only one part of life and must not be overemphasized. It takes its place with work, worship, and love as an important segment of life. Studies, work, and home responsibilities are also part of a well-balanced daily regime. In many communities so many organizations and activities compete for our leisure that careful selection must be made by both children and adults.

All recreation time should not be used for family activities. Each member of the family should have time for individual pursuits or for participation with others of his own age group.

Care must be taken that members of the family do not become addicted to watching television, listening to the radio, or reading frivolous books. These passive forms of recreation must be kept within limits so that they do not crowd out activities that require vigorous mental or physical participation.

What Parents Can Do

For purposes of convenience, we place home recreation activities in various categories. It will be noticed, however, that many overlappings occur.

Every home should provide good magazines and books. With libraries almost everywhere, good reading is available to young and old. Reading aloud, especially at bedtime, is a cherished tradition in many families.

Parents can encourage children to write letters to friends and relatives, keep diaries, or express their thoughts and feelings through original poems or prose. Memorizing poetry may give a measure of satisfaction which will increase with passing years.

Enjoyable conversation, particularly at meal time and shared by all members of the family, contributes to good family relationships as well as to social graces and education. Children are imitators; good grammar, clear enunciation, and a wide vocabulary used by the parents will help the children in their use of language more effectively than constant correction.

Dramatics has its place in home activities. Charades, puppet plays, and original plays written and produced by the children are excellent activities.

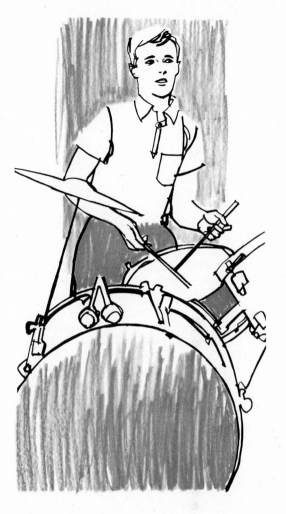

Fortunate is the child whose parents give a willing ear to his fumbling efforts to make music, and encourage his progress. Music enters the home also through listening to good recordings, singing with a group around the piano, singing lullabies to the baby, and playing instruments together. Singing while working makes household chores lighter and dispositions happier. Parents can encourage high standards in music without being stuffy.

Many a happy hour can be spent in various forms of art, ranging from finger painting, crayon coloring, and drawing for the younger members of the family to oil painting, wood carving, and ceramics for the older ones. If space and money permit, a shop for woodworking makes possible the construction of useful objects, adding a practical aspect to esthetic enjoyment.

Weaving need not be limited to homes where large looms may be installed. Children enjoy hand looms on which they can make potholders and mats or looms on which they can make beaded belts. Knitting, sewing, embroidery, crocheting, and basket weaving are additional possibilities for home recreation.

Photography may begin with a five-dollar camera for the young and proceed to a complicated art for the elders. Developing the film and printing the picture is more than half the fun.

Home-improvement projects, such as redecorating a room, offer numerous possibilities for employing the artistic talents of the family.

Fishing, swimming, hiking, gardening, and many other outdoor activities in which families can participate together are discussed elsewhere in this book. To these can be added picnics, cookouts, and camping. Family camping, which has mounted in popularity in recent years, is both a means of seeing new places at small cost and of learning about and appreciating the natural world. Many communities now have family camping clubs through which families learn how and where to camp and what to take on a trip. Excellent books on the subject are available in most libraries.

The backyard may accommodate equipment for badminton, croquet, horseshoes, archery, darts, and many other games which can be played by both young and old, as well as swings, slides, and sandboxes for the children. Jigsaw puzzles, table tennis, cards and numerous table games, many with educational values, add to indoor enjoyment. Many games which require no special equipment are suggested in books on games.

A whole family can share in the pleasure of a collection. Space should be allotted in the home for the display of collected items, be they rocks, shells, leaves, buttons, dishes, or less bulky items such as coins and stamps. Satisfactions from collections are multiplied by learning about the items collected and by arranging the collection logically and attractively. Books and magazines relating to the hobby are choice gifts to family members.

The joys of birthdays, wedding anniversaries, Christmas, Easter, Thanksgiving, Halloween, and other holidays are enhanced when the entire family engages in preparation for them. Special decorations, foods, music, and games can enhance these events.

Other special events, such as graduations, promotions, winning of awards, and similar occasions give the family an opportunity to express its pleasure and pride in the honored one. Events shared with friends, if possible, add to the festivity.

Leisure activities are powerful forces in the home. They can cement family ties, create wholesome attitudes, and foster understanding among members of the family. They can open up new fields of learning and awaken interests which will not only enrich personal life, but may lead to future vocations for the younger members of the family. Many an avocational interest has turned into a career.

CHAPTER TWO

SPORTS AND PHYSICAL FITNESS

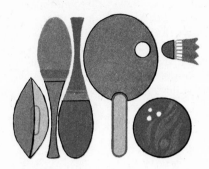

RECREATIONAL ACTIVITIES of all kinds, including sports, contribute greatly to our enjoyment of life. Recreational activities which involve exercise promote physical fitness when they are performed regularly, and the maintenance of physical fitness is an important factor in the maintenance of health.

Schools and colleges recognize that physical education is an important part of a general education. The period of life when we go to school is for most of us the time when we take the most exercise. The problem is to continue throughout our later life a degree of exercise that will help us to maintain a state of good physical fitness and good health.

Exercise and Fitness

Vigorous physical activity helps to develop muscles, and physical strength makes an important contribution to daily activities. Once developed, strength can be easily maintained with little diminution for many years. More importantly, the heart is a muscle. It is strengthened and improved in its function by any form of strenuous exertion. Exercise also enables the lungs to increase their ability to take in air and to utilize more efficiently the oxygen which they extract from this air.

All levels of activity depend on the capacity of one's heart, blood vessels, and lungs to perform with maximum efficiency. And in general, the harder the work, the greater will be the benefit to the body. One way to determine the relative demands which different kinds of exercise place on the body is to compare the number of calories which the body must burn each minute to support these exercises. The calorie is a unit of heat used to measure energy in studies of metabolism and physical activity.

The following table shows calories burned per minute for common recreational sports.

Sport	Cal/min.
Canoeing (2.5 mph)	3.0
Horseback riding (walking gait)	3.0
Volleyball	3.5
Walking (2.5 mph)	3.6
Bowling	4.5
Cycling (5.5 mph)	4.5
Golfing	5.0
Swimming (20 yd/min)	5.0
Rowing (2.5 mph)	5.0
Walking (3.75 mph)	5.6
Skating	6.0
Table Tennis	6.0
Tennis	7.1
Water Skiing	8.0
Horseback riding (trotting gait)	8.0
Skiing	9.9
Squash	10.2
Cycling (13 mph)	11.0
Rowing (race speed)	14.0
Running (10 mph)	15.0

All of the above sports can be played individually with the exception of volleyball, table tennis, tennis, and squash. Volleyball needs a group, but the others only a partner. All of these sports are enjoyed by both men and women. They can be started early in life and continued to an advanced age, sometimes with slight modifications. The secret of success is to play them on a regular basis.

To derive the greatest benefit from exercise, it should be undertaken at least once a week. Some sports are more suitable to one season than another, some are indoor, others outdoor activities, and some are both. In many instances the possibility to enjoy them depends on the existence of nearby facilities. Each person should try to select those recreational activities which are most suitable for his regular participation based on convenience of location, the prevailing climate, and the time and expense involved.

Fashions shape our participation in sports just as they do our choice in cars or clothes. Golf became tremendously popular in the 1920's, suffered a decline just before and during World War II, and now enjoys greater popularity than ever before. Other circumstances affect the popularity of sports. The growth of industrial leagues and the televising of matches has made bowling the most popular participant sport in the United States. Better roads and more powerful cars have made water resorts more easily available to millions, creating a boom to skin diving and water-skiing as well as all forms of boating.

Selecting a Sport

A brief summary of the most popular recreational activities which involve some degree of exercise and which are suitable for men and women of all age groups is presented here as an aid in your selection of a suitable sport or sports. The necessary equipment and facilities, the general type of exercise which is afforded, and any precautions which are necessary for safe enjoyment of each activity are indicated.

The popularity of badminton is based largely on the fact that it can be played with pleasure by the learner as well as the expert. The court is marked like a tennis court on two sides of a net which is raised to a height of five feet off the ground. The court is relatively small and can be easily located indoors or outdoors. The only other equipment required is racquets and a shuttlecock. Complete sets of equipment can be purchased at a reasonable cost.

The player does not have to cover so much ground on this small court, but the fast action builds up his wind. Leg and shoulder muscles get the most exercise.

A common injury to badminton players is an ankle sprain, due to the sudden stops, starts, and turns. Players should wear well-fitting sneakers and wrap their ankles if they are weak. The only hazard is the flying shuttlecock, and it can cause a serious injury only if it hits an eye.

The development of inland waterways for recreational purposes, the creation of many man-made lakes, and the opening up of our thousands of natural lakes and several thousand miles of sea coast have made all forms of boating one of our leading recreational activities. Canoeing, rowing, and sailing all provide vigorous outdoor exercise. Small boats can be put on the luggage rack of the car and larger ones on a boat trailer. There is almost no end to the equipment one can add to a sailboat, but all that is needed for a canoe is a paddle.

Rowing and canoeing exercise the muscles of the back and shoulders particularly, but the legs also come in for their share of activity. Rowing a racing shell exercises just about every muscle in the body and also develops lung capacity and endurance. Sailing provides a more varied but usually less strenuous pattern of activity.

Basic precautions to be observed in all boating activities are simply developments of two cardinal rules; show proper respect for others and use common sense. Don't overload your craft; don't stand up or change seats while under way; watch out for swimmers and floating objects; take along life preservers; don't go too far from shore on a large body of water in a small craft; if your boat overturns, stay with it; and, above all, don't go out in a boat if you can't swim. (See Part VII, Chapter Five.)

More than 30,000,000 Americans participate in indoor bowling each year. Alleys

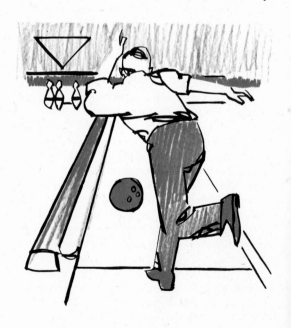

equipped with automatic pinspotting equipment for tenpins and duckpins are within driving distance in almost all parts of the country. Shoes can be rented and balls are supplied in a variety of weights and sizes. The bowler has only to present himself in some loose, comfortably fitting clothes. Lawn bowling is enjoyed by a much smaller number of persons since it requires a perfectly level and carefully tended grass area and is limited to the time of year when the grass is growing.

Bowling provides good exercise for the muscles of arms, shoulders, and back. It is not vigorous enough to give more than very mild exercise to the heart and lungs, but is, therefore, suitable for persons of all ages, and for many for whom other sports are too strenuous.

Bowlers are subject to muscle strains, particularly in the muscles on the inner side of the thigh, to bursitis and inflammation in the tendons around the elbow and the shoulder, and to blisters on the bowling hand. Injury to the fingers can be avoided by not placing the hand in the ball return without looking to see if another ball is arriving.

Once the most popular recreational activity for young and old—as well as a means of transportation—cycling has suffered from the development of automobile travel. Riding today is dangerous on city streets and even on country roads. Very few cycle paths of any considerable length have been built. Competitive cycling is almost unknown in this country today because of lack of interest and the small number of wooden tracks available. Nevertheless over 55,000,000 persons own and ride bicycles in the United States today.

No special equipment besides a bicycle is necessary, although it is helpful to have soft comfortable shoes and loose-fitting clothing. For extended trips, a bicycle with a gearshift is helpful in climbing hills. Hand brakes are also desirable for the experienced rider.

Cycling exercises principally the leg muscles, but the back and shoulders participate as well, especially at faster speeds. Cycling is a great exercise for building up endurance and can be carried out for this purpose on a life-long basis.

The principle hazard besides the traffic is being pitched forward from too sudden a stop or striking an object in the road. If a bicycle is ridden after dark, it should be equipped with a handlebar light and a rear reflector. Competitive cyclists should wear crash helmets. (See Part VII, Chapter Three.)

The possibility of golf as a sport depends on

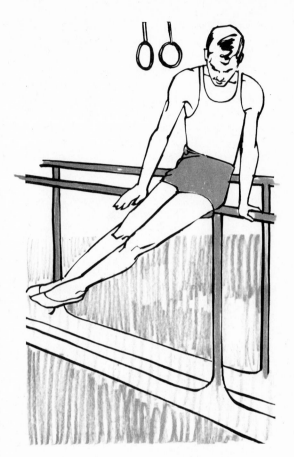

the availability of a golf course. Many persons, however, can practice on driving ranges or play on the short pitch and putt courses which may accompany them. The necessary equipment is a set of golf clubs, which may consist of as few as 5 or as many as 20 clubs, a bag to carry them in, some golf balls, and a pair of sturdy shoes with crepe soles or sport spikes.

Golf provides primarily walking exercise, the average golfer covering about 6 miles on an 18-hole course about 6,500 yards in length. Some exercise is obtained in striking the ball, depending on how hard and how often you hit it. The exercise values of golf are increased if one carries one's own bag. They go down when one pulls a golf cart or rides in one.

Back sprains and blisters of the hands are the chief hazards directly attributable to golf. An occasional golfer is struck by a flying ball. Some deaths from lightning result from taking shelter under isolated trees on the course during thunderstorms.

Relatively few clubs sponsor programs of gymnastics today, but there is a growing interest in this subject in schools and colleges. A great variety of exercises and gradations of exercise are available under the scope of gymnastics, so that a program suitable for either sex at any age can easily be established. Competitive gymnastics requires such a high degree of skill that it remains largely a sport for the relatively few.

Gymnastic equipment for one sport or another is available in school and college gymnasiums, in YMCA's and YWCA's, in athletic clubs, and in other similar organizations. Tumbling requires only a few mats. The trampoline provides a special form of tumbling exercise which has become popular. Light clothing and light rubber-soled shoes are necessary.

The effect of gymnastics on the body is to build strength and endurance, increase the efficiency of the heart and lungs, and to promote coordination, balance, grace, and good posture. A person who continues a program of gymnastics throughout his life is probably getting the best-rounded program of exercise obtainable.

The more advanced forms of gymnastics, including the trampoline, pose a hazard of injury to the inexperienced. They should be undertaken only after instruction and practiced while following the appropriate safety precautions.

About 5,000,000 persons play handball in the United States each year. The cement court with one wall is a common feature of modern playgrounds. Four-wall handball is played in gyms. Beside rubber-soled shoes, the only special equipment required is a pair of gloves and the hard rubber ball.

Handball develops speed and endurance primarily, although it also develops the muscles of the legs and shoulders. It is played primarily by men since most women's hands are too soft for the sport.

The ability to ride a horse is no longer a necessity as it was once. There are three principal forms of this activity: walking or trotting horses in the ring or cross-country, jumping and steeplechasing, and riding to the hunt. Flat racing of horses is almost entirely a professional sport. All forms will always be open to only the select few because the ownership of horses and their equipment is an expensive thing, and outdoor or indoor facilities are not always accessible.

Horseback riding mainly exercises the legs, forearms, and wrists. It does not do much under ordinary conditions for the heart and lungs. The principal hazard is in falling off the horse. One should, therefore, not undertake riding without a suitable period of instruction.

Most of those who adopt running as a form of recreational exercise have been competitors in track or cross-country during school days. Running deserves greater popularity since it is a natural exercise which requires no special equipment other than a pair of light rubber-soled shoes. A place to run can be found almost anywhere and it can be carried on throughout the year. Many people are afraid of it perhaps because they think that the neighbors will think them queer.

Running is the best exercise to develop the functions of the heart and lungs. It also exercises the shoulders and arms as well as the legs. Precautions should be taken not to run short distances at maximum speed without warming up so as to avoid straining the muscles of the thighs. Wearing heavy comfortable-fitting socks and using mineral oil on the soles of the feet will help prevent blisters.

Roller-skating maintains a steady popularity throughout the United States, numbering about 15,000,000 fans. Although skates are the only special equipment needed, it is necessary to have an indoor rink available for year-around use. Ice skating has increased in popularity with the growth of indoor ice rinks around the country, making it a sport for all seasons.

Skating provides exercise similar to running, but less vigorous. It is suitable for all ages, although the hazard of broken bones as the result of falls on the ice is much greater for older persons and the results apt to be more serious.

Snow skiing is a relatively old sport which currently attracts about 3,500,000 adherents in this country. It is relatively expensive, since the cost of good skis is high, special clothing is needed, the best ski areas are remote from where most people live, and the use of lifts and tows is costly.

Skiing is excellent exercise, requiring and promoting strength in the thigh muscles and in the shoulders. If not performed all downhill, it builds endurance. Coaching from a qualified ski instructor is essential to the safe enjoyment of this sport. Injuries to knees and ankles are the chief hazard. Skiers should never ski alone or in areas that are not patrolled. They should have at least eight weeks of exercise for the legs and thighs before the season begins. Never ski when fatigued since falls are more apt to occur.

Water skiers now number about 6,000,000 in the United States. Suitable bodies of water—

lakes, large rivers, and the ocean—are available to the most of the country for a relatively long season. Good skis, which are moderately expensive, and a boat with a powerful motor are necessary. A life jacket should be used.

Muscles in the back, shoulders, arms and legs are developed by water skiing. The skier must be a good swimmer. Injuries due to falls, fouled lines, collisions, and being hit by the tow boat are common. The boat should always contain two persons, one to operate it and the other to tend the line and watch the skier.

A group of four-wall court games played with rackets—which include squash racquets, squash tennis, racquets, and paddle racquets—maintain a small but steady popularity because they are fast, place emphasis on skill, and can be played in all seasons. Rackets and balls are inexpensive. Courts are limited in number.

These court games are excellent conditioners for both men and women, but cannot be played with much pleasure after 50 because of the speed required. Injuries occur chiefly from being struck by the ball or the opponent's racket. Sprains and strains are also fairly common in these games.

Although swimming should seem to be a natural exercise because of man's long association with water, the development of effective swimming techniques is relatively modern. Several million Americans now own private swimming pools, most of them outdoors. These are expensive to build and maintain. Thousands of pools in hotels, clubs, and recreational centers are also available to those who don't own pools or live near a lake or beach.

Some sort of basic instruction is necessary to learn how to swim properly and to maintain

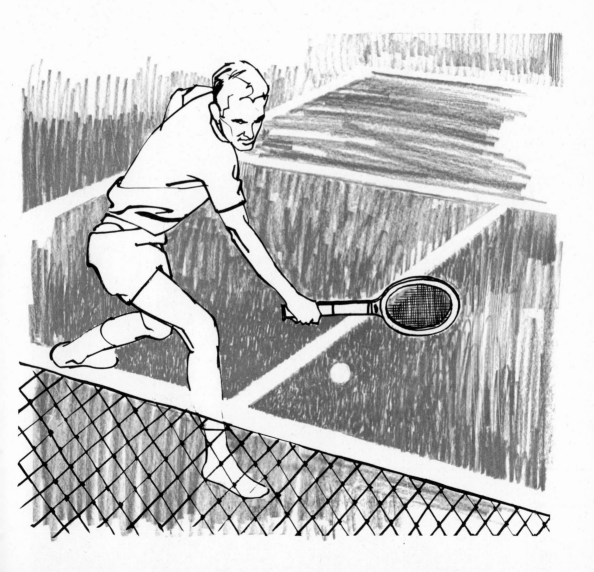

oneself safely in water. Lifesaving courses are given regularly by the American Red Cross, YMCA, YWCA, and other organizations. Swimming is an excellent all-around exercise for conditioning.

Pool owners should keep their pools fenced in, preferably covered when not in use. The water should be filtered and kept clean and chlorinated. Someone who knows the technique of artificial respiration should be around when the pool is in use, a long reaching pole should be handy, and no one should be allowed to swim alone. Roughhouse play around the pool and outdoor swimming during thunderstorms should be barred.

Skin diving as an extension of underwater swimming has come into being only recently, but already attracts millions of addicts. It is called Scuba when Self-Contained Underwater Breathing Apparatus consisting of compressed air tanks are used. This is a hazardous sport which should be undertaken only after a thorough course of instruction by an expert. The equipment is expensive. Only areas where clear water is the rule are suitable.

The most serious hazard of Scuba diving is air embolism due to improper breathing control and surfacing technique. Ruptured eardrums, decompression sickness (bends), and injuries from rocks, shells, and spears are fairly common. Divers should always work in pairs and follow standard procedures to avoid the many possible difficulties which may be encountered.

Tennis is one of the oldest sports still played, although the present form is quite different from the original. Court tennis, which is derived directly from the original, is played by only a few, since it requires a specially-constructed court. About 7,500,000 Americans play other versions of tennis on grass, clay, wooden, or composition courts indoors and outdoors. Outdoor courts of one sort or another are available in most parts of the country. Rackets and balls are inexpensive. Rubber-soled shoes are used. A new variety called paddle tennis is played outdoors on a small wooden-floored court with a paddle instead of a racket. Table tennis is widely played indoors and out.

Speed and agility are required for competitive tennis, but the game can be enjoyed to an advanced age with slight modification of the rules to make it more of a back-court game. It provides good general conditioning exercise if played regularly. The chief hazards are sprains of muscles and ligaments.

Volleyball is used regularly by Y groups and other athletic associations as a general conditioning and recreational exercise for pick-up games with any number of players. It can be played indoors and outdoors, requiring only a ball and two uprights to support the high net. The chief injury sustained is a sprained ankle.

Frequently a matter of necessity but too often neglected in this automotive age, walking can be a very enjoyable recreational exercise. Long-distance walking at a measured pace is frequently referred to as hiking. When undertaken cross-country or in the hills, it is an excellent conditioner, developing the heart and lungs as well as exercising the legs, back, and arms. Good, stout, well-fitting shoes and comfortable socks are essential. The worst injury to be expected, barring tumbles on uneven ground, is a few blisters or shin splints.

CHAPTER THREE

REDUCING THE RISK IN SPORTS

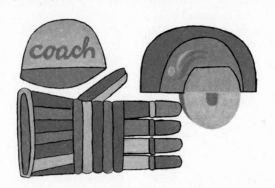

SOONER OR LATER, children are going to begin playing competitive sports, either in the backyard, on the playground, the winter ice, or the polished wooden floors of the gymnasium. They will be pushing around and handling various leather and rubber objects according to certain rules. They will also be pushing each other around, and sooner or later, someone will get hurt.

The playing of competitive sports always raises an important question for parents. Naturally, they do not want their children injured. At the same time, they do not want them to grow up without taking part in wholesome competitive sports. Actually, many situations are far more hazardous than competitive athletics. Accidents in the home and on the highway, many of them preventable, are much more readily accepted as part of the hazards of living than are accidents due to sports.

The value of competitive sports is similar to that of recreational sports. Competitive sports have the additional advantage of enabling the players to learn skills other than the physical ones required to win games. Under proper leadership from a good coach, they can learn sportsmanship. They can learn how to be good losers without being willing to lose and how to accept victory without being objectionable about it. They can learn that hard and strenuous participation does not mean ruffianism. They can learn the value of group and team play as distinguished from individual starring.

Participation in organized sports is steadily increasing. It is being realized that the young *must* blow off steam and the playing field is much to be preferred to the tavern as a locale for doing so.

Acceptance of the value of competitive sports increases the need for working to overcome the problems of prevention, diagnosis and treatment of injuries sustained in sports.

These are no longer relegated to a back room in the gymnasium and a footnote in the annual athletic budget of the school. The home, too, must realize that it has its part to play and that proper precautions can and must be taken to minimize injuries and to prevent their occurrence whenever possible.

Bill of Rights of the Athlete

The medical profession, in conjunction with coaches, has established some principles through a Committee on the Medical Aspects

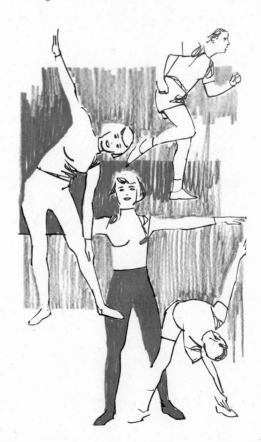

of Sports, appointed by the American Medical Association. This committee has helped establish standards for the medical care of athletes in schools and colleges and has expressed these points of view in a document called the "Bill of Rights of the Athlete." The home can play a part in assuring its junior members that the institutions with whose teams they participate are living up to the requirements of this Bill of Rights. These rights are, in brief, as follows:

1. **Good Coaching**. The coach who teaches unsportsmanlike tactics to win at any price is today almost extinct. Almost all coaches today are competent instructors in the technical aspects of the game, ignorance of which, of course, greatly increases the incidence and severity of injuries.

2. **Good Equipment**. This right, too, can easily be achieved. The manufacturers of equipment take their responsibilities seriously and are continually modifying and improving the various types of protective devices worn in contact sports. The problem lies in the false economy of using worn-out, outmoded, or ill-

fitting gear. The outfitting of a team is no place for penny pinching.

3. **Good Medical Care,** which has three major aspects:

• A thorough pre-season history and a physical examination of each player. These constitute the most important factors in the prevention of injuries. Many of the sports tragedies which occur every year are due to medical conditions—such as heart disease, hypertension, and diabetes—which went unrecognized. For many years at Harvard University, loss of function of one of any paired set of organs also has been cause to bar participation in any contact sport. This rule produces an annual crop of unhappy young men who seem to have played for years in high school with one testicle, one kidney, or one eye, but no exceptions are allowed. Other less potentially dangerous sports are available, and no game is worth the risk of blindness, death, or castration.

Another important part of the pre-season examination, particularly in high schools and preparatory schools, is the proper matching of players. Boys grow at different rates. Some at 15 have mature and well-coordinated musculoskeletal systems. Others are small and soft, having barely entered adolescence; and still others are large-boned, skinny and uncoordinated, being in a period of rapid bone growth, with barely compensated nerves and muscles. To mix these types on a team is to court trouble. This is an area for cooperation between coach and doctor. Well-matched teams are safer and provide much more fun for all concerned.

• A doctor (ideally the same one) should be available throughout the season and should be present at every game. To let a trainer or coach decide whether an injured player should continue to play or be removed from a game, and, if removed, whether he should be carried or walk off the field, is to gamble with a player's future.

• The doctor's authority in medical matters should be absolute and unquestioned. Adherence to this principle is the measure of a good coach. Almost all coaches today are happy to leave medical decisions to the medical profession. They have enough difficult decisions and problems as it is.

It is quite true that the great majority of sports injuries are not serious, will heal despite even bizarre treatment, and will leave no remnant of permanent disability, but the day of regarding this problem as "minor" and beneath

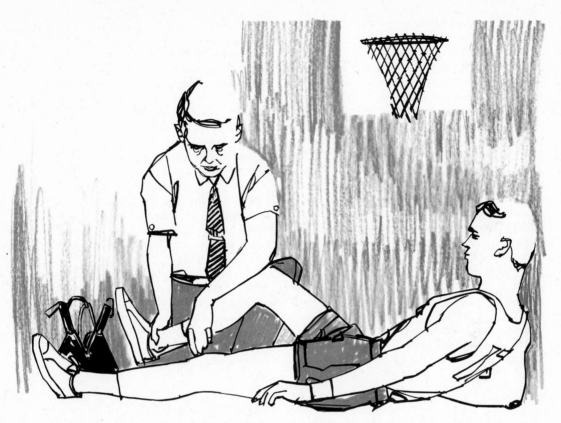

the dignity of a proper doctor is gone. The doctor who assumes responsibility for a school or college team may be greatly helped if he is furnished information from the family physician as a background for his judgment of the capabilities of the players. Athletic injuries differ in no way from other injuries except that they usually occur among athletes.

The home can help to assure the safety, the pleasure, and the profit of its younger members through participation in athletic programs which are soundly conceived and in which proper precautions are taken for the safety of athletes.

Children and Competitive Sports

A further consideration in relation to athletics is its place in the general program of the child. No young person should be without athletic interests. These should be chosen with the preference of the participant in mind and with due consideration for his or her special abilities.

No young person should be pressured into athletics of a particular type because of a parent's special interest. It is a disservice to the child when parents try to get personal satis-

faction out of the success of their children, especially if they place this above the child's welfare. Too much emphasis should not be placed upon winning and, at the same time, too great a willingness to lose should not be encouraged.

Proper control and direction for participants in competitive sports is a part of the general plan for guiding the child in his development. As in scholastic and other activities, the problem is the setting of realistic goals. While a child may need to be stimulated to do his best, he must not be pushed and pressured for the attainment of goals beyond his capabilities. At the same time, he must not be allowed to become slack by the setting of goals too easily attained. Either extreme is destructive; only a wise approximation of the happy medium and a recognition of individual differences among children give the child the best opportunity for self-expression in all of his activities, including sports.

It is obvious that no right-thinking parent will intentionally sacrifice his child to his own psychological needs. However, self-appraisal is one of the most difficult achievements for a human being. The parent who has had great success in competitive athletics must be careful not to expect too much of his child. Some children have felt overshadowed by the outstanding capabilities of their parents and have consequently developed a feeling of inferiority.

Some parents need to be especially careful not to be tempted to achieve belated satisfaction through the success of a child or grandchild. Athletics for children should be judged on the basis of their benefit to the child, rather than on satisfaction to the personal emotional needs of adults, or favorable publicity for school or community such as is derived from winning teams.

An important factor in athletic programs for children and youth is the emotional impact of too much publicity, combined with poorly supervised trips to other communities, late hours, and mingling with unfamiliar young people. Athletics for children under high school age should be limited, in the judgment of many experts, to events within their own communities. At the high school level, regional and statewide events many be defended if properly supervised and intelligently geared to the age level, experience, and emotional stability of the age group involved.

Athletic programs for younger children, or for high school and college youth, are not good or bad in themselves; they are good or bad according to how they are managed. Parents have an obligation to their children to become familiar with the sports programs sponsored in their communities by various organizations. These programs are good if they are so conducted as to provide opportunity for play for many children without overemphasizing the special abilities of the stars. These programs are good if they avoid undue emotional tensions and exaggerated competition. They are good if they keep the children largely in their own community with a minimum of trips and with as little as possible intercommunity rivalry. These cautions are particularly pertinent with young children who may be severely upset emotionally by excessive tensions and too much emphasis upon victory for the sake of the community. The game should be for the benefit of the child and not for the adults.

CHAPTER FOUR

Rx: A VACATION

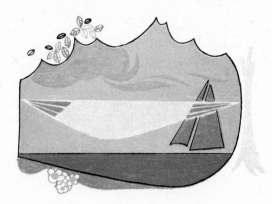

THE VACATION, which used to be a luxury limited to the few, is now among the best health prescriptions for the many. Self-made men who formerly boasted that they never took a vacation now require their employees to do so, because they have learned that properly arranged vacations improve health.

The word "vacation" is related to "vacate," which means to leave, to get out, to go away. That is the key to the proper vacation. One must go away. This may be a physical departure from the home and the community where one lives, or it may be merely going away from the office into the garden, the hobby workshop, the library, the beach, the nearby countryside, the golf links, or the theater. It may be no more than a mental change of scenery from the job environment to the far reaches of the universe through books, museums, or lectures. The vacation should, above all, be a complete change from the usual routine.

The physically-active worker may wish to take a quiet vacation; the desk-bound person may want to get out and stretch his muscles. So long as there is a change, and the vacation is something the person wants to do, it should produce benefits.

Whether a family should vacation together or separately depends in large degree on the members of the family, their likes and dislikes, and whether they have been together or separated all year. A scattered family may want and enjoy a vacation all together; a family that has lived together all year may want to go it alone for awhile, especially if individual tastes differ.

Much debate has gone on about what to do when father wants to climb a mountain, mother would like to sit on a cottage porch in the woods and rest, son wants to fish and daughter insists on dancing, while little brother prefers to stay home and go to the beach or the pool with his pals. An unselfish family settles this by compromise—they go to the mountains with dad one year, where mother can find a porch and rocker and son can fish another. They try to find a place where daughter can dance and the little brother can swim in the motel pool. Maybe they even take one of his pals along to keep him company.

Important to the vacationer is the main purpose of his vacation, rest and *re*-creation, which is not quite the same as *rec*-reation— sometimes more appropriately spelled "wreck-reation." Too strenuous activity may spoil the vacation, and may even bring on serious illness or cause injuries. Strenuous activities should be begun gradually, until endurance is established. They should be held to a sensible level. Even the young and active may find a dip before breakfast, a morning of horseback riding, an afternoon of tennis, a swim before dinner, dancing until one a.m., and watching the moon for another hour to be too exhausting.

Exposure of white indoor skins too long to unaccustomed sunlight may result in painful burns or even generalized illness, especially in high altitudes where the atmosphere does not filter out the ultraviolet rays, or in the tropics. Early morning and late afternoon, the sun is less powerful than at midday.

Automobiles, motorcycles or bicycles, boats, planes, ski lifts, mountain trails, fishing and hunting paraphernalia, riding horses, pools and beaches all are wonderful aids to a good time and a refreshing vacation—when properly used. Misused or abused, they can be dangerous or deadly. When in doubt, it is always better to play it safe than to take a chance and be sorry.

It is usually better not to start a trip the first day of a vacation or to return the last day. This leads to hurry and flurry, adds to fatigue and interferes with the proper planning of the vacation beforehand and the equally important mopping up afterward. One may expect more pleasure even in the shortened time by avoiding pressures before, during, and after the vacation.

Where it is impossible to take a vacation in one parcel of time, the long weekend may be a necessity. Much depends on the nature of the individual's work and responsibilities. Whatever the arrangement, the important point is that every person should have a vacation for the sake of his physical and emotional health and to make him easier for family, co-workers, and friends to get along with.

CHAPTER FIVE

VACATION HEALTH AND SAFETY

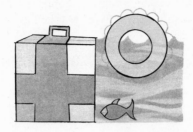

HOLIDAY FUN begins with anticipation. But healthy holiday fun should begin with some good family organization, cooperation, and planning, too. Adequate planning well ahead of time will prevent ruffled tempers at the last minute and will help make your family's vacation a pleasant memory. Accidents and illness don't take vacations, but forethought and planning may prevent them from accompanying you and your family. So you won't need a vacation when you get back, take your time, leave your home and office cares behind, and pace yourself during your holiday.

Before Leaving

A full safety check of your home before you leave may save you worry during your vacation and regret when you return. Plan your safety check well in advance. At the last minute—and during the excitement of leaving—you may overlook potential hazards.

Several days before you leave, cancel all deliveries of milk, laundry, cleaning, and newspapers. Arrange with the post office to hold your mail, or to forward the first-class mail and hold the rest. These steps prevent the house from showing that you are absent and thus discourages burglars. A lighted house is advisable, especially one where the lights go on and off. This is readily arranged with electric timing clocks; one in a bedroom and one in a downstairs room or bath, timed at differing intervals, will make the house look occupied in your absence.

It is also good foresight to notify the police that your house will be unoccupied. If you have relatives or good friends who will look in once in a while, that helps too, but the police should know about it. A friendly neighbor may be asked to keep a key in case of the need for emergency entry in your absence. Valuable objects such as silver and jewels should be stored in your bank.

Remove all accumulated waste from baskets; destroy any oily rags or flammable liquids. Disconnect electric appliances and lamps except those on the time-clocks, including the radio and TV. Be sure stove burners are turned off. Dispose of all perishable food. Close water faucets tightly. Lock all doors and windows. In cold weather, adjust the thermostat on the heating system to maintain a temperature which will prevent freezing of water pipes and toilets.

If possible, arrange for cutting of lawn or shoveling sidewalks and driveway, depending on the season, as a further means of suggesting that someone is at home.

These precautions will put your mind at rest while you vacation and, in that sense, they are real health measures.

Traveling

Whatever the mode of travel, the goal is a sensible trip that takes everyone's comfort, safety, good health, and enjoyment into consideration. Excessive hours of daily travel lead to fatigue, uncertain tempers and, possibly, accidents. More casual travel, without a stiff schedule of things to do and see, will assure a more relaxed and enjoyable trip.

The best time to find out something is wrong with your car is before you leave—not after you are under way. A week or so before you plan to leave, take your car in for a thorough safety check, that includes brakes, battery, tires, headlights, tail and stop lights, directional signals, steering mechanisms, exhaust system, horn, and emergency brake.

When packing the car, keep items which will be used during traveling hours within easy reach. However, leave the rear view clear and guard against flying objects on sudden stops by keeping all objects off the rear window ledge. Leave adequate leg room on the floor.

The trip will be more bearable and relaxing

for small children if pillows and blankets are provided. Books and games will help entertain them on long trips. Make frequent stops—at least every two hours—to refresh yourself and to let the children blow off steam.

Depending on the number in the party, their ages and states of health and vigor, and the

serious than merely an inconvenience if elderly people or children have to be left in a car exposed to hot sun or to severe cold.

Clothing for a trip should be casual and comfortable, and provide for either extremes of heat or cold. At least two pairs of sturdy, comfortable, and "broken-in" shoes are essen-

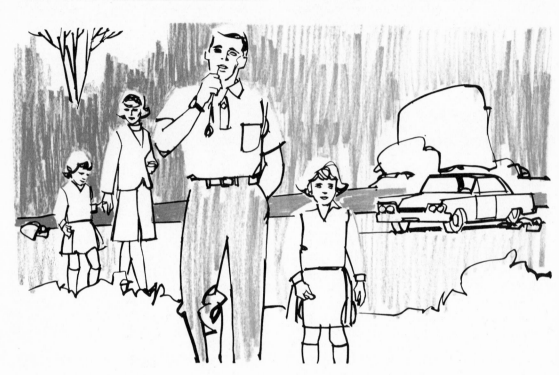

spaciousness and comfort of the vehicle, daily mileage may range from a leisurely 200 to as much as 400 without placing too much strain on the physical and emotional resources of the travelers. Anything above 400 miles a day becomes a burden for many, though some enjoy going farther and faster. An occasional two-night stop at intervals of two or three days helps to provide rest, a chance to see the sights, and time to catch up with the laundry.

In extremely hot weather, travel is most comfortable in the morning, before the sun is high, and in the late afternoon or early evening. In general, safety calls for avoiding night driving, except when deserts are to be crossed. Then the relatively cooler air of the night is an advantage. Air conditioning or drip-cooling of the car adds to passenger comfort and the prevention of fatigue. In dry or desert places, a desert water bag or two may be required, both for drinking and to replenish the radiator. Keeping the gasoline tank well filled may prevent running out of gas; and this can be more

tial for a trip which includes any appreciable amount of walking. So are hats to shield you against the sun, especially in high altitudes, and suitable rainwear. Sunglasses should be available for those who require them and should be of good quality, with ground-in correction where required.

Disposable handkerchiefs, paper towels, disposable diapers also help to lighten the maintenance chores along the way, and contribute to a trip that will be truly restful.

Motion sickness is a sensitivity to movement, acceleration, or deceleration. It can put a damper on an otherwise enjoyable trip by ship, plane, train, car, or bus. Much of the time this miserable experience can be avoided if susceptibility is known. The person who has this difficulty should prepare for a trip by not eating or drinking too much before or during the ride. When traveling by plane or ship, try to get a place where motion is at a minimum— a midship cabin on a lower deck on shipboard or a seat between the wings of a plane. Activities requiring close eye attention such as reading or playing cards may aggravate or even cause motion sickness. Often fresh air will help to relieve nausea. Your physician can tell you about medicines available for motion sickness prevention, and how and when to use them.

The first aid kit—which is a good thing to have in your car at all times, not just on trips—may be purchased ready-packed at many drug stores, or it can be made up at home. It should consist of:

A metal box with a good catch or combination lock (key locks are no good because you may lose the key);

A first aid manual (AMA, Red Cross or Boy Scout);

A bandage scissors or other blunt-pointed scissors;

A fever thermometer;

One or more disposable enema packages;

A roll of one-inch finger bandage;

A roll of two-inch roller bandage;

A tin of finger bandages and "spots" of varying size;

A plastic bottle of tincture of green soap;

A package of double-ended cotton applicators;

A cotton "picker" package;

A package of sterilized gauze squares in envelopes;

A roll of one-inch zinc oxide adhesive plaster;

A plastic bottle of eye-drops as prescribed by your doctor for use after a long, dusty, sunny, drive; and

An 8-ounce plastic bottle of isopropyl alcohol or 70 per cent grain alcohol for skin disinfecting.

Travel by bicycle is not so common in this country as in Europe, primarily because we have no comparable cycle roads and our motor traffic is much heavier. However, bicycle vacations are possible for the young, and for the more vigorous older persons. Cyclists, obviously, must travel light, usually stopping at hostels, motels, or camps. Cyclists should avoid the busier highways; they are not permitted on the turnpikes and toll roads. They should certainly familiarize themselves with bicycle safety. (See Part VII, Chapter Three.)

The Handicapped Traveler

The time may come when a handicapped person must travel. Or he may choose to see the world in spite of his handicap. He then requires special medical advice before he starts, and must do some extra planning in terms of his handicap. He may have to make arrangements in advance for wheel chairs, if required, or he may carry a collapsible one with him. He will need to go by routes and stay in accommodations where attendants are available to assist him. The Travelers' Aid people in most cities can be called upon to help. Hospital arrangements for special services needed may have to be made in advance, or physicians alerted in stopping places or at the destination. In such instances, a good travel agency can be extremely helpful. Where the handicapped person forms one of an automobile party, his needs will readily be met by his companions, presumably relatives or close friends.

Food and Lodging

Travelers and vacationers on the move may be more subject to bodily disorders than are the same persons in their daily routine at home. The places you choose to eat and stay may make the difference between a family of exhausted, deflated travelers and one of comfortable, alert travelers. Although tension and excitement may manifest themselves in stomachaches or headaches, often the changes in food and water will have as much or more to do with the way you feel and how much you enjoy your vacation.

Sub-standard food and lodging establishments should obviously be avoided. Use common sense in selecting a place for your family to eat and stay. Select a clean restaurant, cafeteria, diner, or drive-in; many of these bear well known labels of recognized quality. Health authorities in many states post ratings in a prominent place in the establishment. Such a rating doesn't guarantee excellence in food, but it does indicate that equipment and general sanitation meet minimum standards.

Generally you can tell from the appearance of the establishment whether or not to take a chance on eating there. Have someone in the family go inside first to check out the general appearance, looking for uncovered food or other obvious signs of uncleanliness. These will be a fairly good indication of the conscientiousness of the operator. If your family plans to use the rest rooms, check these out too. It you have any qualms whatsoever, leave and find another restaurant; there is no need to take unnecessary chances with illness. Also, public rejection can do much to raise sub-standard sanitation facilities in food and lodging establishments.

Caution: Food and Water

Travelers are likely candidates for food poisoning and infection. A breakdown in proper safeguards for food preparation and service can cause either during any season of the year. During the summer months, however, the risk is greater, since heat and improper refrigeration may combine to spoil food.

The best safeguard to follow to avoid food infection or poisoning is to avoid certain foods which are more likely to cause such effects, unless you can be absolutely sure of the eating spot. These foods include: ground or mixed combinations of foods not cooked immediately before being eaten such as meat spreads (chicken, ham); potato, sea-food, and egg salads; cream or custard-filled pastries; cold sliced meats, including cold cuts; creamed dishes; undercooked meats—particularly poultry and pork; and custards. Such foods are not dangerous if proper methods of preparation are followed. But even a slight breakdown in preparation, handling, or refrigeration of these foods provides an opportunity for contamination and bacterial growth. If in doubt, always ask if the milk or cream is pasteurized. If it isn't, don't drink it; many serious illnesses can be spread through raw milk and cream. If it is necessary to drink milk or cream in an area where they are not pasteurized, ask for canned or packaged dry milk or cream.

The safety of water supplies in U.S. cities usually can be taken for granted. In some parts of the world, however, or in any recently flooded area, bottled soft drinks are usually less risky than the local water. Typhoid fever and diarrhea are both waterborne diseases which may be avoided by assuring safe water.

Wild plants, including berries and mushrooms, can be particularly dangerous to the traveler making frequent stops along the roadside. Although they may be tempting, wild plants are best left alone. In particular, learn to identify and avoid poison ivy and oak.

A portable icebox that will fit in the trunk of the car or on the floor in the back seat is a good investment for travelers planning to carry their own food. Snacks such as fruit juice, fresh fruits or vegetables, cookies, crackers, and soft drinks make car travel much more fun for youngsters, and are fine refreshment for adults

as well. Take care, however, to avoid bringing meat salads and other perishable foods which may serve as good media for bacterial growth under improper refrigeration. Although portable iceboxes will help keep foods cool, they are makeshift and cannot be relied upon to inhibit bacteria growth. Buy only as much food as you will eat within a relatively few hours and discard any leftovers.

Avoiding Infectious Diseases

Any number of infectious diseases may plague a traveler. For sure protection, see that immunizations for all communicable diseases are up-to-date for each member of your family. These should include immunizations against diphtheria, tetanus, polio, measles, smallpox and, for children, whooping cough. Ask your physician about any special protection you might need before traveling into certain areas.

If a member of the family is taking any special medicine prescribed by a physician, make certain to have an adequate supply for the entire trip. It will be a good idea to ask for an extra prescription, too, in case the bottle is broken or is left somewhere. Most common drugs can be purchased along the way as needed.

Your health and the way you feel during your holiday is probably the most important factor in determining the success of your trip. In the excitement of vacation preparations, do not overlook any aspect of the family's health that may cause problems during the trip. This may mean a trip to the dentist to guard against toothaches, and an extra prescription for eyeglasses, in case of loss. In planning where to go, the family should consider allergies and possible reactions to high altitudes.

High elevations, excessive heat, and high humidity can make a stay uncomfortable for persons with heart trouble or difficulty in breathing. Check with a physician about any special problems concerning a member of the family who has been ill or is an older person. Planning for special limitations in advance will assure everyone of a more enjoyable vacation.

Summer Vacations and Travel

Summer, when children are out of school and the weather is warm, is the most popular time for vacationers to take to the road. With relaxation and recreation foremost, summer vacations offer swimming, boating, camping, hiking, and other outdoor sports. Along with the out-of-doors, however, comes the possibility of accident or disease which may mar or bring your vacation to a sudden and unexpected end. Some thought beforehand may prevent summer accidents from happening.

Swimming, probably the most popular of summer sports, can be a healthful, stimulating part of the summer vacation. On the other hand, swimming can be one of the most dangerous of outdoor pastimes. Healthful swimming should begin with clean, sanitary water. Water furnishes an easy and quick means of transmission for many disease organisms, and inevitably swimmers will swallow some water. Swim only in approved areas where the water is clean and free from pollution.

Swimming can be dangerous. Deaths from drowning can occur at any age. Inability to swim, inexperience, carelessness, poor judgment, or lack of supervision are cause of most water accidents. Infants and toddlers need constant supervision by adults who themselves practice good water safety rules.

The water should be respected and swim-mers should know their limitations. The depth of the water should be checked and hidden rocks and stumps looked for before diving. Swimmers should always have someone else along and, preferably, swim where a lifeguard is near. And remember that salt water and surf can be more tiring than swimming in a quiet pool or lake.

In case of trouble, swimmers should remain calm, assume a face-up floating position, keeping their hands under water and moving their feet and hands slowly. Every member of your family should know mouth-to-mouth resuscitation procedures. (See Part IX, Chapter Two.)

Boating is increasing as a family summer pastime all across the nation. This boom in boating has also increased the potential hazard from drownings. With boat traffic getting heavier, boat operators must understand and practice safe boating practices.

Boating equipment should be checked *before* leaving shore. Essential safety equipment for a boat includes an anchor, a fire extinguisher, oars, a horn, running lights, a mirror, and a first aid kit. A life preserver should be provided for each person aboard; nonswim-mers should wear them at all times. Some states

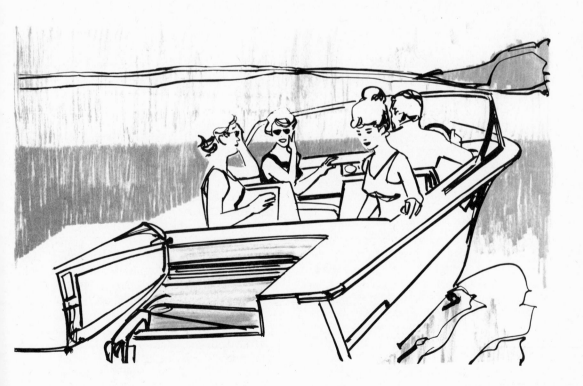

require such equipment before boats can be licensed for hire.

Most boating accidents involve faulty operation, negligence, or ignorance. The operator should know his boat, keep his mind on business, and operate the boat according to nautical rules. And by all means stay ashore in threatening weather.

If water skiing is on your list of water activities, make certain you and other members of your family who might try the sport know how to swim. There should be at least two persons in the boat when pulling water skiers.

Good physical condition is a prerequisite for water skiing, and the skier should practice basic maneuvers before adding new or advanced skills. A life jacket or belt should be worn to conserve energy. In case of a fall, the skier should stay with the skis and signal the observer in the boat that he is all right. Ski only during the daytime, never at night.

Sun and Heat Protection

An attractive, golden tan can not be acquired during the first day on the beach. Begin the first day with about 15 to 20 minutes of exposure, and then extending the period in the sun each day. Painful burns can be caused by wind as well as the sun, and even on cloudy days it is possible to overexpose oneself to the rays of the sun.

Too much exposure to the sun can also cause sunstroke or heat prostration. Anyone can be affected, but older persons, persons with high blood pressure, and chronic drinkers are most likely to be affected. Usually sunstroke or heat prostration can be prevented by wearing head coverings in hot sunshine, avoiding strenuous exercise on hot days, wearing light, loose clothing, and avoiding too much to eat or drink. Take sufficient liquids and salt foods freely.

Swimmer's itch (schistosome dermatitis) is caused by small parasites in the water, usually in lakes. It occurs in all northern states from coast to coast, as well as in the extreme south. Salt water bathers in the seaboard states have also been known to get swimmer's itch. The parasites burrow into the skin when you come out of the water, and may cause a prickly feeling. Welts resembling mosquito bites usually appear within about 24 hours, but may take up to 2 weeks to appear. Often swimmer's itch is mistaken for poison ivy rash or chigger or other insect bites.

The parasites must live part of their life in certain fresh water snails. The best way to avoid swimmer's itch is to stay out of lakes when the parasites are emerging from the snails. Usually these lakes give little trouble in early spring or late summer. If you do swim in parasite-infested waters, swim as far away from the snail beds as you can. Short dips reduce chances for exposure. When you come out of the water, give yourself a brisk rubdown with a towel—you may be able to rub off the parasites before they burrow under your skin.

Many hotels and motels now have swimming pools. It is important in using them to follow the safety rules laid down by the management, as well as those requiring showers before entering the pool. A protection against the fungus infection commonly known as athlete's foot is to wear bath sandals when not actually swimming. It is also a good idea to wear shoes or slippers at all times when staying in hotels and motels, since the athlete's foot fungus is found in carpets and rugs as well as in gymnasiums and locker rooms and around pools. A soap and water shower after swimming is as good a protection as any against fungus infections of the feet. Careful drying of the feet, particularly between the toes after bathing, is also important.

Camping and Hiking

To some, living in the woods is one of the most enjoyable and relaxing vacations. Proper planning and adequate precautions against potential health hazards can make the camping trip relatively hazard-free. The trick is to make the camp a well-managed and safe one rather than a haphazard one.

Consider the equipment carefully, including bedding and tents, also your clothing, cooking equipment, and food. Sleeping bags and air mattresses provide more warmth and comfort than cots; and the enjoyment of camping depends a great deal upon a good comfortable bed. Select clothing with regard to season, freedom of movement, and protection from insects, briar, and heavy brush. Be sure to include rain jackets and proper sleeping clothing.

Adequate meal planning for a camping trip is of paramount importance. The camper's health depends much upon well-selected and substantial foods. Precautions must be taken, however, for safe preservation of all foods taken on the trip. Remember that potential health hazards exist when foods are refrigerated on a makeshift basis, or left exposed to flies or rodents.

Running water is not necessarily clean water. Campers should use water only from springs and wells that have been declared safe. If necessary to use water from creeks, lakes, or rivers, boil it before use, or use water purification tablets.

As in most outdoor summer activities, planning ahead is an important aspect of safe hiking. Good physical health should be a prerequisite. The route to be taken should be selected in advance, and all members of the group briefed. Equipment should include a first aid kit, comfortable shoes, matches in a waterproof container, a compass, rainwear, and an ax or hatchet. Safety practices to be observed by each hiker are: remain with the group; wear proper clothing; carry pure water; avoid eating unfamiliar wild berries or fruit; be able to recognize poisonous plants and animals; know signals and rendezvous points in case the group becomes separated.

Emergency Medical Help

Despite all precautions, there is always the chance that someone in your family may become ill or be injured while you are on vacation. When you need medical help in a strange town or area, call the nearest hospital or look in the yellow pages of the telephone book. For recommendations, call the county, parish, district, or city medical society, or check with the local health officer or public health nurse. Emergency medical services are best procured in a strange community through the hospitals; doing so prevents your falling into the hands of unethical or unqualified practitioners. In larger cities, the local medical society is listed in the telephone directory, usually under the name of the county. It may also be listed under "medical society" or "academy of medicine," and an additional listing may be found under "emergency medical service" or "physicians' telephone service bureau." The local health department is also a source of information. When you do get in touch with a physician, take his advice; don't disregard what he says merely because he is a stranger.

In this country it is not necessary to carry reserves of ordinary drugs, but a copy of any essential prescription is a safeguard in case of loss, breakage, spoilage, or other need for replacement. You should remember, however, that drugs not commonly called for may not be in stock in outlying community pharmacies. Liquids should be carried in plastic bottles rather than glass. A medical identification card may be useful, especially for diabetics or epileptics, and the emblem should be worn if an emergency is likely (see Part IX, Chapter One). Individuals requiring medical services en route, such as blood sugar tests for diabetics, can get them at almost any hospital, usually without prior appointment.

Communicable diseases are less of a problem than they used to be, but families traveling with children may wish to avoid epidemic areas. They can get advance information about these by writing to their own State Board of Health, giving their proposed route or by telegraphing and authorizing a collect reply.

Perhaps the most important factor in successful travel, especially with your family or other groups, is the ability of everyone to take things as they come, make the best of bad breaks, and get fun out of any mishaps that are not serious. A relaxed and happy atmosphere contributes not only to enjoyment but also to safety, especially on the highway. This is doubly important toward the end of the day, when everyone is tired and some are inclined to be edgy.

Insect Bites and Poisonous Plants

An effective insect repellent applied liberally to exposed parts of the body is your best protection against most insects. Available in either liquid or spray form, the repellents are not

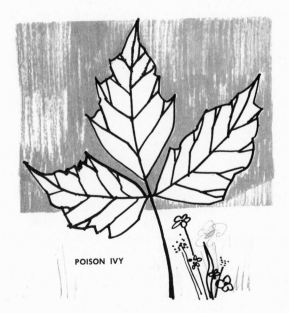

POISON IVY

harmful to human skin or to clothing, but they do produce an odor very disagreeable to mosquitoes. Protective clothing during the day and mosquito netting at night will help, too.

If you camp or hike in areas where ticks abound, cover yourself as well as possible. Tick repellents, usually in powder or spray form, are available to treat clothing. At least twice a day, check your hair and skin. If a tick is attached to your skin, pull it off gently, preferably with tweezers, or use paper or cotton. A drop of turpentine may cause the tick to back out, dislodging itself. After removing the tick, disinfect the bite with alcohol or some other antiseptic. Never crush a tick between your fingers or fingernails.

Adequate clothing is the best protection against bee stings and chigger bites. Try to keep children away from holes in trees and other obvious places where bees gather. A paste of baking soda and water will soothe a single sting, but contact a physician if someone gets many stings or if severe swelling develops. Chiggers are common in grassy and brushy areas, and usually cling to the legs. Wash with soap and sponge with alcohol after hiking in such areas. Do not sit down or be in the grass where chiggers are likely to be found. Refrain from scratching the bites. Include in your first aid kit some soothing ointments to alleviate itching from any insect bites.

To avoid trouble from poisonous plants, teach all members of your family to recognize and be on the lookout for poison ivy, poison sumac, and poison oak. If you know you've come in contact with such a plant, wash exposed parts as soon as possible with soap and hot water.

There are few poisonous snakes in the United States, but some of them are very dangerous. Before venturing on foot into unknown territory, the vacationer should check with a ranger, a licensed guide, or a well-informed local resident about snakes which may be encountered. Snakes are found in deep grass, about rocks, and sometimes in water. High leather shoes and heavy gloves are the best protection against snake bite. When exploring in unfamiliar territory, it is best to "poke around" with a stick rather than with the hands. This is also a safeguard against black spider bites. For first aid information, see Part IX, Chapter Two.

Winter Vacations and Travel

Vacations, holidays, and travel are not limited to the summertime. Ski enthusiasts look forward to the bracing cold air as much as others look forward to sunny, sandy beaches.

Special precautions are needed, however, while driving during the winter. Take along safety gear such as chains, shovel, snow tires, and extra gasoline, and stock the car with warm clothing, and some nonperishable foods, just in case you spend an unexpected night on the road.

Most winter sports require good health and good physical condition. Your comfort, health, and safety depend primarily on advance training and preparation and the clothing you take along.

Inexperience and overconfidence, together with fatigue, probably cause most winter sports accidents. Whichever sport you choose, use common sense, and know your limitations. Dress warmly, but not so you'll get overheated. Wear loose fitting, woolen inner clothing and a windproof jacket. Mittens will keep your hands warmer than gloves. Wear goggles or sunglasses to protect your eyes from glare, and take precautions against sun and wind burn.

CHAPTER SIX

FOREIGN TRAVEL

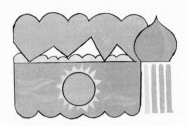

A TRIP ABROAD may help to improve physical and mental well-being if good health precautions are followed. The international traveler should consult a doctor as well as a travel agent. The doctor knows his personal health needs and requirements, and if he can see the travel itinerary, he can see that his health needs are cared for.

A health examination before departing is wise, if one has not been performed within the past few months. Minor medical and dental needs can be cared for, and any lurking major condition which might spoil the trip can be identified. Even if a postponement becomes necessary, this will be better than having illness mar an expensive trip.

Immunization

All travelers entering the United States are required to show an International Certificate of Vaccination. This certificate blank may come with the passport. If not, one can be obtained from a travel agency or local health department.

Travelers who go outside the United States for all but a few destinations are required to prove a successful vaccination against smallpox within the past three years in order to re-enter the United States. Vaccinations for cholera, diphtheria, plague, polio, tetanus, typhoid, and typhus may be required for travelers to areas of special risk. A doctor or the local health department can get information about vaccinations recommended for the traveler's protection, depending upon his itinerary. Each country has its own set of immunization requirements. Vaccinations are for both the traveler's personal protection and for the protection of people around him.

It would be well to give the doctor plenty of advance notice of your trip since some vaccinations can cause discomfort for a short time. Also, there are some vaccines that are not readily available to the doctor or to local health authorities.

Eating and Drinking

Every traveler needs to know about the safety of the water and food in the countries he is going to visit. In past years, food and drink were more of a problem than they are today. Now most countries you will visit have a sanitation code which keeps their own people healthy. In case of doubt, check with the local American embassy or consulate.

Conditions under which natives remain healthy may not be equally healthful for strangers who encounter new foods, new seasonings, and new germs. Except in large cities and well-known hotels, it is often safer to eat only cooked foods, avoiding salads and raw berries, fruits, or vegetables, unless they can be peeled. Even washing is not always a complete safeguard.

A wise traveler does not overindulge in food or drink when he is traveling. It is fun to experiment with foreign delicacies and native foods, but this should be done gradually so that a tolerance can be established.

If the water is unsafe, you can use such chemicals as tincture of iodine or a bleaching solution for sterilizing as follows:

Tincture of iodine: three to five drops (double this for cloudy water) for each quart.

Bleaching solution (sodium hypochlorite): two drops (double this for cloudy water) for each quart.

Commercial water purification tablets can also be obtained at most drug stores with instructions for use.

If there is doubt about drinking water, bottled water or soft drinks or beer may be considered safe. Hot tea and hot coffee are acceptable.

Eating should not be a problem if discretion and moderation are observed. Most major cities throughout the world have restaurants that observe the same standards for food and sanitation that prevail in the United States. However, if you suspect that the food offered has not been cared for properly and washed or cooked thoroughly, don't eat it.

Many travelers suffer from looseness of the bowels which may amount to stubborn diarrhea. When this happens, the diet should promptly be limited to toast and strong tea. If the condition does not improve in 24 hours, medical advice should be sought. Some travelers like to carry a supply of medicines with them to overcome any infection that may have been acquired and halt diarrhea. Such preparations should be discussed with the physician before departure, and the appropriate drugs procured through him, together with instructions for their use.

Locating a Doctor

When the international traveler needs a doctor, he usually desires a good general physician who has a knowledge of English. The traveler's own doctor might know of a physician in the country which is to be visited. Sources to check in a foreign country are the American embassy or consulate, the Red Cross, travel agencies, the police, medical associations, hospitals and clinics, American business or cultural institutions, church and mission groups, American armed forces installations, and the American Express. Wherever one goes in developed localities, he may expect to find a doctor who will be able to take care of his health problem. One need not feel hesitant about consulting a physician in any foreign country. In case of need, your personal physician in the United States is only a telephone call away.

The Traveler's First-Aid Kit

Unless you are going on safari or into the woods or mountains away from population centers, or into remote and underdeveloped parts of the world, don't load yourself down with a first-aid kit that takes space and adds weight, especially if you are flying. Ordinary drugs can be purchased in any major city around the world, and so can such medical supplies as finger bandages. Do take a clinical thermometer, a plastic bottle of 70 per cent grain alcohol or rubbing alcohol, and small vials of the everyday drugs you use.

If you are straying from the traveled paths

of civilization, you do need a first-aid kit. The basic supplies are listed below, but it would be advisable to consult health authorities or experienced travel agents about special needs for particular areas you intend to visit. Carry starred (*) items wherever you travel.

1. A first-aid booklet—American Medical Association or American Red Cross.
2. Scissors—sharp pointed variety.
3. Tweezers.
4. A roll of sterilized cotton.
5. Sterile gauze—two inches wide.
6. Adhesive tape—one inch wide.
7. Adhesive finger dressings.
8. *Toilet paper or cleansing tissues.
9. *Soap.
10. Collapsible enema bag.
11. Fahrenheit thermometer with case.
12. *Flashlight.
13. *Summary of medical history, particularly for those with previous serious illness.
14. Eyeglass prescription.

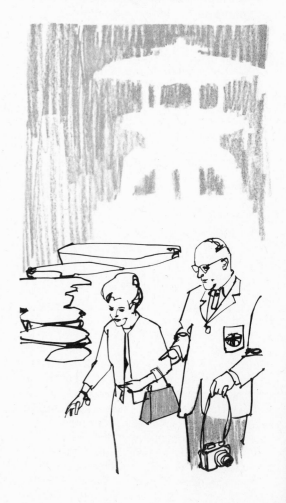

15. *Spare denture, if you wear one.
16. *Spare glasses, if you wear them.
17. *Plastic bottle of 70 percent alcohol.

A basic first-aid kit can be purchased at any drug store or notion counter in a department store. Replacements are available in all parts of Europe and in major cities elsewhere.

Some travelers may want to carry additional medicaments depending on their personal health needs and the conditions in the countries they intend to visit. Certainly everyone should carry any medicaments in current use. That is, patients with specific health problems should carry essential medicines and prescriptions for their refills abroad. A person subject to motion sickness should carry some sort of medication in the event this occurs.

Most important for the traveler who has a past history of illness or in the event of an accident or sudden illness, is an emergency medical identification card and perhaps a medical ID tag. (See Part IX, Chapter One.)

The traveler should check the climatic condition of the countries he will visit before selecting his wardrobe. In the tropics, clothing should be light in weight and color to help combat the heat and moisture. A hat or helmet must always be worn as protection against the powerful direct sunlight. In the colder countries, clothing should help combat cold, dampness, and, in most places, the absence of central heating. The traveler can check with a travel agent or experienced traveler to be sure his wardrobe will fit the temperature variations of the places to be visited. The traveler should always carry a raincoat, sweater, or jacket and comfortable walking shoes.

Sound health practices apply not only at home, but perhaps even more so when traveling abroad, or, for that matter, when touring in the United States. Whether one travels for business or pleasure, the trip will be more enjoyable and relaxing if the traveler remembers that good health and good sense go together.

Chapter Seven

CHILDREN'S CAMPS

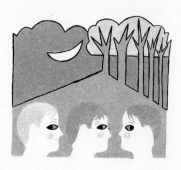

Almost every child has a thirst for adventure—a strong desire for new experiences, an urge to explore open fields, woods, and streams. Few activities, if any, provide greater opportunities for satisfying this urge than camping. The increasing number of school systems providing field trips as a part of the regular school curriculum is ample evidence that school authorities consider camping a valuable learning experience. The fact that the strong appeal of camping is not limited to children is apparent in the tremendous surge in family camping in our state and national parks and forests since the 1950's.

The increasing concentration of our population in large metropolitan areas has made it more and more difficult for a sizable percentage of children to enjoy the great outdoors. This situation has spurred the rapid development of camps which provide a seasonal camping experience for countless thousands of youngsters each year.

Perhaps the most important benefit the child gains from his camping experience is plain enjoyment. Removed from the daily routine of his home and school environment, he can thoroughly enjoy the variety of activities the camp offers. He will develop new interests as well as a new appreciation of many of the activities in which he previously participated.

Camping also helps the child to mature, to develop good sportsmanship, and a capacity for "ruggedness" when the going is hard. Camping makes an invaluable contribution to the child's health. The regular health practices at camp will reinforce those he has learned at home. The returned camper should have a greater understanding of the importance of such habits as eating well and getting plenty of sleep. He should also have learned the value of taking part in physical activities.

The camp offers a living laboratory for learning to get along with others. The child makes new friends and learns to give and take in his daily relationships with his fellow campers. He develops a sense of responsibility in learning to do things for himself and others. He also learns to adjust to a new environment. The city child will find the outdoor life a new and exciting experience, while a child from the country will face social situations not met in his farm home.

Spiritual values are also gained from the camping experience. In his daily contact with the wonders of nature, the child develops an increasing spiritual awareness. In his daily dealings with other campers he can be taught many moral and ethical values.

One of the important values for the camper is the feeling of independence which comes from being away from his parents for the camping period. This separation is good for both the parents and the child. He learns to do things on his own without depending on his parents or brothers and sisters for help.

Another important learning experience to be gained from camping is that of good citizenship. The child lives in a camp environment in which democratic living is a necessity. He learns the importance of being a contributing member of this democratic society and thus learns through actual practice the responsibilities of a good citizen.

The advantages just outlined accrue to most campers, and it is generally agreed that as many children as possible should have the opportunity to attend a camp. However, children differ, and it does not follow that every child should necessarily go to camp. Those who have no interest in going, or have been and do not care to repeat, should not be sent anyway "for their own good." There are other ways in which the desirable influences inherent in camping can be brought into a child's life.

Selecting the Right Camp

In choosing the right camp for a particular child, parents must consider several important factors relating to the camp's equipment and facilities, program and leadership. This is true regardless of whether the camps being considered are private or sponsored by public or voluntary youth-serving agencies.

The most important consideration is whether your child will have healthful living conditions. Parents must be assured that the eating facili-

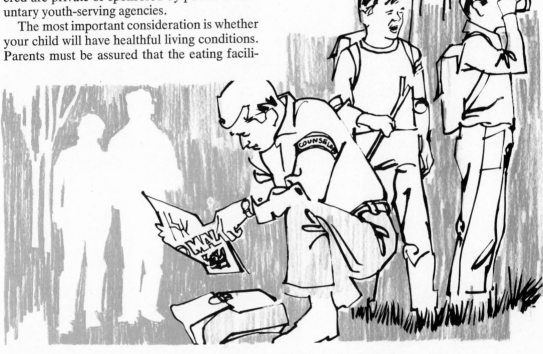

ties are sanitary. The meals must be well planned and the food prepared and stored under safe conditions. The water supply for drinking, bathing, and swimming, must have been determined to be safe through regular testing as required by local or state health authorities. In addition, the camp should employ acceptable sanitary methods for sewage and garbage disposal as approved by state or local health authorities.

The camp sleeping facilities should be well spaced, comfortable, and well ventilated. There should also be assurance that campers are allowed enough time for sleep.

It is most important that there be adequate provision for medical attention. It is highly desirable that the camp employ a registered nurse as a regular member of the camp staff. In any event, the camp should have a well-equipped infirmary and a doctor should be readily available in case of emergency. There

should also be an adequate program of communicable disease control.

The camp site should be free from serious physical hazards such as unprotected cliffs, swamps, and dangerous waters. Adequate safety equipment should be available to cope with a fire or waterfront accident. The camp staff should be trained to use this equipment and should know the latest and most effective accident-prevention methods.

The kind of leaders the child will have at camp is a very important consideration. The camp director should be a person of integrity, with a sound background of good camp experience and an understanding of children. The counselors should be mature (at least 19 years old), well-trained, and of high moral character. Each counselor should be the type of person to whom a child will turn readily for guidance. The camp standards suggested by the American Camping Association should be observed.

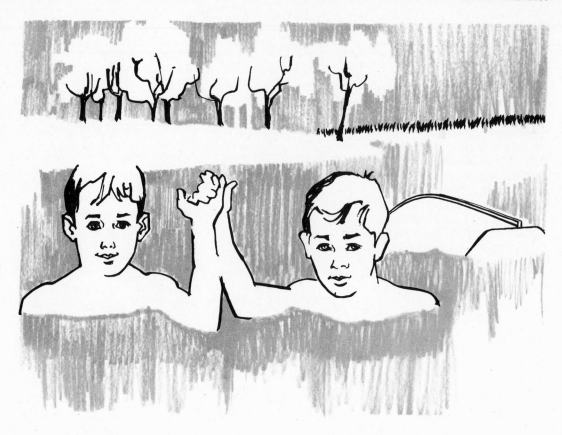

Each counselor should be responsible for no more than eight campers.

Parents should be concerned about the kinds of opportunities and experiences the child will have at camp. The camp program should be varied, well planned, and flexible enough to fit each individual camper's need for self-expression. There should be opportunities to learn new skills not possible at home and also to develop further any skills already acquired. There should also be sufficient opportunity for comradeship with the other campers. The living groups should be small enough to give each child a sense of "belonging."

The camp should offer new and exciting experiences in outdoor living. They should be selected so as to maintain a high level of physical and emotional well-being. There should also be ample opportunity for the child to develop leadership.

Parents should concern themselves about the standards used for the selection of campers, since they determine the types of influence to which the child will be exposed.

The general spirit of the camp is important. It should be a happy place. One of the best

ways to evaluate this factor is to determine whether or not the campers want to return next year.

One practical consideration is the cost of sending the child to camp. The parents should have some assurance that the child will receive a full measure of experience commensurate with the financial outlay. There are good camps at many price levels, the cost dependent upon length of stay, facilities available, and cost of leadership. Remember, however, that it costs money to operate a good camp.

Preparing the Child

In choosing the right camp, parents should assess carefully the child's needs and capacities. An important consideration is his readiness to leave home. He will be better prepared for the camping experience if he has already had a number of short stays away from home.

Perhaps the child has a special need for security, for discipline, for a group living experience, for independence, or for group awareness. Perhaps he needs special consideration because of some physical condition. The parents must decide whether the child's needs may be best met in a regular camp or in a camp especially designed for children with similar needs.

Before making the final choice of camp for a child, parents should make every effort to visit the camp and talk with its director or counselors. This firsthand observation can provide a much clearer picture of the camp, its objectives, strengths, and weaknesses than will any number of brochures. It is also well to talk to some of the campers themselves and, if possible, their parents.

Parents should make sure the camp is a member of the American Camping Association and that it is sponsored by an organization which has high standards of its own, or has an established reputation. Such membership insures that the camp has been visited by the ACA Standards Committee and has been accredited under its National Standards Program. The Association publishes a national directory of its accredited camps, which may be obtained for a nominal fee.

Parent Responsibilities

The responsibilities of the parents do not end with the selection of the camp. If the child is to have a pleasant camping experience, he must be prepared emotionally and mentally, as well as physically. One important part of this preparation is to talk with him about camp as a happy adventure.

Parents should follow closely the directions for preparation of the clothing and equipment the child will take with him. It is most important that he have a thorough physical examination before leaving for camp. Parents should also give the camp personnel any information about the child that will help them enrich his camping experience.

While the child is at camp, parents should write cheerful letters. It is important to follow the camp policy relating to such matters as visiting the child, sending food packages, and providing spending money. Following the rules regarding gift packages is important. Limits must be placed upon them because of space required for storage of extra articles. Food stuffs may spoil or may upset dietary practices in the camp. And if some campers have many extras and others have few, a feeling of inequality may be created.

Some metropolitan newspapers and national magazines provide a referral service or carry advertisements to assist parents in locating camps for their children. A few department stores in large cities also maintain school and camp bureaus or camp departments which offer assistance relating to camps.

Sections of the American Camping Association also provide information about camps in their areas. A list of these sections can be obtained from the American Camping Association, Bradford Woods, Martinsville, Indiana. Organizations in your own community which maintain camps can also be helpful in reviewing standards and selecting camps for children or for whole families.

CHAPTER EIGHT

HOBBIES

"EVERYBODY SHOULD have a good hobby for when he retires." This statement sounds like good advice, and it can be heard at almost any time when retirement is being discussed. But it isn't good enough advice. It is lacking in several important respects.

The statement seems to suggest that hobbies are all one needs for successful retirement, and that isn't so. It implies that hobbies can be postponed until retirement is right around the corner. It suggests that hobbies are more important than they really are for better health.

A good hobby is perhaps a help to better emotional health, because it helps to release the tensions created by an active life. But it is not a cure-all; it is not enough in itself to satisfy an active-minded person in retirement, and it is just as valuable before retirement as afterward. Moreover, it cannot be picked up when one retires, like putting on an old jacket instead of dressing up for the office.

What is a good hobby? It must be something one likes, not something that somebody else suggests one ought to like. What may be an excellent hobby for one person may be exactly wrong for somebody else. It must be worth doing. Mere wasting of time by going through the motions of some useless activity does not constitute a good hobby. This does not exclude doing things for fun, because fun is important to good emotional health. But it does rule out making things that cannot be sold or even given away, unless the procedure gives the individual real pleasure and deep-down satisfaction. A good hobby must do the following things:

It must help one to relax and put his problems and perplexities into the background for the time being.

It must give real satisfaction in the activity itself.

It should be more than a mere time waster.

It should produce something worth producing, either tangible or intangible.

It should increase one's knowledge and skills.

It should cost no more than one can afford; it may even produce revenue.

Hobbies are as varied as people. Some can play games and be happy—they enter shuffleboard tournaments, marathon bridge games, checkers, chess matches, or play bingo. Such activities are fine, if they fill the objectives outlined above. But if play gets to be a bore, it isn't any good any more. Some go for more active sports, in or outdoors—bowling, swimming, boating, fishing, volleyball, handball, golf, tennis, hiking, biking, gardening. All are good if they contribute to satisfaction with life. All are useless if they do not.

Collecting offers a great field for developing a hobby, although some forms of collecting may be expensive. The collector may save anything from precious jewelry to pocket matchbooks. Some collectors' items emphasize antiquity, some beauty, some rarity, some utility, and some just the collector's personal interest—which is after all the best reason there could be for collecting.

Just one topic may offer a variety of opportunities for collecting. The music lover may collect records, musical instruments, original scores of famous compositions, programs of operas or concerts attended, or books about music and those who make it. He may play an instrument for his personal amusement or with a group in church or elsewhere, or sing in a chorus, a church choir, or a barbershop quartet. He may even learn to compose.

Other collecting areas offer similar variety. Developing skills may be a fine hobby, as in the case of the woman who learned to play a piano and to speak French. She never played in public and had no great need to know French, but she enjoyed making music for her own pleasure, and mastering a language fascinated her. Many people train themselves in skills outside their business and professional lines. Doctors, lawyers, and statesmen paint, invent mechanical gadgets, play musical instruments, or study ancient history. Three prominent modern novelists, Somerset Maugham, A. J. Cronin, and Frank Slaughter, were doctors who found their best creative outlet in the writing of novels rather than in their basic profession. They began to write as a hobby, but the hobby took over.

Making things of beauty or utility is often a satisfying hobby, providing there is a real use for what is made—either through sale or by giving it away. Craftsmanship can be developed in wood, metal, leather, plastics, or other materials. The almost lost arts of embroidery, lace-making, and weaving can be a source of great satisfaction, as proved by the wife of an English dentist. She weaves all the materials for her family's woolen clothes, including her husband's and sons' suits, and has even woven material for export. She enjoys the satisfaction of seeing her family clothed by the work of her hands. This is a genuinely intelligent use of a hobby.

Among the best hobbies is service to others. This can be personal in nature, as was the case with the retired man who loved to tinker with things that needed repair. He went about among his neighbors doing repair jobs around their homes and would never accept any remuneration except thanks and a cup of coffee. He prepared for this by learning the necessary skills in his spare time before he retired. Service is needed by many organizations—churches, neighborhood houses, voluntary health agencies, and social service organizations. This may be almost anything from stuffing envelopes for an education or fund-raising campaign to preparing meals or serving refreshments, or even to ringing doorbells. People with time on their hands have a great opportunity to serve the political party of their choice by assisting at candidates' headquarters or in the field.

The aging and the shut-in offer a wide field for service by those who have time to spend in a constructive and heart-warming manner. These unfortunates can be visited; small and helpful services can be performed for their comfort and convenience; their loneliness can be cheered by playing games with them or reading to them. By helping some one else, the individual helps himself more; he may even find in unselfish service the key to better emotional adjustment for himself as he observes the sufferings of others and how they meet them.

An important opportunity for service exists in hospitals, out-patient medical services, public health clinics, and immunizing stations. Here the shortage of trained and practical nurses can be eased by nurses' aides, Gray ladies, and clerical volunteers. Varying amounts of training and experience are needed for these activities, but a good hobby includes the learning of new skills.

A hobby need not be profitable financially, but there is no reason why it should not be. A skilled photographer can find outlets for his talents by entering photo contests, submitting pictures to newspapers, magazines, and photograph syndicates. He can take candid pictures at social events, picnics, weddings, and conventions. Other hobbies too may open the door to profitable adventure.

A hobby cannot be picked up overnight. It should be the logical outcome of developing interests, which may be expanded when there is leisure time during vacations or when retired. A good hobby can be an emotional lifesaver during times of unemployment or work slowdowns. It offers a means of relaxation when pressures threaten to build up too much, and it may help to cushion the shock of crises or bereavements. In short:

It is important that a hobby be something worth doing.

It is important that it be chosen and started before the need for it is urgent.

It is important that a hobby give satisfaction, relaxation, and contentment to the one who practices it.

It is unimportant what other people think of your choice of a hobby. It's your life, not theirs.

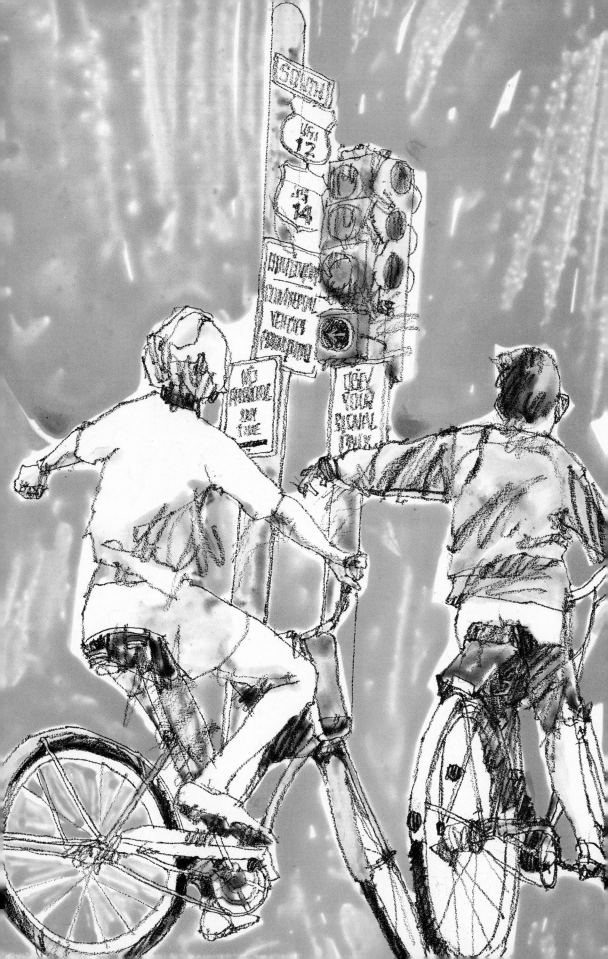

PART VII

Safety

CHAPTER ONE

SAFETY IN THE HOME

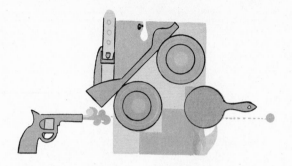

ACCIDENTS RANK fourth as a cause of death in the United States each year. Most important for parents, is the fact that more children between the ages of 1 and 14 years die as a result of accidents than of the next six causes of death combined. And accidents *in the home* each year are responsible for more deaths than tuberculosis, diphtheria, polio, syphilis, rheumatic fever, appendicitis, and murders *combined*. This is a startling fact often overlooked in the barrage of popular literature on health. During the past 15 years, while medical science has made astonishing strides in the reduction of deaths from certain diseases, there has been only a slight reduction in the death rate due to accidents.

Parents naturally want to protect their families from disabling and fatal mishaps, and parents are in a key position to do so. In fact, they occupy the key position. No teacher, no physician can do as much to promote home safety as parents can.

Safety is Common Sense

Let us suppose that the homemaker is cooking dinner. She is working from the stove to the sink, from the refrigerator to the dining room table. She fills a pan with water and sets it on the stove to boil. She sets it down just as she holds it—the handle jutting out dangerously over the edge of the stove. She doesn't give the procedure a moment's thought. She has always done it that way.

Along comes a two-year-old. Like all two-year-olds, he's curious. He talks in that semi-jabber, semi-understandable speech of his while his mother dashes around murmuring, "huh, huh, yes Johnny" at odd moments.

It's natural for him to want to see what's going on. It's just as natural as for the cook to have one ear open for the sound that warns her the water is boiling. Johnny hears it too. He reaches for the pan, pulls it towards him to see —and over it goes.

What would be the common-sense safety practice in this instance? Turn the handle of that pan slightly inwards from the edge of the stove so that Johnny can't reach it.

This common-sense attitude, consistently maintained can make the day—every day—free of accident. It is nothing more nor less than plain horse sense to keep a wary eye out for the multitude of big and little things that somehow manage to get left on the floor or stairs each day when there is a house full of youngsters.

But isn't it more sensible to keep those tripping hazards off the floor and stairs? This can be done, of course, by making the mother a semi-martyr who picks up after her family constantly all day long. Adults expect to pick up after themselves, of course, but why should parents not enlist the aid of the whole family and make them a party to this safety idea?

In many situations children can share in adult activities by working alongside their parents. Men who are handy at the work bench can let their sons work along with them. Mothers can give their daughters opportunities to work in the kitchen with them as they grow up. In situations like these, parents can find natural ways to teach lessons in the safe handling of tools and equipment. For instance, if a girl spills a little water or grease on the floor, mother can teach her to wipe it up immediately to prevent a fall. If adults do this as a matter of course when they are working in the kitchen, the chances are children will do likewise, for children are imitators.

If parents make sure that their own ways of doing things are reasonably safe, their children will be more likely to develop safe practices.

Of course, parents cannot prevent every mishap. Even if they could, they would succeed only in making a child timid and dependent.

But the large majority of serious accidents can be avoided if parents know where the common dangers lie and take steps to eliminate them.

Falls

Not only for the children's sake, but for adult safety as well, it is best to start at once by making the home as safe as possible. Each year some 27,000 persons are killed in home accidents. Nearly half of these deaths are caused by falls. What can be done to eliminate hazards that might produce a fall? A good start can be to make a tour of the house and yard and list all the things that need correction. Then, as soon as possible, correct the hazards.

What to look for? Starting with the yard, one should see that no fallen branches lie across the pathways, that the sidewalks are in good condition, that the back and front porches and steps are in good repair.

Window screens should be securely fastened when they are set in place for the summer season. Ladders used to put the screens up should be kept in good repair and checked periodically for loose or broken rungs.

Basement steps should have a handrail, preferably on both sides. Dim lighting on stairways should be replaced with better light.

Tripping hazards such as unanchored small throw rugs should be corrected. Handrails belong on all stairways with more than two steps, either on the grounds or in the house. Stair lighting should be controlled from both top and bottom.

Highly polished floors can be a very serious hazard. When wax is used on floors, it should be rubbed in thoroughly. This tends to make the small globules of wax harden in tiny beads which offer a traction surface. Repeated coatings of wax will gradually fill in these little beaded particles until there is a very smooth, highly slippery surface. Therefore, it is wise to remove all the wax about every fifth coating or so and start from scratch again.

Hands should be kept free and vision unobstructed in hazardous or unfamiliar surroundings. In the event of a slip, it is more difficult to avoid a fall if the arms are full. Hazards cannot be detected if the load which is being carried is piled too high.

Stairs and ladders should be climbed slowly and one step at a time with at least one hand kept free for support. Ladders should always be used rather than chairs or boxes, and should be firmly set and well supported.

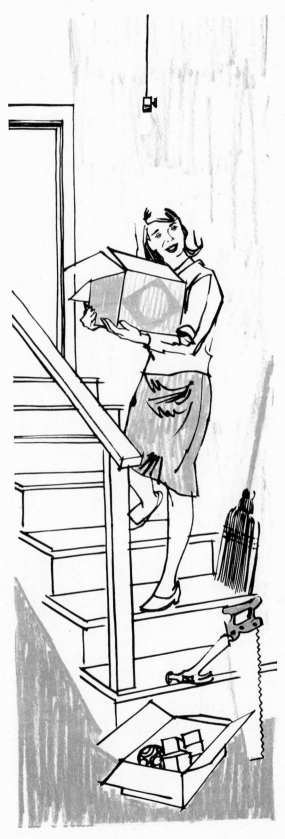

Sensible footwear, comfortable yet providing enough support for the activity engaged in, adds to safety. Wearing only stockings in the house may be quite comfortable, but could be very hazardous on slick floor surfaces, especially stairs. To wear out old and delapidated shoes can be dangerous.

Fire

Fires and burns are caused in numerous ways. Many people die each year in home fires caused by hazards such as faulty electrical equipment and wiring, smoking and misuse of matches, defective or overheated heating equipment, accidents with oil stoves, spontaneous ignition of rubbish, misuse of flammable liquids, hot ashes, and the placing of combustibles too near heaters.

Wiring in older houses is often inadequate for the increased loads placed on the circuits by modern appliances. Overloaded circuits, defective wiring, poor insulation, defective switches, and improper use of appliances contribute directly to fires from electrical sources. The overloading and consequent overheating of a circuit may be produced by trying to operate too many lamps, motors, or other appliances on one circuit. Wires with current-carrying capacities too small for the load sometimes become overheated and cause fires.

When electrical installations have loose or improperly made connections in wires, switches, or sockets, dangerous heating or sparking may occur at these points, even when currents are not excessive. The habit of using a penny or other permanent "bridge" for a fuse can be disastrous. So can the habit of using fuses of larger size than proper. Automatic circuit breakers are the safest form of fuse.

The entire family should assist in making the home safe. A hunt for hazardous rubbish can be made into a game. This is a project in which the whole family can take part, helping to clear out all rubbish in the basement, closets, garage, and attic. While removing one hazard, it is important not to produce another, such as running up and down stairs with loads so big that they obstruct your vision.

One inspection a year is not enough. No matter how much good it may do, it isn't going to eliminate fire hazards completely. Fire safety requires daily attention.

One must:

● Learn to see cigarettes that aren't completely snubbed out.

● Learn to see piles of oily rags left in the corner of a closet or the garage.

● Learn to see rubbish baskets left too near the furnace.

● And most of all, make fire safety practices a part of everyone's daily habits.

The following points will improve your chances of avoiding burns:

Everyone should know by now that pot handles should be turned parallel to the front of the stove but not over a hot burner—it's a habit that must be formed.

Because hot grease ignites readily, keep a pan lid ready to smother a possible fire; water added to it will cause it to splatter with explosive force.

Smoking and matches are still the number one fire hazard. Smoking in bed or when extremely tired should be taboo.

Enough large ashtrays should always be at hand. Matches should be out of children's reach at *all* times.

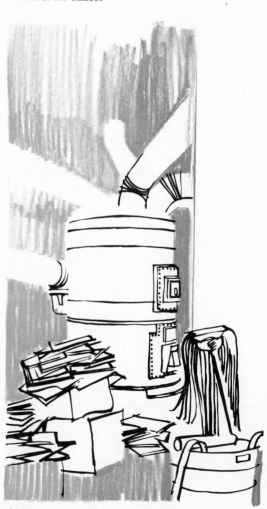

Flammable liquids (gasoline, oil, paint, etc.) don't necessarily need open flames near by to "flash." Their fumes are often flammable and can travel some distance; therefore, they should be both stored and used outdoors whenever possible and never used around flames, sparks, or anything hot. They must *never* be used for starting fires indoors.

Combustibles (paper, cloth, leaves, rubbish, wood shavings, etc.) should be kept away from heat and such ignition sources as heaters, fireplaces, furnaces, ranges, and electrical equipment including light bulbs. Special care should be taken in handling heat-producing electrical appliances since they continue to hold heat for some time after they have been turned off.

Any kind of fire should be kept where it belongs, in proper containers with spark screens and well away from buildings. It is wise to avoid getting too close to heat and flame since many injuries result from accidentally ignited clothing. Girls' and women's clothing fire most easily because of their loose and flimsy nature. Men's casual wear ranks second in danger.

Homes should have adequate emergency fire-fighting equipment such as fire extinguishers (with the Underwriters' Laboratories label). Several garden hoses with strategically located outlets are valuable.

When using torches, soldering irons, or other heating devices in the home workshop, a sturdy, noncombustible rack for holding them should be provided and a supply of water kept available to douse any uncontrolled fire.

Space heaters have caused many severe fires. Kerosene heaters should be of the type that won't tip over easily. Fuel lines for gas and kerosene heaters should be of metal tubing or rigid pipe (never rubber) and should be protected against damage. Electric heaters should have a safety switch on the bottom which will turn them off if they are tipped over. Gas and kerosene heaters should be vented to the outside of the house.

Home Heating Systems

Each year, especially during the winter months, deaths occur from poisonous gas. A typical instance was the death of a mother of a family of four. She and her family were overcome when a defective flue leading from a hot water heater filled their apartment with fumes and steam. Her husband and children, aged four and one and one-half, were revived by firemen and taken to the hospital. Firemen found the flue clogged—they scraped out half a bushel basket of rust particles.

Defective heating equipment can cause death from carbon monoxide gas poisoning and can also cause fire. Therefore, every home owner should check the following annually:

All flues and chimneys should be inspected and any corroded or cracked sections or linings should be replaced or repaired.

All furnaces and heating appliances should be inspected by qualified service personnel to be sure they are in proper adjustment and repair. Proper adjustment assures that the fuel will be completely burned and there will be no dangerous amounts of carbon monoxide in the flue gases.

All fuel-burning equipment, flue pipes, and chimneys should be checked regularly and maintained in good condition.

The type of fuel burned in the heating appliance should not be changed unless a qualified serviceman has made the necessary adjustments in the equipment to be sure of proper fuel combustion.

No furnaces, fireplaces, space heaters, or water heaters should be operated without an adequate supply of fresh air for continuous replacement of the air lost or exhausted through burning. (Local authorities and utility companies are the best sources of standards for adequate air supplies.)

Automotive Gas Poisoning

Many accidental deaths are due to faulty automobile exhaust systems. These should be checked regularly for blown-out gaskets, loose manifolds, leaking exhaust pipe connections, and holes in the mufflers. The objective, of course, is to be sure that the exhaust fumes are carried completely to the end of the tail pipe and away from the car.

When an automobile motor is running in a garage or any enclosed space, the garage doors should be open, and even then the motor should be run for only a few minutes. If it is necessary to run the engine indoors for any period of time, an extension such as used by commercial garages should be placed on the exhaust pipe and run directly outside.

When you sit in a parked car for more than a few minutes, shut the engine off unless the windows are open. While traveling through tunnels, or in slow-moving and closely-spaced traffic, you should close the air intakes of your

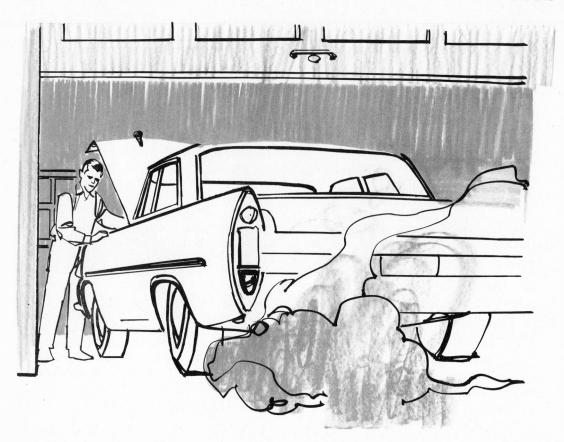

car to be sure that the carbon monoxide from the exhausts of automobiles in front of you will not collect in significant amounts within your automobile.

Electricity

Electricity is the most convenient form of energy used around the home. However, when improperly used, it presents a serious hazard to both life and property. In addition to death from electric current, it can also cause burns, fires, and shocks.

A three-year-old girl in a small midwestern city recently was left alone for a few minutes at the breakfast table. She grabbed a fork and tried to spear a slice of bread from the electric toaster, as she had seen her parents do. With adult skill this common, though ill-advised, practice seldom results in electric shock. In this case, however, the girl happened to have her other hand, which was moist, on the metal casing of the toaster—a perfect conductor for electricity. When the mother returned to the kitchen, she found her daughter unconscious from burns and shock. Despite immediate treatment, the child could not be revived.

Deaths from electric current indicate the need for adults and children to understand the dangers of electricity. Electricity should be a friend—and it can be if one follows the following safety rules offered by safety experts:

Too many lamps or appliances on a single circuit may cause a fuse to blow; this is a danger signal. The cause (usually overloading) should always be corrected before you replace the fuse.

Lamp or appliance cords should not cross over radiators or pipes; one should not touch such grounded metal when handling cords or appliances.

An electric appliance, radio, or light switch (even the phone) should not be touched when one is in the bathtub, is standing in a puddle (as on a laundry floor), or has wet hands.

Electric cords should not run in door jambs or under rugs. Constant closing of the door will damage the insulation, as will walking on the cord—and when it is under a rug, the damage will not be seen.

Convenient outlets in walls should be used for connecting appliances.

An electric iron should never be left connected and unwatched even for a few minutes.

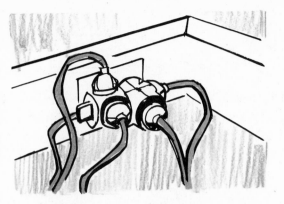

Plugs should not be pulled out of sockets by the cord, but by pulling on the plug itself.

A lamp, appliance, extension cord, power supply cord, or cord set should always bear the words, "Inspected, Underwriters' Laboratories, Inc." This is proof of a tested, electrically safe cord or appliance. Since the two are tested separately, both cord and appliance should have this label.

Cords with frayed or cracked insulation should be replaced. Sharp corners of furniture, twisting, or pulling on cords can cause protective insulation to wear out.

Repairs or additions to home wiring require the attention of a qualified electrical contractor. Electrical jobs do not constitute "do-it-yourself" projects.

Poisoning

Deaths from accidental poisoning in the home have been rising since 1956, as much as seven per cent a year. More than 1,500 Americans die from this cause each year.

Here is a flight in fancy. In a little town in Ohio, it's morning. The older children have gone off to school. With only four-year-old Johnny at home, mother is free to do some housecleaning. Johnny watches her for a while and then decides to play "doctor" with his toy animals. He goes to the bathroom and climbs up on the washbowl to reach the medicine cabinet. He takes down a bottle and samples some of it. Soon he's yelling in terror and pain. He is rushed to the hospital. It is a close call, but he survives.

Today his mother has all poisonous medicines, household cleaners, insecticides, and other poisonous items locked away where her children can't get at them. Even aspirin and laxatives, too often regarded as harmless, can cause severe trouble if a young child consumes

a quantity of them. And sleeping tablets are a deadly menace at all ages.

While children are all too often victims of accidental poisoning, the surprising fact is that more than two-thirds of all such accidents happen to people older than 14. Now is the time to take stock of practices around your house to determine just how likely your family is to suffer a tragedy of this kind. The following checklist should help you make this evaluation and point out where you could improve. Do I:

Read *all* labels carefully so that I know exactly what I'm taking or working with, its hazards, dosage, antidote, etc.?

Protect labels from damage so that I'll always know exactly what is in the container, especially in case someone takes the contents accidentally?

Know that many medicines change with age and become either stronger or weaker, and discard them when they are old or no longer needed?

Keep medicines for internal use entirely separate from those to be applied externally?

Avoid taking medicines in the dark and read labels at least twice when taking medicines or using hazardous products? (Nurses are trained to read them *five* times.)

Avoid transferring potentially hazardous or poisonous substances into other containers even temporarily, without first labeling them and NEVER put them into kitchen utensils, soda bottles, or the like?

Keep medicines and pills in separate containers, not mixing them?

Wash all fruits and vegetables thoroughly before using?

Never allow insect and rodent poisons in the kitchen, and know which ones can be used with relative safety in food storage and preparation areas?

Know where the local poison control center is and how it can be contacted?

Naturally, with children in the house, additional precautions are necessary. Kids can get into the darndest things. The householder should be aware that common household products like detergents, waxes, kerosene, mothballs, hair sprays and dyes, match heads, and many others can be lethal and that it takes a lot less poison to kill a child than an adult. Therefore, these things should be kept locked up or well out of reach of little ones. Lockable medicine cabinets are now available.

Since children love to imitate adults, medicines should not be taken in their presence if

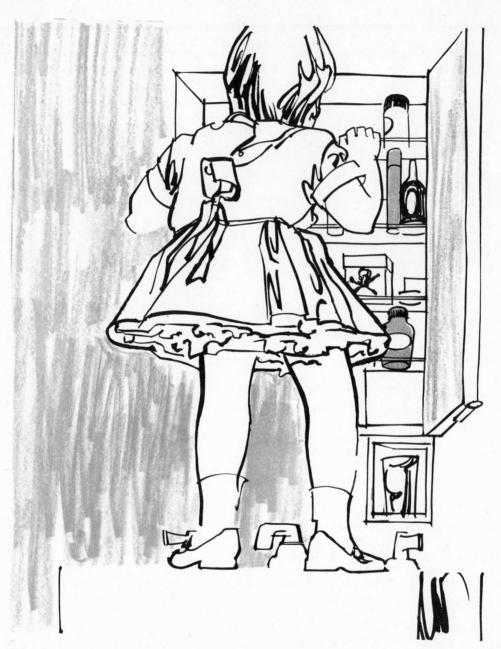

this can be avoided. Aspirin is the number one child poisoner. Medicine for children should always be called just that, never "candy."

The preceding check list should be used to make a *room-by-room inventory* of your home. It is amazing how many potential poisons will be found within easy reach of everyone in the average home.

Cuts

Everyone gets cut from time to time—some people more often than others. For the most part these injuries are passed off as among the hazards of enjoying life to the fullest. But what about the next cut? Will it be just another small nick that requires only a little do-it-yourself first aid? Or will it be one that causes severe pain, costs you time away from work and play, and perhaps leads to blood poisoning, tetanus (lockjaw), or a severe infection requiring removal of a finger, hand, or leg?

Perhaps there will be partial crippling because of a cut tendon or too much loss of blood. These things don't always happen to the other fellow. It is possible to avoid that bad cut or avoid cuts altogether by following a few simple general safety rules. The following checklist will help you and your family improve your safety habits.

Use of Cutting Implements

• Keep them sharp. Because dull tools usually require more force to do the same amount of work, hands using them tire more quickly and slip more easily.

• Keep them in good repair. Handles should be sound and solid to provide a proper, safe grip. Blades and metal parts should be sound and not in a weakened condition.

• Store them in a safe place. Knives, hand tools, and utensils should be kept in racks or drawers completely separate from other tools. Larger tools, such as axes and sickles, should be so stored that they cannot topple or fall when bumped.

• Transport tools in a safe manner. Generally when carrying tools, you should hold them with their points and cutting edges away from your body. However, turn them around, blunt-edge first, when handing them to someone else.

• Use them as they were intended to be used. Generally cut away from the body or use a cutting block or board. Don't use knives as hatchets or razor blades as knives (except with proper holders).

• Broken pieces of glass, porcelain, ceramic, etc, should be swept up and wrapped in several thicknesses of newspaper before discarding. If broken glass falls into water, the container should be first drained and the pieces removed using several pieces of cloth to protect the hands. (This operation is particularly hazardous when washing dishes.) Small slivers are easiest to pick up with damp paper towels. Specific items beside bottles and tableware which often cause severe cuts are: broken porcelain lavatories, glass table tops, glass door handles, and porcelain faucet handles.

• A relatively new hazard is the large glass areas in modern buildings, especially glass doors and window walls. Such hazards should be protected with furniture, planters, or other barriers or well marked to reduce the possibility of "walking through." (At a little extra cost, safety glass is now available for replacements or new installations.)

• Despite the well-known hazards of razor blades, people still get cut by them. A special container should be provided for their disposal, preferably with a slot in the top which can be sealed over when the container is discarded. Another safe way to dispose of blades is to wrap them in toilet tissue before putting them in the trash container.

• Sheet metal in all its various forms can always present a hazard especially when broken, torn, or improperly finished off. It should always be promptly repaired, protected, or discarded when unsafe.

• Tin can lids should be accorded the same respect as broken glass. Older can openers should be replaced with modern, safer implements.

• The improper use of steel wool has caused many a deep gash. It should never be separated into smaller portions by tearing, but should be cut with shears. Better yet, buy it in the single-portion "pads."

Firearm Accidents

More than half of all fatal firearm accidents occur at home rather than in the field under actual hunting conditions. And the greater part of these accidents do not happen to the younger set, but are almost equally divided on either side of the 25th year of age. Older, supposedly experienced persons have plenty of gun accidents. "Why so many gun accidents at home?" This question will probably answer itself in the following gun safety rules:

Know your firearm. Know what makes it fire, what its potential hazards are, and what special safety features it possesses.

Treat every gun as if it were loaded.

Always keep a muzzle pointed in a safe direction (usually up or down).

Never load a gun unless you intend to shoot it at something.

Break, open the bolt, or otherwise make a gun safe when leaving it unattended.

Keep the safety catch on but don't trust it.

If possible, keep others away when handling or cleaning guns.

When storing, keep unloaded guns away from children and irresponsible adults and in a different location from the ammunition. (Ideally, guns and ammunition should be locked up.)

When demonstrating your gun to others, insist that they use proper safety precautions when handling it.

Keep guns in top condition by cleaning, lubricating, and inspecting them according to the manufacturer's recommendations.

Never leave obstructions, such as patches of dirt, in the barrel.

"Collectors" and antique guns, if still operable, should be checked by a competent gunsmith to determine whether they are safe to use with today's high-powered ammunition and if they may be fired with safety. If no longer operable, they should be made safe by removing the firing pin and destroying the ammunition intended for them.

The backyard or other populated areas are generally not acceptable for target shooting since adequate backstops are not available for protection against ricochet. If basement shooting is to be pursued, only small caliber weapons should be used under proper conditions which include a steel plate backstop and a sandpit for receiving the slugs. Local gun clubs can probably supply all the information needed for an installation of this kind.

Pellet guns, whether powered by compressed air or gases, can also be extremely hazardous and most of the same rules for gun safety should be applied to them. These guns, however, are probably better suited for basement target shooting since they do not require such elaborate installations.

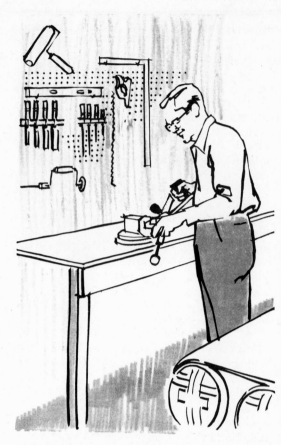

Gardening

Almost every home has its gardening "bug." And even if you have none, you still have dozens of little jobs to do to maintain your yard and garden. Such activity can be an interesting as well as a profitable form of recreation, and one which is comparatively safe.

Experience proves that yard accidents occur more frequently to amateurs and younger gardeners than to experts or adults. Most accidents are caused by unsafe practices or conditions, or a combination of both. Gardeners should be aware of the dangers that exist and observe the following suggestions to insure safety in the garden:

Select garden tools with care. Good tools are safe tools. A few well-chosen tools are better than many chosen haphazardly.

Use the right tool for the task at hand. Tools misused are tools abused. The right tool is a safe tool.

Avoid throwing any tools.

Keep garden tools in good condition. Safe cutting tools are sharp and clean. Tool handles should be smooth and strong. Shovels, spades, trowels, and forks should have points that are smooth and properly shaped.

Avoid use of dull, dangerous, and broken garden tools. Dull tools are unsafe—sharpen them. Broken tools are dangerous—repair them.

Rusty tools are difficult to use—clean them. If tools are beyond repair, discard them.

Store garden tools in a safe place. Tools lying on the ground cause accidents—pick them up. Tools piled in a corner carelessly are inaccessible and dangerous; arrange them.

A place for every tool and every tool in its place is a safe rule to follow.

When rakes are on the ground, be sure that teeth are down. Be sure the sharp edge of the hoe is always down.

Garden spray materials are dangerous. Handle spray materials with care as directed on labels. Study directions for their use and follow them carefully.

Know the nature of the material used, the danger of being poisoned, and the antidote.

Thoroughly cleanse your hands and face and all objects contaminated by poisonous materials. Store poisonous materials in a safe place.

Label poisons plainly as such. Substitute nonpoisonous insecticides whenever possible.

Be able to recognize poisonous vines, shrubs, fruits, and insects. Avoid contact with poison oak and ivy. Destroy permanently all poisonous growths.

Wash hands thoroughly but gently after working in the garden. Insect bites should be properly and promptly treated; serious infections can result from insect bites.

Guard against cuts and infections. Protect all cuts and scratches with proper antiseptic covering. Remove all foreign matter, such as glass, metal, wire, etc. from the soil.

Use gloves if skin is tender or susceptible to rash. Wear sturdy shoes and appropriate garments for protection.

Observe the fire laws. If they require it, secure a permit from the fire department for an outdoor fire. Bury garden refuse; it is a valuable source of fertilizer.

Avoid accidents caused by fatigue. Set an attainable goal. Limit the size of the garden. Avoid sudden or sustained periods of activity.

Power Tools

Power tools are a boon to weekend gardeners. But they can also deal the user or an innocent bystander a serious or even fatal injury if proper safety precautions are not followed. Below are some suggestions for safe use of power tools.

Because these tools are usually smaller and lighter than power tools used on farms, many people seem to have the mistaken notion that they are safe for children to operate. Never allow children, immature youths, or uninstructed adults to operate them.

An examination—before using—for leaks, loose connections, loose fittings, etc. will often prevent troublesome or dangerous situations from arising during operation.

Always shut off power before cleaning, adjusting, oiling, or refueling.

Always store tools and accessories so that there is no chance they will trip or cut persons passing in and out of garage or shed.

Store only small quantities of fuel in approved containers, kept tightly capped and plainly marked.

Mowers and Garden Tractors

Follow manufacturer's manual of directions in operation.

Make sure power mower or tractor is not in gear before starting motor.

Keep chain shields or belt shields in place at all times.

Keep blade shields in place. (The hand-propelled lawn mower with a power-operated horizontal rotary blade usually has a removable shield, which must be removed in order to cut weeds and tall grass. Use extreme caution during this operation.)

Keep children and pets well out of way when mower is being used.

Check lawn for all debris which could be thrown by the mower.

Do not mow up or down slopes. Mow crosswise to avoid foot injuries.

Always disconnect the spark plug before making repairs or adjustments.

Never attempt to unclog a power mower while it is running.

Never refuel while engine is running or is excessively hot.

Avoid pulling a power mower backwards.

Shut off motor whenever leaving the job temporarily, in case children happen to be playing around.

Stand firmly with feet clear of the blade while starting the mower.

Keep gasoline only in an approved marked container.

Operate power mowers at reduced speeds whenever possible.

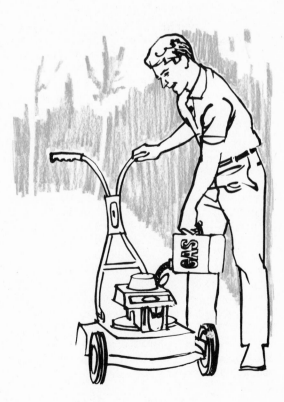

When riding mowers, keep your feet on the foot rests.

Keep your mower in good repair.

The usual injuries involving the use of electric hedge trimmers are amputated fingers, serious cuts on fingers and hands, and cuts on knees and legs incurred while lowering the trimmer to rest the arms. Shocks and short circuits from frayed cords or use of inferior or indoor extension cords also occur.

Make sure you have long enough heavy-duty cord and extension (never use ordinary indoor extension cord).

Rotary type trimmers (with whirling circular blades) may throw cuttings and twigs into space. Always wear safety goggles when using this type.

Hold clippers in position ready for use before switching on current. Use both hands to hold and guide clipper.

Always shut off current when resting arms, picking off cuttings, before changing direction of cut, etc. If trimmer becomes jammed or fails to start, always turn off switch before attempting to free the jam or before looking for the trouble.

When leaving the scene, even for a couple of minutes, always shut off current and disconnect plug. If there are children nearby, carry clipper with you.

Always keep children well away from the scene while clipper is in operation.

All portable electrical equipment should contain a built-in ground wire with a polarized plug and receptacle. This protection is necessary in the event that the equipment is used in wet grass or hedges. It is recommended that the new "U" shaped grinding slot receptacle and plug be used.

Home Dry Cleaning

While many housewives do some of their own dry cleaning, few realize the dangers involved. Many cleaners are made from flammable liquids. The word *in*flammable means flammable—not *non*flammable. Inflammable cleaners are flammable!

The fumes of these liquids can travel throughout the house. The fumes from flammable liquids are heavier than air and will seek a lower level. Homes have been blown to bits when these fumes have reached the pilot light in the basement hot water heater or on the stove in the kitchen. The tiniest spark of static electricity caused by rubbing textile materials together can set it off, too. The common-sense answer to using flammable liquids is obviously —*don't do it*.

Some nonflammable cleaners have been put on the market, but the fumes from these cleaners can be toxic. The labels on containers of cleaning fluid should be read—and heeded! The directions are there for a reason. If there is a possibility that the fumes will be toxic, the directions will call for adequate ventilation while using the liquid.

The best safety precaution for home dry cleaning of clothing is simply "don't do it"— especially since garments may be cheaply and more effectively cleaned by commercial establishments, or by coin-operated machines.

In case you insist on dry cleaning at home, however, take these precautions:

- Use only a nonflammable fluid. (A fluid may be marked "nonexplosive" and still be flammable.)
- Avoid doing anything that will set loose fumes from the fluid in any building.
- Do the cleaning outside of the house, where all toxic and other vapors will be quickly dissipated.
- Keep hands out of the solvent by using a suction washer.
- Keep children and pets at a safe distance.
- Never use gasoline, naphtha, or kerosene for cleaning garments.

Accidents are Preventable

Most accidents can be prevented. From the blinding of an infant who gets into a cleaning compound to the scars from kitchen burns, accidents can be prevented. It is not, however, just knowing what causes accidents that prevents them. It is rather a daily, hourly awareness of the dangers inherent in the simple details of living, and a constant habit of "doing something about it" that prevents them. It takes the cooperation of every member of the family, but it can be done.

One reason why so many accidents occur in our homes is because we don't believe they can happen to us. It is always the other fellow. We fail to recognize that we *are* the other fellow. The sooner we start believing that accidents can happen to us in our own cozy homes, the quicker we can make our home a safer—and happier—place in which to live.

CHAPTER TWO

SAFETY ON THE PLAYGROUND

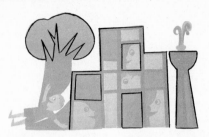

USE OF THE PLAYGROUND and play field facilities has increased because of both the national "population explosion" and greater neighborhood use of public and school playgrounds. While a most desirable trend, this has however, resulted in more playground accidents.

Unfortunately, only limited statistics on playground accidents are available. A number of schools, however, do report their school jurisdiction accidents to the National Safety Council. Of the reports received and analyzed, organized play activities, such as baseball, football, etc., accounted for about 23 per cent of the accidents. Playgrounds not under school jurisdiction produced 5.5 per cent of the accidents. Nearly half of the accidents that occur have a contributing factor of an environmental hazard such as a fence, uneven turf, etc.

Parents have a primary responsibility to know about the area or areas that serve as playgrounds for their children.

Recreation officials should consider "building into" play areas conditions that will assure the greatest protection and safety. Parents should insist that they follow these principles:

A play area should be near the population center of the district it is designed to serve. The most dangerous and heavily traveled streets should serve as district boundaries.

An important factor is the safety of the children going to and from the playground. Safety patrols should be established at definite periods during the day.

The playground should be in clear view when approached on the street from any direction. If it is impossible to provide open approaches, warning signs of standard design should be displayed in prominent locations.

It would be best for playgrounds not to be located near such features as railroads, taverns, or industries, although there are excellent playgrounds which are near these.

Regardless of the size of the area, parents should use their influence to assure partial separation for children into groups of different ages or physical development. The types of games played, the nature of some sports, and the size and weight of older youth often contribute to hazards for younger children.

Where ball diamonds, football fields, and courts for various games are included as part of the playground, exits and entrance areas should be located to minimize congestion and its associated hazards.

Some local school or public officials do not concur with the policy of enclosing the playground area with a smooth wire fence to keep activities confined. Whether there is a fence or not, parents must assume responsibility for teaching their children about the dangers of running into streets or other adjacent hazardous areas.

Playground Equipment

It is better to concentrate apparatus in one section than to scatter it over the playground, although overcrowding must be avoided. Whenever possible, apparatus should be in a well-defined area, such as between a fence and a path.

Rules for the use of apparatus should be understood. Supervision and education will also encourage proper use of equipment. Age groupings should be noted in connection with certain pieces of equipment and strongly adhered to.

Existence of public playgrounds should not discourage parents from providing their own backyard play space with apparatus and parental supervision wherever space permits. Children are more important than lawns or gardens.

Swings. Swings should be set firmly and the frames should be securely braced. Hooks, hangers, clamps, and connections should be examined regularly. Swings should be set at different heights for different age groups. Children should not be allowed to stand up or kneel on swings, or to jump from moving swings. Children should be discouraged from

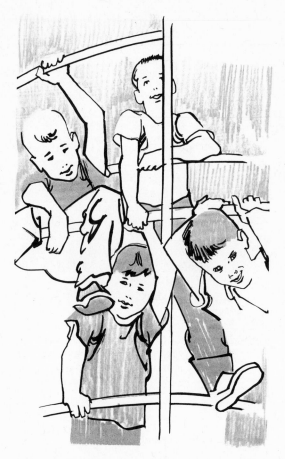

from broken glass and other debris. The frame of the box should be inspected frequently to see that there are no protruding nails or screws and that it is free from split portions or slivers. Bottles and sharp utensils should never be permitted in sandboxes. Boxes should be covered at night so that unnecessary moisture will not accumulate in the sand and to keep out dogs and cats.

Ladders and Bars. Ladders of various heights should be available, depending on the age of the children using them. Children should take a firm grip before swinging, and traveling should be in one direction. Heads and feet should never be put through rings. Benches and boxes should not be used as take-off boards.

Wading Pools. Water should be kept clean by frequently emptying the pool. Children should not stay in the water too long or enter it with a skin disease.

Drinking Fountains. Fountains should be free from paper, stones, and rubbish, and should be kept clean and sanitary in accordance with local health standards and regulations. Pushing near the fountain should be discouraged; broken teeth may result.

Baseball. Face masks, body, and shin guards are necessary for the catcher if accidents are to be avoided. Bases should be of such material that a player sliding into one will not be injured. Basic rules should be observed as to how close spectators or players stand near the batter.

Football. Properly fitted protective equipment is vital in this sport. Overexhaustion is common, especially in warm weather. Adult supervision is considered a "must" in some playground areas and considered advisable where bodily contact is in evidence. The playing field should be carefully checked for broken glass and other debris.

Toys and Play Equipment. Parents or supervisory personnel have a responsibility to check the equipment regularly for any defects and to assure its being safe to use. Certain toys and equipment associated with sports should be restricted to use at home or under adult supervision—guns, bows and arrows, darts, javelins, slingshots, etc.

All sports and recreational activities have a certain element of danger. However, hazards can be greatly reduced if parents guide their children in their choice of activities. Frequently an underdeveloped youth will try to "keep up" with a big brother or an older pal who is able to compete safely in a given activity. Many serious accidents have resulted from a child be-

holding smaller children in their laps while swinging. Playing or standing near swings or climbing on frames should not be allowed, especially when swings are in use.

Slides. Whenever possible, slides should be placed in the shade, since the chute becomes hot from exposure to the sun. This is especially true of metal slides. Soft clean sand, or sand and sawdust, should be placed at the bottom of the slide and replaced or added to at regular intervals. Crawling or running up the slide, sliding down backwards, and sliding in wet bathing suits should not be allowed.

Teeters. Teeter board fulcrums should be protected to prevent children from smashing their fingers. A block should be placed under the end of the board so children will not catch their hands or feet under the board if it descends too rapidly. Children should be instructed to warn the person on the other end before they get off, and to stay away from a teeter board when they are not using it.

Sandboxes. Permit only small children to use the sandbox. Sand should be checked at regular intervals to make sure that it is free

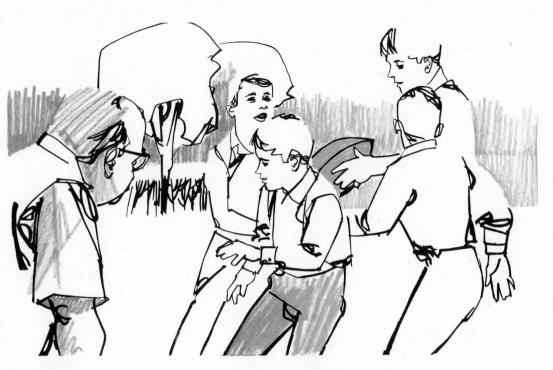

coming involved in a sport or game that was beyond his mental or physical capabilities.

Unauthorized Play Places

While parents know of many permanent hazards in their neighborhoods, they frequently fail to take heed of hazards which are either temporary or seasonal in nature. Some common dangers of this type are:

- Bodies of water, irrigation ditches, and excavation projects.
- Eroded or rotten equipment.
- Underground holes or shafts from mining.
- Highly combustible or explosive substances.
- Empty houses and buildings or new construction sites.
- Railroad property.
- Dumps and junk yards.

Children have a natural desire to explore, take chances, exert, and excel. Effort on the part of all adults to help create and maintain safe playground areas will help satisfy these desires while reducing needless accidents and resulting suffering and injury.

CHAPTER THREE

SAFE BICYCLING

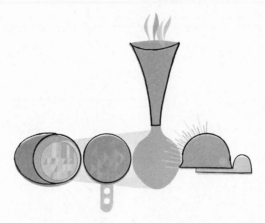

BICYCLE RIDING is a pleasant part of the American scene, and each year more and more people "take to the wheel" for recreation or transportation. But there is a less pleasant side to bicycling; each year many people are seriously injured or lose their lives in bicycle accidents.

Data on the number, seriousness, and circumstances of bicycle accidents are scarce because reporting of such accidents is seldom required, except when motor vehicles are involved. But even the meager data available points up the bicycle problem as one that should receive the serious attention of parents and community leaders. In recent years, from 400 to 500 deaths and 25,000 to 30,000 injuries a year have occurred in collisions between bicycles and motor vehicles. By far the greater number of these deaths and injuries were suffered by children from 5 to 14 years of age.

Much can be done at the community level to promote bicycle safety. Many cities and towns have adopted ordinances providing for the regulation and registration of bicycles. Bicycle licensing facilitates the identification of the rider and of the bicycle, the tracing of lost or stolen bicycles, and increases the sense of responsibility of the rider.

However, parents cannot rely on these requirements alone to promote safe cycling. They must assume the major responsibilities for the safety of their children. These cannot be "shrugged off" onto the local school officials, police, or other youth leaders. Among these responsibilities are the following:

- Teaching riders when and where bicycling is safe.
- Helping riders get their bicycles in safe condition.
- Promoting a more friendly attitude toward law enforcement officers.
- Developing an understanding among riders of the purposes of traffic regulations.

Safety Programs

Further, parents can do much to strengthen both official and voluntary bicycle safety programs conducted in their community. These programs are concerned with most aspects of cycling safety and include inspection programs, the establishment of bicycle routes, proper parking and storage, education programs, and the development of cycling skills.

The primary purpose of bicycle inspections is, of course, to insure their safe mechanical condition. In addition they have an educational effect in making the owner think definitely about safety at least at the time he reports for the inspection. It is very important to make maximum use of this aspect in conducting a bicycle safety inspection campaign. The inspectors should be carefully trained to realize that their job is to promote safety—not simply to make inspections in a mechanical way. Everything possible should be done to make the bicycle rider feel that the inspection is not a nuisance but a real service to him. All defects should be carefully explained.

A compromise regarding the use of sidewalks and roadways by bicycle riders is generally necessary for maximum safety. Riding on sidewalks might be prohibited in business districts and in other localities where the pedestrian movement is heavy. Along residential streets where the pedestrian movement is light and where the volume and speed of vehicular traffic make bicycle riding in the street both dangerous and annoying, bicycles might be prohibited on roadways and limited to sidewalks. The accident experience and circumstances should govern the solution of this problem for each community.

Homestead, Florida, a small city just south of Miami, has found a practical and highly successful answer to the problem by setting up Bicycle Safety Routes. Secondary traffic routes connecting housing areas with schools, playgrounds, shopping centers, ball parks, and other centers of activity have been designated Bicycle Safety Routes, and so marked with large, easy-to-read signs.

The safety routes generally parallel the most heavily traveled roads, and the peace of mind afforded by their safety seems to more than make up for the few extra minutes it takes the cyclist to get to where he's going. Homestead's Bicycle Safety Route Program, the first in America, was the brainchild of the Dr. Paul Dudley White Bicycle Club, long active in

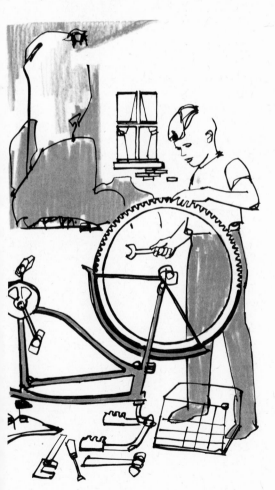

Homestead which is known as "The City of Bicycles."

Club members, with the aid of the local Chamber of Commerce, convinced the city fathers of the need for and the feasibility of the project. Working with traffic engineers, they laid out the routes, then raised the $1,000 necessary for the manufacture and installation of the 300 blue-and-white metal signs.

Then, enlisting the aid of the police department and the board of education, the club members launched a city-wide indoctrination and education campaign to acquaint everyone in the community with the program. Descriptive leaflets were sent to homes, and police officers lectured at schools, PTA, and service club meetings.

Finally all was ready, and on February 8, 1963, Dr. Paul Dudley White, famed heart specialist and bike enthusiast for whom the club was named, came to officially open the routes by leading a parade of more than 300 cyclists over them.

The program appears to be a great success. Motorists instinctively slow down when they see the blue signs. Many avoid the routes entirely, leaving them to the cyclists. Bikers avoid the busier streets, and the parents of the more than 600 youngsters who bike to Homestead schools each day rest more easily. They know their children are getting good, health-giving exercise by biking to school in the safest way possible.

Bicycle riders using the roadways are subject to the same regulations, responsibilities, and privileges as motor vehicle drivers. When operated on the roadway, bicycles belong on the right side, moving *with* traffic, in both urban and rural areas. A number of factors make riding on the right-hand side desirable:

• Crossing and turning at intersections from the right-hand lane is an easier and more natural movement; and it is less confusing to motor-vehicle drivers.

• Bicycle riders cannot be expected to yield the right-of-way on the pavement to every approaching vehicle. Raised curbs, rough or soft shoulders, guard rails, and other obstacles often make leaving the pavement hazardous for bicycle riders.

• It is possible for a motorist to adjust the speed of his vehicle to that of a bicycle moving in the same direction and wait for a safe time to pass, but he must pass, regardless of circumstances, when meeting a bicycle moving in the opposite direction.

When there are systems of parks or parkways, bicycle paths can be easily established. These are particularly attractive where they follow rivers, canals, and other scenic routes. Such bicycle paths should be considered as a part of every comprehensive recreational development plan.

For boys and girls, especially those who are just learning to ride, cycle paths can easily be established around the edges of playgrounds. In certain parks or other recreational centers, circular or elliptical tracks with properly banked corners can be provided for fast cycling. In these "bowls" youngsters can exercise without endangering themselves or others.

Serious injuries are caused, particularly at night, by persons stumbling over bicycles which have been left lying on the ground or sidewalk. Many bicycles left lying in a driveway or roadway are damaged by being run over by motor vehicles. In all homes in which there are bicycles, special places should be arranged for storing them. The garage or basement is best. Arrangements should be made to hold the bicycle firmly in an upright position.

Suitable bicycle racks should be provided at schools, post offices, newspaper offices, playgrounds, theaters, and other places where children, messenger boys, workmen, or others wish to leave bicycles. If the bicycles are to be parked for a considerable time, the racks should be protected from rain by some sort of roof. Racks have the advantage that bicycles may be locked in place and thefts avoided.

Because the majority of bicycle riders are children, every effort must be made to reach them by education rather than punishment. Children are more receptive to safety education and will develop a safety consciousness more readily than adults. Consequently, every consideration should be given to the teaching of bicycle safety rules in the schools, the spon-

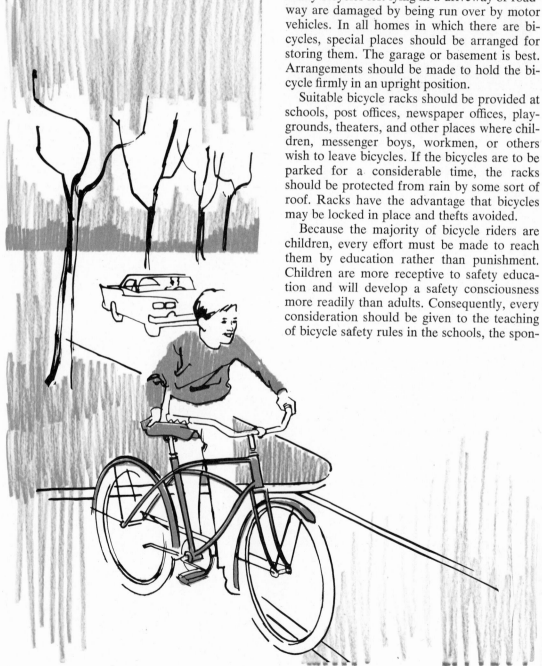

soring of juvenile safety meetings, the showing of bicycle safety films, and the distribution of literature on bicycle safety.

Parents who have a proper appreciation of the bicycle safety problem will undoubtedly encourage safe riding practices and attitudes in their children. The adult bicycle rider, too, should not be overlooked.

Safety Rules

The Bicycle Institute of America offers the following "Bike Riders' Safety Rules":

1. Observe all traffic regulations—red and green lights, one-way streets, stop signs.

2. Keep to the right and ride in a single file. Keep a safe distance behind all vehicles.

3. Have a white light on front and a danger signal on rear for night riding. Wear white or light-colored clothes at night.

4. Have a satisfactory bell or horn to warn of approach. Always ride at a safe speed.

5. Give pedestrians the right of way. Avoid sidewalks, if possible; use extra care when riding on them.

6. Look out for cars pulling out into traffic. Keep a sharp lookout for the sudden opening of car doors.

7. Ride in a straight line. Do not weave in or out of traffic or swerve from side to side.

8. Always use proper hand signals for turning and stopping. Park your bicycle in a safe place.

9. Slow down at all street intersections and look to right and left before crossing.

10. Be sure that your brakes are O.K. and keep your bicycle in perfect running condition.

11. Never carry other riders—carry no packages that obstruct vision or prevent proper control of your bicycle.

12. Never hitch on other vehicles, "stunt," or race in traffic. Never ride two on a bicycle.

Families and neighborhood and community groups have a wealth of opportunities to develop cycling skills and appreciation. Simple as well as more complex bicycle safety programs can be administered with limited resources. Some of the more common program activities are as follows:

- Bicycle riding skill tests
- Bicycle obstacle courses
- Rules and laws matching tests
- Bicycle inspection lanes
- Bicycle rodeos
- Bicycle clubs
- Bicycle safety contests
- Bicycle reflectorization programs
- Bicycle courts

Building the proper attitudes among bicycle riders will serve as the foundation for a sound, effective program in the education and training of automobile drivers in the years ahead. Skills, knowledge, and attitudes developed at the bicycle rider age have been found to have a positive influence on driver behavior. Parental example and respect for constituted authority likewise has great influence on the bicycle rider's general acceptance of responsibility.

CHAPTER FOUR

SAFE AND SANE MOTORING

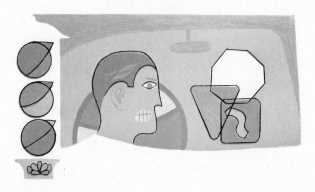

THE AUTOMOBILE has utterly changed the way of life of the whole world, and especially that of Americans. We are now a mobile society and a significant part of the country's economy is devoted to the automobile and related industries. Making automobiles and maintaining them, building and maintaining streets, roads, highways, and parking areas all provide millions of jobs. Service and housing of automobile travelers similarly account for great numbers of jobs.

Unfortunately, the automobile has been a mixed blessing. Along with its many benefits has come a tragic record of loss of life, disabling injury, and property destruction. There were 41,000 traffic deaths and 1,500,000 injuries which were disabling beyond the day of the accident in 1962. Minor injuries numbered about 3,000,000.

Accidents of all kinds are the leading cause of death up to the age of 36. Motor vehicle accidents outrank all other causes of accidental death for all age groups except the under 1 and over 75 categories. Traffic accidents constitute one of the nation's major unsolved health problems.

Motor vehicle travel increases each year. Travel totaled 767,000,000,000 miles in 1962, an increase of 29,000,000,000 miles over 1961. There were about 79,000,000 vehicles in 1962, a four percent increase from 1961, and about 91,000,000 drivers, an increase of slightly more than two percent over 1961. Predictions for the future show continuing increases.

The death rate per 100,000,000 vehicle miles has shown a rather steady decrease over the past 40 years. The total number of annual traffic deaths, however, has remained relatively the same because of the yearly increase in the number of miles driven.

Age and Accidents

Since traffic accidents are the leading cause of accidental death among young people, special attention needs to be focused on the young driver. The young adult (16-24) has the best reflexes, the fewest physical disabilities, the highest visual acuity, and in general, the least illness of any of the groups of driving age. The accident record of this age group, particularly males, however, shows a disproportionate number of accidents. Many traffic safety people attribute this high accident rate to the fact that many young drivers have not acquired the mature judgment needed for continued accident-free driving.

This judgment can be developed only through driving experience. Parents and adults responsible for teenagers' learning to drive should make every effort to provide as much supervised driving experience as possible. The purpose of driver training is not just to get a driver's license but, more importantly, to teach safe driving habits. It is unfortunate perhaps, that the aggressive attitudes which many feel are important to business and social success and which many parents attempt to instill in their children, are not the attitudes which lead to the safest possible operation of an automobile.

At the other end of the age scale, there is a disproportionate number of traffic accidents involving those above age 65. The infirmities of age, slowed reflexes, and physical disabilities all play a part in this increased accident incidence.

While there is an increased frequency of accidents in this group, it is certainly true that many elderly people can operate an automobile in complete safety. Therefore, it is not practical to establish an upper age limit for drivers. Rather than an arbitrary age limit, driver's licenses should be renewed for elderly people after a reasonable examination and a road test in which driving ability can be adequately demonstrated.

Human failure is the principal cause of traffic accidents. Poor judgment, faulty attitudes, emotional disturbances, and physical disabilities are basically responsible for most accidents. Thus the greatest potential for accident prevention programs lies with the driver—his intelligence, his sense of personal and social responsibility, his reactions to various stimuli

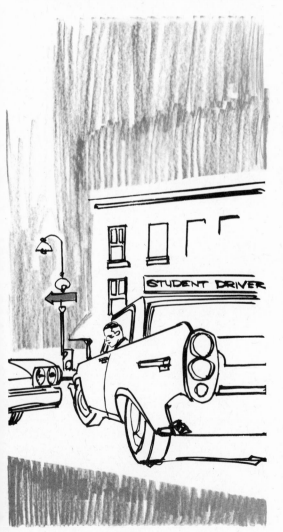

in normal conditions and under stress, and his driving ability in good health and in bad.

Drugs, Alcohol, and Accidents

Many persons of driving age take drugs and medicines, hopefully under the direction of a physician, but sometimes self-administered. Many drugs produce reactions that temporarily impair the ability to drive an automobile. The degree of impairment varies tremendously depending on the severity of the reaction and individual susceptibility to the drug. Drugs likely to impair driving ability include central nervous system depressants; hypnotics, sedatives, and anesthetics; tranquilizers; central nervous system stimulants; antihistamines and drugs preventing motion sickness; and anti-infective agents.

The use of alcohol is responsible for many automobile accidents. Studies show that approximately half of all fatal accidents involve a drinking driver.

Many people incorrectly think of alcohol as a stimulant. Its true effect on humans is in all phases and stages a depressant. Driving performance begins to be impaired when the concentration of alcohol in the blood reaches about 0.05 percent, or 50 mg. alcohol per 100 cc. blood. Studies using individuals accustomed to drinking point up that two 12 oz. bottles of 3.2 percent beer or 2 oz. of 100 proof whiskey consumed within one hour will impair the driving ability of the average moderate drinker.

Alcohol is oxidized in the liver and eliminated through the kidneys and the lungs. The average person of 150 lbs. can oxidize and eliminate about one-third fluid ounce of alcohol per hour. It is best not to drink at all for several hours before driving. However, a practical rule for drivers to follow is: One drink may be tolerated, two drinks impair driving ability for about two hours, three drinks are too many for safe driving.

Safety Factors

Automobile accidents rarely result from a single cause. The multiple factors involved make it very difficult to obtain statistical evidence on accident causes or to isolate the effect of one factor. There are, however, some positive steps which can be taken to reduce the chance of injury when an accident does occur. Chief among these is the use of seat belts.

Several states now require that all new cars

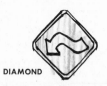

DIAMOND

THE WARNING SIGNS MEAN GET READY FOR DANGEROUS OR UNUSUAL ROAD CONDITIONS AHEAD, SUCH AS CURVES, INTERSECTIONS, HILLS, DIPS, SCHOOL ZONES. OBEY THEM.

ROUND

THE RAILROAD ADVANCE WARNING SIGNS MEAN A RAILROAD CROSSING IS AHEAD. BE PREPARED TO STOP. MAKE SURE ALL TRACKS ARE CLEAR BEFORE CROSSING.

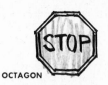

OCTAGON

THE STOP SIGN, RED WITH WHITE LETTERING, MEANS WHAT IT SAYS —COME TO A FULL STOP. BE SURE THE WAY IS CLEAR BEFORE PROCEEDING.

RECTANGLE

THESE WHITE SIGNS STATE THE LAW, SUCH AS "NO PASSING" OR "SPEED LIMIT 50." THEY TELL YOU WHAT TO DO AND GIVE INFORMATION.

TRIANGLE

THE TRIANGLE YIELD SIGN REQUIRES A DRIVER TO YIELD — SLOW DOWN OR STOP—TO GIVE THE RIGHT OF WAY TO CROSS TRAFFIC.

CROSSBUCK

THIS IS THE TRADITIONAL SYMBOL AT RAILROAD GRADE CROSSINGS. ALONE, OR WITH A BELL, LIGHTS OR GATES, IT IS THERE TO WARN YOU TO BE ALERT.

have two seat belts installed in the front seat prior to sale. The evidence is clear that the use of seat belts will materially reduce the number of fatalities and the severity of injury in automobile accidents. Other safety features available are crash padding for dashboards, visors, and ceilings, collapsible steering wheels, and head rests.

The car and the road on which it travels are important elements in safe transportation, and much attention is quite properly given to the engineering design of automobiles and roads. But it should never be forgotten that the driver is the most important safety factor of all. If the driver performance can be improved, there will be fewer accidents.

One way to improve driver performance is to expand driver training and safety education programs. No beginning driver should be permitted to drive unaccompanied by an experienced driver until he has shown himself to be competent in the handling of the vehicle and knowledgeable of the rules of the road.

Good Driving Habits

Good driving, like many other skills, can be reduced to a habit pattern which permits the individual to react quickly and correctly in an emergency. Some good driving tips are:

1. Keep your car in good condition, with special attention to tires, brakes, steering, and engine operation.

2. Keep the car as clean as possible, especially windshield and windows.

3. Fasten seat belts before starting the motor.

4. Drive at a speed suitable for road and traffic conditions.

5. Keep the car under control at all times.

6. Signal all starts, stops, and changes of direction, using hand signals when necessary in addition to automatic turn and stop signals.

7. Drive only when fully alert.

8. Drive only when you are not fatigued; if sleepy, stop and nap.

9. Drive only when you have not had alcohol or any medication which might make you sleepy or interfere with good coordination.

10. Drive only when you are mentally and emotionally calm.

11. Keep your temper when other drivers irritate you.

12. Keep your mind on your driving.

13. Refrain from smoking while driving.

14. Wear glasses at all times if you need them while driving.

15. Avoid arguments or distracting conversations while driving.

16. Keep the inside of the car uncluttered, especially the back window ledge.

17. Keep children and pets away from you while driving; children should be restrained by seat belts or harnesses, and pets should be trained to lie down and be quiet or should be put in a cage.

18. Think and look ahead, behind, and all around—keep yourself fully oriented to traffic conditions and be ready to meet changing situations whenever they occur.

19. Be patient when delays occur—trying to run up the shoulder to get ahead in the line can be dangerous.

20. Look before you back up, especially out of a drive where children may be playing—a "back-up horn" is a good investment.

Overconfidence, the feeling that accidents can happen only to the "other fellow" is possibly the most deadly of all the driving booby traps, leading to carelessness and recklessness. Good drivers are defensive drivers—anticipating and reacting to potentially dangerous situations. They realize that the stop light which suddenly flashes far up the road, or the siren that sounds behind, may affect them and they respond accordingly. Other situations that may produce trouble include:

Sand blowing off trucks. This can cover your windshield—don't follow too closely.

Trucks carrying heavy machinery. These are often wider than normal, and the load may project behind; watch for red flag signals.

Deer crossings. The signs should be heeded, especially at night; the eyes of the deer may reflect the headlights.

Old and battered cars, especially if they are losing rubber from tires; a blowout might affect your car.

Two cars passing in opposite directions at high speed near you; slow down in case they crash or side-swipe.

Carelessly loaded trucks which may drop crates in your path or send a heavy plank crashing into your windshield.

Fumes in station wagons near the back window, especially when it is open; be alert for the smell of exhaust fumes and avoid carbon monoxide gas poisoning. For the same reason, stay far enough back from other cars so that their exhaust fumes do not enter your car.

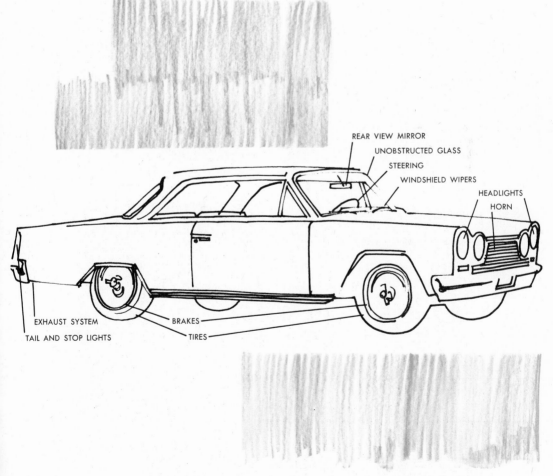

REAR VIEW MIRROR
UNOBSTRUCTED GLASS
STEERING
WINDSHIELD WIPERS
HEADLIGHTS
HORN

EXHAUST SYSTEM
TAIL AND STOP LIGHTS
BRAKES
TIRES

Give frequent checks to the points designated above to be certain your car is safety sure.

CHAPTER FIVE

BOATING AND SWIMMING SAFETY

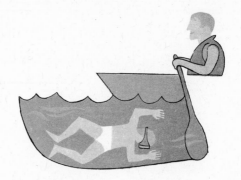

BOATING OFFERS American families a great opportunity to get outdoors in a sport which can be enjoyed by almost every age group. Every year, 40,000,000 people engage in this healthful and fun-filled activity using at least 8,000,000 boats. Accompanying this activity are a number of safety considerations which cannot be overlooked—especially by the person planning a family outing.

Boats range from large cabin cruisers to small boats with outboard motors and canoes. Most precautions herein pertain especially to small boats, but some refer to boats of all sizes. One fundamental rule takes precedence over all others: Persons using boats for the first time should familiarize themselves thoroughly with all phases of boating, including how to cope with engine failure in power boats. They should understand weather warnings and develop a basic ability to judge weather trends for themselves, at least to the extent of recognizing circumstances which suggest they should head for shore.

Among the more common boat hazards are overloading, incorrect loading, improper movement of passengers, horseplay, and poor trip planning.

Drowning is the principal concern in all water activities, as more than 90 per cent of the approximately 1,200 boating fatalities that occur in the United States each year belong in this category. Thus, the prevention of drowning is the first concern for anyone planning a boating trip.

The best precaution to take is to "drown-proof" your entire family by insuring that everyone knows how to swim. This requires considerable forethought, for just a little swimming skill may not be enough in a boating emergency. Preferably all family members should be schooled in survival-type swimming —the ability to stay afloat—and how to swim while wearing clothes. The Red Cross or YMCA normally provides this type of training.

For the family going on a boating outing, especially for the first time, a number of other preliminary precautions should be taken. Appropriate dress guarding against sun exposure should be worn. On a sunny day one can expect the sun's rays to be compounded by their reflection on the water surface. Every boater, especially persons highly sensitive to the sun, should regard a hat as essential.

Basic Training

There can be no substitute for training for the novice boatman. The nearest U.S. Coast Guard Auxiliary can be consulted for courses in boat handling. Local boating clubs and the Red Cross also frequently provide such training. This training is essential before taking the responsibility for the safety of others. The greatest single cause of boating collisions is failing to obey the right-of-way rules. There is really no excuse for ignorance, since copies of these rules are readily available.

The Federal government and a number of states have laws covering boat ownership, operation, and registration. The Recreational Boating Guide published by the U. S. Coast Guard (U. S. Printing Office, Washington 25, D.C.—40c) should be studied by all boaters. The Outboard Boating Club of America, 307 N. Michigan Ave., Chicago, Ill., also publishes an excellent handbook of state boating laws.

The condition of your boat and its equipment is of basic importance. A must for every boater is a safety inspection each year by a competent agency, such as the U.S. Coast Guard Auxiliary or local Power Boat Squadron. Inspections are normally offered without cost and involve no obligation to the boater.

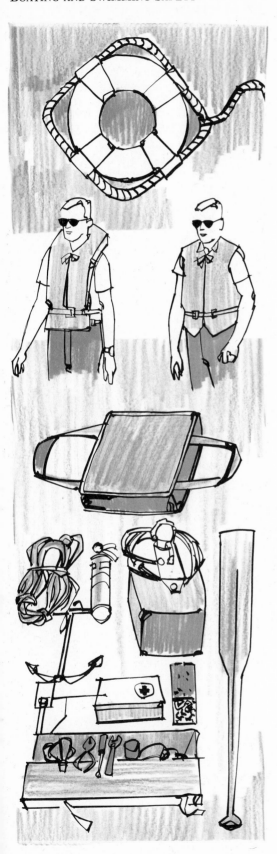

All craft should be checked thoroughly for leaks and other defects prior to casting off on any trip. Any water that may have accumulated in the boat must be removed. Even a small amount can become a slipping hazard. On all small boats, it is a good idea to carry an extra oar or paddle and a bailing can. Motor-driven boats should carry a fire extinguisher and tools or equipment for minor motor adjustments or repairs. A first-aid kit is always good equipment on any type of boat.

There should be life jackets for each passenger with appropriate sizes for all ages. Life jackets should be put on children before they board any craft. This in itself can add fun to a boat outing if you borrow some of the expressions, known to all children, such as "count down," "check your equipment," "prepare to shove off," etc.

Never hesitate to have "all hands" wear life preservers whenever the weather or any other unusual circumstances cause the slightest doubt of safety. Make sure all life preservers carry the U. S. Coast Guard approved label. A good idea in selecting life jackets or buoyant cushions is to pick a bright color such as orange which will contrast with the normal color of water and can be a significant aid in search and rescue.

A briefing session, or "boat drill," for all passengers is vital before casting off.

This can be something of a challenge, where children are concerned, with their excitement running high and anticipation clouding most other thoughts. Nonetheless, it is sound practice and better than trying to issue instructions when an emergency occurs.

Briefing normally covers such specifics as:

• Seating arrangements and the necessity for each passenger to stay in his assigned place.

• Instruction to stay with the boat in the event of capsizing, because it usually will not sink entirely beneath the water surface and people can be located and rescued more easily.

• Assignment of "buddies"—the person to look to in case of emergency.

Total safe load, including passengers, outboard engines, and any other heavy equipment placed in the craft must not be exceeded. Determining the safe passenger load capacity for a small boat involves a number of technical considerations for which competent and specific advice should be sought in advance. The obvious danger in overloading is that it reduces freeboard—the distance from the waterline to the gunwhale or edge of the boat. Thus the craft can take water easily and even overturn.

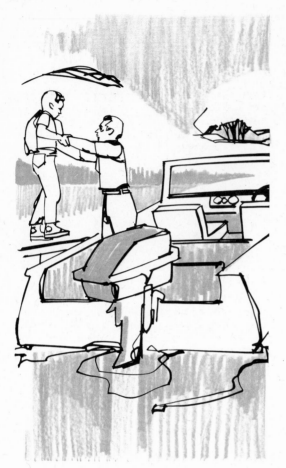

moving barges can weigh thousands of tons, need lots of room to turn, and often can't stop in less than half a mile. Avoid standing or drifting in the channels frequented by these large vessels; they frequently have a blind spot just in front of the lead tow which makes a small boat invisible to the pilot. Courtesy as well as common sense requires any boater to keep in plain view at all times.

The wash of such large craft, or for that matter, of speed boats, can swamp or overturn a small boat caught broadside. Before large swells reach your boat, turn and head into them, slowing down so that they will slide under you from end to end. Conversely, when operating a boat which leaves a high wake, courtesy demands reduced speed when passing small craft and their docking areas.

Passage through anchorages must always be at a minimum speed since a wake can rock other boats violently, spilling dishes and hot fluids and causing other nuisances.

The standard distress signal for boaters in the event of disablement or when help is otherwise needed is a slow and repeated raising and lowering of the arms outstretched to each side. A boater can increase the visibility of his signal by holding a handkerchief, towel, or shirt in each hand.

The difference between a fun-filled, safe

At best it will be awkward to handle.

Rough water requires even lighter loading. Stability of small craft is aided by keeping loads as near the bottom as possible. Sitting on the seat or thwarts of a canoe makes the craft less stable. It is far better for paddlers to kneel and all others to sit on the bottom.

Even on brief cruises it is always a good idea to check the weather forecast before departing. Offshore winds can make the center of a lake dangerously rough even though the water near shore is calm. In addition to sufficient fuel in the tank, it is a good idea to carry an emergency supply in a clean can with a safety spout. Never attempt refueling with the motor running.

Boat Handling

Many small-boat operators fail to realize the power exerted by a strong current or the difficulties of maneuvering large craft—especially the commercial barge type frequently encountered on open waterways. These slow-

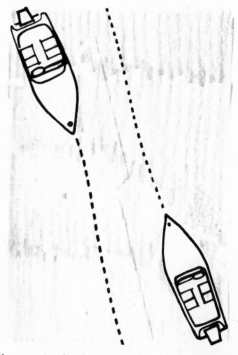

When meeting head on or nearly so, keep to the right.

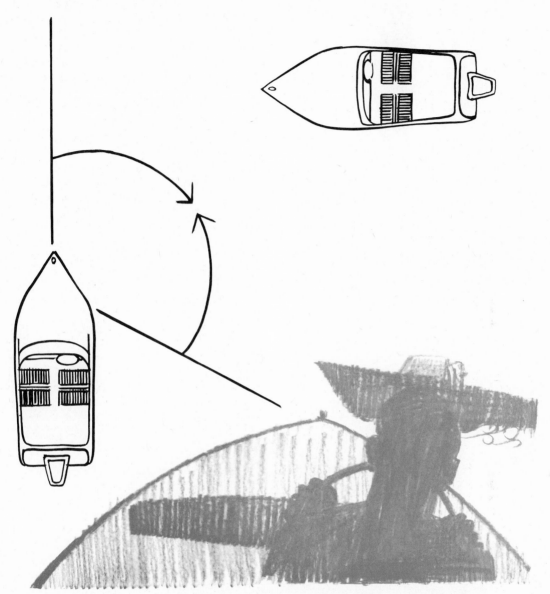

When crossing, the boat on the right has the right of way, and the boat on the left must make adjustments.

boating adventure and a tragedy rests with the boat operator. In the tradition of the sea captain, a boat owner must be responsible for all that occurs aboard his vessel. So it behooves every boater—actual or potential—to learn all he can about this wonderful sport so that he and his family can have maximum enjoyment of our wonderful water resources.

Falls are a prime cause of injury afloat as well as ashore. Tripping hazards should be eliminated whenever possible, or marked conspicuously if they must remain. Shoes that grip the deck are essential.

Good housekeeping is even more important afloat than ashore. There is less room on a boat for storage, and in an emergency some article may be needed in a hurry. There should be a place for everything—and everything should be kept in its place. This practice also makes for cleanliness and helps reduce the chance of fire aboard ship.

Water Sports

A boater may engage in many related water activities. Fishing, one of the most common, requires only a few special precautions:

1. Don't stand up or jump around in the

boat—control your enthusiasm even when netting a big fish; this can be a special problem when very young "sailors" are in the party.

2. Cast overhead, not side arm.

3. Make sure that back casts do not hook others on board.

Water skiing is another popular activity which any good swimmer can enjoy. The sport is easy to learn and does not require a large degree of athletic ability. Because skiing should never be done in less than five feet of water, a novice swimmer should improve his ability before he puts on skis. The flotation device worn by all knowledgeable skiers is no substitute for swimming ability. But no skiing should be done without a life vest or jacket which will keep the skier's head out of the water in case the splash of impact leaves him breathless. Devices can be obtained which meet Coast Guard specifications; they can be used as boat equipment as well as for water skiing. A skier who falls should recover his skis quickly since they also will help keep him afloat.

When operating in an area frequented by Scuba (Self-Contained Underwater Breathing Apparatus) divers, boaters must be mindful of the flags which indicate that a diver is in the water. This flag is square with a red background and diagonal white stripe from the top of the hoist to the bottom of the fly. By staying clear of such an area you will avoid striking a submerged diver or cutting his line.

Swimming Safety

The National Safety Council estimates that only about half of the American people swim well enough to take care of themselves in the water. And one doesn't have to go swimming or boating to get into trouble in the water.

Of 6,500 drownings in a recent typical year, only 2,500 took place while victims were swimming. The others fell into the water from docks, piers, boats, or while fishing, and most of them were clothed. If they had learned nothing more than how to stay afloat with clothes on, they might have been saved.

The first thing any prospective swimmer should learn is how to float. The body floats naturally because of the air in the lungs. Trouble comes when the swimmer becomes panicky and tries to get too much of his body out of the water. Then he starts to flounder. Even very small children can learn to float, with clothing or in bathing suits. Treading water and dog-paddling are easy first steps in learning to swim.

Swimming instruction is available in almost every community for those who need it. Many children take to water naturally and learn to swim without instruction, but they must be

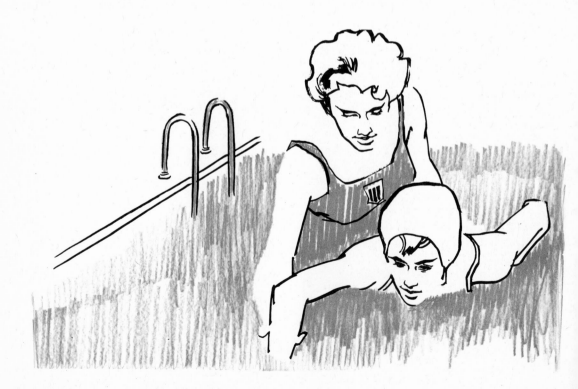

supervised until they learn. For lessons, one may consult the community facilities where swimming pools exist—the schools, playgrounds, gymnasiums, and YMCA. The American Red Cross has published standard instructions for formal lessons, and the local chapters provide the instruction in many communities. Many schools now make swimming an integral part of their physical education program. It is recommended that children expecting to spend a summer at a camp learn to swim during the previous winter or spring.

Learning to swim is a basic necessity for anyone who ever goes in, on, or near water. But even experienced swimmers can drown if they forget or ignore the principles which make swimming safe. Some of these warnings, which too often go unheeded, are as follows:

Don't swim at a beach or pool that is posted as dangerous.

Always swim with a buddy, never alone.

Don't swim at night except in lighted and attended pools.

Don't go swimming without letting some responsible person know where you are going.

When swimming across a lake or river, or performing other endurance tests, have a boat accompany you.

Pay attention to posted depth signs if you are not a good swimmer.

Don't swim in the surf unless you are a strong swimmer.

Don't dive into strange waters where rocks or stumps may be concealed.

Don't call for help unless you mean it—remember the boy who called "wolf" so often that nobody paid attention when he really needed help.

Don't let children float into deep water on wings or inflated toys.

Don't indulge in swimming races or endurance tests immediately after a meal.

Don't dive or jump into extremely cold water; the shock may cause muscle cramps; it is better to ease in gradually; also avoid swimming long distances in cold water.

Cramps are due to cold or tired muscles; if you get a cramp while swimming, draw your knees up to your chest while floating, and massage the cramped muscle.

Water games should be played according to the rules; rough-house in the water and especially ducking non-swimmers should be strictly avoided.

Questions have been raised about the dangers, if any, involved in swimming after a meal; at some schools, parents have protested against swimming instruction immediately following lunch. The swimmer caught with a "cramp" is the bogeyman of the small boy being warned against going beyond his depth. Studies have shown that simple swimming, without competitive urge and in the absence of emotional disturbance is not interfered with by the process of digesting a recent meal, nor does swimming affect digestion.

The practice by apprehensive mothers of keeping their children from even wading after a meal is unnecessary and has no medical justification. Swimmers should not, however, plunge into cold water after being overheated by a ballgame on the beach.

Scuba Diving

A sport of increasing popularity is Scuba diving. This is a sport for experienced swimmers only and for persons in good physical condition and of a courageous and calm temperament, since there is more than a little danger involved.

Special safety sugestions for Scuba divers pertain to the equipment which assures the diver of pure air to breathe, and from which the sport takes its name—*Self-Contained Underwater Breathing Apparatus*. These are:

1. Use water-cooled compressors only; never air-cooled.

2. All compressors should have an outside intake located at a height of at least 20 feet.

3. In order to insure maximum freedom from air pollutants such as carbon monoxide from automotive or boat engines, air should be compressed in the early morning or at night.

4. There should be regular (monthly) inspections by state authorities to be sure that sellers of air for Scuba divers are delivering air of the requisite purity; such suppliers should be licensed.

5. Those who train beginners in Scuba diving should be licensed by the state to require that they are familiar with symptoms due to bad air, and with the right safety procedures if that situation occurs.

CHAPTER SIX

SAFETY ON THE FARM

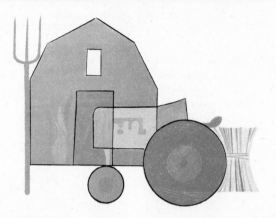

SEVERAL THOUSAND farm residents die in farm, home, and highway accidents each year. Many hundreds of thousands suffer disabling injuries and are often permanently crippled. The human and economic costs are enormous. This is why farm leaders are so concerned about accidents, why they often ask for help in the big job of preventing accidents.

The farm has many hazards. The entire farm family, because it lives on the worksite, is exposed to farm or farm-work dangers. Farmers must operate many kinds of machinery and handle many different jobs requiring a variety of skills.

Farm safety is up to the farm family—no safety consultant comes out to help the farmer as is the case in industry. In the factory or office, the boss or a safety supervisor sees to it that everyone is trained for his job, that machines are properly guarded, and that everyone works safely. It is much easier to keep the number of accidents low in places where work habits and work areas can be checked often. Because of this fact, industry and business (except mining and construction) have a much better safety record than does agriculture.

Individuals are to blame in 9 out of 10 accidents. There are many reasons why farm people have accidents; often a combination of things lead up to them. For example, let's take the case of John Smith who lost an arm in a corn picker trying to unclog the picker with the power "on." But what happened before the accident that got John into trouble? He was usually a safe operator.

A week ago, John and his neighbor had an argument over some bad fencing. Last night they met in town and John came home boiling angry. He lay awake half the night. The morning went badly—his wife was grouchy, the trac-

tor wouldn't start, and the neighbor's cows had gotten into his yard. He was in no mood to go to the field that day. He was sleepy and tired and so occupied thinking about what he'd tell Brown about those cows that he wasn't paying much attention to his job. His reflexes were slower. The accident stage was beautifully set—a tired, angry, preoccupied man . . . a powerful tractor and a potentially dangerous machine . . . then a bad clog to anger him further. He jumped off the tractor, not turning off the power, and attacked the mass of stalks and weeds. Then, it happened!

The point of this story is that no accident is simple. Many things contribute to an accident. Here are some of the "human" factors behind most farm accidents:

• Fatigue, working while sleepy, or while taking strong medicines—not feeling well. The farmer should take breaks during the work day to prevent fatigue. If he doesn't feel well, he should take it easy and not try dangerous jobs until he's back to normal. Some medicines make persons drowsy or less alert. Hazardous activities such as operating machines, climbing, fixing roofs, driving, and heavy labor should be avoided while taking medication.

• Anger, emotional upsets, being "down in the dumps," grief, worry, tension. Take time to calm down. Count to 10. Anger is a leading cause of accidents.

• Lack of skill or knowledge of the job at hand. Learn the safe way, which is usually the right way. When tackling a job or activity new to you, get someone to help or show you how. Ask questions. When using new or unfamiliar farm machinery, read the instruction manuals. Read the labels on farm chemicals.

• Hurry, taking chances, using unsafe short-cuts such as not shutting off the power before unblocking a machine. A little time might be saved, but an accident will cost far more time. The odds are against anyone when haste makes him forget to be safe.

• Boredom, monotony, day-dreaming or thinking of something else while working at jobs needing full attention for safety. Sitting on a tractor all day or driving on a super-highway, such routine tasks can be dull. Admittedly, it's hard to make some jobs or activities interesting enough to hold the worker's whole attention. Varying the routine sometimes helps. Seeing new things or new angles about the job may help.

• Age—being too young or too old for activity—physical defects or limitations, poor vision, slow reaction time, dizziness, poor health, being easily hurt by accidents. Young children and infirm elderly people are vulnerable to accidents. Persons with poor vision or slow reaction time cannot safely perform certain activities.

• Hunger (low blood sugar), extreme heat or cold, vibration or noise of machines, dust, fumes from engines or chemicals, alcohol. Farm accidents increase toward lunch and in the late afternoon—times when the blood sugar is down. Midmorning and midafternoon snacks during busy times will help prevent let-down, will help carry on the work at top efficiency and safety. Avoid either extremes of hot or cold if you can. Dust and fumes from engines or chemicals affect safety. If necessary a respirator should be used.

• Panicking, inability to cope with situations, reacting wrongly to danger, "freezing" with fear or surprise. Be prepared for the unexpected. Learn how to cope with possible situations by study and by practice.

• Putting off fixing something, not removing or correcting hazards, overlooking or ignoring small things that could cause trouble, forgetting to put shields back on machines if removed. The hazard you may put off fixing now may hurt you months or even years later. Survey farm and home periodically for hazards that might hurt someone, cause a fall, start a fire, entice children into trouble. Check wiring, steps and stairs, heating system, machinery guards, chemical or fuel storage, clutter, wobbly ladders.

• Negative attitude toward safety, thinking that accidents are someone else's problem. "It can't happen to me" attitude, not caring, not respecting the hazards of farm life, disregard for other people.

• Failing to protect and train children, not anticipating their behavior, letting them ride on machines or tractors, not keeping them away from dangerous places or farm activities, not looking to see if they're safely out of the way.

• Pace—some people are faster or slower than others. The important thing is to accomplish the most in a reasonable period of time with safety.

Farm Machinery

Of all farm machinery, the tractor is involved in the most injury-producing accidents, but it is considerably safer than several other machines (cornpicker, baler, combine, etc.) in terms of man hours of use. The major factors in tractor accidents are: tractor tipping

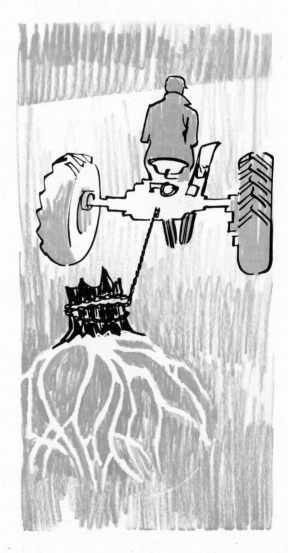

or flipping (both on and off highway), falling from tractor (often extra riders), collision (on highway), and getting caught in exposed power take-off shaft. Also, many farmers get burned while trying to refuel a hot or running engine or when smoking while refueling. Nasty wounds can result from trying to make repairs with inadequate or improper tools. Slick, muddy shoes can cause slips and barked shins.

Here are some tractor hazards and suggested safe practices:

Driving too fast or turning sharply at high speeds causes many upsets. Keep your speed at a safe level.

Be extra careful to prevent backward flips when going up or down slopes, crossing slopes and ditches, or pulling heavy loads. For heavy loads that push down on the drawbar, set the drawbar at its lowest position and weight the front end.

High hitches, such as to the axle or seat bracket to get more traction, can cause a backward flip when pulling or trying to pull a heavy load. Always hitch to the drawbar.

When attempting to start pulling an extra heavy load, such as stump pulling or moving a small building, apply the power gradually. If the front end feels as if it is going to come up, stop.

If the wheels stick, such as in deep mud, or if you put chains or wooden block on the drive-wheels for more traction, something will turn when full power is applied. If the wheels won't, the chassis will revolve around the axle—on top of the operator. If you can't back out of trouble, get help.

Watch for hidden obstacles such as rocks, stumps, or logs. Watch also for holes when going through weeds, grass, or crops. All can throw you.

Have power take-off shield in place before using power take-off. Unguarded, it is extremely dangerous. Disengage engine power to the power take-off when leaving tractor seat.

When stopping the tractor, lock the brakes and put the gears in neutral. Hang onto the keys yourself if youngsters might attempt to start the tractor. Recheck to be sure gears are in neutral when starting the engine.

Don't refuel hot or running engines. Don't smoke while refueling, either. Keep engines free of old grease. Fix fuel leaks immediately. Get a fire extinguisher for your tractor (CO_2 or dry chemical).

Don't wear loose or torn clothing or shoes that could catch on something or cause slips.

Shoes with good soles and close-fitted clothing are both safer and more comfortable.

When on roads, use legal warning devices (flags, a slow moving farm vehicle emblem, lights, reflectors) that can be seen by drivers. Be courteous. Pull over to let traffic pass. Always signal for your stops and turns.

Modern farms are equipped with one or more power-driven machines for harvesting grain, hay, silage, cotton, soybeans, and other crops. Some are driven by the tractor power take-off. Some are tractor-pulled but self-powered. Lately, many are self-propelled. There are several danger spots common to all of them.

These machines have systems of belts, pulleys, gears, chains, shafts, arms—things that whirl, rock, and revolve moving with speed and power. Keep all guards in place; they are put there to protect you. Watch cuffs, sleeves, and gloves when around moving parts.

Machines have "mouths" into which goes the plant material for husking, threshing, grinding, cutting, shredding, crushing, or compressing. These can't be guarded because the machine couldn't do its work if they were. When these machines have cutter bars, extra care must be taken in the field to avoid obstructions as well as children or pets. Annually, thousands get tangled or pulled into running machines. Children fall into them. Or people try to adjust, service, or unclog the machine with the power on. Two good rules are: 1. Always shut off the power before adjusting, servicing, or unclogging machines. 2. Keep youngsters and unauthorized persons off and away from working machines.

The back end of machines can cause trouble too. Hay bales are ejected into wagons; combines have rapidly spinning blades to spread straw. Spreaders, blowers, choppers, and many other machines can be dangerous from any angle.

Chemical Safety

Many agricultural chemicals are now being used in farming operations to kill weeds, insects, disease agents, or rodents and to improve the fertility of the soil. They can be used safely and effectively if a few simple basic safety rules are followed.

Read the label and follow the directions on the label. If the label is not clear, call the chemical dealer, county agent, or health department and ask for someone who can explain

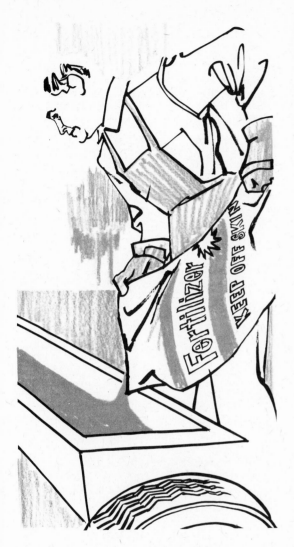

it clearly. You must know what's in the container, what it's for, how to use it safely, what special equipment may be needed, how to store it, how to dispose of unused portions and the container, and what to do if toxic chemicals get on or in the body.

Use as directed, using only the amount recommended on the label. The old adage that if a little is good, a little more must be better is not true with chemicals. Companies spend much money and effort testing chemicals to determine the amount, time, and method of application for maximum effectiveness, safety, and economy. No layman can match that.

Some chemicals can be safely handled with just a few precautions; others of a potentially toxic nature may require special handling and protective devices. Avoid contact or inha-

lation. After their use, wash up before eating or smoking and change clothing when you come in from the job. If the chemical fails to give results, consult an expert first rather than trying out heavier applications or your own "mudpie" mixtures with other chemicals made for other purposes.

Store chemicals in the original or approved container, labels intact, in a suitable storage area. Chemicals should be locked up or otherwise stored beyond the access and ingenuity of children, animals, and unauthorized persons. Never put chemicals in unmarked containers where youngsters have access to them. Many children are poisoned each year because people put chemicals in pop bottles, milk bottles, or cider jugs.

Dispose of unused chemicals and empty containers. Odd bits of chemicals and nearly empty containers clutter up many a barn, shed, back porch, or cellar. These should be disposed of. Burial is best, especially for toxic materials. Unless the label says so, chemicals and containers should not be burned because they might give off harmful fumes, leave poisonous ashes, cause intense fire, or even explode. Toxic chemicals should never be poured on the ground or into a stream.

Rural Traffic

Rural roads and highways are the site of three out of every four traffic fatalities. Traffic safety in general is discussed in Chapter Four, but several points apply especially to farm people.

Slow moving farm vehicles, (SMV), such as tractors, self-propelled farm equipment, and animal-drawn vehicles, present problems in traffic safety. Many rural accidents are collisions between them and cars or trucks. Often, the driver of the faster-moving vehicle didn't see the SMV in time to slow down or the driver misjudged the difference in speed until he was on top of the SMV. Often farm vehicles are too wide or the operator fails to pull over to the side to let traffic pass safely. Drivers who must follow slow farm equipment for some distance, being unable to pass because of oncoming traffic or road conditions often get angry and take chances in passing.

Farmers should be courteous enough to pull over when possible to let traffic pass. Proper and legal warning devices should be used to help the other fellow see you and what you are operating soon enough to slow down and

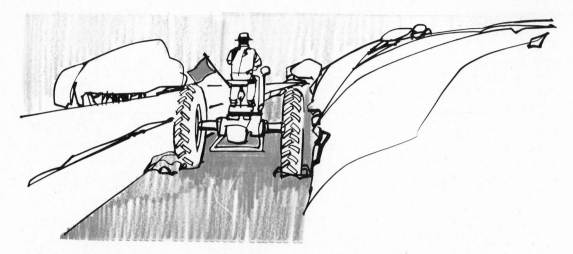

get around you safely. When coming out of a driveway or field, stop and look. Make certain oncoming or following drivers get your signals when you wish to turn or slow down.

Farm trucks should be maintained in good condition. There's a real difference between the acceleration of an empty or lightly loaded farm truck and the same truck heavily laden. This difference must be compensated for when trying to pass or accelerate after pulling onto the road. Lights, tires, brakes, and engine should be checked periodically. Care must be taken in loading farm trucks with high, heavy, or bulky loads so that the truck will not be hard to handle and so the load won't fall off on the road.

Because country roads don't usually have heavy traffic, drivers often become slack in following safe driving practices. Rural roads are often narrow, have sharp rises and dips, high banks and curves, and frequently are rough or poorly surfaced. Many intersections have no stop signs and sometimes high crops or weeds obstruct vision. Yet farm people, perhaps too familiar with their local roads, will speed along in the middle of the roadway, not stop for intersections, and whip around curves or up and down hills with hardly a thought that someone else (maybe a neighbor or a stranger) may be approaching in like manner.

Good driving practices are just as important on country roads as they are on highways. Country roads may force slow driving; many rural "old timers" drive at horse-and-buggy speeds. This practice can cause some trouble for city folk who aren't used to the slower pace.

Farmers who rarely use fast highways or who just prefer a leisurely rate of speed can also be a menace on these highways by driving much slower than the traffic. The safest way is to drive at a pace about average for the traffic. If one's car or truck is unable to keep up, it's wiser to stay off of the highways with heavy, rapidly moving traffic.

Fire Prevention

Fire consumes between $150,000,000 and $200,000,000 worth of farm property annually. Many farm families watch their homes, livestock, crops, keepsakes, and possessions—and sometimes their hopes—destroyed by the flames of unnecessary fires.

Farmers can't always rely on community fire protection. Often, a farm fire is out of control before aid is able to arrive and begin battling the blaze. If rural roads are especially bad, the fire department may not make it through at all.

Prevention is the answer to the farm fire problem, plus protective devices and measures to keep a small fire, if one accidentally starts, from growing into a big fire. Farm fires can be prevented. Here are some suggestions:

● Remove paper, rags, rubbish, and other unused combustibles from house and other farm buildings.

● Keep heating systems in good shape—check out flues, chimneys, stoves, furnaces, kerosene heaters, space and barn heaters.

● Use care with gasoline and kerosene. Never pour them into stoves to get a fire going. Keep fuels stored out of the house in sturdy, well-marked containers.

● Check the electric wiring periodically. If lights dim or fuses blow, you're overloading the circuit or have a short. Check the trouble.

If it's overloaded, lighten the load. Or better, install wiring with greater capacity to handle all your needs. Use only the fuse size called for in the circuit—never substitute a heavier-rated fuse. Periodically check wiring which is exposed to weather or to flexing and physical stresses.

• If hay is stored in the barn, use a hay thermometer daily for signs of heating. If hay is heating (180 degrees and over), cut slices through the center or move it around into smaller piles or out of the barn.

• Fuel to power farm machinery should be stored in overhead or underground tanks made for this purpose, preferably 40 feet from nearest building. One should be able to refuel with minimum spillage.

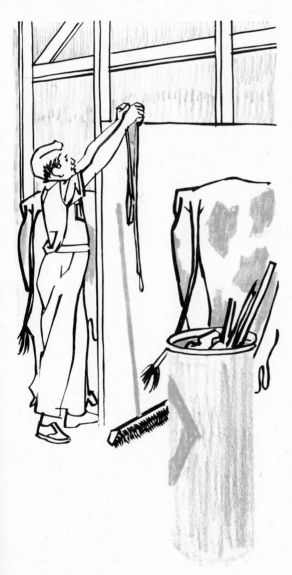

• Make certain lightning rods are well grounded and insulators are in good shape.

• Watch smoking habits. Provide plenty of ashtrays or receptacles in the house and work areas. Don't smoke in buildings where flammable liquids or chemicals are stored or where hay, straw, or litter is present. Keep matches away from children. Don't toss away lighted matches or cigarettes—be sure they are out. Don't smoke when you're apt to doze.

• Repair or replace worn power cords, plugs, or switches.

• Keep proper and adequate fire extinguishers handy in all buildings and on trucks and tractors. Read the instructions; know how to use extinguishers immediately and note recharging information.

• Keep buckets, sand, and ladders handy.

• Have a good supply of water available and easily accessible. Special couplings for water systems help the fire department hook up its equipment.

• Develop a home drill and fire escape plan so that the family can quickly evacuate a burning house or barn. Farm families especially need this plan, as help may be delayed and early escapes will be up to the family itself. Each bedroom should have a rope ladder or means of getting from windows to the ground. Learn how to break and leave a window safely, how to test a door for heat before opening it. Smoke and heat are usually the killers, not flames. Have a meeting place outside and insist that everyone go there for "head count" (hundreds have rushed back into flaming houses and died to save someone who was already out but out of sight).

• Keep phone numbers of fire department, police, and nearest neighbors handy. When fire strikes, get persons out and away from the danger area. Don't risk life. Call or send for help.

A delaying action may be possible if the fire is small enough to put out by an extinguisher or other means used quickly. Class A fires—those involving such combustible materials as wood, paper, or hay—should be cooled off. Use water.

Class B fires are caused by grease, oil, paint, gasoline, etc. They burn only on the surface. When the flame is out, the fire is out. These must be smothered by shutting off the air. Use dirt, sand blankets, and sacks soaked in water or dry chemical, carbon dioxide, or vaporizing liquid extinguishers. Water may spread the fire (oil and the blaze will float on top of the water). Never pour water on kitchen grease fires. The hot grease will spatter. Use baking soda instead.

Class C fires involve electricity and electrical equipment. These must be smothered. Use dry chemical, dioxide, or vaporizing liquid extinguisher. Never use water because shock danger is very great and potentially death dealing. Extinguishing agents must be non-conductors of electricity. Don't use vaporizing liquid extinguishers in confined places—they need ventilation.

Farm Homes

The section on home safety (Chapter One) discusses ways to prevent most home accidents. These apply equally to farm homes. Some special hazardous conditions often found in farm homes are the results of age, weathering, neglect, unsafe design, and use of antiquated household equipment. A large number of presently used farm homes were built by farmers themselves with families or neighbors pitching in, or by local carpenters. Little attention was paid to providing safety features. They often are firetraps and easily set ablaze. Many farm homes have very narrow and hard-to-climb stairs and steps. Rather than basements, low-ceilinged cellars with rough, uneven floors were made.

Remodeling has made many old farm homes quite modern and considerably safer to live in. In some areas, however, many farm homes still have no electricity, indoor plumbing, or running water. Wood, coal, or oil stoves are used for heating and cooking, thus increasing the fire danger or danger to small children. Lighting is by lamps or lanterns, another fire hazard.

If some of the "built-in" hazards of older farm homes can not be eliminated, the dweller should learn to live safely, with them. Extra care is needed to prevent fire. Strong handrails are needed on narrow or steeply rising stairways along with plenty of good light. Flooring and porches should be checked often for rotting or loosening boards. Outdoor toilets should be kept sanitary and free of stinging insects and spiders.

Farms can be safe if a little time, effort, and interest are given to learning the rules of safety. It is up to the individual farm family who, as a group, are unmatched in independence and responsibility for their own safety and progress.

CHAPTER SEVEN

ON-THE-JOB SAFETY

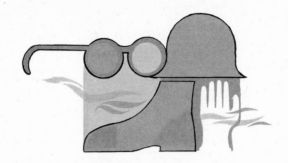

TWO WORKERS are killed and 220 are injured each hour in the U.S. Who pays the price of these accidents? The cost, estimated to be about $300,000 per hour, is paid by every American family. Accidents lower production rates and lessen the quality of products. Accidents, by increasing production costs, raise the prices of commodities purchased by the public. The injured worker, however, pays most through the loss of an arm, leg, or eye, or perhaps the loss of his job or his life.

Most accidents are caused by unsafe conditions, unsafe acts, or both. Some simple common-sense rule has either been ignored, forgotten, or misunderstood.

Lifting

The major cause of injuries, disabling about 500,000 workers a year, is the mishandling of materials. Most injuries are to the back as a result of improper lifting. Stooping with the back arched and with the load out at the end of the arms causes the injury. Lifting in this manner puts the whole strain at the point of the bend of the back where the muscles lack the strength to bear the load.

There are simple rules for lifting which must be understood and practiced. The object to be lifted should be inspected for weight and size. Help should be secured if the load is too heavy or awkward. The worker should plant his feet firmly, well apart. He should then squat with his knees bent and get a good grip on the object. He should keep his back as straight as he can and lift slowly, without jerking, by pushing up with his legs. The strong leg muscles should do the work rather than the back muscles. The body should never be twisted with the load. The way to lower an object is essentially the reverse of lifting it.

There are tricks that can help the handling of odd shapes. Sacked material should be grasped by diagonal corners and swung to one shoulder with a boost from the knee. Long objects should be carried over the shoulder with the end held as high as possible to prevent striking other employees or damaging property. Carboy boxes should be handled by hand trucks. Cylinder dollies should be used to move compressed gas cylinders.

Falls

The second greatest number of on-the-job injuries results from falls, which disable almost 400,000 workers a year. As many happen on the level as from elevated places. Falls may be the result of stumbling, slipping, or loss of balance. Usually they are caused by plain carelessness—objects left in the middle of the aisle or on stairs, spilled oil, grease, or water, waxed floors, or icy exterior walks. Rushing up or down stairs can throw an individual off balance. Stairs should be walked up and down slowly with feet firmly planted on each step and the handrail used. Jumping from trucks or loading docks has caused serious injuries.

Falls from ladders have permanently disabled many workers. Ladders should be inspected for cracks or loose rungs. They should be long enough so that it is not necessary to stand on the top rungs. The ladder should have safety feet. A board should be used on soft earth to level the feet. The ladder should be set one foot away for every four feet up to the point of support. Since the rungs are one foot apart, it is very easy to figure the distance. Climbing up the ladder should be done with both hands holding the rungs. One should never overreach from a ladder.

Protective Equipment

The third major cause of work injuries is falling, moving, or flying objects. More than

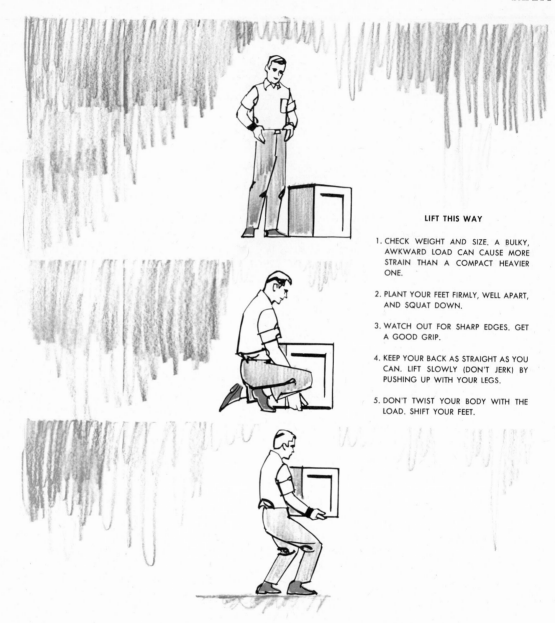

LIFT THIS WAY

1. CHECK WEIGHT AND SIZE. A BULKY, AWKWARD LOAD CAN CAUSE MORE STRAIN THAN A COMPACT HEAVIER ONE.

2. PLANT YOUR FEET FIRMLY, WELL APART, AND SQUAT DOWN.

3. WATCH OUT FOR SHARP EDGES. GET A GOOD GRIP.

4. KEEP YOUR BACK AS STRAIGHT AS YOU CAN. LIFT SLOWLY (DON'T JERK) BY PUSHING UP WITH YOUR LEGS.

5. DON'T TWIST YOUR BODY WITH THE LOAD. SHIFT YOUR FEET.

260,000 workers are seriously injured in this manner each year. In most cases, the injured worker has failed to wear protective equipment when the job calls for it.

Safety glasses or shields will protect the eyes from small particles that can penetrate them and cause permanent blindness. Safety glasses can be equipped with corrective lenses for those who need them, but they are of no value unless worn. Many tragic eye losses have occurred to workers who made a habit of removing their eye protection for just a few minutes.

Safety hats should be worn on certain jobs, especially around overhead work or where there might be falling objects. Such industries as construction, petroleum, or steel have zoned areas in which hard hats must be worn by all personnel, workers, and visitors.

Safety shoes are one of the greatest inventions in the history of accident prevention. The steel toe box, made to specifications, is strong enough to support a load of 2,500 pounds and to withstand the impact of a 50-pound weight dropped on the foot. The hidden steel cap often means the difference between a crushed foot or an injured toe and no injury at all.

In addition to wearing required protective equipment, the worker must stay out from under cranes, suspended loads, or overhead work. He should stand clear when bells or horns warn him of passing power trucks and overhead equipment. He should stay clear of barricaded areas. To protect others, he should prevent tools or materials from falling from overhead work and warn unauthorized personnel away from danger zones.

Machinery

Machinery mishaps are the fourth major cause of work-related injuries. About 200,000 workers are disabled each year because of misuse of machines, disregard of guards, failure to dress properly when operating machines (no jewelry or loose clothing), not locking or tagging main power switches during repairs, or letting machines run unattended.

These four major causes of on-the-job injuries cause 13,700 deaths and 2,000,000 disabling injuries annually. We have mentioned only a few of the common-sense precautions all workers should naturally take because, in addition to preventing injuries, they are the best way to do the job. Other precautions are advisable in special jobs.

The reduction of accident and death rates in industry over the past half century has been remarkable. During this period, the work force has been doubled and the gross national product has increased five fold, still the industrial accident death rate has been cut in half. Occupational health and safety programs with emphasis on prevention have been primarily responsible for this reduction. These programs have not only included technical know-how and engineering to reduce mechanical and health hazards, but also educational programs to train workers in practices designed to prevent injury to themselves and their fellow workers.

Both American industry and American labor are still concerned with the disastrous effect of accidents on the worker and his family and the accompanying increase in the cost of production. They have combined forces to reduce further and even eliminate accidents on the job. It is only with cooperation and understanding of the fundamental concepts of occupational health and safety by both management and labor that this goal will be achieved. Safety teamwork needs everyone's cooperation.

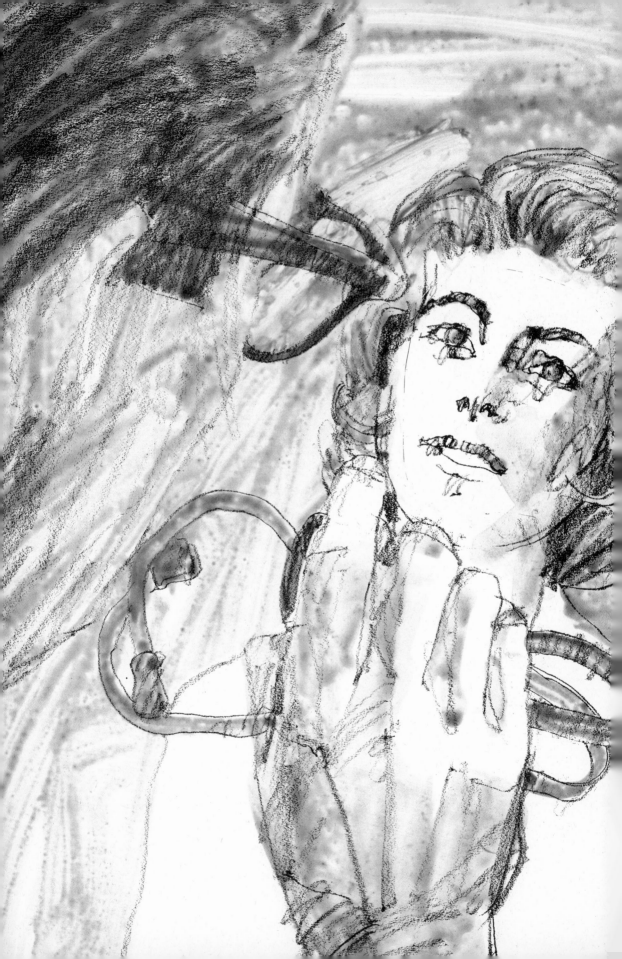

PART VIII

Medical Services for the Family

Chapter One

DOCTORS AND PATIENTS

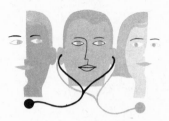

Physicians believe that the most important factor in good medical care, assuming that well-trained physicians and adequate facilities are available, is the personal relationship between doctors and their patients. This is sometimes strained under present-day conditions. Factors that especially cause strain include changes in community structures, dispersal of families, increased mobility of the population, and trends toward medical specialization.

The word communication in its various forms is much in vogue today. Webster defines communicate as "to make common to both parties. . .the knowledge or quality concerned." Psychologists often stress the importance of communication as the only basis on which satisfactory human relationships can be built. It is necessary for the patient and his doctor to be able "to make common to both parties" the knowledge each has to impart.

In this book, of course, the term *doctor* refers to an M.D., a doctor of medicine. Unfortunately the title *doctor* is one of the most misused and misunderstood in the world. Too many people believe that chiropractors, naturopaths, and practitioners of other cults who call themselves doctors are also qualified to treat disease—and the cultists do their best to encourage this belief. As this chapter was written, the local morning paper carried a two-column advertisement by a chiropractor who claimed to "correct" such serious disorders as "diabetes and other kidney diseases (diabetes is primarily a disease of the pancreas rather than the kidneys), high blood pressure, female disorders, rheumatism, heart, liver, stomach, spleen, and nervous diseases." A few weeks earlier, another advertisement claimed that "chiropractic results with convulsions are excellent." Many otherwise intelligent people believe such statements, and with tragic frequency fail to seek medical attention for some organic disease until they have made the round of the cultists. The result is much unnecessary suffering and, sometimes, even death.

The Importance of the Family Doctor

While some speak slightingly of the doctor-patient relationship, a statement made by the late Dr. Francis Peabody many years ago is still true:

"With the exception of the relationship that one may have with a member of one's family or with the priest, there is no human bond that is closer than that between physician and patient (or patient's family), and attempts to substitute the methods of machine or organization, be they ever so efficient, are bound to fail."

The sort of doctor-patient relationship described by Dr. Peabody cannot be expected to blossom in the course of a single physical examination or even a single illness. It comes to full flower in the bond that develops between persons and families and the doctor who has advised them in medical matters over a period of many years—"in sickness and in health."

One of the first things a family or individual should do upon moving to a new town is to select a medical adviser, family doctor, or personal physician, and then write or call him, *before illness occurs,* to ask if he is willing to serve in that capacity. A still better idea is to visit the physician of one's choice for a routine physical examination before making a final decision. If the patient is not satisfied with the way the physician conducts the examination, or if the rapport necessary for a good doctor-patient relationship seems to be missing in that initial contact, the patient would be wise to search further.

A family doctor may be a general practitioner or an internist (a physician who specializes in diseases of the internal organs). General practitioners in small towns often deliver babies, set broken bones, and perform routine surgery. In larger cities, however, they usually limit their work somewhat. Since most ailments for which patients consult doctors are medical rather than surgical conditions, the family doctor, whether general practitioner or internist, is able to care for about 85 percent of them himself.

He usually lacks the facilities, however, to carry out such special procedures as fitting glasses, looking into the bladder, or making complicated x-ray studies. If such specialized attention is required, the family doctor will recommend one or more reliable specialists in the appropriate field, and in most cases will arrange for the patient to see the one the patient prefers.

It should strengthen rather than weaken the patient's confidence in his family doctor to hear him admit that he cannot do everything and that he wants the patient to have special attention for a particular problem. The family or personal physician is rather like a general contractor, who has over-all responsibility for building or repairing a house, but calls on electricians, plumbers, or painters to do special jobs.

Some excellent family doctors like to treat the children in their patients' families. Others refer responsibility for the care and feeding of infants and young children to a pediatrician, whose business it is to keep up with changing trends in infant feeding and immunization, and in the treatment of pediatric diseases. A pediatrician in his relationship with children fills the same role as the family doctor does for the adult.

Periodic Physical Examinations

The patient who expects to receive prompt attention from his family physician in times of sickness should not neglect regular visits to the doctor when he is well. It is a good idea to let each birthday serve as a reminder to make an appointment for a physical checkup. In addition to helping the doctor and patient become better acquainted, such examinations serve two important purposes: They permit the doctor to detect and treat chronic disorders in their early stages and to advise the patient about problems he has or habits that need correction; and they provide information about the patient's usual state of health which may prove invaluable when illness occurs.

Because of the time required to take an adequate "history," most family doctors allow at least an hour for the first examination of a new patient. An individual's medical history begins with that of his ancestors, and includes all information which might have a bearing on the state of his health:

● Any possible hereditary diseases in the family, the ages of his parents (if they are living) and of any living brothers and sisters—or their ages at death and the causes of their death.

● Any noteworthy features of the mother's pregnancy and the patient's birth.

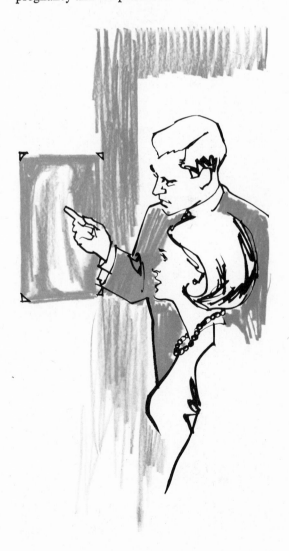

- All operations, childhood diseases, and major illnesses and accidents.
- The date of marriage and the number of children, as well as their state of health.
- The patient's domestic situation, habits, and living and working conditions.
- Any symptoms which might point to trouble in any of the body's organs and systems.

Unless the patient is senile or a small child, the most satisfactory history is obtained directly, when no third party is present. A patient can help the doctor by answering questions as clearly and concisely as possible, and by "staying on the track" instead of rambling off on conversational detours. He should be prepared to give a clear-cut description of any symptoms he may have, preferably in the order of their relative importance. He may wonder at some of the questions the doctor asks, but there is a reason for every one.

The patient should not object to being asked very personal questions about his domestic life, habits, and possible sources of anxiety or worry. He should answer these fully and truthfully, for this information plays an important part in the evaluation of his health. It is hardly necessary to say that the doctor is bound by tradition, training, and the Hippocratic oath to keep in confidence all information given him by a patient.

After the history comes the physical examination, which usually begins with taking the patient's temperature and blood pressure and examining his eyes, ears, nose, and throat. Since blood pressure may be elevated by excitement, the doctor will often take two or three readings during the examination in an effort to determine its usual level. One should not be alarmed by repetitions of this procedure. After the patient has removed his outer clothing, he is weighed, and his height and often his chest expansion are measured. If the patient is a woman, the doctor's nurse or office assistant will help her to undress and will stay in the room during the examination. Obviously, one should not allow undue modesty to interfere with the examination.

In addition to the history and physical examination, certain laboratory tests are usually carried out as part of a routine checkup: blood studies, urinalyses, and possibly some x-ray studies and an electrocardiogram. The doctor orders these, not necessarily because he suspects trouble, but often because he wants to establish a baseline to use for future comparison.

After the examination and tests are completed, the doctor is ready to talk to the patient, and possibly to some member of the family, about his general physical condition. He will often advise the patient about his diet, exercise, recreation, and sleeping habits, and about immunizations needed. This advice is as much part of the treatment as the drugs which the doctor will prescribe if they are needed. Because of the length of time required to make the necessary explanations and answer all the questions that arise, it may be necessary for the doctor to give the patient a second appointment to talk over the findings of the first examination and the results of laboratory studies.

Prescriptions

Most prescriptions today could not have been filled 20 years ago, and probably not more than half could have been filled even 10 years ago. The so-called "wonder drugs" have accomplished such miracles of healing that patients have come to expect a quick cure for every illness. Unfortunately the virus infections—which include influenza and the common cold—are not influenced by any sulfonamide or antibiotic now known. The eventual hope for controlling these diseases lies in immunization or vaccination. Yet many patients demand that doctors give them "a shot of penicillin" or other antibiotic for simple colds or other virus infections. The doctor who yields to such pressure not only adds an unnecessary item to the patient's drug bill; he also exposes the patient to the unwarranted risk of sensitization to a drug which he might urgently need to survive some future illness.

Since Congress passed the Harrison Act in 1918, druggists have had to keep copies of prescriptions for narcotics (cocaine, opium derivatives such as morphine and codeine, and certain other pain-relieving drugs) in a separate file open to inspection by government officials. Every practicing doctor is required to have a narcotics license, and his individual license number goes on each narcotic prescription he writes. If a doctor is found to be prescribing an unusual number of narcotics, he must give a satisfactory explanation or run the risk of having his narcotics license, and possibly his license to practice medicine, revoked. The reason behind these regulations is a good one, and a doctor is seldom hampered in prescribing narcotics when they are needed.

Any powerful drug is a potentially dangerous one if it is misused. For this reason, most prescriptions given today cannot be refilled without the doctor's permission. The number of times that a prescription may be refilled is indicated in the lower left-hand corner of most prescription blanks.

Preventive Medicine

Reputedly, the early Chinese doctor was paid while his patient was well, but not when he was sick. This probably legendary method has at least two modern counterparts—the principle of voluntary health insurance and the emphasis placed on preventive as opposed to curative medicine.

The idea of preventive medicine is for the private practitioner, the public health officer, and the public to cooperate closely in their efforts to keep people well. The private physician's responsibility in the field of preventive medicine lies in giving his patients a thorough physical examination—supplemented by any special diagnostic procedures that are indicated—when they come to him for routine checkups. In addition, the conscientious family doctor will recommend the necessary immunizations and will give his patients advice about their health habits. It is the patient's responsibility to go to his doctor for checkups at regular intervals and to follow the advice his doctor gives him.

Perhaps the most important single piece of advice that the doctor will give most adult patients is to keep their weight at its best level. Many doctors follow up this advice with a reducing diet for their obese patients. Anyone who needs to reduce should consult his doctor, rather than the nearest bookstand, about diet. Unfortunately, many best-selling books on diet have no scientific foundation, and many give advice that may actually be dangerous.

Public health personnel have an increasingly important position on the medical team. While private doctors are interested in the individual patient, public health physicians are concerned about the health of a whole community—city, county, state, or nation. The traditional public health program includes the control of disease, sanitation, quarantine for contagious diseases (seldom needed now), immunization against preventable communicable disease, the mass application of certain diagnostic procedures (for example, chest x-rays) to large segments of the population, public health nursing services, and the dissemination of general health information.

Thanks to public health measures, smallpox, typhoid fever, diphtheria, polio, dysentery, and many other diseases that once claimed many lives are now medical curiosities. Tuberculosis, which led all causes of death at the beginning of this century, is now near the bottom of the list of major killers.

In recent years public health agencies have conducted a vigorous campaign to make the public conscious of the necessity for detecting cancer in its early stages. This campaign may have succeeded in lowering the mortality from this dread disease, but it has also had the unfortunate side-effect of frightening scores of people into an acute anxiety state. Many clinicians will agree that a cancerphobia—the morbid fear of cancer—is often harder to eradicate than a genuine cancer.

States with progressive health departments are now conducting mental hygiene and birth control clinics, in addition to the usual prenatal and "well baby" clinics. Educational campaigns and certain diagnostic programs among adults, especially among the elderly, are aimed at prolonging and enriching adult lives.

The "Nervous" Patient

One of the most famous surgeons of a bygone day often said that every patient with indigestion should be operated upon. That statement is a far cry from Dr. Walter Alvarez's oft-repeated dictum that more than half the patients who come to him with digestive complaints have no organic basis—that is, no disease of any bodily organ—to account for their symptoms.

The number of patients who come to the doctor with vague physical symptoms and the complaint of "nervousness" seems to be increasing. Most of these patients are suffering from some emotional disturbance, often characterized by abnormal anxiety or depression, or both. In recent years the term *psychosomatic illness* has been coined to describe those conditions in which one or more functions of the body are upset by emotional disturbances. The word psychosomatic comes from two Greek words meaning mind and body. Solomon proved his wisdom by being one of the first writers to note the effect the emotions can have on bodily functions, especially the digestion: "Better a dinner of herbs where love is than a stalled ox and hatred therewith."

The disturbances produced by emotional stress are just as real and just as painful as those caused by a diseased organ—though the ultimate results are far less serious. When a physician is unsympathetic toward a patient with such disturbances, the patient often goes from one doctor to another in the hope of being told that some correctable physical condition is responsible for his symptoms.

Eventually, he is sure to find a doctor (or a cultist) unscrupulous enough to tell him what he wants to hear, and then to carry out some unnecessary therapy—perhaps surgical—to "cure" him. Unfortunately, such "cures" are seldom permanent and the treatment may have serious consequences.

Some patients with depression and anxiety states require more psychotherapy than their family doctor can give in the time at his disposal, and will need to be referred to a psychiatrist. The psychiatrist will often be able to treat them as office patients, with the aid of the modern drugs available; in other cases, however, he will want the patient to spend some time in a hospital for more intensive therapy.

A Doctor's Training

The practice of medicine has changed since the turn of the century. In 1910, when Abraham Flexner made his survey of the medical schools of the country, in collaboration with the American Medical Association's Council on Medical Education, there were more than 160 medical schools in the United States. Many were mere diploma mills, with only the most meager equipment.

As a result of the information given in Flexner's report, more than half the existing schools were closed, or merged with others to form stronger facilities. Now the United States has fewer than 100 medical schools, all approved by the American Medical Association's Council on Medical Education and Hospitals and the Association of American Medical Colleges. Their requirements for admission ensure, so far as is humanly possible, that only competent candidates enter the study of medicine and that they receive the best medical education possible.

Most medical schools require three years of college as a minimum, and a number require a four-year premedical course. After another four years in medical school, the student is graduated with the M.D. degree, and begins a one to five-year period of training as an intern,

or hospital house officer. The true physician continues to be a student as long as he is in practice: reading medical journals and books, attending medical meetings and hospital staff meetings, and conferring with his colleagues.

In view of the decrease in the number of medical schools, the increase in population, and the growth of voluntary health insurance plans during the past 50 years—together with the stringent requirements for admission to medical school and the long and arduous period of training required before the doctor can begin to practice his profession—it is not surprising that some parts of the country are beginning to experience a shortage of doctors. The shortage is still more a matter of maldistribution than an over-all lack of doctors. However, it is likely to become more acute as more and more young doctors are lured into the glamorous and increasingly lucrative field of research, and as the sciences related to the conquest of space attract more and more high school and college graduates of the caliber sought by medical schools.

Understanding Your Doctor

Doctors are not immune to criticism, nor should they be. However, the common criticisms of doctors should be objectively reviewed. Some of these are:

1. Doctors do not give the patient enough time to tell his story.

2. Doctors keep patients waiting too long.

3. Doctors do not explain the reasons for diagnosis and treatment.

4. Doctors will not make house calls.

5. Doctors charge too much.

6. The doctor's secretary will not let a patient talk to him on the phone.

Unfortunately, there is sometimes justification for many of these criticisms—but it may help the person who reads this chapter if he understands the doctor's point of view.

1. It is too often true that doctors do not give the patient enough time to tell his story. Doctors are human, and when they know they are far behind schedule and have several patients waiting to see them, are apt to show impatience with undue wordiness. Many patients repeat their complaints over and over, instead of giving a clear-cut description of their symptoms. It requires unlimited patience and vast amounts of time to "get to the bottom" of such a patient's trouble. One such patient can disrupt a doctor's schedule to such an extent that

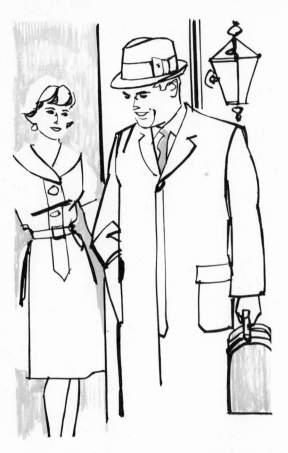

he feels rushed for the rest of the day, and fails to give any of his patients the sympathetic, unhurried attention he knows they deserve.

2. That doctors keep patients waiting too long is, perhaps, the complaint most frequently heard and, probably, the one most justified. Many physicians are genuinely concerned about this problem, which is closely tied to the one just discussed. The doctor who gives all his patients all the time they would like to have is sure to get far behind with his appointments.

About the best a doctor can do is to work by appointment, allowing a reasonable amount of time for each patient. He should instruct his secretary to give new patients more time than those who are making return visits. The patient, in turn, should cooperate by being on time for appointments and by giving his history as clearly and concisely as possible.

Occasionally an emergency will throw a doctor so far behind schedule that the best solution is to have his secretary cancel as many appointments as she can—giving each patient another one at the earliest possible date.

3. Doctors do not explain the reasons for diagnosis and treatment. No matter how busy a doctor is, he should take time to explain to his patients, in the simplest words possible, the nature of their ailments and the results to be expected of the treatment recommended. This explanation is particularly important when the symptoms are caused by emotional stress. The assurance that no cancer or serious organic trouble is present, followed by an explanation of the autonomic nervous system and its effects on physical functioning, is often all that is necessary to effect a cure, or at least considerable improvement.

Sometimes the breakdown in communication between doctor and patient is partly the patient's fault. Some people are unwilling to admit that they don't understand medical language and to ask the physician to translate into "plain English." Since doctors are not mind readers, it is the patient's responsibility to ask the doctor any question about his problem that may seem important. This is part of the "collaboration of candor" that is an essential part of the doctor-patient relationship.

To help the patient understand and save the doctor's time, he may suggest articles for his patient to read which give basic facts and can lead to more understandable discussion.

Patients who have a serious organic disease should be told about it in the least alarming terms possible. Patients can be told they have had a stroke or damage to their heart, without being greatly upset. Many a patient, in fact, is relieved to know that the closure of a small artery in his brain has caused digestive symptoms that he had feared, perhaps secretly, were due to cancer. In most such cases, it is also important for the doctor to discuss more frankly and fully, with some responsible member of the family, the patient's condition, the treatment recommended, and the probable outlook.

4. Doctors will not make house calls. In most cases the doctor's preference for seeing patients in his office rather than going to their homes is justified. His office is much better equipped for making the necessary examinations and tests than the traditional black bag. In emergencies, treatment can often be obtained more quickly by taking the patient—in an ambulance, if necessary—to the emergency room of the nearest hospital than by waiting until the doctor can be located and can get to the patient's home. Treatment can be begun at once by the doctor on duty in the emergency room and continued by the family physician when he arrives.

In cases of acute illness, when the patient

needs to be kept in bed but not necessarily hospitalized, most family doctors will go to the home. Before choosing a personal physician, it is wise to ask him if he is willing to make house calls if necessary. Realizing the value of the doctor's time, however, patients should not insist that he come to the house if they are able to get to his office without undue hardship.

If modern doctors were required to make as many house calls as physicians did a generation ago, an acute shortage of doctors would result. The horse-and-buggy doctor spent 70 per cent of his time in going from one patient to another, leaving only 30 per cent to be devoted to his patients. The average doctor today spends only 10 per cent of his working day in transit, leaving 90 per cent for his patients.

5. Doctors charge too much. While it is true that a few doctors are more commercial-minded than others, most are reasonable in their fees. A doctor's education represents a great deal of money, time and energy. The same amount of cash and brain power invested in some business would usually bring him much greater financial reward than the practice of medicine.

Perhaps this comparison is pertinent: In 1920 the charge for a house call by a physician ranged from $3 to $5. Today they vary from $7 to $10. During the same period the price of potatoes went from 39 cents a bushel to $5.40. Yet we hear few complaints about the present price of potatoes. In the past 20 years physicians' fees have risen about 95 per cent. But per capita incomes during this period rose 290 per cent. The real cost of medical care—in terms of hours of work to purchase it—is less today than it was 20 years ago.

6. The doctor's secretary will not let one speak to him on the phone. Except in a real emergency, no thoughtful person would expect the doctor to interrupt his interview with a patient to answer the telephone. Certainly any person who did make such a demand would resent it if the physician were interrupted a number of times while he himself was a patient in the office. The secretary tries to shield her doctor from as many interruptions as possible while he is concentrating his attention on a patient, and will usually ask the caller to leave his name and number so that the doctor can phone him later. If a real emergency arises, however, the experienced secretary will sense it and put the call through. She knows most of the patients well enough to know which ones are considerate and which ones are not.

Some doctors set aside a period of time between or after office appointments for returning telephone calls. The person who has left a message for the doctor to call should do his best to keep the phone free during the time the return call might be expected.

Many patients resent being asked by the doctor's secretary about the nature of their difficulty. Reluctance to discuss intimate problems with a third party is understandable, but the patient should realize that the secretary has been instructed by the doctor to ask for this information. It isn't necessary to give a detailed report of symptoms, but only to let the doctor have some idea of what the trouble is, so that he will be prepared to deal with it when he returns the call or sees the patient in his office.

CHAPTER TWO

YOUR DOCTOR, THE AMA, AND YOU

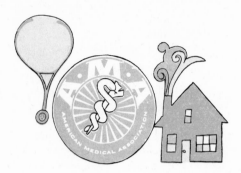

THE AMERICAN MEDICAL ASSOCIATION may seem a remote and somewhat mysterious organization to you. You see its name in the newspapers, and you hear discussion of its public declarations and actions. Often you don't understand them; sometimes you disagree.

Actually, the Association is as close to you as your family doctor or the consultant or specialist to whom you are referred. The Association has over 200,000 physician members, practically all doctors who are eligible to belong. They hold their membership in county medical societies, which in turn are organized into state medical societies and the American Medical Association. The Association is governed by a House of Delegates elected to represent the members; one delegate per 1000 members or fraction thereof in each state society. All important policy decisions are made by this representative body. The Association is supported entirely by the dues of its members and the earnings of its publications; it never asks for public funds nor seeks contributions.

The Association works for "the improvement of the science and art of medicine and the betterment of the public health." These purposes are accomplished in many different ways. The Association has no legal power to compel anyone to do anything, has never sought such power, and does not desire it. It prefers to work through education and cooperative endeavor. While it cooperates with government at all levels, it is not a governmental body. It cannot make or enforce laws, issue licenses or revoke them, or punish offenders.

The Association's main concern has always been educational; when it was first organized in 1847, medical education was among the important topics of discussion. Education of the public came somewhat later, but interest in it was expressed very early in the history of the Association.

The growth of the Association was greatly stimulated by the establishment in 1883 of its Journal, which has grown into what is generally recognized as the world's leading medical periodical. It is published weekly, and goes to every member as a part of his membership privilege, bringing him articles, abstracts, editorials, book reviews, case reports, a question and answer column, and carefully screened advertising of medical products, books, appliances, and other such items to keep him up-to-the-minute in medical progress.

The Association also publishes 10 specialty journals in important medical areas. There are also 32 state or regional medical journals published by state societies or groups of such societies. A bi-weekly newspaper sent to all member physicians keeps them abreast of current events of medical interest.

An important adjunct to the Journal and the specialty journals is the library of the American Medical Association. Here more than 1,500 medical journals from all parts of the world are received. The doctor's membership entitles him to whatever information is available in the form of tear-sheets or photocopies of articles, or lists of references which he can use to help him search local medical libraries for material. Medical schools have good libraries; so do many of the state and urban medical societies.

Medical Meetings

Medical meetings are among the important ways in which your doctor stays abreast of the fast-moving world of medicine. The American

Medical Association holds two principal meetings each year—one in June and one in early winter. The former is the official annual convention, held in one of the nation's major cities; the latter is a regional clinical session held in various parts of the country, giving doctors in the vicinity an opportunity to attend with a minimum loss of time.

At both conventions, the Association's House of Delegates deliberates over the medical problems and issues of the day.

At these same two conventions there are extensive medical exhibits, where outstanding clinical and laboratory researchers demonstrate new methods, new appliances and new studies, giving your doctor not only fresh information, but the stimulus of personal contact with leaders in the medical and allied sciences.

Also at these conventions, foreign medical guests of distinction contribute their findings and are available for personal conversations.

In addition, the Association holds a number of special meetings and conferences on topics such as medical education, mental health, school health, environmental health, rural health, and others. State and local medical societies also hold annual meetings, and local medical societies meet once a month or oftener. The national Association assists and participates in many of these meetings. Hospital staff meetings and many local and clinical con-

ferences round out the program which helps your doctor keep up-to-date; these are encouraged by the Association in every possible way.

The American Medical Association and state societies have always encouraged the improvement of medical education, which is obviously fundamental to good medical care. The Association cooperated in the sweeping reform of medical education which occurred just after World War I, during which the large number of inadequate medical schools was reduced by mergers, affiliation with recognized universities, or discontinuance. At the present time the nation's medical schools all meet the minimum standards for educating capable physicians. Other organizations have cooperated in this program, but the Association has always maintained a role of leadership.

While it is not a governmental agency, the Association has maintained a lively interest in

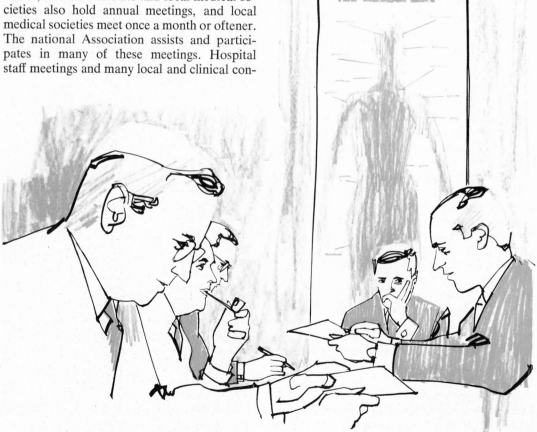

legislation bearing upon medical education, especially the organization of state medical licensing boards and the passage of basic science requirements as a prerequisite for medical school attendance and licensure. Such basic sciences as anatomy, physiology, chemistry, physics, biology, and bacteriology are necessary to an understanding of medicine.

The American Medical Association encourages a high standard of doctor-patient relationships. This relationship, as you have seen from the preceding pages, is a very private and personal one, demanding the highest standards of integrity. The Association has no way of compelling specific conduct by physicians, except through encouraging a careful selection of candidates for medical schools, or by denying membership to any who in later years fail to live up to the ideals they have learned from their teachers and associates. The profession is proud that the number of such unworthy members is very, very small.

Medical ethics have sometimes been misunderstood as a sort of mutual protection among physicians in the event of dissatisfied patients. This is by no means the case. Indeed, the medical societies, encouraged by the American Medical Association, have established local committees in virtually all areas where a patient may take a complaint about his doctor, and be assured of a fair and impartial hearing. Of course, the doctor is entitled to present his case, too. Such committees do not hesitate to admonish a physician, or even proceed more severely against him when the misunderstanding cannot be resolved by conference and discussion.

Health Legislation

Most laws governing medical practice are state laws, since the states license the physicians. Exceptions are the Harrison Narcotic Act, legislation governing interstate matters and international topics, and certain forms of federal aid such as the Hill-Burton Act, governing construction of hospitals and other facilities with federal financial aid. The Association has always endeavored to guard the public health in these matters, and as a result has sometimes taken a stand which proved unpopular at the moment, but later turned out to be wise and sound.

The question has been raised, sometimes by sincere and unbiased persons, why the American Medical Association so often opposes and so seldom supports health legislation in the Congress. The facts are that the Association more often supports than it opposes—as in the case of President Kennedy's mental health legislation, the fluoridation controversy, aid to hospital construction, and many other issues. Support, however, is not news. It gets a mere paragraph on an inside page. Opposition, especially to a proposal which is medically unsound but politically popular, is quite another matter. That is controversy, and so it gets on the front page.

When the medical profession, through the American Medical Association, opposes a medical or public health proposal, its reasons should be understood before its actions are judged. The Association believes in local responsibility in preference to reliance upon federal benevolence, and on personal initiative before outside help is sought.

In the matter of health insurance, for example, the Association is commonly represented as having been opposed to health insurance in the beginning, and only later changing its stand. This is partly true. The first health insurance proposals were so poorly conceived that disappointment was inevitable, both for patients and doctors. The Association opposed these proposals. But it laid down principles to be embodied in acceptable health insurance plans. These principles are now the basis for health insurance which the Association vigorously supports.

The Association also supports federal aid, with appropriate safeguards, for the construction of hospital and medical school facilities, but not for current operating expenses. The distinction is made to avoid federal control of activities which are essentially local, and which the Association is convinced should be kept under local control. This, among other reasons, also explains the Association's opposition to medical care for the aged tied to Social Security taxes, instead of to state and locally controlled programs with federal aid when necessary.

Community Services

The Association is looking to the future of medicine through its encouragement of the Student American Medical Association, a nationwide organization of medical students with its own headquarters, with student officers, and its own medical journal. The young men and women who form this organization are your doctors for tomorrow.

The Association pursues its quest for information to serve you by aiding your physician through a number of scientific councils and committees. These deal with the evaluation of drugs, with foods and nutrition, with medical physics, mental health, occupational health, governmental medicine (including disaster care, military, and governmental services), with international health matters, the medical aspects of sports, rural health, cost of illness, and the work of the voluntary health agencies.

Doctors are located for communities needing them, and physicians are helped to find a suitable place to practice. The problems involved in maternity and child care receive attention, as do school health problems, health of the aging, environmental sanitation. The social and economic aspects of medicine are studied. The Association endeavors to supply information to the physician without attempting to do his thinking for him. Policies are formed and enunciated, however, when medical organization leadership seems to be required. State and county medical societies and individual physicians usually support such policies, but they enjoy complete freedom of thought and expression, and dissenting opinions are respected.

The doctor needs a hospital in which to care for his patients; hospitals are also needed for the training of nurses, the continuing education of medical graduates, the advanced experience required by physicians for specialization, and for clinical research to keep medical knowledge constantly growing. The standards for acceptable hospitals have been steadily advancing, as a result of efforts by the hospitals themselves—with the aid of medical, nursing, and surgical organizations. In these efforts the American Medical Association played a pioneer role for many years, and now serves as a member of a four-organization Commission for Hospital Accreditation, with special reference to the education of internes and resident physicians.

The foregoing activities of the Association represent a brief summary of its most important efforts to improve the quality of medical care through maintaining and raising the standards of medical education, both in the medical school and after the doctor starts his practice. The real beneficiary of this extensive activity is the patient.

Health Education

Turning to its public service activities, the Association's history goes back a long way to an interest expressed at its first annual meeting in 1847, where the delegates discussed health and sanitary conditions in institutions and prisons. Among the most recent expressions of this concern is the Association's interest in convalescent and nursing homes, some of which have turned out to be no credit to the many reputable members of this class of facility, for which the need grows day by day. In conjunction with the American Association of Nursing Homes, the American Medical Association is working toward the improvement of the better homes and the elimination of those whose management is unable or unwilling to progress in the right direction.

Prompt medical care in an emergency is essential. This is of special importance to people who have no family doctor or who become ill in a strange community. The medical profession provides an emergency service in most urban centers through an answering service operated by the local medical society. Closely related to this service is the need for a means of recognizing the requirements of a person suddenly ill, and acting promptly and properly if the individual is unconscious, dazed, or incoherent, or too young or too old to respond. The Association convened a conference of the many organizations interested in this problem. Subsequently the Association developed and is promoting the use of a recognition emblem and a wallet card which will inform the first aider or other Samaritan of any medical conditions which might affect the treatment of sick individuals. (See Part IX, Chapter One.)

The Association established its health magazine, first called *Hygeia* after the mythical Greek goddess of health, in 1923. It is now known as *Today's Health*. It is subsidized by the Association, supplied to all member physicians for their waiting rooms, and open to subscription by schools, libraries, and families. The AMA publishes, and distributes at nominal cost, a wide and varying selection of up-to-date pamphlets on medical and health topics. It provides a nationwide speakers' service, with the cooperation of local medical societies, for all sorts of organizations on numerous medical and health topics. From time to time the Association conducts radio and television programs, and consults with the broadcasting industry about the portrayal of medical situations in entertainment programs.

The Association has actively promoted the widest possible use of both kinds of polio vaccines. It is now encouraging the immunization

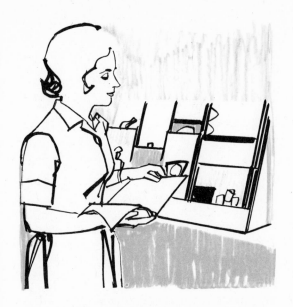

of more adults against tetanus, and cooperating in the introduction of the new measles vaccine. It is publicizing, through a series of press releases and radio spot announcements, such important medical information as the hazard of German measles to the expectant mother and the life-saving possibilities of automobile seat belts. It has courted unpopularity, in the conviction that its stand is right, by supporting fluoridation of public water supplies for cutting down tooth decay.

The Association has been vigorously exposing the quack and the charlatan—inside the profession and out—for many years, having acquired a formidable history of lawsuits in the process. It has lost only one, and was required to pay damages of one cent—but the plaintiff had to pay the costs of the suit. As a result of this activity, many of the worst cancer quacks have been driven out of business. Too often, however, it seems that two quacks spring up wherever one is knocked down. As in other areas, the Association has no legal powers to control quackery, nor does it desire any.

The school health program of the American Medical Association is among its most important community services. Through a Joint Committee on Health Problems in Education established in 1911, and a series of conferences with the National Education Association, dealing with physicians and schools, the Association and related organizations with similar interests, have established standards which have been adopted by most elementary and secondary schools in the United States. These standards are published in books, pamphlets, resolutions, and declarations. There is hardly a school system where these materials are not known.

Woman's Auxiliary

Doctors' wives contribute to the services rendered by the Association, through their organization, the Woman's Auxiliary. This is organized, like the AMA, on a local, state, and national basis. It has over 100,000 members. It raises funds for the American Medical Association Education and Research Foundation, and renders numerous community services. An example is its G.E.M.S. program, standing for *Good Emergency Mother Substitutes*—in other words, babysitters. This program instructs youngsters in the proper babysitting procedures.

Locally, Auxiliary members have served the health interests of community health agencies, acted as hospital volunteers, and supported community causes aimed at improving the health or serving the social needs of the community. They have given the Association and its programs the essential "woman's touch."

The Association is interested in you and your welfare. If you see a warning about danger on a pesticide, the Association had a part in putting it there. If your community has a poison control center, or has built facilities to attract doctors to come and stay, or has a new wing on its community hospital, or if you hear health hints on your radio, or your child brings home a notice about health examinations in school—the Association probably had a hand in bringing it about. This may have been due to a publication, to testimony before a Congressional committee or information furnished a State legislature, or to attendance by one of your local physicians at a meeting or conference, or the influence of a teacher who has been at an AMA health workshop, or a newspaper story that moved someone to action. These indirect influences cannot readily be measured, but they are at work all the time.

The influence of an organization representing substantially all actively practicing physicians, including public health and hospital personnel, cannot help being felt. If it were suddenly disbanded, it would be missed.

In your community, the local medical society is the American Medical Association. In your family and personal life, the Association is your capable and respected family doctor.

CHAPTER THREE

COMMUNITY HEALTH AND MEDICAL SERVICES

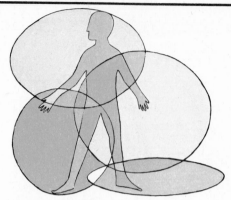

THE STRENGTH of any nation is directly related to its health. The nation's health is the sum of the health of the people in its various communities. And the health of a community depends on the network of facilities available for ministering to its residents.

Their needs are basically the same, though they vary in detail from community to community according to geographic, racial, age, economic, population, and other factors.

Community health is a composite of the health of many individuals. Each person is responsible for his own personal medical care. When he cannot provide this care for himself, the responsibility should properly pass to his family, the community, the county, or the state, and only when all these fail, to the Federal government, and then only in conjunction with the other levels of government, in that order.

The family doctor and his counterpart in allied professions are the hub of the health program of any community. When a family needs health care, it turns first to its doctor for treatment and counsel. When the services of other health facilities are advisable, the doctor should recommend their use.

Community health facilities include both individuals—physicians, dentists, nurses, therapists, and technicians—and organizations—hospitals, nursing homes, health departments, and voluntary agencies. All are involved in the prevention of disease and the diagnosis of specific diseases and ailments. Some include treatment of certain diseases and ailments in specific patients and restoring the patient after treatment to a useful role in the community.

Doctors

Responsibility for medical care centers upon the doctor. Health facilities within a community may provide services that assist the doctor

in carrying out this responsibility, and doctors will be found working in such facilities. They are there because these facilities need medical skills to direct their programs and to coordinate the activities of other personnel into a meaningful pattern of health care. Thus, doctors will be found specializing in public health, directing the medical care activities of hospitals, acting as consultants to nursing homes, serving on the boards of voluntary health agencies, and assisting in church-sponsored welfare work and other agencies.

Basic family medical care is provided by the family physician. Most frequently he is a general practitioner or an internist, who specializes in diseases of the internal organs. When the condition of his patient calls for different knowledge or skills than he possesses, the family doctor will call for the aid of specialists.

The technology of medical care has advanced with such speed in recent years that it is impossible for each physician to have at his fingertips all available knowledge about each part of the body, or to gain familiarity with each new tool and skill of all the various specialties. This fact has led many a physician to narrow his field of interest so that he may maintain intimate acquaintance with the developments in a single area.

Doctors wishing to specialize following graduation from medical school and after one or two years of internship, enter residency training in a teaching hospital for three years or more. During this period, the doctor is trained under skilled specialists in the field of his choice.

The following are the fields of medicine which the American Medical Association has approved for specialized residency training:

Anesthesiology. Administration of anesthetics and other drugs that produce loss of sensation or consciousness, operation of heart-lung machines, and the monitoring of the patient's reactions.

Colon and Rectal Surgery. Operative correction of conditions and diseases of the colon and rectum.

Dermatology. Treatment of diseases of the skin and scalp.

General Practice. Treatment of the whole body, largely through non-surgical means.

General Surgery. Operative correction of conditions and diseases of the body, not limited to specific areas thereof.

Internal Medicine. Treatment of nonsurgical diseases and illnesses. Among subspecialties are gastroenterology, allergy, cardiovascular disease, and pulmonary disease.

Neurological Surgery. Operative treatment of conditions of the brain, spinal cord, and peripheral nerves outside the brain and spinal cord.

Neurology. Diagnosis and therapeutic management of diseases of the nervous system.

Obstetrics and Gynecology. Management of pregnancy and childbirth and the treatment of women's diseases, especially of the reproductive organs, the urinary tract, and the rectum.

Ophthalmology. Surgical and medical treatment of diseases of the eye; refractions.

Orthopedic Surgery. Operative correction of deformities, fractures, and other disorders and diseases of the skeletal system and related structures.

Otolaryngology. Operative and therapeutic treatment of disorders of the ear, nose, and throat.

Pathology. The identification of disease through the analysis of body tissues, fluids, and other body specimens.

Pediatrics. Management and treatment of children from birth to the teens. Subspecialists include pediatric allergy and pediatric cardiology.

Physical Medicine and Rehabilitation. Treatment and restoration of the convalescent and physically handicapped patient.

Plastic Surgery. Reparative operations on the scalp, face, eye sockets, nose, mouth, neck, trunk, and extremeties.

Preventive Medicine. Study, prevention, and control of epidemic, environmental, and occupational diseases and hazards. Special affiliated fields include aviation medicine, general preventive medicine, occupational medicine, and public health.

Psychiatry. Interpretation and treatment of mental and personality disorders. A subspeciality is child psychiatry.

Radiology. Diagnosis and treatment of diseases by the use of radiant energy, for example, x-ray and radioactive isotopes.

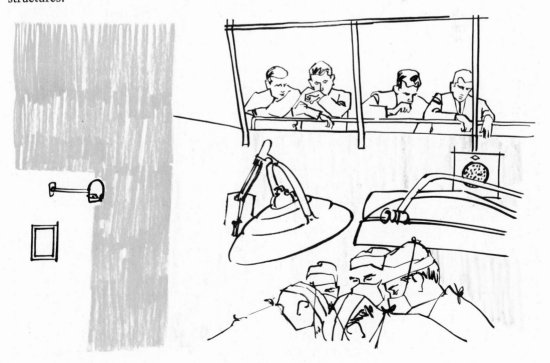

Thoracic Surgery. Operative treatment of diseases of the lungs, esophagus, and related organs.

Urology. Diagnosis, therapy, and operative treatment of diseases of the urinary tract, including the reproductive organs in the male.

Dentists

Allied with the nation's physicians in the care of the health needs of the American public are the dentists. Like the practice of medicine, dentistry is divided among general practitioners and a number of specialists.

A dentist in general practice may concentrate only on the cleaning, filling, and extraction of teeth, or he may have an internship and perform work in one or several of the speciality areas. The main specialty areas in the field of dentistry are:

Orthodontics. The straightening of irregularities of the teeth and corrections of malocclusions of the jaw.

Periodontics. The treatment of diseases of tissues around the teeth.

Oral Surgery. Surgical treatment and repair of teeth involving cutting into the jawbone.

Pedodontics. Treatment of the dental ills of children.

Prosthodontics. The construction of special appliances to compensate mechanically for such deficiencies as a cleft palate.

Proper family dental care involves periodic visits to the dentist. The American Dental Association recommends that such visits be made at least every six months. At the time of these visits the dentist will clean the teeth, removing tartar formations at the gum level, and will fill any cavities that have developed since the last visit. The dentist will also advise whether x-rays are needed to determine if there are infections of the roots of the teeth which may be treated to help prevent extractions.

Where the community does not fluoridate its water, the dentist may recommend and apply a fluoride solution to the outer surfaces of children's teeth. When the services of a dentist skilled in one of the specialty areas are required, the general practicing dentist will advise the family.

Nurses

Nurses may serve in hospitals, nursing homes, doctors' offices, public health departments, industrial plants, or with visiting nurse associations. The registered nurse is a graduate of high school or college and a course in nursing conducted by a teaching hospital. This course of training usually lasts about three years. The duties of the registered nurse in giving the patient medications and treatments are prescribed by the physician under all circumstances. The nurse is not qualified to diagnose or to prescribe a course of treatment for any disease.

Registered nurses are in short supply. Their numbers are supplemented by practical nurses. In most states, practical nurses are licensed, and it is usually required that they be high school graduates and have completed a one-year course of study and training. The duties of the licensed practical nurse are to care for selected chronically ill and convalescent patients and to assist the professional nursing team in the care of acutely ill patients.

Therapists

Therapists are involved in the rehabilitation of patients who are recovering from an attack of an acute short-term illness or are subject to a long-term or chronic disease. Included in the category of therapy specialists are:

Speech Therapists, who aid in correcting speech deficiencies and in helping the patient cope with speech problems following illness, such as stroke.

Physical Therapists, who provide skilled treatment, under the direction of a doctor, involving heat therapy, massage, exercise, and certain muscle stimulation which, together with proper medications, improve the muscle tone and increase coordination.

Occupational Therapists, who are involved in the care of chronically ill patients to help them maintain a proper mental outlook through the devising and assignment of various tasks which help the patient build his sense of self esteem.

Vocational Therapists, who help patients recover their functions and regain their capacities through projects in which the patient performs tasks that use the physical functions which need development, and which help restore their mental and emotional status.

Technicians

Technicians perform a wide range of services which are essential in the diagnosis and treatment of disease. Among these are x-ray

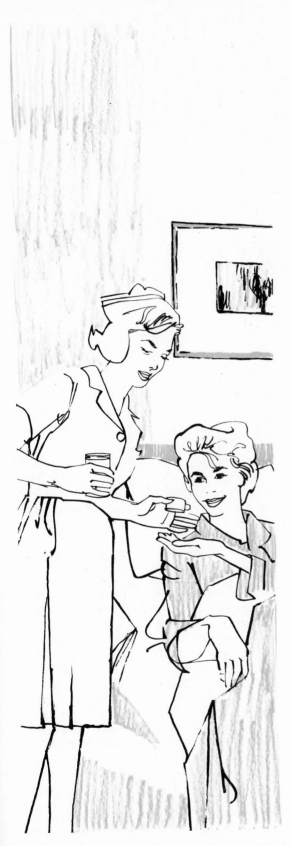

technicians trained to operate x-ray machines under the direction of a physician. The technician takes the pictures and develops the film for reading by the radiologist.

The laboratory technician is also concerned with health care. Working under a physician's direction, he makes tests upon blood, tissues, urine, etc., and reports the findings to the doctor for use in diagnosis. Laboratory technicians are usually required to have at least two years of college and more than a year of hospital laboratory training. Their work demands a knowledge of chemistry, bacteriology, and hematology.

Hospitals

A hospital may be operated by a local governmental body such as a state, county, or city; it may be operated by the Federal government such as an Army, Navy, or Air Force hospital, or one operated by the Public Health Service or by the Veterans' Administration. Voluntary or nonprofit hospitals may be either church-related or operated and organized under community sponsorship. Hospitals may also be proprietary; that is, operated for profit.

Hospitals may be either short-term or long-term. By common definition, in the former the average stay is under 30 days; in the latter, the average stay is 30 days or over.

A hospital may provide a wide range of services (a general hospital) or it may limit its services to psychiatric, tuberculous, maternity, eye, ear, nose, and throat, orthopedic, chronic disease or convalescent, children's diseases, mental retardation, epilepsy, alcohol or drug addiction.

The hospitals with which most families will come into contact are voluntary, short-term general hospitals. The organization of even the smallest of these is complex. It involves the labors of many different types of personnel and provides a wide range of services to a constantly changing public. For this reason, the hospital is structured somewhat as a business organization. At the top is a board of directors which oversees the financial operations of the hospital and which is morally and legally responsible for all phases of hospital operation. The responsibility for the quality of medical care in a hospital is the function of the medical staff. This staff is composed of doctors of the community who are appointed by the board of trustees on the

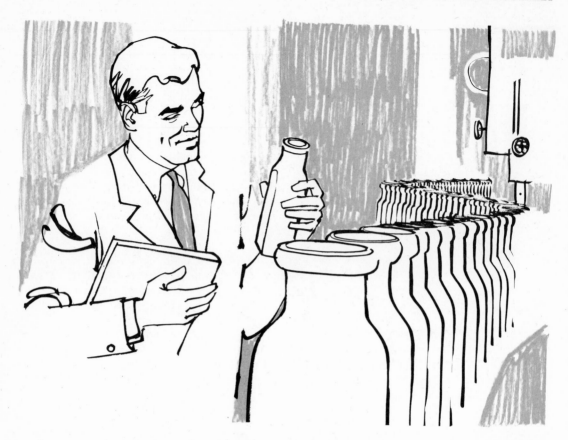

basis of their qualifications, and who are granted the privilege of using the facilities of the hospital to treat their patients.

Depending upon the size of the hospital, the medical staff is organized in varying degrees of complexity to provide control over the quality of medical care provided. Through rules and regulations established by the staff, the type of care and/or operations that may be performed by any member of the staff is delineated. Various committees of the staff provide a way to check the type of care that staff members are providing, both individually and as a group. Through the supervisory activities of these committees, the quality of medical care is maintained at a high standard.

Authority over the various housekeeping functions of the hospital is vested in the hospital administrator. The administrator will have charge over all personnel in the hospital with the exception of the doctors. It is his responsibility to see that all the various departments of the hospital are run efficiently so that patient care is of a high quality and costs are kept as low as possible.

In its care of patients, the hospital divides its services into in-patient and out-patient care. In-patient care is that rendered to patients who occupy beds in the hospital. Out-patient care is that rendered to patients who come to the hospital for treatment which does not require their being placed in bed. They usually come to the hospital at the direction of their own physician, who has scheduled them to receive various diagnostic tests, or who treats them in the out-patient clinic while he is present at the hospital.

Out-patient care may also be given to a patient who comes to the hospital of his own volition, or is brought there without referral by his own physician, because of an accident or other emergency. Such patients will either be treated and sent home, if the emergency is not serious, or assigned to a bed in the hospital if hospitalization is required, and the personal physician of their choice is notified.

Staffing of the hospital emergency department is the responsibility of the members of the medical staff. In most cases this is accomplished by assigning the members of the medical staff emergency call duty of 24 hours' duration on a rotating basis. A doctor on emergency call will either be present at the hospital or can be summoned by the head nurse to arrive within a few minutes after the emergency patient has come to the hospital. In the meantime, a resident physician or intern looks after the patient.

Nursing and Convalescent Homes

Once considered a one-way street where the aging patient was made more or less comfortable in his last days, nursing homes today are coming to be places in which to live and get well. Emphasis is being placed on skilled nursing care, rehabilitation through physical, occupational, and psychiatric therapy, recreational programs, and healthful diet.

Nursing homes serve as a link between the hospital and home. The convalescing patient may no longer need the intensive care provided by the general hospital, but may still require care that he cannot secure at home. He can obtain it in a nursing home at a cost lower than that of a hospital.

A properly staffed nursing home will have a registered nurse in charge. Essential medical care, as well as physical and other therapy, will be performed under the supervision of the patient's doctor.

While there are numerous progressive homes, unfortunately there still are many substandard homes. Families faced with the decision of placing a convalescing or aging relative in a home should visit several of them to determine where to get the best care possible for the funds available. Advice can be secured from the physician, minister, or local welfare council.

Efforts are being made to upgrade the quality of all nursing home care. In 1963, the American Medical Association and the American Nursing Home Association jointly established a program for the accreditation of nursing homes. In order to secure accreditation, nursing homes will have to meet established standards and maintain care at a satisfactory level.

Health Departments

The American Medical Association has defined public health as "the art and science of maintaining, protecting, and improving the health of the people through organized community efforts. It includes those arrangements whereby the community provides medical services for special groups of persons and is concerned with prevention or control of disease, with persons requiring hospitalization to protect the community, and with the medically indigent."

Each state has a health department. In addition, there are at local levels single- and multiple-county health units, city health departments, and state health districts. According to the United States Public Health Service, in 1960 only 5.6 per cent of the total United States population lacked local organized health services. The services provided by public health departments normally include at least the following:

● Recording of births, deaths, and sickness; tabulation of these to provide meaningful data so that problem areas can be determined, needed services provided and later evaluated.

● Environmental sanitation, such as the controlling of water and milk supplies; food sanitation; air pollution, including radioactive fallout; inspection of trailer camps, motels, and swimming pools; garbage and sewage disposal, etc.

● Provision of public health laboratories for the supervision of sanitation and the control of communicable diseases.

● Prevention and control of communicable diseases; sanatoriums with both in-patient and out-patient care for persons affected with tuberculosis, together with testing programs to uncover persons unaware that they have the disease, may be a health department service, but often is administered otherwise.

● Education of the public on health matters.

● Hygiene during maternity, infancy, and childhood, covering services both before and after birth for those who cannot afford the services of a private physician. Well-baby or well-child clinics for children under school age provide health supervision of the child and parental instruction in proper health care.

In addition to these basic programs, state and local health departments may provide hospital and medical care for special groups; services for crippled children, including mechanical devices and rehabilitative therapy; dental health programs, and mental health clinics. The health department may also conduct a school health program, including physical examinations, dental checkups, and screening programs to help in the early detection of chronic diseases. Frequently, school health programs are the direct responsibility of the school system itself, with or without the assistance of the health department. When medical care is indicated, parents are requested to take their child to the family doctor. Financial problems in connection with such care are often alleviated or assumed by the local welfare agency or by a voluntary health agency interested in the particular problem.

The number of public health services available will vary from community to community, according to the awareness of need and the amount of tax money available to support governmental health services.

Closely allied to the health departments are the state and local welfare departments. These tax-supported agencies arrange for medical, dental, hospital, and nursing care for families who are on the welfare rolls or whose incomes are too low to include such care within their budgets. Allied societies in the medical-care fields work closely with these agencies, and frequently fee schedules are reduced to provide as extensive coverage as possible from available funds. Working arrangements are also made with local pharmacists for drugs needed to combat specific illnesses. Hospitalization of indigent families is provided in city or local government hospitals, and in the ward service of teaching hospitals.

Voluntary Health Agencies

Supplementing other health services within a community are a number of voluntary health agencies, each of which ordinarily focuses its attention upon a specific disease (for example, The American Cancer Society) and is financed by private contributions. At the national level, such organizations engage in research aimed toward greater knowledge in the management of disease. At the local level, they may establish diagnostic and treatment clinics, provide financial assistance for afflicted persons, train doctors, nurses, and therapists in methods of care and treatment, and engage in educational activities. A detailed discussion of these agencies is presented in Part XIV, Chapter Two.

CHAPTER FOUR

DIAGNOSING DISEASE

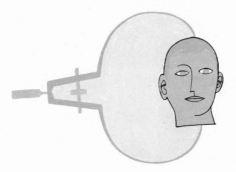

"I KNOW NOTHING IS WRONG with my heart. I had an electrocardiogram and it didn't show anything. . ."

"My chest x-ray shows nothing the matter there. . ."

"My BMR test proves that I have thyroid trouble. . ."

Patients make statements like these every day, but in many cases they are far from the truth. Laboratory and x-ray tests and the other specialized mechanical adjuncts to diagnosis are among the most valuable tools the physician has, but they do not have the accuracy of precision measurements. One can measure the characteristics of a piece of steel with some exactitude, but measuring the human body is much more complex and subject to error.

The most dangerous heart disease is one that affects the coronary arteries, the vessels that supply the heart muscle with blood. Changes in these arteries themselves are not shown on the electrocardiogram. When one of the vessels closes, the area of heart muscle which it usually supplies is suddenly cut off from the general circulation and no longer has an adequate blood and oxygen supply. When this actually happens, electrical changes occur which show on the ECG. But until there is an actual change in circulation there will be no visible alterations in the electrocardiogram even though the arteries are diseased and there is possibility of serious trouble ahead. To say that a negative electrocardiogram means that no heart trouble exists can be a totally false conclusion.

Does this mean that the test is worthless? Not at all. Many difficulties can be diagnosed with accuracy by means of the ECG. It does mean, however, that the test alone, without other information, is of little use.

The trained clinical judgement of the physician supplemented by the electrocardiogram and other tests is the only way to approach accuracy in diagnosis. It is a fallacy to have the test alone and to base predictions solely on the results. In the final analysis, the expert physician is really the best diagnostic instrument available.

There is a popular belief that a white blood cell count is an excellent way to diagnose appendicitis. This is only indirectly true. The white count is a good indicator of the presence of infection, but it is in no sense specific for appendicitis. For example, an infected toe will send a person's blood count from its normal 7,500 or so white cell count up to as high as 13,000 or 14,000. If at the same time one gets a pain in the right side, appendicitis may be suspected. In such a case, the white count is of little use. Which infection caused it to rise, that in the toe or in the appendix? This is a decision the doctor has to make.

We have no positive, error-free techniques of medical testing. The measures we have provide estimates, some crude and a few accurate. None is perfect. Each test has to be judged in the light of the entire clinical picture.

Sometimes it takes two or three x-ray examinations to find an ulcer, or to be absolutely certain that none is present. By evaluation of symptoms the doctor can decide whether or not the hunt should continue.

This is not meant to imply that tests are no good. The point to remember is that they are not perfect. Each year some progress is made and accuracy is increased.

Some doctors feel that there has been an overselling of the American people on the advantages of mechanical tests. People are in-

319

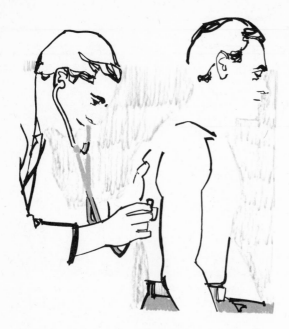

clined to believe that if something is done with scientific machinery it is better than can be accomplished with the human brain alone.

Actually this is not at all true in medicine. The best medical instrument we have is the intelligent and thorough physician.

An educated young woman may come in to her doctor and say, "I have been feeling a little off lately. I want to get a blood count to see if my blood is up to normal." Unless she has a great deal of special medical training, this girl knows little or nothing about interpreting a blood count or whether she needs one.

Perhaps she knows that 4,500,000 is a normal red blood count in women. If hers turns out to be 4,300,000 she may think, "I need some iron and vitamins. I thought I felt a little anemic."

Actually, the difference between 4,300,000 and 4,500,000 lies within the standard error of the count. The young lady may have no anemia at all. Her doctor can explain this and save her from being fooled by the wrong interpretation of the test.

Millions of people have read of the wondrous tests available in medicine and the superb work done with the help of these tests, but they do not realize that laboratory determinations are worthless by themselves. It is only in the light of proper interpretation that they become of value.

The development of new medical procedures in recent years has been almost unbelievable, yet all require someone to direct and chart their course. Perhaps some day doctors will mechanize themselves out of business and design doctorless hospitals, but that date lies far in the future, if ever.

The results achieved in medicine are exactly proportional to two things— the intelligence used by the physician and the degree of cooperation and understanding the patient brings to him.

Laboratory tests are supplemental things, not perfect measurements. They are of no service to the average patient until interpreted by a physician who has close and intimate knowledge of the case under study.

CHAPTER FIVE

MEDICAL QUACKERY

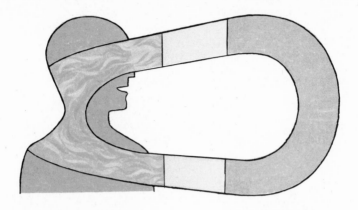

MEDICAL QUACKERY is the practice of deceit. It persists with a fervor equalled perhaps only by the sincere quest for more effective cures for more and more diseases.

Quackery in medicine probably is as old as, if not older than, civilized man. It was Voltaire who said that the quack was born when the first knave met the first fool.

It has been said that the first recorded prescription for a hair grower was that made up for the Egyptian Queen Ses, mother of King Teta, in about 3400 B.C. It consisted of a mixture of dog toes, date refuse, and asses' hooves. Mixtures promoted today that are claimed to grow hair are no more effective than that concocted for Queen Ses.

The word "quack," is an abbreviation of the earlier form "quacksalver." The word quack has as its first meaning the cry of a duck. The word "salver" means to save or heal. Thus the original word quacksalver described one who pretends to be a saver or healer and who makes noisy pretenses to medical skill not based on real knowledge.

There are many persons today who claim they can treat organic disease by a special method or by a certain product. They pretend to have the skill to cure cancer, arthritis, feeblemindedness, diabetes, tuberculosis, and many other serious conditions. Through faddism, fraud, deception, and delusion, the unknowing are led to seek non-existent short-cuts to health. Knowing only what they are told by a "pitchman" or "health lecturer," millions each year attempt self-medication for self-diagnosed symptoms. Others, some with confirmed illnesses, are beguiled with assurance of a quick cure, even for incurable diseases. Honest medicine cannot always give such assurances. The quack, unhindered by ethics or concern, can.

Quackery can negate much of the good that medicine can do. It can steal precious time—that early period of a disease when prompt, efficient treatment can often make the difference between life and death.

The cancer patient who infuses himself with expensive bottled sea water or a secret remedy is, in reality, only withholding from himself surgery, chemotherapy, or radiation which might arrest the disease.

Quackery can also mask diseases with telling effect. The non-prescription potion that soothes a persistent stomach upset may serve only to delay a trip to the doctor by a man with an undiagnosed ulcer—a delay that often leads to serious consequences.

As with most serious medical problems, the solution is not simple. The prosecution of frauds perpetrated in the guise of medicine is extremely difficult. Just as the hypochondriac imagines disease, so can the gullible imagine cures, even when disease still exists.

State and federal law enforcement alone cannot do the job, although it certainly can help, as we have seen in the past few years. Before we can hope to make major progress toward the eradication of quackery, however, the public must gain a wider understanding of what quackery is and how it flourishes.

Accurate figures are difficult to obtain, but some experts estimate that Americans spend $1,000,000,000 each year on useless cures, mechanical gadgets, fad foods, and other quack remedies. Breakdowns of the cost of quackery in this country include $500,000,000 for vitamin preparations, self-prescribed or sold house-to-house, and other nutritional nonsense; $1,500,000 for self-prescribed laxatives, which can be harmful; $250,000,000 for arthritis and rheumatism treatments with claim of cure; more than $100,000,000 annually for "patent medicines," and more than $50,000,-000 for cancer "cures" and treatments.

How to Identify a Quack

What does a quack look like? Quacks are generally well-dressed, neat, healthy, kind, patient, and sympathetic with the people they deal with. They give the patient sufficient time to tell his troubles.

Beware of the person or institution in the healing arts that advertises directly to the public. In the daily newspapers, in certain magazines, and over the air there are those who advertise their alleged skills in the treatment of serious disease. Such advertisers also use privately printed pamphlets, booklets, and even newspapers, wherein appear testimonials of persons, with pictures "before and after" the alleged treatment.

Medical testimonials are a very poor source of information to their readers. The files of the Department of Investigation of the American Medical Association contain examples of newspaper testimonials by individuals whose obituaries appear in the same issue.

The AMA Department of Investigation lists six simple indicators for spotting a quack:

1. He uses a special or "secret" machine or formula he claims can cure disease.

2. He guarantees a quick cure.

3. He advertises or uses case histories and testimonials to promote his cure.

4. He clamors constantly for medical investigation and recognition.

5. He claims medical men are persecuting him or are afraid of his competition.

6. He tells you that surgery or x-rays or drugs will cause more harm than good.

Drugs, devices, and fad foods labeled as quackery fall into one or more of three major classifications:

• Those dangerous to health or life when used without proper supervision.

• Those worthless for the purposes for which they are offered.

• Those offered for conditions for which they alone do not constitute competent treatment, and where unwise self-treatment may permit the conditions to progress so far that the damage cannot be repaired.

Official agencies such as the Food and Drug Administration, the Federal Trade Commission, and the Post Office Department, many state departments of public health and pri-

vate voluntary agencies, including the American Medical Association, the American Cancer Society, and the Arthritis and Rheumatism Foundation, have cracked down hard on the first two groups. They are not so widespread as they were 25 years ago. Products in the third group are still common and constitute a major health problem today.

The Department of Investigation of the American Medical Association has been functioning for more than 50 years. The department originally was formed to combat "patent medicine" advertising, and was a regular department of *The Journal of the American Medical Association,* revealing to the medical profession the ingredients of the many secret nostrums then on the market, and exposing the many false claims made by their promoters. The department maintains voluminous files of information available to any person who has a legitimate reason for inquiry.

In maintaining such an activity, the American Medical Association recognizes that education of the public is a potent weapon in the fight against medical quackery. With this in mind, meetings on medical quackery have been held and methods for combating it discussed.

The first Pure Food and Drugs Act was passed in 1906. This afforded a degree of protection, particularly in the area of adulteration of foods and drugs, by requiring that certain information be placed on the labels of drug products. This was a great step forward, because the patent medicine industry was vocal, and for a long time successful, in its resistance and objection to such an "impairment of liberty." Such liberty, however, was not in the public interest, and, as a result, Congress recognized its obligation to the public by passing the law.

In 1937 a series of deaths occurred in some of the Southern states because a manufacturer of a certain drug, a sulfa elixir, had substituted a poisonous ingredient for glycerin. The Federal law at the time was not sufficient to protect the public from such a tragedy, and, as a result, Congress passed in 1938 the Federal Food, Drug, and Cosmetic Act.

Advertising of drug products, however, was not placed under the jurisdiction of the Food and Drug Administration; rather, it was assigned to the Federal Trade Commission.

The Federal Food, Drug, and Cosmetic Act has been amended on several occasions to strengthen the law. Thus, today, if a manufacturer wishes to market a new drug, he must

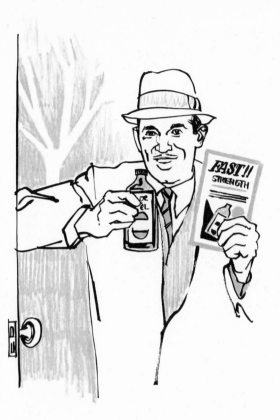

The Post Office Department also engages in protecting the public by watching over the mails, and, in case of medical fraud, proceeds against sellers of a variety of products which are sold and promoted by mail. These may include vitamin pills, reducing preparations, "hair restorers," "rejuvenators," and similar products appealing to the vain, the old, or the sick. That agency reports its findings, after hearings, to the postmaster of the city in which the goods are mailed, directing him to return to the senders all remittances, stamping the envelopes "Fraudulent." If the firm agrees to stop the solicitation, the remittances are returned to the senders with the envelopes stamped "Out of Business."

These federal agencies are extremely active, although most people know very little about their operation.

Food Supplements

The housewife is not generally aware that her food supply is the best on earth from the standpoint of adequate nutritional quality. So far as residues from pesticides are concerned, government tests show the food supply to be entirely safe. The American citizen who goes into the marketplace to purchase his groceries, his meats, his vegetables, and the rest, can be reasonably sure that they are safe, wholesome, and nutritionally adequate.

The United States, the best-fed nation on earth, certainly does not need to waste $500,000,000 annually on vitamin pills, special dietary foods, and dietary monstrosities such as rose hips, fenugreek tea, and a host of other so-called health foods. But the American public does waste approximately that amount of money each year—more than is spent in a year on medical education in the United States.

Within the past decade there has arisen a wholly new class of pretenders to medical skill. These are the persons who come to your doorstep with a wonderful multi-vitamin and mineral product which they will sell to you as an insurance policy against poor health if you are well, or as a sure cure if you are sick.

Since these sales people claim benefit in the area of health and disease, they come under the jurisdiction of the Food and Drug Administration, and many have been fined, placed on probation, or otherwise discouraged by Federal regulatory action. The firms behind them have had their stocks seized, their literature impounded, and their officers prosecuted.

demonstrate to the satisfaction of the governmental agency that not only is the product safe for use when used as directed, but also that it is effective for the purposes for which it is sold.

The Food and Drug Administration proceeds to bring violations of the law to the attention of the Federal courts, obtains court orders calling for the seizure of goods and secures the prosecution of the firm or person who is responsible for the violation. The government may also move to stop the violation of the law by the individual or firm involved.

The Federal Trade Commission, which evaluates advertising of drug products, proceeds by hearings. When violations are brought to its attention, the commission proceeds by written complaints charging that the manufacturers or distributors of certain drug products are advertising such products in a false or misleading manner. The firm may deny that its advertising is not truthful, and hearings are then scheduled and held, wherein the matter is heard and disposed of. An order or a consent may be issued by the commission, directing the firm to comply with the requirements of the order. This is also published in the *Federal Register*. The advertiser may appeal rulings of the commission to the Federal courts.

Because of our ample food supply, better methods of processing, and alert federal agencies, the average American in reasonably good health obtains the essential nutriments from his diet—provided, of course, it is fairly well balanced. The body excretes the excess of vitamins and minerals (except for the fat-soluble vitamins A and D, which are retained), so a person taking vitamins under such circumstances is simply wasting money.

It is, of course, another matter if the family physician finds that a patient needs special vitamin or mineral supplementation. Rarely, however, is it advisable for the individual to supplement his diet on his own. It is always best to obtain the advice of a competent doctor, who can determine any need for vitamin or vitamin-and-mineral supplementation.

Quack Remedies

Beware of advertisers who market alcoholic mixtures for sluggish blood, for anemia from iron deficiency, for a run-down or tired feeling, or lack of youthful pep and vigor. If a person is feeling tired or run-down, he may be suffering from serious organic disease. Here again he should be in the hands of a competent physician, because the tonic may well mask symptoms which could lead to serious chronic diseases or disability.

Persons should not rely on cure-all methods to overcome disease. Spinal manipulations and colon irrigations have been widely promoted as systems of medicine that can correct serious conditions and diseases. Suffice it to say that if such methods had merit, they would have withstood the scrutiny of competent scientific observers, and the likelihood is that they would be widely used by doctors of medicine.

Beware of persons who have a special or exclusive treatment for cancer. Here is an area of human suffering that has been exploited by heartless, scheming, and clever individuals. Even in this enlightened day, it is estimated that $50,000,000 a year is wasted pursuing non-existent cancer cures and treatments. They are described as "non-existent" because, while they may be administered by kindly, apparently well-intentioned people who may even be doctors of medicine, they nonetheless have no established merit in the treatment of cancer. When anyone, whether he is a doctor or not, appeals to the public claiming that he has a substance, a method, or a system of treating cancer adequately, it is virtually certain that he does so because the medical profession has evaluated his treatment and found it wanting. Doctors of medicine die from cancer, some lose members of their families to this dread condition. Thus one can rest assured that the medical profession, which continuously searches under both private and governmental auspices for a cure for cancer, would use without hesitation any such product that had demonstrated promise.

When the promoter of a cancer treatment demands a "fair test" publicly, or accuses medicine of treating him unfairly, or appeals to the public through newspapers, books, magazine articles, and radio and television programs, it is safe to say that he is a quack. Anyone interested in the history of medicine will find these signs as common to all who have falsely claimed, both in the past and at present, to have a cure for cancer.

The American Cancer Society maintains a standing committee which evaluates claims made for cancer treatments and publishes informational articles on the various treatments and their promoters.

An Arthritis and Rheumatism Foundation survey a few years ago estimated that 14,000,000 arthritics in this country waste $250,000,000 dollars each year in their fruitless effort to return to relative bodily comfort and freedom from pain. From time to time, when the need arises, the Foundation publishes informational bulletins to let people know the truth about the claims made by those who pretend to have peculiar skill in the treatment of arthritis.

Any institution which advertises that it has a treatment for arthritis should be avoided. Persons who go to such places usually will find the methods to be no different from such ordinary physical treatments as heat, light, colonic irrigation, and vitamin therapy, none of which is an adequate treatment, either singly or in combination. Persons also find these institutions demanding high fees, payable in advance.

Beware of glorified aspirin tablets which cost so much more but which actually are no better as pain-relievers than ordinary aspirin, a standard drug of recognized merit as an analgesic.

Specific Types of Quackery

Other major areas in which quacks operate fall into these categories, as listed by the Boston Better Business Bureau:

Alcoholism. Advertised "cures," "remedies," or "treatments" for this disease are worthless. There are no "easy" or "secret" treatments for alcoholism, or any drugs conclusively demonstrated to remove or overcome addiction to alcohol permanently and safely, or to make it possible for the alcoholic to drink normally. Recovery from this disease is dependent upon the individual's sincere desire to stop drinking, and his willingness to accept mental and spiritual help, as through psychiatry, Alcoholics Anonymous, etc.

Baldness. There is no known drug, preparation, device, or method of treatment recognized as a cure, remedy, or competent treatment for baldness, or as capable of growing or aiding the growth of hair, preventing baldness, or feeding or nourishing the hair or scalp. Hair does not have "roots" like a plant and cannot be "fed" by any external application.

Breast Developers. There is no known preparation, system of exercise, or mechanical device which may be properly offered to the public to increase the size of the female breast. Estrogenic (hormone) preparations cannot be used with safety except under a physician's supervision, and then may produce satisfactory results only in a minority of cases.

Diabetes. Diabetics should be under the care of a physician for periodic examinations and possible adjustment of control measures. Derivatives of the sulfanilamides are being used effectively in some cases. With this exception, diet and diet with insulin injections are the only recognized treatments for controlling this disease. Reliance upon advertised treatments may cause early death.

Diagnostic Devices. Devices have been promoted by quack practitioners as possessing magical properties in the diagnosis and sometimes the treatment and cure of serious ailments. The sick person who relies on quack practitioners and their devices is gambling with his life, and is causing needless damage to his pocketbook.

Epilepsy. Certain drugs help to control the seizures of epilepsy, but they are not a "cure" for the condition, the cause of which is unknown. Epilepsy is too complicated and serious a condition for self or mail-order treatment.

Eye Diseases. The human eye is a complex and delicate mechanism, and should not be tampered with by the unskilled. No known medical preparation may be truthfully offered to the public as a cure, remedy, or treatment for pathological conditions of the eye or to correct errors of refraction. Properly compounded eye drops and lotions may, however, be used to help cleanse the eyes and allay irritations due to minor local conditions. Defective vision has many causes. Eye glasses cannot be accurately or safely fitted by mail, nor can mail-order courses in eye treatment be truthfully offered to the public to correct defects of vision.

Hair Dyes. Most hair dyes on the market today will not harm the majority of people when properly used, but they are potentially dangerous when misused. Some represent greater danger than others. The best and safest results are obtained when the hair is dyed by a qualified operator. In dyeing one's own hair, one should follow directions exactly and make all the prescribed skin tests to determine possible allergy to the dye. No one, as yet, has discovered a means of "restoring" color to gray hair or achieving permanent coloration results. Consumption of vitamin products is worthless for these purposes. (See Part III, Chapter Eight.)

Hair Removers. Electrolysis, in expert hands, is the only known method of removing superfluous hair permanently and safely. Misused by inexperienced people, electrolysis can cause tragic disfigurement. There are many chemical depilatories, epilators, abrasives, etc., which, when used according to directions, will temporarily remove hair in a satisfactory and reasonably safe manner, but the results are not permanent and these products do not retard growth of hair. Bleaching creams or lotions, including those alleged to generate oxygen, will not remove hair, even temporarily. X-ray machines, generally under fanciful trade names, have been advertised for hair removal, but such treatments are extremely dangerous.

Health Foods. The term "health foods" is a misnomer, since it implies that the products have health-giving or curative properties, when, in general, they merely possess some of the nutritive qualities to be expected in any wholesome food product. More specifically, and contrary to what has been advertised, *maté,* or Paraguay tea, has no more healing properties than ordinary tea; kelp is not a cure for stomach ailments or obesity; honey is not a cure for whooping cough; root beer is not a tonic for the nerves; baking soda does not cure colds; grape juice will not reduce weight; gelatin does not prevent fatigue; blueberry juice is not a cure for diabetes, and olive oil will not prevent appendicitis.

High Blood Pressure. High blood pressure,

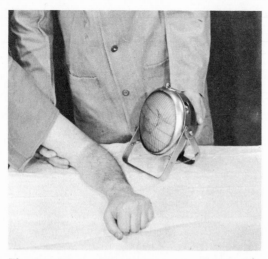

The Depolaray—claimed effective in treating over 100 diseases—was essentially a weak electromagnet.

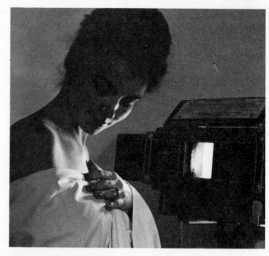

Spectrochrome, said to cure many diseases, treats patients with color lights—at certain moon phases.

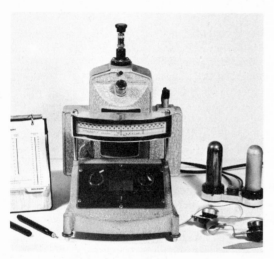

Micro-Dynameter was sold as a general diagnostic device, but it actually measures only skin moisture.

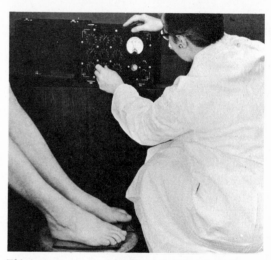

This instrument was said to permit diagnosis and treatment of patient, even when not physically present.

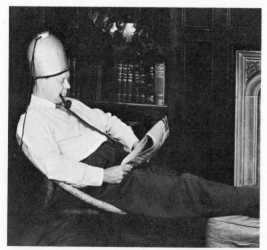

Manufacturers of Cel-O-Ray claimed the Christmas tree light bulb inside would grow hair on bald heads.

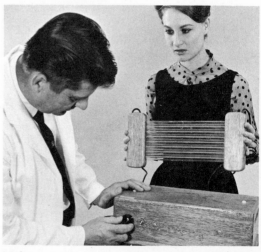

Makers of this ozone-producing device made false claims that the gas would cure 38 different diseases.

or hypertension, is not a disease, but it may be a symptom of various diseases or disorders. There are no known substances which may be properly advertised for self-treatment of high blood pressure. Garlic tablets have been offered for that purpose. Although credited with magical properties by the ancients, garlic has no value in the treatment of hypertension.

Hormones. The value of male hormones in the treatment of impotence is very limited, and the potentialities for danger in such products are so great that they should not be used in self-treatment. The Food and Drug Administration conducted an extensive investigation of the use and abuse of female and male hormones, and concluded that such hormones could not be safely used for therapeutic purposes, except under medical supervision.

Influenza. There is no known effective home treatment that may be truthfully advertised to the public as a cure, preventive, remedy, or treatment for this contagious and extremely serious disease. Proper treatment of influenza requires the personal attention of a physician.

Kidney Disease. No known preparation may be truthfully advertised as a cure, remedy, or treatment or relief for "kidney trouble," "bladder trouble," "kidney disorders" or diseases of the kidney or bladder. These are serious ailments, not amenable to self-treatment.

Mole Removers. Tampering with a mole may encourage its development into a dangerous growth; hence advertised preparations should be avoided. Only a physician should remove a mole.

Reducing Schemes. The essential cause of obesity is overeating. Lack of exercise may be a contributing cause. Reduction of the amount of food consumed by careful and proper eating is therefore essential. This may involve some discomfort and requires willpower. Stringent dieting should be considered in relation to one's physical condition, and therefore should be done only under the direction of a physician. Reducing plans which call for adherence to low-calorie diets and endurance of the hunger consequent thereto should not be offered to the public as "easy" or "pleasant," or as enabling reducers to eat "plenty," "eat what they want," etc. Too hasty reducing may be unsafe. Products advertised to reduce weight by curbing the appetite, and to enable users to adhere to low calorie diets without experiencing hunger and its attendant discomforts, should be avoided unless approved by your physician.

Laxative products have no value in reducing weight. Massage is not recognized as having any fat or weight-reducing value. Massage devices will not "reduce in spots" or remove "bumps" or "bulges," nor are creams of value except as lubricants. Belts, girdles, etc., may cause the wearer to appear slimmer, but they do not remove fat or reduce weight.

Obesity is not effectively and permanently reduced by sweating. Rubber garments, perspiration-inducing baths, or devices and soaps, creams, and other external preparations have no value for fat or weight reduction.

Pep Pills. Stimulant drugs such as Benzedrine, Dexedrine, and other brands of amphetamine sulfate are prescription drugs and have valuable medical uses. But they are also habit-forming, and may be dangerous if improperly used. They should not be employed as a substitute for rest, especially on the highways. Serious accidents have resulted from their use.

Hemorrhoids. Ointments and other external applications may be of value in relieving soreness, itching, or burning caused by piles or hemorrhoids, but they do not constitute a cure, remedy, or competent treatment for the condition. Serious cases require surgery or other specialized treatment. One should not attempt self-treatment of bleeding piles, because bleeding may indicate a serious condition requiring prompt medical attention. Laxative preparations should not be used for the self-treatment of piles.

Pitchmen. "Pitchmen" or "barkers" posing as health lecturers may have a selfish interest behind their talks—selling courses of instruction or books or other products on which they make a profit. Many of them attack well-known foods and products in order to sell their own preparations at "special" prices. Many "health fad" lecturers are in this class.

Prostate Gland Disorders. Devices designed to permit the application of heat to, or massage of, the prostate gland have been advertised for prostatitis, hypertrophy, and other prostate gland disorders. Even in skilled hands, such implements have limited value, and their use by untrained persons, to the neglect of more competent measures, may be attended by serious consequences. Prostate gland disorders may include many disease conditions, such as cancer, which are too serious for self-treatment.

Radioactive Products. Most of the waters, drugs, and other allegedly "radioactive" or "atomic" preparations and devices offered to the public for the treatment of numerous ailments contain insufficient radium or none at all, to justify their consideration as therapeutic agents. A genuinely radioactive or atomic water or drug would be extremely dangerous to use except under a physician's constant supervision. It would be illegal to sell a strongly radioactive product to the general public. Such a product would probably not be in the proper form to be of value, as well as being dangerous for unsupervised use.

Rupture. Surgery is generally necessary for the successful treatment of rupture or hernia in an adult. A well-constructed truss, when properly fitted, may provide palliative treatment for reducible rupture, but advertising should not encourage unskilled individuals to fit themselves. No truss, or any other method of self-treatment, may be truthfully advertised to cure or heal hernia or enable the patient to engage in unlimited activity. Use of a truss for a rupture which should be otherwise treated, or without competent advice and prescription, may delay and complicate proper treatment. A rupture should have competent diagnosis and prescription by one having specialized knowledge and the license to do so.

Sinus Disorders. Sinusitis is an inflammation or infection of the sinuses or internal cavities of the skull. It may be associated with numerous other afflictions. While certain products may afford temporary relief of symptoms such as nasal congestion, pain, or discomfort, the cure or successful treatment of the condition requires medical attention. Short-wave diathermy devices should not be used for the self-treatment of sinus disorders.

Skin Blemishes. There are preparations which will relieve itching and certain symptoms of superficial skin blemishes. However, in adopting any treatment for diseased or abnormal conditions of the skin, the only sensible thing to do is to consult a physician, preferably one who specializes in the treatment of skin conditions. Self-treatment may seriously delay proper medical treatment and unnecessarily prolong the condition. Conditions diagnosed as psoriasis, impetigo, and acne should be treated by prescription based on the diagnosis.

Stomach Ulcers. An antacid preparation may help relieve pain incident to stomach ulcers caused by hyperacidity, but a person suffering from an ulcer should be under the observation of a physician. In many cases the early symptoms of stomach cancer are similar to those of stomach ulcers. A stomach ulcer is a serious matter, and its proper treatment requires a competent medical appraisal of the condition and a careful regimen of diet, rest, and other corrective measures if one is to achieve substantial relief or eventual healing of the ulcer. Proper medication is but one of the necessary measures of treatment.

Tobacco Habit Cures. No known drug or combination of drugs can be truthfully offered to the public to cure or overcome the tobacco habit, or permanently eliminate the' desire for tobacco. A simple determination to stop, backed up by will power, is the best way to moderate or abstain from smoking.

Tuberculosis. For many years no drugs were known which would have any effect upon tuberculosis, other than the alleviation of symptoms when judiciously prescribed by a physician. Nevertheless, many products have been offered for the treatment of this disease, and in years past they have undoubtedly hastened the death of many a tuberculosis victim, or impeded his recovery. Until very recently the arrest of tuberculosis depended entirely upon rest, proper diet, and judicious surgery. Neglect of such measures and attempts to treat the disease with home or advertised remedies often proved disastrous. There are now some drugs useful to physicians in hastening the recovery of the tuberculous, but these cannot be used safely by non-medical persons. Also, there has been a shift in the prevalence of the disease, and now many elderly persons who have tuberculosis mistake it for "chronic bronchitis" or just "chronic cough." Not only should all remedies recommended for "chronic coughs" be looked upon with suspicion, but old people with "chronic coughs" should be examined to make sure they do not have tuberculosis.

The AMA and Quacks

The American Medical Association, at its first meeting in Philadelphia in 1847, called attention to a need for a constant and increased effort against the medical quack. The Association has continued the pledge of unceasing educational effort, both to the medical profession itself and to the lay public. Keeping the public informed, urging it to beware, and alerting federal and state officials to violations of law is a continuing effort by organized medicine to be a force for public good.

CHAPTER SIX

BUDGETING FOR ILLNESS

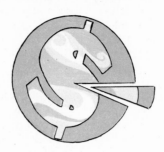

WHEN DOCTOR AND HOSPITAL BILLS are discussed, they are usually called the costs of medical care. Actually, it would be more accurate to call them the costs of *illness*. Even then, medical and hospital care are only a part of these expenses, and often a relatively small part at that.

Unless an illness is minor in nature and short in duration, it extensively disrupts family life. When the homemaker cannot do her work, help must be procured, often at considerable expense. A wage earner who is ill may lose some of his pay. A key provider's disabling illness may permanently lower the family's standard of living. Homes may be sacrificed and extensive other adjustments have to be made. Educational plans may have to be abandoned or altered. Costs of appliances, medicines, special foods, and nursing services may be heavy. These items, seldom considered in estimating the costs of illness, may far outweigh the medical and hospital bills which have occasioned so much dispute.

Paying the expenses of illness is an individual or family responsibility and one which should be planned for along with such other necessities as food, clothing, and shelter.

Before the industrialization of our society and economy, medical care costs received relatively little attention from anyone other than those who had to pay them. When people became ill, they paid for their professional care when they could or if they could; and physicians then, as they do now, provided a great deal of professional care for those in need, regardless of their ability to pay for it.

Some fairly reliable predictions can be made regarding the frequency of certain types of illnesses among a large number of people. To a large degree, this is also true regarding the number or percentage of persons who will incur medical expenses of certain amounts. A recent analysis of medical expenses per year per person in the United States among those who incurred any such expense, reflected the following:

- 68 per cent incur medical bills of less than $100 per year.
- 15 per cent have bills between $100 and $200 per year.
- 6 per cent have bills between $200 and $300 per year.
- 6 per cent have bills between $300 and $500 per year.
- 2 per cent have bills between $500 and $1,000 per year.
- 3 per cent have bills over $1,000 per year.

The above figures indicate that 83 per cent of the people in the United States incur medical expenses totaling less than $200 per year, and 89 per cent incur total medical expense in an amount under $300. The 68 per cent of the people whose medical expenses were less than $100 per person spent 26 per cent of all medical expenditures during a year. At the other end of the scale, while only 3 per cent of the people have medical expenses in excess of $1,000, these persons incur 19 per cent of all medical expenses.

What these figures do not and cannot indicate is which persons or families will fall into what category of medical care expenditures in any given year. A substantial number of families have the financial capacity to pay for the more or less routine medical expenses as well as unexpected expenses of modest proportions. For many, such expenses can be taken care of either out of savings or current income, others can borrow the sum needed for payment on a short-term credit basis without serious disturbance to their budgets and without recourse to insurance or similar financing mechanisms.

Budgeting for Illness

Budgeting for ordinary living expenses is a daily routine, whether it is done formally on paper or merely in the mind. It includes the expenses that come up every month or every week, and the well-managed household takes care of its obligations promptly. One item that seems to be left out most often is the possible costs of illness. Yet it is quite probable that a family will have minor illnesses, especially when there are children.

There will also be dental bills, immunizations, periodic check-ups, drugs and medicines, and medical supplies. These are as regular and predictable as food, household repairs, time payments, rent or mortgage payments. All such items should be considered a part of the running budget, week by week or month by month. The self-supporting family can afford these as well as it can other necessities.

The more costly illnesses are those that require extensive medical or surgical procedures, prolonged hospital or nursing home care. Long-term or sometimes permanent disability and consequent heavy expenses and loss of earnings seriously disrupt the budget of all but the well-to-do. These items should be covered by insurance.

But insurance can work only if it provides the necessary assistance at a cost which is not in itself too great to be borne. This means spreading the risk over a group of persons or families. The least expensive insurance for the heavier costs excludes the smaller items which the family can bear itself, out of current revenues. This is familiar in the automobile field as deductible insurance. The first $25, $50, or $100 of accidental damage are excluded from coverage in order to provide greater protection at less cost against the more expensive accidents.

A prominent actuary has estimated that the premium required to finance medical expenses through insurance to a limit of $175 per person per year would purchase coverage that would cover all medical costs *without limit* for persons whose medical expenses exceed $175 in any year. In other words, it costs as much to insure the first $175 of medical costs as it does to insure all such costs, without limit, in excess of that amount.

It could be said, then, that any attempt to finance small medical costs by an insurance program is a wasteful use of that mechanism.

Voluntary health insurance of some type now protects more than 75 per cent of the non-institutionalized population of the United States. It is sold by a large number of orga-nizations, most of which offer their programs on either an individual or a group basis.

Insurance companies, Blue Shield plans, Blue Cross plans and many independent plans offer a variety of health insurance coverages. The term "independent" is applied to those plans and programs which are not normally identified with insurance companies and are not affiliated with the National Association of Blue Shield Plans or the Blue Cross Association. As might be expected, such plans have a variety of organizational patterns, but several of them attempt to combine the features of group medical practice with an insurance arrangement whereby professional services are financed by periodic payments.

In terms of numbers of persons as well as in dollars of premiums collected and benefits paid, the Blue Shield plans, Blue Cross plans and insurance companies are the three general classifications of insurers that protect the greatest number of persons. For the most part, the certificates and policies issued by these organizations do not contain provisions which restrict either the choice of hospital or physician, although some agreements provide a lesser degree of coverage if the subscriber or insured is admitted to a non-affiliated hospital or is treated by a non-participating physician.

Insurance Plans

Most persons protected against the costs of hospital, surgical, or medical expense are insured under group coverage. These programs are usually arranged to insure all (or certain categories of) employees of one employer. However, this underwriting approach has been and is being extended to groups of employers, to members of unions, as well as to members of associations and other organizations not related directly by employment. Group insurance may cover the employee or member only, although the majority of programs include protection for the spouse and dependent, unmarried children.

Insurance purchased individually is a contract between the insured person and the insuring organization. It usually involves an enforceable contract which spells out the complete details of the privileges and obligations of both the company and the insured person.

In between these two specific types of coverage there is another marketing approach identified by terms such as franchise or wholesale insurance. This is a method of selling by which the insured person enjoys some saving in the premium charge and each person receives an individual contract or policy. This arrangement has some of the elements of both individual insurance and group insurance and is used by many Blue Shield and Blue Cross plans as well as by some insurance companies when making coverage available to persons who do not qualify for true group insurance.

For those who are protected under a group plan through their place of employment, it may usually be assumed that the coverage was arranged by persons who understand insurance. To this extent the employer, trustee, or personnel officer undoubtedly reviewed several proposals and selected the one that would best serve the needs and the budgets of the majority of persons in the group. In addition to this initial screening, those responsible for group health insurance purchase and administration may be expected to review their programs periodically in light of changing conditions and needs.

Although the person protected under a group program may have the advantage of an experienced person or committee working toward his best interests, this fact by no means relieves him of all responsibility with regard to his health insurance program. While group insurance has the advantage of somewhat broader protection at a somewhat lesser premium cost per person than individual coverage, it does not and cannot accommodate everyone's entire insurance needs. Everyone must thus understand fully what health care expenses are covered by his group insurance and, equally important, those that are not. He can then avoid buying unnecessary coverage in some areas and be certain he is not unprotected in others.

Health insurance purchased on an individual basis serves two primary needs: One is to provide satisfactory protection for those persons, such as the self-employed, who are not members of a group. The second is to supplement or complement group insurance.

In planning or evaluating a health insurance program, each individual or family should consider certain factors. The first question should be what kinds or what amounts of medical care expenses can be paid out of current income or otherwise handled without unduly unbalancing the budget. An answer to this question will determine those types (or amounts) of potential medical expense against which insurance is desired.

It is generally agreed that the basic purpose of health insurance is to alleviate undue financial hardship. Insurance is at its best when it provides protection against those situations which are not likely to occur but, if they did, would have severe or catastrophic financial consequences. Overemphasis on covering relatively small bills and routine medical care is an uneconomic use of insurance.

The American Medical Association has been and continues to be interested in the successful operation of the various voluntary mechanisms designed to help the American people finance their health care. The phenomenal growth of plans in the last 10 to 15 years is a dynamic demonstration of American enterprise and repudiates those who say that only the Federal government and a compulsory program can do the job. The Association, believing as it does that voluntary plans fulfill a useful and a necessary function in the total health care by removing or minimizing economic barriers, encourages experimentation in this field so that more people and more services can properly be brought within the scope of this kind of protection.

Buying Health Insurance

As we have said, experienced personnel usually screen various group health insurance proposals before they are offered to the group's employees or members. But when an individual undertakes to arrange his own protection for himself or his family, he has to take upon himself the responsibility of evaluation and selection.

Before deciding upon a particular individual (non-group) voluntary health insurance plan, the purchaser should consider the type of health care expenses he desires to be protected against and the extent to which he wishes these expenses insured.

The types of expenses which can be insured against include hospitalization, physicians' services, and services rendered by technicians and/or paramedical personnel.

Hospital expenses are charges for hospital room and board, drugs and dressings, use of operating or delivery rooms, routine nursing care, and use of recovery rooms.

Professional services are those performed by physicians licensed to practice medicine and surgery. In addition to the diagnosis and treatment of medical conditions, the term includes surgery, radiology (x-ray), anesthesiology, physical medicine, and laboratory services.

Paramedical services include those performed by laboratory and x-ray technicians as well as by physical therapists and private duty and visiting nurses. The services of such personnel are generally either supervised or prescribed by a physician.

Hospitalization and surgical operations lend themselves more readily to the principles of insurance than do routine home and office calls. The costs of hospitalization or surgery are greater, and thus less predictable, than those of an office or house call. However, some people maintain that the cumulative financial effect of home and office calls can be as great or greater than the cost of hospitalization and surgery.

Many insurance authorities believe that home and office calls are more properly the subject of budgeting than of insurance since the cost of processing claims is too large in proportion to the benefit paid. This is the principle that distinguishes the so-called "catastrophe" or major hospital and medical expense benefit coverages from the so-called "basic" plans.

Not all persons want to insure the probable total costs of health care. Some wish to insure a certain portion while still others want to pay for certain kinds of costs or a stipulated initial amount.

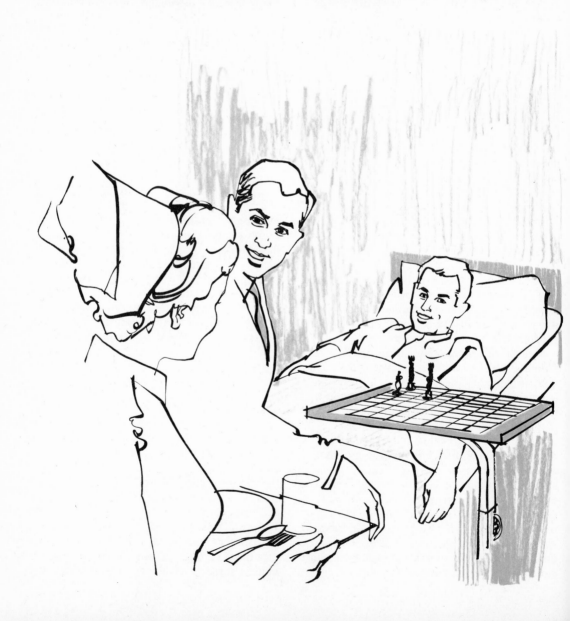

It is necessary to learn what the costs usually amount to. With respect to hospitalization, you should attempt to determine what the prevailing charges are in your community for hospital room and board. Such costs may be obtained from the hospital in smaller communities, while hospital councils may provide such data for urban or metropolitan areas. Usually the charges differ according to whether the patient desires private, semi-private, or ward accommodations. In addition, published data may summarize "prevailing charges" either on a regional or local basis.

Determination of professional charges is somewhat more difficult since these services are primarily personal rather than institutional in nature. However, your family physician should be able to advise you on these matters. A physician takes several factors into consideration when he establishes his fees for the care of individual patients.

Among these are: the degree of specialized knowledge either needed or applied, the nature and number of complications encountered, the length of time involved in the care of the patient, the economic level of the community, and the financial ability of the patient to pay for health care. With respect to the latter, the American Medical Association has maintained that physicians should reduce their bills when the patient cannot afford normal charges. This is irrespective of the existence of insurance, since insurance does not create any new wealth.

Although determinations of charges for professional services are not generally "standardized," such information is available in many areas. If you have a personal or family physician, you should be familiar with his charges for current and past services. In such instances you are in a favorable position to discuss his charges in advance for any "unusual" service such as surgery or other procedures. Physicians generally are willing to discuss fees prior to rendering care—especially when the patient desires it or when extended or expensive treatment may pose financial problems for the patient. In addition, physicians and medical societies in certain areas have established schedules of suggested "minimum" charges, "usual" charges, or relative values for professional services.

Among the more important considerations in selecting an insurance organization are: 1. Is the company or prepayment plan licensed to do business in your state? 2. What is the general reputation of the organization in discharging its obligations to its subscribers or policy holders? 3. What is the reputation of the organization for prompt and efficient service on claims?

In selecting a company, you should be satisfied that the organization has the appropriate charter power to do business in the state and a license, if it is required. The state insurance commissioner can provide information regarding insurance companies and Blue Shield and Blue Cross plans if the laws provide for his supervision. For obvious reasons such officials are sources of information rather than recommendation. Depending upon the state, other possible sources of information include the secretary of state, the corporation and securities commission, and the state board of health.

The agent, solicitor, or salesman should be of good local reputation and also present satisfactory evidence or credentials to the effect that he is an authorized representative of the organization for which he is soliciting.

You should also satisfy yourself regarding the general reputation of the company or plan. Frequently this can be done by contacting others in your community who are subscribers, members, or policy holders. Additional sources include your local chamber of commerce, better business bureau, local credit bureau, and similar reputable organizations.

The Contract, Policy, or Agreement

When you buy insurance or join a prepayment plan you are entering into a business arrangement. This arrangement is usually formalized by contract or agreement. The contract normally will include both privileges (benefits) and obligations. It is reasonable to expect that the framers of these contracts have protected their own interests. You should, in turn, make every reasonable effort to see that you understand the contract's terms, conditions, and exceptions as well as your obligations.

If a company or plan is licensed and supervised by your state insurance department (or other regulatory authority), it is usually the responsibility of that authority to protect the interests of the policy holders or subscribers. The department is frequently required to review contract forms and determine their conformity with state laws before such contracts may be sold to the public. Moreover, the department as further protection to the public, may require that the rates (premiums) charged are reasonable in relation to the risk assumed and that they do not discriminate unfairly. This responsibility of the state official is primarily that of a screening nature in the public interest; but the actual understanding of the terms, conditions, and provisions of the contract or agreement is largely your own personal responsibility.

For the most part, insurance contracts are considered upon the basis of an application. Another principal consideration is the periodic payment of a premium or membership fee. In applying for the policy or agreement, you may be required to give evidence of your insurability or eligibility. This may include questions about your present health status, past illnesses, and treatments, if any. If these questions are asked, it is your responsibility to provide true answers to the best of your ability. If a policy or agreement is issued on the basis of incorrect or false information, it may be sufficient ground for voiding or nullifying the contract.

The Insuring Clause. One of the more important portions of your policy stipulates the scope of coverage by telling what types of expenses or "losses" are being assumed by the insurance company or prepayment plan. You should be satisfied that the insuring clause includes the types of benefits you desire before considering the company or prepayment plan.

Exclusions or Conditions Not Covered. Most policies or agreements have exclusions which state those conditions which are *not* covered by the insuring clause. Some exclusions should be expected, but all should be thoroughly understood. Some contracts contain more exclusions than others and their number and nature are determined largely by the amount of premium and other factors.

Examples of exclusions are occupational accidents and illnesses which are frequently covered by workmen's compensation, conditions resulting from acts of war or riot or injuries and illnesses sustained while serving in the armed forces.

Waiting Periods. Most insurance company or prepayment plan contracts include certain "waiting periods." These clauses indicate the interval that must elapse between the time the contract is issued and the date certain benefits are payable. For example, a policy may provide that benefits are not payable during the first 90 days after issue date for appendectomy or hernia operations. Another may provide that benefits are not payable during the first six months for any condition for which the applicant received medical treatment or advice prior to purchasing the policy.

These waiting period provisions are included because the insurance company or prepayment plan usually agrees to cover only those conditions that commence after the insurance is written. They do not normally assume liability for already existing illnesses under non-group contracts. Such clauses together with the health statement of the applicant are frequently used in underwriting in lieu of a physical exam.

Benefit Reductions. Some policies or agreements specify conditions under which a benefit may be reduced below the amount otherwise payable. For example, if a contract is predicated either on the basis of a contracting hospital or a participating physician and the policy holder is hospitalized in a non-contracting hospital or treated by a non-participating physician, there is a possibility of a benefit reduction. Although such provisions are not found frequently, they are a possibility that should be understood.

Who is Covered? If you want your eligible dependents (usually defined by law as spouse and unmarried dependent children) insured, are they included in the policy or program you buy? Actually the policy holder or subscriber is usually insured "on behalf of" the covered health expenses of his dependents. If the policy does not specify such coverage, in all probability the policy holder is insured only against his own personal health care costs.

Age Limits. Some policies and agreements specify minimum and maximum age limits. In this type of insurance, minimum ages may be specified for dependent children in order for them to be included in a family policy. Maximum age limits may be of two types. One may be a maximum age stated for an adult policy holder or covered spouse. The other may state the maximum age to which a child will be included as a dependent under a family policy.

In an increasing number of instances, maximum age limits, such as 65 or 70, are either being raised or eliminated entirely as they pertain to adult policy holders or covered spouses. If such a provision is included in your policy or contract, it should be fully understood.

Cancellation and Renewal Provisions. Many policies or agreements are cancellable by the company or plan. Some provide that the company or plan, although it cannot cancel the contract, can elect not to renew the policy at any premium due date. Still others are both non-cancellable and guaranteed renewable to a specified age. Each type of contract has its merits and each may be subject to differing premium charges or rates since the non-cancellable and guaranteed renewable-type would be more expensive.

Choice of Physician or Hospital. If the insurance or prepayment plan imposes more than the usual limitations with respect to the selection of either the physician, hospital, or both, this should be understood clearly and fully at the time the contract is purchased. Should the subscriber be limited to a panel of local physicians and/or be entitled to hospitalization only in a specified hospital or list of hospitals, he should determine what benefits would be available should a need arise while he is away from his home area.

Many people travel extensively in the course of their employment and others travel during vacations and holidays. Medical emergencies may make it difficult or impossible to get to a designated physician or hospital.

Although most plans which normally limit choice of physician or hospital make some provision for benefit payment under such circumstances, this information should be known and understood in advance.

By keeping these points in mind, you should be able to make a wise selection of health coverages that will best suit your own and your family's needs. If you have any further questions regarding specific policies and coverages, consult with your insurance counselor, your local Blue Shield and Blue Cross representative, or some other source in which you have confidence.

Public Care Facilities

There will always be some families which are temporarily or permanently unable to care for costs of prolonged or serious illness involving heavy expense. There is no reason why any such family should suffer, or any patient remain uncared for, by reason of inability to pay. Provisions exist in every community for the care of such patients. The principal channels through which such care can be procured are:

● Veterans' hospital facilities available to veterans of all wars.

● Public hospitals operated by cities or counties for the care of the needy.

● Free beds in most private hospitals, with medical care either by the patient's own doctor or by the hospital staff.

● Medical care under provisions for assistance to the aged.

● Medical care under the provisions of the Kerr-Mills Act, by which older persons obtain care at state expense, with federal aid.

● Medical assistance provided under private auspices such as lodges, unions, and denominational groups.

The medical profession has always guaranteed care for those unable to pay without charge or obligation, and will continue to do so. The hospital and other out-of-pocket expenses must be provided from other sources as here indicated.

There is no shame attached to poverty; it is a misfortune which might happen to anyone, even to those presently in good financial "health." Sick persons should not be allowed to go without medical care because of reluctance to ask for aid.

The sources of information about where medical assistance can be had in a given community include the local medical society; social service agencies such as welfare organizations, community chest or fund; hospitals and voluntary health agencies.

A family that has a family doctor can rely on him to bring all available resources into play as they are required.

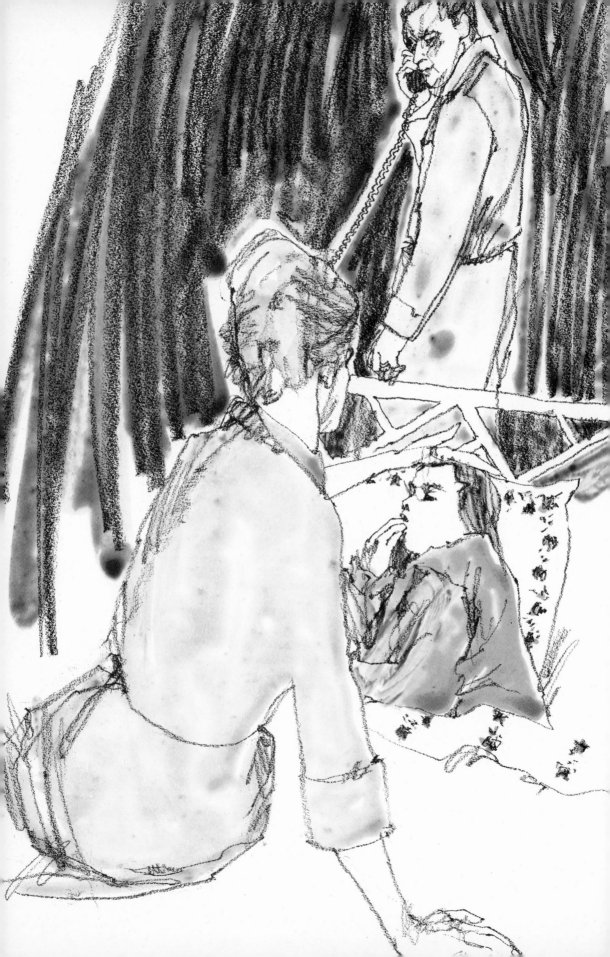

PART IX

When You Need a Doctor

CHAPTER ONE

EMERGENCY MEDICAL IDENTIFICATION

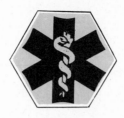

WHEN ONE SUFFERS an injury or sudden illness, those who offer medical help should know about any health problems that need special consideration. But how can this be done? By a medical identification card and a signal device bearing the universal symbol of medical identification. With these, a person who is unconscious or for some other reason cannot make known his needs, still can tell whoever helps him that his safety depends on their doing or not doing certain specific things.

The special kinds of care a person may need when he becomes ill or injured and which can be made known by signal or identification devices, can be illustrated by a few examples. Some diabetics who have been in an accident or have developed diabetic coma have gone for long periods without the essential insulin because no one knew about their need. Another problem of the diabetic is insulin shock. This condition, the result of an overdose of insulin, makes a person appear to be intoxicated and is as dangerous for a diabetic as not getting enough insulin. In both cases, a signal device bearing the emergency medical identification symbol and the word "diabetic" would start action in the right direction.

A fair proportion of the people who have had a coronary heart attack take drugs that prevent the blood from clotting as a way to avoid further coronary occlusion. If they are cut or internally injured in an accident, they may bleed profusely unless drugs are given to help the blood clot. Words on a signal device such as "taking anticoagulants" with more specific detail on an identification card would speed treatment to stop such bleeding.

Tetanus antitoxin is the usual preventive treatment for wounds that might harbor tetanus bacilli. It contains horse serum, and some people are violently allergic to horse serum. To be sure that they receive no horse serum in an emergency, they should wear a signal device saying "allergic to horse serum" or otherwise indicate that antitoxin is to them a serious hazard. Ideally, active immunization against tetanus would permit a booster dose of toxoid, rather than tetanus antitoxin, to be given at the time of injury. Every person's identification card should list the date of his original tetanus immunization and the most recent booster.

Inability to speak clearly, or at all, can be a problem. Those who speak no English should note the language they understand. Persons with aphasia—the inability to speak—and the deaf or hard of hearing need some recognition of their problem during an emergency.

These few examples illustrate the basic idea —a person who could be harmed by what would normally be done, or not done during emergency care, should use this simple and effective way to let others know his needs at a time when he can't tell about them himself.

Over the years several national health organizations have designed cards for purse or pocket which inform first aiders that the bearer is a diabetic, is taking anticoagulants, is an epileptic, or has some other condition in which the organization is interested. A score of manufacturers make and distribute metal or plastic signal devices to alert first aiders to the needs of the wearer. At least three organizations have programs by which information on their members' needs can be made available by telephone in emergencies. But these are all isolated unrelated activities.

Universal Symbol

In an attempt to unify these many efforts, the American Medical Association held a conference in April, 1961 at which representatives of many interested organizations discussed ways to identify a person's medical needs in an emergency. Later, a symbol was designed by the American Medical Association and offered to all who publish cards or make signal devices. It is hoped that this will become the universal symbol of emergency medical identification. Wherever it is seen, it means that in conjunction with it or on the person wearing it is information important to that person's health in an emergency.

The symbol consists of the star of life—a six-pointed asterisk type of device—on which appears the snake-entwined staff of Aesculapius—the mythical Roman god of medicine and healing—taken from the seal of the American Medical Association. The whole is framed in a hexagon.

The techniques of emergency medical identification are also helpful in keeping track of the very young and the very old. Children not yet old enough to know their name, address, and phone number often wander from home and become lost when they go shopping with mother or become separated in a crowd. A metal or plastic tag worn about the neck or wrist and carrying a phone number, an address,

and a name would make it easy for these lost youngsters to be reunited with their family.

Oldsters, too, become lost. Many have periodic lapses of memory, or become confused and are not sure where home is or how to get there. A similar device with address, phone number, and name could save many worrisome hours.

The AMA's Committee on Emergency Medical Identification has recommended that everyone carry an identification card whether he has a health problem or not. The fact that a person has no health problems is in itself valuable information to the physician in the emergency room of a hospital. A card that could be used by everyone has been designed by the AMA and is being widely distributed.

This AMA committee has further recommended that in addition to a card, the young

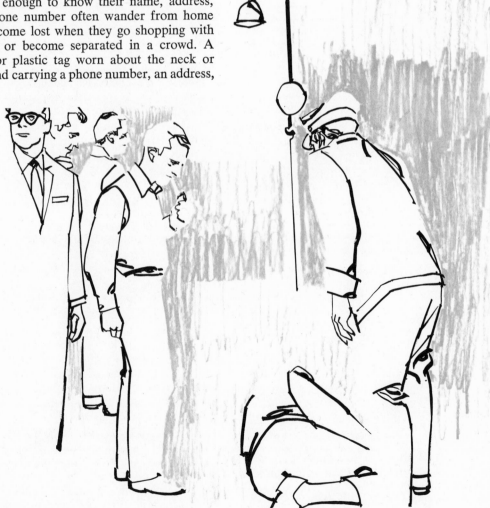

MEDICAL INFORMATION
(with date of notation)

Present Medical Problems_____

_____

_____

Medicines Taken Regularly_____

_____

_____

_____

_____

Dangerous Allergies_____

_____

_____

Other Important Information_____

_____

_____

Last Immunization Date

Tetanus Toxoid_____ Polio: Salk_____
Diphtheria_____ Sabin _____
Smallpox _____Typhoid _____
Others_____

REMEMBER: This is the minimum medical and personal information needed by those who help you in an emergency. It is not designed to be a complete medical record. Check its accuracy with your doctor.

Why You Should Carry Emergency Medical Identification

An emergency medical identification card is your protection in an emergency. If you are not able to tell your medical story after an accident or sudden illness, the information entered on this card can save your life.

You may have health problems which can affect your recovery from an emergency. You may have a problem which is no emergency but often is treated as one, such as epilepsy. Even if you do not have a health problem, the information on this card can be of valuable assistance to the first aid attendant.

Why You Should Wear an Emergency Medical Signal Device

In an emergency, you may be separated from your pocket card. Possibly you are one who has a medical problem so critical that it must be immediately known to those who help you. If so, a signal device of durable material should be worn around your neck, wrist, or ankle in such a way that it can be present at all times—even while swimming.

The device should be fastened to the person wearing it with a strong nonelastic cord or chain so designed that it does not become an accident hazard in itself.

On this device there should be:

• The universal symbol of emergency medical identification
• The name of your major health problem
• For children and the aging, the name and address of a responsible relative and a telephone number, including area code

Carry Your Card and Wear Your Signal Device at All Times!

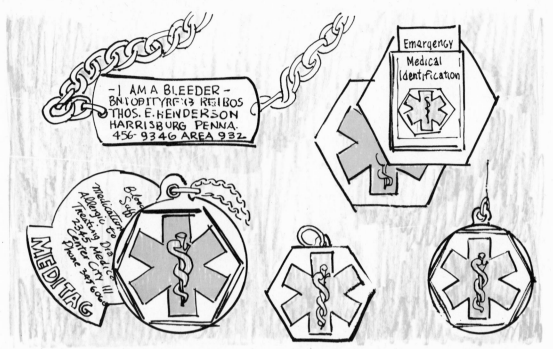

These pendants and bracelets, marked with AMA signaling device, give emergency medical information.

and the old and all who have significant health problems should wear a durable signal device bearing the information their individual circumstances suggest.

Unfortunately, it is difficult to convince many of the need for wearing a signal device. When they are persuaded, it may be equally difficult to put them in touch with sources of supply. Even when a device has been purchased, it may not be worn at all times. This is especially true of women who may find their necklace or bracelet unattractive.

Occasionally a person who should wear a signal device does not wish to be identified as having a problem. In some cases, such identification might interfere with employment. Epileptics are torn between the need for identification during a seizure to avoid unnecessary hospitalization, and the fear of labeling which could affect both their social and occupational acceptance.

A problem peculiar to children is their love of exchange. In typical Tom Sawyer fashion, they will swap the contents of their pockets for the treasures in someone else's. A signal device is good trading material. Unfortunately, this can mean that a tag saying "Joe Smith is a diabetic" may end up around Bob Brown's neck, and Joe Smith may have a tag with someone else's name and affliction on it. Children who wear signal devices or carry cards should be given sound instruction about their purpose and checked daily or oftener.

In spite of these complications, the safety of a large portion of our population will be improved when everyone carries an identification card and the wearing of a signal device becomes accepted.

Chapter Two

EMERGENCY FIRST AID

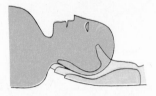

THE DIRECTIONS that follow represent simple, concise recommendations for first aid in common emergencies. They supplement but do not replace instruction in first aid techniques. Every person should receive basic first aid instruction if possible. Knowing *what to do* and *what not to do* in an emergency can help to avoid further injury, ease pain, and possibly prevent disability and death. First aid can be a lifesaving skill.

First aid is the immediate and temporary care given the victim of an accident or sudden illness until the services of a physician can be obtained. The first objective is to save life. With this in mind, the first aider must try to prevent heavy loss of blood, maintain breathing, prevent further injury, and prevent shock. The first aider must also communicate with a physician, avoid panic, inspire confidence, and do no more than is necessary until professional help arrives.

Common sense and a few simple rules are the keys to effective first aid.

Preventing Bleeding

Heavy bleeding comes from wounds to one or more large blood vessels. Such loss of blood can kill the victim in three to five minutes. Don't waste time. Use pressure directly over the wound.

- Place pad—clean handkerchief, clean cloth, etc.—over the wound and press firmly with your hand or both hands. If you haven't a pad or bandage, close the wound with your hand or fingers.
- Apply pressure directly over the wound.
- Hold the pad firmly in place with a strong bandage. Raise the bleeding part higher than the rest of the body unless bones are broken.
- Keep the victim lying down.
- Call a physician.

At this point look to the needs of other accident victims, if any. Try to control bleeding and maintain breathing for as many of the victims as possible. Then go back to the victim whose bleeding has been controlled and do the following:

- Keep the victim warm. Cover with blankets, coat, etc., and put something under him if he is on a cold or damp surface.
- If the victim is conscious and can swallow, give him plenty of liquids to drink (water, tea, coffee).
- Do not give the victim alcoholic drinks.
- If the victim is unconscious or if abdomi-

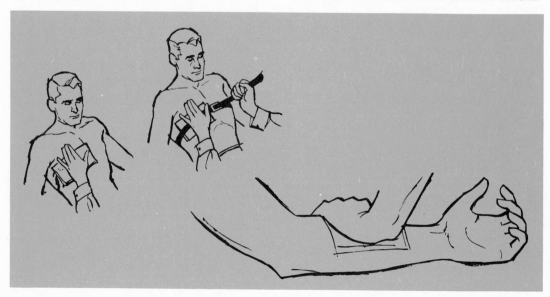

nal injury is suspected, do not give him fluids.

A tourniquet should not be used to control bleeding except for an amputated, mangled, or crushed arm or leg. Use only a strong, wide piece of cloth. Never use wire, rope, twine, or other narrow material. Wrap the tourniquet around the upper part of the limb above the wound. Tie a half-knot; place a short stick on the half-knot; tie a full knot over the stick; twist the stick just tight enough to stop bleeding. Mark the letters "TK" and the time on the victim's forehead with crayon, pencil, soot, or other substance. Do not cover the tourniquet. Loosen the tourniquet for a few seconds every 15 minutes.

Maintaining Breathing

When breathing movements stop, or lips, tongue, and fingernails become blue, there is need for help in breathing. When in doubt, begin artificial respiration. No harm can result from its use and delay may cost the victim his life. Start immediately, for seconds count. Check the mouth and throat for obstructions, place the victim in position, and begin artificial respiration. Maintain a steady rhythm of 15 breaths per minute. Remain in position. After the victims revives, be ready to resume artificial respiration if necessary. Call a physician. Do not move the victim unless absolutely necessary to remove him from danger. Do not wait or look for help, and do not stop to loosen clothing or warm the victim. Don't give up.

Directions for the mouth-to-mouth breathing method of artificial respiration follow:

- Place victim half-way between a faceup and a side position.
- Lift victim's neck with one hand and tilt his head back by holding the top of his head with your other hand.
- Pull the victim's chin up with the hand that was lifting the neck so that the tongue does not fall back to block the air passage.
- Take a deep breath and place your mouth over the victim's nose or mouth, making a seal.
- With adults, pinch the victim's nose shut.
- Blow your breath into the victim's mouth or nose until you see the chest rise. The air you blow into the victim's lungs has enough oxygen to save his life.
- Remove your mouth and let the victim exhale while you take another deep breath.
- As soon as you hear the victim breathe out, replace your mouth over his mouth or nose and repeat the procedure.
- Repeat 15 times per minute.

For mouth-to-nose breathing, make a leak-proof seal by holding the victim's lips closed with your thumb. Be sure your lips do not close the victim's nostrils. In mouth-to-mouth breathing, seal your lips around the victim's mouth. Pinch his nostrils closed with your thumb and finger.

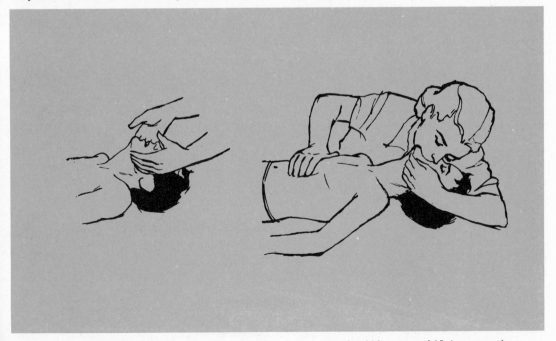

Mouth-to-mouth breathing for infants and small children, as shown, should be repeated 15 times per minute.

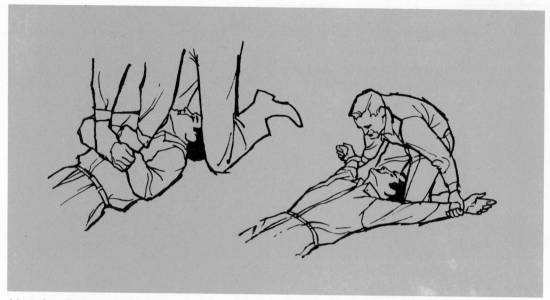

Manual method of artificial respiration, shown above, should also be maintained at 15-per-minute rate.

Poisonous gases in the air or lack of oxygen can stop breathing. If this happens, move the victim to fresh air and begin mouth-to-mouth breathing. Control the source of poisonous gases if possible. Keep others away from the area, and do not enter the area yourself without respiratory protection unless rescue can be accomplished during one holding of the breath. Never enter the area alone.

In cases of drowning, begin mouth-to-mouth breathing as soon as possible. It can be started as soon as the rescuer in a boat reaches the victim or as soon as the rescuer in water has carried the victim to shallow water. In case of suffocation by plastic bag, tear or remove the plastic bag and begin mouth-to-mouth breathing immediately.

In electric shock, do not touch the victim until he is separated from the current. Do not try to remove a person from an out-of-doors wire unless you have had special training for this type of rescue work. Or you can use a dry wooden pole or board to slam the wire away from the victim or to roll the victim off the wire. Begin mouth-to-mouth breathing as soon as the victim is free of contact with the current.

If concussion results from explosion or blows to the head or abdomen, begin mouth-to-mouth breathing immediately. If poisoning from sedatives or chemicals halts breathing, begin mouth-to-mouth breathing immediately. If constriction from a cave-in interferes with breathing, begin forceful mouth-to-mouth breathing while efforts are being made to free the upper body.

Foreign bodies in the air passage can cause choking. If this happens to an infant, hold the baby by his ankles, letting the head hang straight down. Open the baby's mouth, pull his tongue forward, and let the obstruction fall out. Begin mouth-to-mouth breathing if the infant still has difficulty breathing.

If the choking victim is a small child, hold the child, head down, over your arm or leg and apply several sharp pats between the shoulder blades. Clear his throat quickly with your fingers and pull the tongue forward. Begin mouth-to-mouth breathing if the child still has difficulty breathing.

For an adult who is choking on a foreign body, place the victim on his side so that the head is lower than the trunk, or have the victim lean over the back of a chair. Apply a sharp blow between the shoulder blades. Clear the victim's throat with your fingers and pull the tongue forward. Begin mouth-to-mouth breathing if he still has difficulty breathing.

Shock

Shock usually accompanies severe injury or emotional upset. It may also follow infection, pain, disturbance of circulation from bleeding, stroke, heart attack, heat exhaustion, food or chemical poisoning, extensive burns, etc. Signs of shock are cold and clammy skin with beads of perspiration on the forehead and palms of hands; pale face; complaint by the victim of a chilled feeling, or even shaking chills; frequently nausea or vomiting; shallow breathing.

To save life by preventing or overcoming shock:

- Correct cause of shock if possible (for example control bleeding).
- Keep victim lying down.
- Keep his airway open. If he vomits, turn his head to the side so that his neck is arched.
- Elevate the victim's legs if there are no broken bones. Keep his head lower than the trunk of the body if possible.
- Keep the victim warm if the weather is cold or damp.
- Give fluids (water, tea, coffee, etc.) if the victim is able to swallow. The following formula can be used if available: 1 quart water, 1 teaspoon salt, ½ teaspoon baking soda (sodium bicarbonate).
- Never give alcoholic beverages. Do not give fluids to unconscious or semiconscious persons, and do not give fluids if abdominal injury is suspected.
- Reassure victim.
- The lessening of the effects of shock should be considered with every injury and illness discussed in this series.

Poisoning

Poisoning may be suspected if a characteristic odor can be detected on the breath, (almond in cyanide poisoning for example); if there is discoloration of the lips and mouth; if there is pain or a burning sensation in the throat. Also, if bottles or packages of drugs or poisonous chemicals are found open in presence of children, if there is evidence in the mouth of eating wild berries or leaves, or if there is unconsciousness, confusion, or sudden illness when access to poisons is possible.

What to do in case of poisoning until your physician takes charge is highly important to know:

- Speed is essential. Act before the body has time to absorb the poison. If possible, one person should begin treatment while another calls a physician. Know the poison center in your community. Such centers are usually located in hospitals. Some are treatment centers for physicians only. Consult your physician about the center in your community, and if it is a treatment center, put its telephone number where you can find it in an emergency. Always call your doctor first. If your community poison control center is a treatment center, you may have to call it if your doctor is not available.
- Consult your physician about preparing

for a possible poisoning emergency by having on hand one half ounce of tincture of ipecac, for use as he advises while you wait for his arrival. Some physicians also advise having on hand a few ounces of activated charcoal recommended by the poison control centers. This must be *activated* charcoal; ordinary charcoal and burnt toast are not effective antidotes. These preparations are to be used only when, and as, the physician directs.

- Save and give to the physician or hospital the poison container with its intact label and any remaining contents. If the poison is unknown, bring along a sample of the vomitus for examination.
- The nature of the poison will determine the first aid measure to use.

When poison has been swallowed, do not induce vomiting if the victim is unconscious, or is already vomiting or is in convulsions. Vomiting should not be induced when there are symptoms of severe pain, a burning sensation in the mouth or throat, or when the patient is known to have swallowed a petroleum product (kerosene, gasoline, lighter fluid), toilet bowl cleaner, rust remover, drain cleaner, acids for personal or household use, iodine, styptic pencil, washing soda, ammonia water, or household bleach.

In dealing with poisoning, call a physician immediately. Begin mouth-to-mouth breathing if the victim has difficulty breathing. Give water or milk. If safe (see above), induce vomiting. Induce vomiting by placing your finger at the back of the victim's throat or by use of two tablespoons of salt in a glass of warm water. When retching and vomiting begin, place the victim face down with his head lower than his hips. This prevents vomitus from entering the lungs and causing further damage.

Poison Prevention

Obviously, it is much wiser to prevent poisoning than to treat it. Some suggestions for household safety are:

Keep all drugs, poisonous substances, and household chemicals well beyond the reach of children.

Do not leave discarded medicines where children or pets might get at them.

Do not store nonedible products on shelves used for storing food.

Never tell your children that you are giving them candy when you are actually giving them medicines.

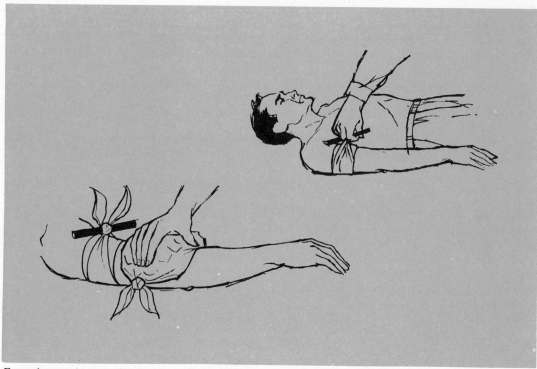

For poisonous insect and reptile bites, a constricting bandage should be applied but loosened every 15 minutes.

Never give or take medicines in the dark.

Read labels before using chemical products.

Do not keep unneeded or unlabeled drugs and chemicals in the home.

Never re-use containers of household or other chemical substances.

Do not transfer poisonous substances to unlabeled containers.

In dealing with inhaled poisons, carry or drag the victim (do not let him walk) to fresh air immediately. Apply artificial respiration if breathing has stopped or is irregular. Call a physician. Keep victim warm and as quiet as possible. If the victim is having convulsions, keep him in bed in a semidark room. Avoid jarring or noise. Never give alcohol in any form. Do not become a victim yourself by exposure to the same poison. If skin contamination from poison occurs, drench the skin with water (shower, hose, faucet) and apply a stream of water on the skin while removing the clothing. Cleanse the skin thoroughly with water. Speed in washing is most important in reducing extent of injury.

In cases of eye contamination (foreign material in eye), immediately hold eyelids open and wash eyes with gentle stream of running water. Delay of even a few seconds greatly increases extent of injury. Continue washing until the physician comes. Do not use boric acid or any other chemicals; they may increase the extent of the injury.

Poisonous Bites

In treating snake, scorpion, and black widow spider bites (injected poisons), make the victim lie down as soon as possible, and apply a constricting bandage around the arm or leg above the bite, if it is on an arm or leg. Use a strong, wide piece of cloth. Wrap the bandage around the limb and tie a half-knot; place a short stick on the half-knot; tie a full knot over the stick; twist the stick. The pulse in blood vessels below the bandage should not disappear, as it does when a tourniquet is used, nor should the bandage produce a throbbing sensation. Loosen the bandage for a few seconds every 15 minutes. Apply an ice pack over the bite if possible. Carry the victim to a physician or hospital. Do not let the victim walk, do not give alcohol in any form, and do not use wire, rope, twine, or other narrow material for the bandage. Don't cover the bandage.

Burns

Burns can result from heat (thermal burn) or from chemicals (chemical burn). Every burn, even sunburn, can be complicated by shock and the patient should be treated for shock. Prevent shock, prevent contamination, control pain—these are the objectives of first aid for burns.

The amount of the body burned is the guide for action. Even skilled physicians find it difficult to evaluate the depth of a burn immediately, but it is possible to estimate quickly the amount of body surface burned to determine action. If the burn covers all of one leg, all of one arm and the head, front of the trunk, or back of the trunk, each means about 18 per cent of the body surface is burned. A person with 25 per cent of his body surface burned can develop "burn shock" and may die unless he receives first aid. In burn shock the liquid part of the blood is sent by the body into the burned areas. There may not be enough blood volume left to keep the brain, heart, and other organs functioning normally.

In cases of extensive heat burn:
* Place the cleanest available cloth material over all burned areas to exclude air.
* Have victim lie down.
* Call physician. Keep victim lying down until physician comes.
* Place victim's head and chest a little lower than the rest of the body.
* If the victim is conscious and can swallow, give him plenty of non-alcoholic liquids to drink (water, tea, coffee, etc.).

In treating small heat burns, soak a sterile gauze pad or clean cloth in a solution of two tablespoons baking soda (sodium bicarbonate) to a quart of lukewarm water. Place the pad over the burn and bandage loosely. Do not disturb or open blisters. If the skin is not broken, immerse the burned part in clean, cold water or apply clean ice to relieve pain. All burns, except where the skin is reddened in only a small area, should be seen by a physician or nurse.

For chemical burns:
* Immediately flush with water. Speed in washing is most important in reducing the extent of injury.
* Apply stream of water while removing clothing.
* Place the cleanest available material over the burned area.
* If the burned area is extensive, have the victim lie down. Keep him down unless a physician advises otherwise. Place his head and chest a little lower than the rest of his body (raise legs if possible). If he is conscious and can swallow, give him plenty of non-alcoholic liquids to drink.

* All burns, except where the skin is reddened in only a small area, should be seen by a physician or nurse.
* Burns from chemicals used in certain technical procedures may require different first aid techniques. These techniques should be investigated in advance of need by anyone working in such areas.

Head Injuries

Consider anyone found unconscious to have a possible head injury. This is particularly true for the unconscious person who smells of liquor. Call a physician immediately. Head injuries require prompt medical attention. Keep the victim lying down. It is better to keep him lying on his side so that his tongue does not fall back into the air passage and so that the airway can be drained of blood, vomitus, and/or other fluids. The neck should be arched by tilting the head back. Keep the victim warm if weather is cold or damp. Control bleeding from a head wound by applying a pressure dressing. Use common sense in regard to using pressure over a possible skull fracture. *Do not move the head or any part of the body if there is bleeding from the nose, mouth, or ears. Do not move the victim unless absolutely necessary until professional help arrives. Do not give the victim anything by mouth.*

Look for emergency medical identification around the victim's neck or wrist that could suggest a cause for unconsciousness. Keep the victim lying down if he regains consciousness.

An epileptic seizure (convulsion) is not a medical emergency. The seizure usually ends by itself after a few minutes. If the seizure should last longer than 15 minutes, however, call a physician. Do not restrain an epileptic during a seizure. Do not slap or douse with water; do not place a finger or hard object between the teeth. Remove objects that might injure the patient.

Bone and Joint Injuries

If there is injury to the spine or neck, do not move victim or allow him to be moved until proper stretchers are available. A physician should supervise moving the victim if possible. Call a physician immediately. Keep the victim warm and quiet. Dispel crowds of onlookers. Watch the victim's breathing and be prepared to start mouth-to-mouth breathing, but do not move the head.

First aid for broken bones should not extend beyond preventing further injury. There are two types of fractures:

1. Closed, when the bone is broken but the skin has not been punctured.

2. Open or compound, when the skin is broken as well as the bone.

Fracture should be suspected if the part does not have a normal appearance or function. Do not move the injured person until the suspected fracture site has been splinted unless the victim is in imminent danger. Call a physician.

For a closed fracture, place the limb in as natural a position as possible *without causing discomfort* to the victim. Apply splints. They must be long enough to extend well beyond the joints above and below fracture. Any firm material can be used: board, pole, metal rod, or even a thick magazine or thick folded newspaper. Use clothing or other soft material to pad splints to prevent skin injury. Fasten splints with bandages or cloth at minimum of three sites: below joint below break; above joint above break; and at level of break. Bind broken bones in the hand or foot with a pillow or blanket bound around the limb.

For an open fracture, apply a pressure dressing to control bleeding. Place a pad—clean handkerchief, clean cloth, etc.—over the wound and press firmly with your hand or both hands. If you haven't a pad or bandage, close the wound with your hand or fingers. Apply pressure directly over the wound. Hold the pad firmly in place with a strong bandage— neckties, cloth strips, etc. Keep the victim lying down, and call a physician; apply splints as outlined in procedure for closed fractures without trying to straighten the limb or return it to a natural position.

Treat dislocations as closed fractures. Place arm in sling for shoulder dislocation. Be sure that the opposite shoulder supports the weight of the arm.

Apply the same care for sprains and strains as for fractures if there is any doubt that the injury is really only a sprain or strain. Place the injured part at rest, and elevate the part if possible. Apply *cold* compresses or an ice pack for several hours. Consult a physician. Do not apply heat in any form for at least 24 hours. Heat will increase swelling and pain.

Cuts and Bruises

In the home care of minor wounds, it is most important to prevent infection. Never put your mouth over a wound. The mouth harbors germs that could infect it. Do not breathe on the wound either.

Do not allow fingers, used handkerchiefs, or other soiled material to touch the wound. Do not use an antiseptic on the wound. Immedi-

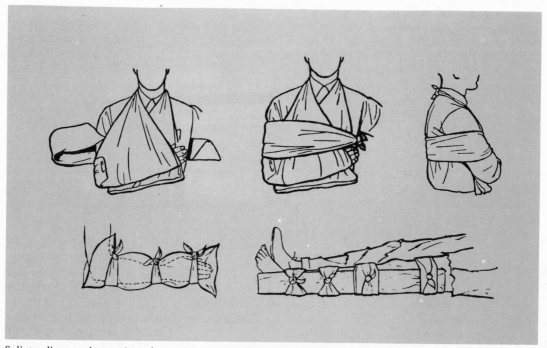

Splints, slings, and wrappings shown should be applied to closed fractures without causing undue discomfort.

ately cleanse wound and surrounding skin with soap and warm water.

Hold a sterile pad firmly over the wound until the bleeding stops. Then change pad and bandage the wound loosely with a triangular or roller bandage. Replace sterile pads and bandages as needed to keep them clean and dry.

In gaping abdominal wounds, first call a physician. Follow the next steps only if professional treatment is not available. Cover the wound with a damp dressing. Hold the dressing firmly in place with a bandage. The object is to control bleeding with a pressure dressing. The bandage should be firm, but not tight.

In deep chest wounds, it is important to prevent air from passing through the wound. The lung will collapse unless this is done. Place a gauze or cloth pad over the wound. Hold the pad in place with firm pressure. A belt drawn snugly around the chest should be effective in holding the wound closed. The band around the chest should not unduly restrict breathing.

When to See a Doctor

Knowing when to see a physician is most important in first aid. See a physician if:
- There is spurting bleeding (this is an emergency).
- Slow bleeding continues beyond 4 to 10 minutes.
- There is foreign material in the wound that does not wash out easily.
- The wound is a deep puncture wound.
- The wound is long or wide and thus may require stitches.
- A nerve or tendon may be cut (particularly in hand wounds).
- The wound is on the face or wherever else a noticeable scar would be undesirable.
- The wound is of a type that cannot be completely cleansed.
- The wound has been in contact with soil or manure.
- The wound is an animal or human bite.
- At the first sign of infection (pain, reddened area around wound, swelling).

Unexpected reactions to heat, cold, insect bites, and stings, or food and plant allergies such as poison ivy—all these can present serious problems.

Heat Exhaustion

Heat exhaustion is a not uncommon occurrence. Its symptoms are pale and clammy skin, rapid and weak pulse, and complaints by the victim of weakness, headache, or nausea. The victim may have cramps in abdomen or limbs.

In giving first aid for heat exhaustion, have the victim lie down with his head level to or lower than his body. Move the victim to a cool

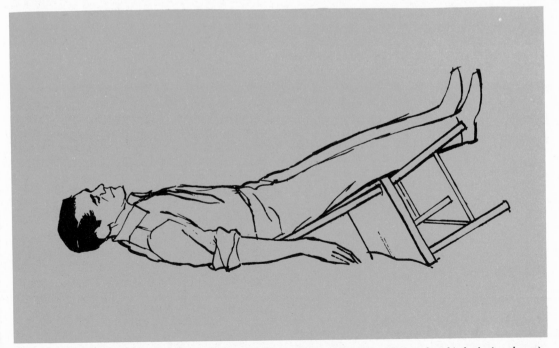

In cases of heat exhaustion, have the victim lie down with his head level to or lower than his body (as shown).

place but protect him from chilling. Give the victim salt water (1 teaspoon of salt to 1 quart of water) to drink if he is conscious. Call a physician.

Heat Stroke

Heat stroke is completely different from heat exhaustion. Its symptoms are a flushed and hot skin and a rapid and strong pulse. The victim is often unconscious.

In cases of heat stroke, call a physician. Then cool the body by sponging it with cold water and by cold applications. If the victim is fully conscious and can swallow, give him salt water (1 teaspoon of salt and 1 quart of water). Do not give alcohol in any form.

Frostbite

The symptoms of frostbite are a pink skin just before frostbite develops which changes to white or greyish-yellow as frostbite develops. The initial pain quickly subsides and the victim feels cold and numb. He usually is not aware of frostbite.

In giving first aid for frostbite, cover the frostbitten part with a warm hand or woolen material. If fingers or hand are frostbitten, have victim hold his hand in his armpit, next to his body. Bring the victim inside as soon as possible.

Place the frostbitten part in lukewarm water. Gently wrap the part in blankets if lukewarm water is not available or is impractical to use. Let circulation re-establish itself naturally.

When the part is warmed, encourage the victim to exercise fingers and toes, if they are involved. Give the victim a warm, nonalcoholic drink.

Do not rub frostbitten parts with snow or ice. Rubbing frostbitten tissues increases the risk of gangrene. Do not use hot water, hot water bottles, or heat lamps over the frostbitten area.

Insect Stings

Persons who have experienced severe and/ or generalized allergic reactions from previous insect stings should receive desensitization treatment from a physician. An insect sting can endanger the life of a sensitized person.

To treat a sting, apply a constricting bandage (not a tourniquet) to the arm or leg above the sting. Use a strong, wide piece of cloth. Wrap the cloth around the limb just above the sting.

Tie a half-knot; place a short stick on the half-knot; tie a full knot over the stick; twist the stick. A pulse should be present below the bandage, and the bandage should not produce a throbbing sensation. Loosen the bandage for a few seconds every 15 minutes. Apply an ice pack or cold cloths to area; remove stinger with tweezers; seek medical attention as soon as possible.

Generalized reactions from food allergy can make the victim seriously ill. Symptoms are difficulty in breathing and possibly hives and skin swelling. In meeting this problem, call a physician. Keep the victim quiet in whatever position is most comfortable.

Poison ivy (and other plant poisoning) should be suspected after known or possible contact with poison ivy, oak, or sumac; itching, redness, or blisters on the skin are early signs. In giving first aid for plant poisoning, cut clothing from the exposed area so that contaminated clothing is not dragged across unexposed areas of the body; wash the exposed area thoroughly with mild soap and water. Repeat lathering and rinsing several times; sponge rubbing alcohol gently over the area; if blisters occur on the skin, see a physician.

Mental Disturbances

Mental disturbances call for a different type of emergency assistance than physical injuries. Here are some suggestions:

Call a physician or relative of the disturbed person immediately. If the person is in danger of harming himself or others and a physician or relative is not available, call a policeman.

Treat the person with respect, however he reacts to you. Divert the person's attention from anything that might be harmful to him or others; for example, try to shift his thinking from destructive to protective acts, from antagonism to cooperation. Be patient, kind, and reassuring. Be firm in your attitude toward the person.

Restrain the person physically only if he seems likely to injure himself or others. Do not argue with the disturbed person. Do not assume a harsh, authoritative role with him. Do not physically hold the person unless he seems likely to injure himself or others.

Childbirth

Childbirth is a natural and normal act. There are only a few things to remember if you are in

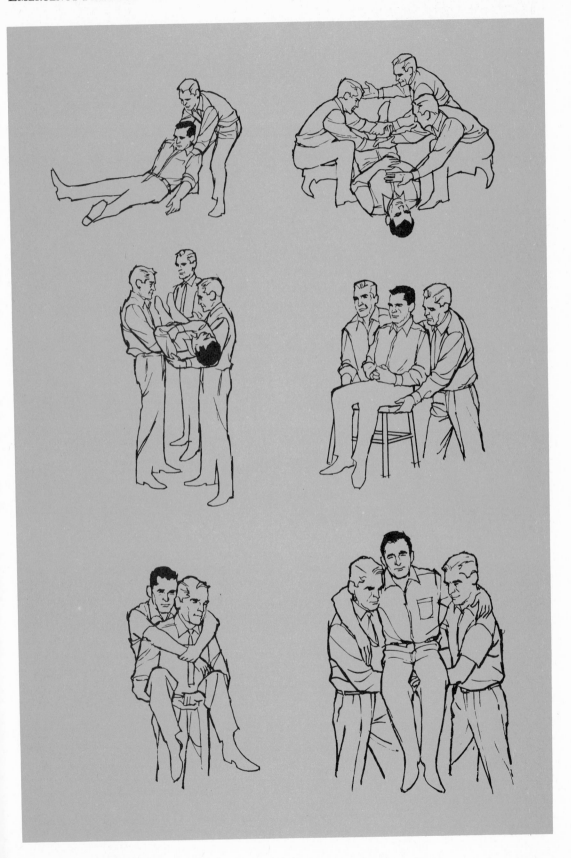

the emergency situation of helping a mother deliver her baby.

● Let nature take its course. Be patient. Wait for the baby to be delivered.

● Wash your hands. Keep your hands and surroundings as clean as possible.

● During the birth process, only support, do not pull the emerging baby.

● When the baby has been delivered, put the baby on the mother's abdomen, his head slightly lowered. Cover the baby to keep him warm.

● If the baby is not breathing, gently use mouth-to-mouth breathing.

● Keep the baby on the mother's abdomen until the afterbirth has been expelled.

● Gently massage the mother's abdomen to help uterus contract.

● Boil or clean scissors with alcohol. Tie a clean tape or cloth in a square knot around the umbilical cord about four inches from the baby to stop circulation in the cord. Tie a second tape around the cord six to eight inches from the baby (two to four inches between the knots). Cut the cord between the two tapes with clean scissors.

● Keep both baby and mother warm. Keep people away from baby and mother. Handle the baby gently and as little as possible. Notify the mother's physician.

● Keep hands and tools out of the birth canal. Do not hurry birth. Do not interfere with birth. Do not hurry to cut the cord. Wait until afterbirth has been expelled. ·

● Do not wash white material off the baby. It protects the skin. Do nothing to eyes, ears, nose, or mouth.

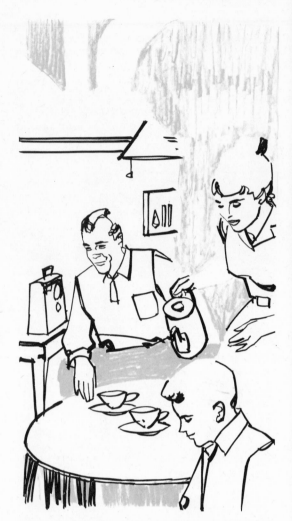

Moving Injured Persons

Do not move an injured person before a physician or experienced ambulance crew arrives unless there is a real danger of his receiving further injury by being left at the accident site. If possible, control bleeding, maintain breathing, and splint all suspected fractures sites before moving. If it is necessary to pull the victim to a safe place, pull him head first or feet first, not sideways. Be sure the head is protected at all times.

If he must be lifted before a check for injuries can be made, every part of the body should be supported. The body should be kept in a straight line and should not be bent.

In carrying the injured person to an area where a stretcher can be manipulated, use either the one, two, or three-man carry method, depending on the type and severity of the injury, the available help, and the physical surroundings (stairs, walls, narrow passages, etc.). The one and two-man carry systems are ideal for transporting a person who is unconscious from asphyxiation or drowning, but are unsuited for carrying a person suspected of having fractures or other severe injuries. In these cases always use the three-man carry method.

An effective stretcher can be made by buttoning two shirts or a coat over two sturdy branches, or by wrapping a blanket in thirds about the branches or poles. If the victim must be moved, a stretcher is the best means for transportation.

Nuclear War Injuries

Most injuries sustained in nuclear warfare would be the same as those already discussed:

heavy bleeding, burns, fractures, and shock. First aid techniques would not change. Consideration for survival from radioactive fallout would be an added concern.

Radioactive fallout is dangerous, but many scientists now believe that it will not cover the world and kill everything. Proper shelter will greatly increase your chances of living and the longer you stay in a shelter, the safer you will be. Radioactive fallout decays rapidly. The first few hours are the most dangerous. People do not become radioactive from fallout. Radioactive dust can be washed off like dust or dirt.

The need for protection in a shelter is determined by time, distance, and shielding. The longer you stay protected, the safer you will be. The center of a large building is safer than an outside room. The greater the mass of material you put between yourself and the source of radiation, the safer you will be. In contaminated areas stay in a shelter for at least 12 hours (or until the area is declared safe); tune in any channel on your AM radio dial for correct information on the amount of radioactive fallout; wash off areas of the body that have been exposed to radioactive dust with soap and water; do not try to diagnose possible illness. If ill with nausea, headache, or vomiting, treat the symptoms. Remember that nervousness and apprehension produce similar feelings.

Purify water when in doubt. Add one drop of household bleach to each quart of clear water, or add three drops to each quart of cloudy water. Let water stand 30 minutes before using. Use only food that has been protected from fallout and disease. Wash it thoroughly, peel carefully, or remove container carefully before eating food that may have come in contact with fallout. Cook food thoroughly to kill germs; do not drink water from an unprotected source, do not throw away good food, but do not eat rotten food. If food cannot be cleaned of all radioactivity, or if food may be contaminated by disease germs, do not eat it. It is better to go hungry than to eat contaminated food.

The most important thing to do is to learn survival techniques *now*. Contact your local civil defense authorities for more specific information.

First Aid Supplies

The emergency first-aid supply items listed below can be wrapped in a moisture-proof covering and placed in an easily carried box. Quantities specified are for a family of four or less. The supplies can be kept on hand at home or carried on family outings.

Useful also for family trips would be several jars of water and a stack of clean newspaper. In any emergency situation, clean newspapers are one of the best ground and surface covers. Spread newspapers under and around the victim to prevent contamination.

When other first aid measures have been taken and as time allows, the first aider should note the following information:
- Identity of the victim.
- Those persons the victim would like notified (including clergy).
- Circumstances of the injury or illness.
- Any special first aid measures taken (mouth-to-mouth breathing, administration of fluids, application tourniquet, etc.)
- Any disease or disability existing prior to the injury or illness (diabetes, heart trouble, allergies, etc.).

FIRST AID ITEM	QUANTITY	USE
1. Sterile first aid dressing in sealed envelope 2 in. x 2 in. (5 cm. x 5 cm.) for small wounds	Box of 12	For open wounds or dry dressings for burns. These are packaged sterile. Do not try to make your own.
2. Sterile first aid dressing in sealed envelope 4 in. x 4 in. (10cm. x 10 cm.) for larger wounds and for compress to stop bleeding	Box of 12	
3. Roller bandage 1 in. x 5 yds. (2.5 cm. x 5 m.)	2	Finger bandage

FIRST AID ITEM	QUANTITY	USE
4. Roller bandage 2 in. x 5 yds. (5 cm. x 5 m.)	2	To hold dressings in place
5. Adhesive tape	1 roll	To hold dressings in place
6. Large bath towels	2	For bandages or dressings. Old soft towels and sheets are best. Cut in sizes necessary to cover wounds.
7. Small bath towels	2	Towels are burn dressings. Place over burns and fasten with triangular bandage or strips of sheet.
8. Bed sheets	1	Towels and sheets should be laundered, ironed, and packaged in heavy paper. Relaunder every 3 months.
9. Triangular bandage 37 in. x 37 in. (94 cm. x 94 cm.) square, cut, or folded diagonally, with 2 safety pins	4	For a sling; as a covering; for a dressing
10. Mild soap	1 bar	For cleansing of wounds, scratches, cuts. Antiseptics are not necessary.
11. Table salt	small package	For shock — dissolve 1 teaspoon salt, ½ teaspoon baking soda in 1 quart water (5 gm. salt, 2 gm. baking soda, 1 liter water)
12. Baking soda	small package	
13. Paper drinking cups	25	
14. Flashlight	1	
15. Safety pins, 1½ in. (4 cm.) long	15	
16. Scissors with blunt tips	1 pair	For cutting bandages or clothing
17. Tweezers	1	To remove stingers from insect bites
18. Eye dropper	1	For rinsing eyes
19. Splints ¼ in. thick, 3½ in. wide, 12 to 15 in. long (6 mm. x 9 cm. x 30 to 38 cm.)	12	For splinting broken arms and legs
20. Tongue blades, wooden	12	For splinting broken fingers and for stirring solutions
21. Measuring spoons	1 set	
22. Tourniquet. Wide strip of cloth, 20 in. (50 cm.) long	1	For use in severe injuries when no other method will control bleeding
23. Short stick	1	To use with tourniquet
24. Essential personal prescriptions		

CHAPTER THREE

WHEN TO CALL THE DOCTOR

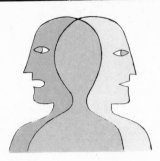

IF EVERYONE were to call the doctor for every cut or scratch, bruise or bump, twinge or burp, the doctors would be so busy with little things that they would not have enough time to take care of the big illnesses. In other chapters we have told how you can care for minor situations. In this chapter we want to tell about the times when it is important to call the doctor without delay.

The following four points are a general guide to help you decide whether medical aid should be sought at once:

1. When the patient's complaint or symptoms are too severe to be endured, such as abdominal pain common to a gall bladder or appendicitis attack or kidney colic, sudden chest pains; immediate relief is then the purpose of calling the doctor without delay.

2. When an apparently minor symptom or symptoms persist for more than a few days or a week and do not appear to be due to some easily identified cause. A bleeding nose from being struck is one thing; a nose that bleeds constantly or frequently in the absence of injury is quite a different matter, and demands medical attention.

3. When the symptom or symptoms return repeatedly for no readily recognizable cause. Digestive disturbances due to repeated overindulgence are one thing; constant digestive distress despite great care and moderation in eating is another. It requires medical investigation without too much delay.

4. When in doubt, it is safer to call the doctor than to take a chance.

Thus the four indications calling for immediate medical attention are: severity, persistence, repetition, and doubt. Any one of the four is sufficient; a combination of two or more adds to the urgency.

The following circumstances, listed alphabetically, have each specific indications as to whether a doctor's help is needed.

Accidents require immediate medical attention when the victim is unconscious; when bleeding is severe or cannot be controlled; when the victim is confused or groggy; when there are signs of shock—pale cold skin, sweating, and weak pulse with or without loss of consciousness; when there is breathlessness and great thirst; when there are signs of broken bones; when pain is severe; when there are signs of poisoning; when serious or extensive burns have occurred; when the victim is "out of his mind"; when persistent severe vomiting is present; when vision is suddenly lost or blurred.

Alcoholic Addiction. Either simple drunkenness or true alcoholism suggest the probability that medical care is needed.

Appetite Changes. May range from complete loss of appetite to excessive hunger and thirst. Unless such conditions are temporary (a few days or a week), they should have prompt attention. Included in this category are the so-called "cravings" of pregnant women, and the common childhood habit of eating plaster, dirt, and other unsuitable substances.

Feelings of insecurity may be masked by persistent indulgence in overeating; this usually calls for medical advice.

Blackouts. Periods when memory is gone but consciousness may exist; afterward the individual remembers nothing of what has happened or where he has been. These occur in alcoholism and in some nervous and mental conditions. They always call for immediate professional investigation.

Bleeding. May be of several kinds. Large sudden hemorrhages are more alarming than slow continuous bleeding, but both are important and require medical investigation. The most common bleeding is the well-known nosebleed. If this happens occasionally, it is nothing to worry about; but if it happens often or continues for a long time, the cause should be investigated. Most often it is a small bleeding point in the nose; sometimes it may have more serious causes.

Bleeding may also occur from the bowels. This is usually due to hemorrhoids (piles), but may be due to intestinal polyps, ulcers, or cancers. When stools are a black, tarry color, bleeding in the upper intestinal tract may be responsible. Under no circumstances should suspected bleeding in the intestines ever be neglected or treated with home remedies or advertised preparations.

In women, change in the length of the menstrual period or in the character of the bleeding should have attention if it is more than occasional. Bleeding, even a "spot" on the clothing, after the menstrual cycle has ceased (menopause) should always have prompt investigation, since it may be due to more significant causes than merely a prolonged period of "change." "Spotting" between menstrual periods is not normal. Neither are prolonged periods or very heavy flows.

Blood in the urine may appear as red blood or as a smoky color in the urine. Traces of red or brownish discoloration in the sputum may indicate bleeding.

Unless there has been an injury which accounts for it and which is receiving care, the appearance of blood in any amount in any of the body secretions or excretions should never be ignored. Prompt attention to these symptoms would result in the saving of many lives now sacrificed to cancer.

Bowel Changes. May involve the appearance or consistency of the stools, or their frequency. Gassy or watery stools, fatty stools, pale stools, or tarry black stools—any of these calls for study of the digestive function. So does persistent diarrhea or diarrhea alternating with constipation. Inability to perform bowel functions normally also requires attention.

Breathlessness. Everyone gets spells of breathlessness from exertion or emotional experiences, but the normal person should be able to climb a flight of steps without puffing too much, and should recover his wind in a few minutes after heavy physical effort. When there is breathlessness after ordinary exertion or when it becomes difficult to breathe even without apparent cause, it is time to assume that something has gone wrong, and to make a date for a medical examination. There are many causes for breathlessness; all of them can be treated more successfully if they are discovered promptly.

Breathing difficulties may be due to obstruction in the nose or throat, pressures on the windpipe, various conditions in the lungs, weakening of the heart muscle, anemia and and other changes in the blood, allergic asthma, disturbances in brain and nerve function, or emotional causes.

They may also be due to poor physical condition, the beginning of heart and blood vessel disease, or a variety of other more or less serious conditions. All demand investigation and most can be helped if caught in time and properly treated. The sooner the cause is discovered and remedied, the better.

Common Cold. Symptoms are important because they may or may not indicate a common cold. In children the runny nose, watery eyes, sore throat, cough, and muscle aches may be the beginning of one of the communicable diseases. These symptoms also are often due to allergies. At any age, they may be the first signs of influenza. If they persist, they may mean involvement of the breathing tubes, the lungs, the sinuses, and sometimes the ears in infections which may prove serious. Colds should not be neglected, nor dosed with home remedies, especially if they last more than three days or are accompanied by fever.

Constipation. Should be a rare symptom because the bowel regulates itself, if given a chance, through proper diet, sufficient fluids, exercise, and good habits of elimination. Because of a false idea that "regularity" requires daily bowel action, many persons suffer from artificial constipation induced by laxatives. Constipation is not usually an emergency, but when it has become a problem, it is better to get proper attention than to fool around with home remedies and advertised preparations, which may tend to make the matter worse instead of better.

Convulsions. A convulsion is an attack of unconsciousness accompanied by twitching muscles. Convulsions in children used to be quite common. Now, with modern feeding methods, they are rare, and are usually due to fever. In acute infections a child may frequently have a "convulsion" when an adult under similar circumstances would have a "chill." Either calls for medical advice. A common cause of convulsions at other ages is epilepsy, which always requires medical care. Convulsions should never be ignored, even if they happen only once. A medical investigation to find the cause and prevent further occurrences is required.

Cough. A protective device which helps to keep the breathing passages clear of secretions and foreign objects. Coughing is a common symptom during a cold; such a cough disappears with the passing of the acute condition. A cough that hangs on is a different matter. This may indicate too much smoking, allergies, chronic infections in the breathing tubes, changes in lung structure, tuberculosis or fungus infection, a lung cancer, or weakening of heart action. Early diagnosis and proper treatment for a persistent cough improve the chances of recovery.

Diarrhea. Consists of frequent loose, watery stools with mucus. It may be due to eating spoiled food, to drugs, to laxatives, or to conditions in the bowel requiring medical or even surgical attention, such as polyps and cancers. A common cause is so-called colitis. Occasional diarrhea due to obvious causes is not alarming; continuous diarrhea or alternating diarrhea and constipation indicates the need for professional attention.

Discharges. Any discharges, including blood, from any body opening should have prompt investigation; they may indicate the breakdown of tissue from infection or malignancies. The most important sources of such discharges are: nose and throat ("phlegm"); lungs; breast (either sex); ears; urethra (penis); vagina; skin sores; bladder; wounds; and rectum.

Dizziness. Practically everyone has an attack of dizziness once in a while, often due to digestive disturbance or so-called "biliousness." This is no cause for concern unless it persists or returns. But continuous or frequent dizziness with no apparent cause may be due to significant changes in blood pressure, disease in the middle ear, failure of fusion of visual images right and left, changes in the brain caused by hardening of the arteries, or more rarely, brain tumors.

Ear Symptoms. Pain and loss of hearing should not be taken for granted, especially in children. This is particularly important if they are accompanied by head noises and dizziness. Running ears demand immediate care. Early treatment gives the best results.

Eye Symptoms. May be an indication that the eyes themselves need help, or they may be signals that conditions in the body as a whole are doing harm to the eyes. Eyesight is so important that signs of abnormal vision should never be neglected. The most urgent symptom is sudden and severe pain in the eyes, spreading over the head; this may be a sign of glaucoma, which can destroy vision in just a few hours. It is more common in older persons, but can occur at any age. Other signs that the eyes need attention, or that something is threatening them, include: dimming of vision; halos around lights; loss of side vision; distortion of objects; crossed or "walled" eyes; frequent need to change glasses; inflammation of the eye; double vision; drooping eyelids; excess of tears; unequal pupils; excessive blinking; red eyelids; sties; and burning sensation of eyelids.

Fatigue. Getting tired is a universal experience, and not an unpleasant one if there is good reason for it, such as a good day's work or an exciting and pleasurable experience. Rest and a good night's sleep usually take care of that. When fatigue is too great, or recovery from it is too slow, or when one is always tired, or arises tired from what should have been a good night's rest, the condition is abnormal. There may be many causes for such chronic fatigue, ranging from poor nutrition to overwhelming emotional problems. The remedy does *not* lie in eating vitamin supplements or in self-medication with advertised preparations, but in medical investigation getting at the cause and proper treatment for it.

Fever. When body temperature is above 98.6° F. taken by mouth or 99.6° F. by rectum, the patient is said to have a fever. It is a protective reaction which helps the body to overcome infection. High fever, and fever which persists for more than 24 hours, indicate involvement more severe than the body can handle without professional help. Low fever which persists over periods of days or weeks may indicate a chronic infection, such as tuberculosis, rheumatic fever, mononucleosis, or one of many other causes.

Forgetfulness. Normal to some extent with everyone, and may grow worse in older persons. It may take the form of loss of memory of word meanings. Memory of isolated events, of events in the past, or those immediately preceding the memory loss, may occur. Events may be misplaced in time, as in older people who commonly confuse memories of the past with events of the present. Inability to recognize printed or written words, or to identify objects by touch, is also observed. As with any other symptom, this requires attention when it is severe or prolonged sufficiently to interfere with the welfare of the individual and his ability to support and to care for himself.

Headaches. Everyone has headaches from time to time, due to such common and easily identified causes as getting too tired, staying in a stuffy room, eating or drinking too much, suffering from a cold, or dealing with a frustrating problem. The occasional headache yields readily to a rest in a quiet, darkened room, an aspirin tablet or two, and a nap or a night's sleep. There are, however, headaches which are more severe, or which return again and again, or are accompanied by other symptoms such as nausea or vomiting, eye symptoms, and other abnormal experiences. Such headaches should not be endured and repeatedly dosed with pain-killers. They are not diseases in themselves, but they are symptoms of deeper causes which should be identified and, where possible, removed.

Hiccups. Due to spasms of the muscle dividing the abdomen from the chest. They are commonly due to eating or drinking too much or too fast, and they ordinarily recover by themselves, which explains why there are so many hiccup remedies. They all work when the hiccups were ready to stop anyhow. Hiccuping which lasts for days, however, is exhausting and can indicate disease. This symptom should therefore have medical attention if it does not yield within a few hours to home remedies.

Hoarseness. May be due to a cold or other throat infection; if it disappears promptly it is no cause for concern. Persistent hoarseness may be one of the signs of a tumor on the vocal cords, and may or may not be cancerous. In either case, it should be investigated and treated promptly. Chronic hoarseness may also occur with tuberculous infection of the larynx.

Indigestion. Except when it is obviously due to overeating or drinking, indigestion may be a symptom of many things, ranging from dietary indiscretions to serious conditions such as ulcers and cancers. It should never be accepted as a mere annoyance, or attributed to dietary factors or other vague causes if it occurs more often than rarely. It requires investigation as to cause in order to make proper treatment possible. Among common manifestations of "indigestion" are: nausea; vomiting; diarrhea; constipation; belching; heartburn; alternation of diarrhea and constipation; blood in stools (see Bleeding); "acid stomach"; and intestinal gassiness.

Home remedies, especially antacids, are not cures; they may relieve symptoms temporarily, while permitting the underlying disease to progress, perhaps beyond help.

Swelling of the abdomen may indicate liver disease, circulatory disturbances, or other abdominal conditions requiring prompt attention.

Itching. Closely related to pain, and may be even more annoying. It may be due to dry skin, excessive bathing, local irritation from soaps, detergents, or cosmetics, skin infections, parasites, or to nerve involvements. It is often made worse by scratching. Usually the quickest and best way to get rid of itching that persists is to get medical treatment.

Jaundice. A yellowing of the skin and white of the eyes due to collection of bile in the blood. It is always a symptom requiring prompt medical action, especially in the newborn baby.

Jaundice accompanied by abdominal pain requires immediate medical advice; jaundice without apparent cause also demands prompt attention.

Loss of Sensation. An indication that there is interference with nerve trunks or pain receptors in the skin which transmit sensations to the brain, or to abnormality in the brain itself. It always calls for prompt attention. Neglect not only postpones proper treatment, but may cause tissue destruction through inability to feel contacts which may be injurious, such as heat, cold, or cutting.

Loss of Taste and Smell. Occurs not uncommonly following severe colds. The senses usually return in time without treatment. When loss of one or the other sense occurs in the absence of apparent cause, it is best to have a medical examination.

Mental Symptoms. Those which are persistent or recurrent and are not adequately explained by illness, bereavement, or other emotional shock of temporary character, indicate the possible onset of mental illness, deterioration due to aging, or diseases affecting the brain. Among such symptoms which call for medical and possibly psychiatric attention are: confusion; depression; suspiciousness; aggressiveness; refusal to eat; crying spells; wild spending; memory changes; antagonisms; withdrawal; sleeplessness; excessive excitability; excessive talkativeness; changed personality; disorientation as to time and place; abnormal imaginings; abnormal fears; tantrums and rages; delusions of grandeur; self-centeredness; and destructiveness.

Mouth and Tongue Soreness. May be due to temporary causes such as too hot food, rough fillings, ill-fitting dentures or broken teeth, local infections, cold sores, too much smoking, or chewing tobacco. If a sore mouth or tongue persists, it may be due to nutritional causes and, especially in older people, to a form of anemia caused by a deficiency in blood-forming tissues. Early medical treatment is required for this or any other persistent abnormality in the mouth.

Muscle Symptoms. Stiffness and cramping are normal up to a point for well-known reasons, such as sitting still too long or getting into uncomfortable positions. When these symptoms become seriously annoying, they should be considered abnormal and should have medical attention.

Stumbling, fumbling, and dropping things are other common indications that muscle action or nerve coordination is not normal.

A common form of spasm is twitching of small muscles, often about the eyes and face. If these do not go away by themselves they require treatment. Spasms, cramps, pains, wasting away, or weakness may be due to various causes, as yet poorly understood, which may be nutritional in basis or due to defects in nervous functioning. These include multiple sclerosis, myasthenia gravis, and the muscular dystrophies. (See Part X, Chapter Five.) Muscle wasting may also be due to interference with a specific nerve function caused by injuries, pressures from scars or tumors, and nerve inflammations (neuritis).

Nausea or Vomiting. Ordinarily obvious results of dietary indiscretions or excessive drinking, allergies, onset of acute illnesses, or poisoning. Both are almost universally present in early pregnancy. They may also be expressions of emotional distress. Severe forms of vomiting may be symptoms of serious internal disturbances or brain involvement. When the symptoms persist or occur frequently, a medical search for the cause is necessary. Exceptionally forceful or "projectile" vomiting is always an emergency.

Nervousness. One of the most misused and misunderstood medical terms, as is "nervous breakdown." These terms were formerly applied to many vague and indefinite conditions for which the cause was not apparent; the popular term was "it's all in your head." More modern diagnostic methods have identified definite causes for many experiences formerly attributed to "nervousness." It is now recognized that emotions play a large part in illness, with or without definite physical disease. Even without physical cause, disturbed functioning can be a very real source of distress and disability. The expression "it's all in your head" tells us nothing and should be promptly forgotten.

Nervous disturbances of emotional origin, popularly referred to as "nerves," should be

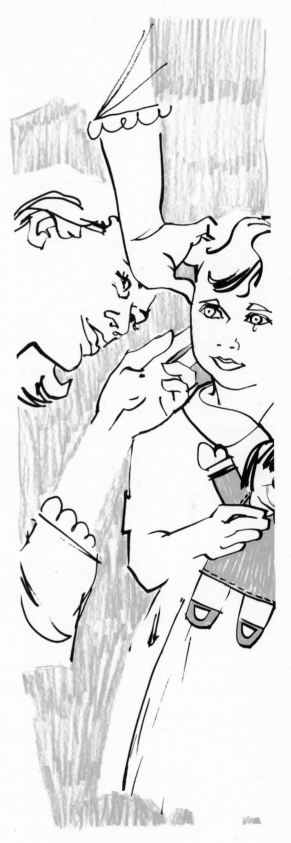

distinguished from physical disease of the nervous system such as tumors, strokes, paralysis, neuritic pain, muscle-wasting diseases, and Parkinson's disease.

Emotional disturbances can now often be helped and should have attention.

Numbness and Tingling. These and other disturbances of sensation are common experiences, often described as a limb "going to sleep." They are no cause for concern if the reason for them is obvious and recovery is prompt. Continuous or persistent tingling or loss of sensation, however, may have deeper significance and should be investigated.

Pain. It is often called a blessing, because it sends the patient to the doctor for treatment. A lesser form of pain may be described as discomfort or aching. The occasional mild pain which is the experience of practically everybody, usually yields to simple home care. But when pain is severe, or when it continues for more than two or three hours, or when it comes back again and again in the same way, or when it is a continuous ache, it is time to have it investigated. It may be due to something more serious than a temporary cause. Some of the more common types of pain which may be indications of serious need for attention, include the following:

Earaches, especially in children, require prompt medical care in order to protect against hearing loss.

Toothache always calls for immediate attention by a dentist.

Abdominal pain may soon identify itself as just the ordinary "bellyache" from too much food or the wrong kind. But if it persists or grows severe, or is accompanied by nausea, vomiting, diarrhea, or constipation, it is no longer safe to use home remedies or to "wait and see what happens." When there is abdominal pain, the taking of food or drink should be discontinued, except for small sips of water. Laxatives should never be given where there is abdominal pain.

Joint pains, especially in children, always require medical attention. They may indicate the beginnings of arthritis, or of acute rheumatic fever, either of which requires medical attention.

Muscle pains may be due to strains, sprains, rheumatic conditions, nervous or circulatory disturbances.

Eye pains, especially if sudden and severe and radiating over the head, always constitute an emergency. If they are due to glaucoma,

vision may be lost or seriously impaired in only a few hours. While this is uncommon, it is very serious.

Chest pains may be due to conditions in the chest muscles, to heart or lung diseases, pleurisy, overexertion when out of condition, or injury. They should always be investigated. "Growing pains" are important because normal growth is painless, and so-called growing pains should always arouse suspicion of something wrong. Often the cause is rheumatic fever or related conditions.

Colicky pains in babies are not usually serious; in adults they may indicate stones, especially in the kidney and the gall bladder.

Cramps may affect muscles anywhere in the body, or may occur in the intestines, the gall bladder, or the uterus. The underlying cause must be sought in order to administer appropriate treatment.

Painful feet may indicate arthritis, overweight, badly fitted shoes or hose, gout, poor circulation, corns, calluses, diabetes, or simply too much standing.

Palpitation. This or flutter in the chest, changes noted in the heart action in terms of speed and regularity, sensations as if the heart had stopped, choking sensations and breathlessness—all these always demand examination. Often these symptoms are unimportant and the examination acts as a reassurance. Sometimes these symptoms indicate a serious heart condition requiring immediate care.

Paralysis. A sudden weakness or progressive loss of function, strength, or coordination is always an indication that something is going seriously wrong in either the nervous system or locally. Perhaps some unsuspected poisoning is taking place, such as occurs from exposure to lead, arsenic, and some other chemicals used in industrial processes.

Skin Rashes. These have many causes, including communicable diseases, skin diseases, irritations from detergents, industrial chemicals or cosmetics, and allergies. Some are of nervous origin and others indicate some general disease which includes skin symptoms. Unless a rash fades promptly when a suspected cause is removed, it should have professional attention. Applying home remedies or advertised preparations may not only fail to improve the condition, but may mask it or convert a simple irritation into a chronic inflammation very difficult to overcome. Pigmented (colored) spots on the skin, whether elevated or not, may become malignant (cancerous). They are particularly dangerous if the color changes or darkens, or if they bleed or grow.

Sleep Disturbances. Include both excessive sleepiness and the opposite, exaggerated wakefulness. Sleepiness and drowsiness due to such obvious causes as lack of sleep, poor ventilation, overeating or drinking are obviously temporary. But when such experiences occur without apparent cause and persist or occur frequently, it is time to be sure that unrecognized diseases which may be causing them are identified and treated.

Wakefulness beyond the common experience of an occasional difficulty in getting to sleep has similar significance, and should have comparable attention. Much so-called insomnia is of little significance.

Sores. Those that do not heal may be due to chronic infections by germs or fungi, to circulatory disturbances, or to cancerous degeneration. Experiments with home remedies or advertised preparations merely postpone proper treatment, increase suffering and expense, and occasionally endanger life. Persistent sores should have medical attention if they are not healed in two weeks. Any sore that returns after healing should be seen by a physician at once.

Swellings and Lumps. May be due to insignificant causes such as wens or fatty tumors, but they should always be investigated in order that one may be sure that they are not of more serious nature. One of the warning signals of a possible cancer is the appearance of a lump or mass where it does not belong. The most common example is the prevalence of lumps in the female breast and in lymph nodes in the armpit. Many of these are not cancerous and are simple to remove; others require removal of the entire breast, and this must be done in time if life is to be saved. Wherever an abnormal lump appears in the body or on it, in either the male or the female, it should be identified without delay, and the physician's advice about treatment accepted.

Swelling in the limbs, especially of the legs at the end of the day, may indicate gathering of fluid in the tissues, and may call for examination of the heart, kidneys, blood, or internal secretion glands. When footwear feels tight at the end of the day, or the flesh "pits" on pressure, it is time to see the doctor.

Bad Tastes. This and sensations of smell or loss of the sense of smell may be due to local and temporary conditions. If persistent they have more serious significance.

Trembling. Most commonly due to simple weakness, or may follow vigorous activity. If it is temporary it is of little significance. If it persists, it may indicate conditions in the brain or nervous system, or of the thyroid gland, or in the body's calcium utilization, all of which require attention. It may be an early symptom of Parkinson's disease, and as such would benefit from early recognition. It may also have emotional connotations.

Urinary Changes. May include greatly increased amounts of urine; necessity for frequent urination, especially at night; burning and discomfort upon urination; changes in the appearance of the urine, especially bright red blood or a smoky appearance indicating oozing of blood somewhere along the urinary tract. Inability to urinate, especially in the elderly male, is common. "Dribbling" of urine frequently troubles older women who have borne many children. Pain in the urinary tract may be due to kidney or bladder stones, infection, acid urine, or cancerous growths.

Warts, Moles, and Birthmarks. Usually can be ignored with safety unless they are located where clothing tends to irritate them. Any skin growth which bleeds, becomes sore, starts to grow, or change in color or appearance should have immediate medical attention. Home remedies in such situations are dangerous, and advertised preparations or treatments are worse.

Weakness. Weakness may present itself as a loss of strength in the body as a whole or in certain of its parts. Frequent tripping, stumbling, dropping things, or difficulty in performing ordinary actions are indications of weakness (or failure of coordination). In some cases it may amount to a partial paralysis; in others it may appear as clumsiness or poor coordination. Everyone gets tired out from time to time, but continuous weakness or poor coordination almost always has a deeper explanation. This should be sought and remedied if possible without losing too much time.

Weight Changes. Those which are not brought about intentionally should be considered significant if they are large, rapid, or progressive in the absence of obvious cause. Such changes may indicate underlying bodyfunction changes or the insidious onset of serious disease.

Yawning and Sighing. These are normal ways of getting more air and more oxygen. They are usually signs of fatigue or of poor ventilation. Yawning may be induced by seeing others yawn. If such symptoms occur to an annoying extent, or happen frequently without apparent cause, they may indicate circulatory or respiratory or nervous-system conditions requiring attention.

Importance of Symptoms

It will be seen from the foregoing that a symptom is not equivalent to a diagnosis. Many patients expect the doctor to prescribe immediately for their principal complaint, which is often only a symptom. Except in emergencies he has to find out what causes the symptom before he can do this intelligently. One symptom may have many causes.

In the home, an understanding about symptoms and what they may mean can be a great help in deciding when to call the doctor. You can avoid the expense of unnecessary calls and at the same time not neglect to get the best possible medical care promptly when it is required.

The following circumstances will give a general guide to help you decide whether medical aid should be sought at once:

• When the patient's complaint or symptoms are too severe to be endured, such as abdominal pain of a gall bladder or appendicitis attack or kidney colic, or sudden severe chest pains; immediate relief is then the purpose of calling the doctor without delay.

• When the symptom or symptoms persist for more than a few days or a week, and do not appear to be due to some easily identified cause. A bleeding nose from being struck is one thing; a nose that bleeds constantly or frequently in the absence of injury is quite a different matter, and demands medical attention.

• When the symptom or symptoms return repeatedly for no readily recognizable cause. Digestive disturbances due to repeated over-indulgence are one thing; constant digestive distress despite great care and moderation in eating requires medical investigation without too much delay.

• When in doubt, it is safer to call the doctor than to take a chance.

Well, that's *When* to call the doctor. Now we will tell you *How*.

CHAPTER FOUR

HOW TO CALL THE DOCTOR

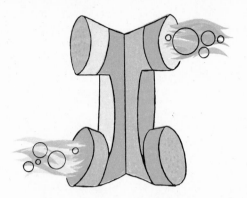

IT WOULD HARDLY SEEM necessary to tell anyone how to call a doctor properly. The experience of doctors, however, is that patients actually do have such a problem. Here is an all too typical call! "Hello. Is this Dr. Jones' residence? May I speak to the doctor?"

"He is not in at the moment. Will you give me the message, please?"

"I need him to see my husband."

"What is the trouble, please."

"If I knew the trouble, I wouldn't need to call the doctor."

This is certainly not the best way to call the doctor. When the doctor's wife or his secretary asked what the trouble was, she did not, of course, expect a diagnosis. She merely wanted to know what the patient complained of, whether he had pain, fever, chills, or other symptoms.

Remember that the physician's wife or his office attendants are his trusted helpers and that they have more than an average knowledge of the nature of illness and are quite capable in most instances of judging the urgency of a situation. Often they are able to offer helpful and reassuring advice while they find the doctor for you. Remember also that they probably can find the doctor or, if he is unavailable, locate another suitable physician much more quickly than you can.

Anyone who receives calls in a doctor's office, home, or answering service knows that there is often little understanding on the part of patients of a physician's unpredictable schedule. Office hours, hospital rounds, surgery, baby deliveries, emergency calls, teaching obligations, medical and staff meetings can turn any doctor's schedule into a maelstrom. Often he has little time for necessary reading of medical literature, no time for relaxation. and not enough for regular meals and sleep. On the other hand, the medical profession exists solely for the care and service of patients, and a doctor's comfort and convenience are secondary when there is a real emergency.

Some years ago there was a big fuss in one of our major cities about the inability to get a doctor when an elderly man was struck by an automobile. He was removed to a home nearby and efforts were made to get medical help. For some reason, no call was put in for an ambulance. Seven doctors were called; none was available. The press made this a big story, and much public indignation was directed against the medical profession.

When the matter was thoroughly investigated, however, the facts were as follows: of the seven doctors called, one was making house calls, one attending a woman in childbirth, and two out of the city at medical meetings. One doctor called was an eye specialist who suggested calling a general practitioner or a surgeon. One doctor was attending another emergency in a hospital, and the seventh was confined to his home with a broken leg.

Of course, such a situation is not a common occurrence, but it illustrates several points about calling a doctor properly. In this instance, just one call to the emergency service maintained by the local medical society would have brought a physician promptly. A call to the police department would have brought an ambulance. It is obvious then that the people who tried to be helpful either didn't know how, or they panicked.

The first error made was, of course, in moving the patient to a home rather than allowing him to lie in the street and bringing a blanket for cover. Moving a severely injured patient might have done him great harm. Most ambulance drivers are trained to handle patients in such a way as not to do further harm.

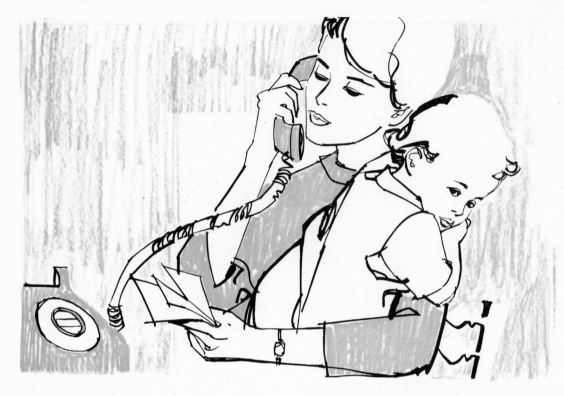

In a center where the local medical society maintains no emergency service, it would be wise to call one physician, either a general practitioner or, in the case of an accident, perhaps a surgeon, or to call either a private ambulance service or the police to take the patient to the nearest hospital emergency room. If he was not seriously injured, he would be sent home. If he had any serious injury, he would be where he belonged.

Who, Where, and What

When a physician is called, the *who,* the *where,* and the *what* are important. State at once who you are, give your address and telephone numbers if the doctor doesn't have this information, and then briefly state what the problem is. Try to have information about symptoms or complaints of the patient, the nature of the illness or accident, whether the patient has pain and where, whether there is difficulty in breathing, unconsciousness, mental confusion, severe bleeding, rash, swelling, lumps, weakness, coughing, diarrhea, vomiting, or other signs of trouble.

If you don't reach the physician immediately and he is to call back, try to keep your line open. Frequently when a physician tries to call back on an urgent call, he will find the line busy for a prolonged period because the family is calling everybody else to tell them about the situation.

If the doctor must come to the patient, finding the place may become a real feat of exploration for him in these days of suburban living, with circles, lanes, terraces, winding roads, and dead-end streets. Therefore, give specific directions to whomever you talk with at the physician's office or home.

The pet peeve of a doctor's wife or secretary is the caller who states, "Oh, never mind. I just wanted to talk to the doctor. I'll call again, it is not important." Please say who you are. You may call a dozen times and never find the doctor in, and what you considered important enough to call about in the first place probably remains important at least to some degree. It will be easier for you and for your physician if you leave your name and phone number the first time and let him call you back. Another common practice under stress and usually in some major emergency, is to call several doctors. Try to restrain yourself from doing this. If one has said he can come, wait until he arrives.

There are four chief reasons for calling a physician:

1. To make an appointment to see him in his office. This call should always be made to the office, for he cannot carry his appointment

book with him and would not know when to give you an appointment without it. Talk to his secretary or receptionist at the office and make your appointment.

2. In an emergency due to an accident or sudden severe illness.

3. For an ordinary illness.

4. To ask a question, to get information, or to discuss a problem.

In any of the above circumstances, call the doctor's office first if you are calling during hours when his office should normally be open. It is the office force that will be keeping track of the doctor's whereabouts at such a time. If it is outside of office hours, call his home. If there is no answer, look in your telephone directory and you will probably find listed with his other telephone numbers a notation such as "Answering Service" or "If no answer call." The number listed under such a notation will be that of a telephone answering service which keeps track of the doctor. Call this number, and if he is unavailable, he will probably have left word as to who is taking his calls.

In the case of many emergencies, it is best to take the patient to the emergency room of a hospital at once, if the patient can be easily transported. Many physicians believe that if there is a stroke or a heart attack, the patient should probably be seen first at home by a physician and then moved only if the physician feels that it is safe to do so. Real emergencies are such things as severe injuries, hemorrhage, severe burns, suspected poisoning, convulsions, sudden onset of high fever, stroke, chest pain, or severe abdominal pain.

Few physicians would deny that these are actual emergencies, and few physicians in active practice would hesitate to see such a patient at home or to supply help for him. On the other hand, for an illness which is not quite so impressive, such as recurrent headaches, persistent dull pain or repeated attacks of dizziness, certainly a little more leisure may be exercised in their care.

The doctor of your choice is probably a busy man, and may not be available at once, or even for some time. In such an instance you should be willing to accept a temporary alternate, if one is suggested by the physician's office or the answering service. The same applies to night calls. Such doctors usually provide a competent alternate to meet any emergency. In the morning, they themselves take over. Often they consult with the alternate by telephone from the patient's home or the hospital.

If you are calling a doctor whom you have never consulted before, you can scarcely expect the same consideration as his regular patients. While no doctor would knowingly neglect a serious emergency, patients and families who have not made arrangements in anticipation of an emergency should not blame the doctor if he is unable to respond. Choosing a doctor is dealt with in Part VIII, Chapter One.

When you wish merely to ask a question of your doctor, to get information, or to discuss a problem, call him at a reasonable hour. Try to avoid disturbing his dinner if you can. Instead, call him at his office or leave word for him to call you at his convenience. An emergency, of course, is not governed by this suggestion.

Certainly, one important factor in calling the doctor properly is to prepare in advance for the time of need. It is well to have the doctor's telephone number or numbers and that of an alternate physician in a handy list of fre-

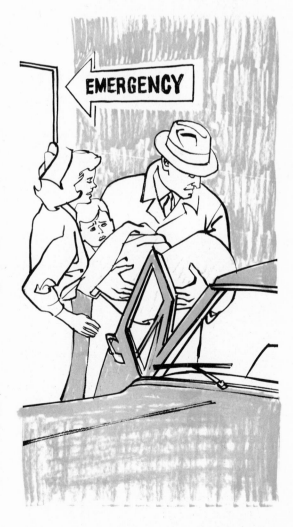

quently called numbers. Here the physician's numbers, along with the numbers of the police, fire departments, the local poison control center if one exists, the hospital of your choice, and the emergency call number of the county medical society (if there is such an emergency service in your area), might well be listed. These should be reviewed once a year so that you do not find yourself with a telephone number which has long since been changed.

House Calls

It is true, of course, that some physicians do not make house calls. On the other hand, most doctors still do, especially pediatricians, internists, and general practitioners. If the physician you happen to like does not make house calls, he usually has someone available to do so. His assistant or associate may make the house call and, if you need hospitalization or further office care, you will be sent back to the physician of your choice.

Try not to get a reputation with your doctor as a "false alarm" person. If your doctor frequently finds after you call that there is no genuine need for him, he will naturally become somewhat wary. This might, in turn, lead to unfortunate delays in a real emergency. Remember the story of the shepherd boy who called "wolf" too often. At the same time, while your doctor does not want you to overdo calling him, he also does want you to remember that you *must* call when there is real trouble.

The medical profession prides itself on the pledge it has made that no person shall go without needed medical care regardless of his ability to pay for service. It intends to keep that pledge. At the same time, your doctor asks that you try to understand some of his problems and that you cooperate in their solution. To do so not only helps the doctor, it gives you better service at less cost and with greater promptness, and it assures the patient of relief from pain and recovery from disability as rapidly as circumstances permit.

CHAPTER FIVE

GOING TO THE HOSPITAL

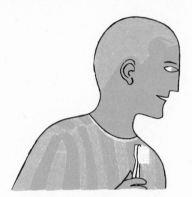

EACH PERSON will react differently to the prospect of going to the hospital. But the more each person knows about hospitals in general, the better prepared he will be—both mentally and physically—for the experience.

Broadly speaking, there are two main types of hospitals in which you may be a patient: the voluntary nonprofit hospital, operated by and for the community; and the proprietary hospital, privately owned and operated for profit.

The voluntary nonprofit hospitals comprise the largest group of hospitals in the country. They exist for the welfare of all the people in their communities. Any profit they make is returned to the hospital for its improvement or for charitable service. It is likely that when you or a member of your family becomes a hospital patient you will go to a voluntary nonprofit community or church, city, county, or state hospital. In some instances, these hospitals may receive some help from governmental sources.

A governing board of representative citizens of the community is in charge of the voluntary hospital. These men and women donate their time and service to insure that the hospital is operated in the most efficient and economical manner possible.

The hospital administrator directs the work of the hospital for the board of governors. He is familiar with the work of every department; his over-all task is to assure the best possible patient care.

Proprietary hospitals are privately owned, often by a group of doctors. They should not be viewed with suspicion simply because they are operated for profit. Any hospital, regardless of type, which is accredited by the Joint Commission on Accreditation of Hospitals, provides high quality care.

Government hospitals are operated by cities, counties, states, or the United States government. This group includes Veterans Administration, Army, Navy, Air Force, and Public Health Service hospitals that serve members and families of the military services, veterans, and other persons as authorized by Congress.

General hospitals care for patients with all types of illness or injury. There are more general hospitals in the United States than any other kind.

Special hospitals provide care for only one type of illness such as tuberculosis, mental illness, cancer, chronic diseases, and the like.

Hospital Accommodations

The family's physician will usually be a member of the medical staff of one or more hospitals, and he will recommend a particular hospital. He will also arrange for admittance and for the type of room to be selected.

Hospitals have three types of accommodations: private rooms; semiprivate rooms with two to four beds; and wards (more than four beds). Regarding accommodations, it is advisable to follow the doctor's advice. There are several factors to consider. A private room is more expensive than the semiprivate room or ward, but some circumstances require it. A day in a private room may seem longer without another patient or patients to talk to. Nursing care is the same in all accommodations; the private room patient does not get more attention. Some persons, however, prefer to be alone when ill, and consider the advantage of having a private bathroom worth the extra cost. Bath and toilet facilities are shared in semiprivate and ward accommodations.

Your hospitalization insurance plan may be a factor in the type of accommodations you choose, since most plans provide for semiprivate accommodations except in special circumstances. The costs of hospitalization, and types of insurance available, are discussed in Part VIII Chapter Five.

A hospital employs many health specialists and serves many other functions besides patient care. Many hospitals operate a school of nursing. Here, the student nurse learns to care for patients under the supervision of graduate nurses. Doctors just out of medical school serve in the hospital as interns. More experienced doctors, serving as residents, receive advanced training and experience in a medical specialty. Medical schools operate hospitals in connection with the training of doctors, technicians, and nurses.

Hospitals are ready to give service 24 hours a day if necessary. In the event of an accident or sudden acute illness, patients are generally admitted through the emergency room of a hospital. Many patients treated in the emergency room are then released and sent home.

The time of day for nonemergency admissions may vary. The doctor will tell the patient what time to arrive at the hospital. The patient is asked to go into the admitting office of the hospital on the day before treatment or surgery. This provides the time necessary for the staff to chart the patient's medical history and make the necessary physical, laboratory, and, where indicated, x-ray examinations. By the following morning the patient should feel comfortably settled and ready for treatment.

The out-patient clinic is a section devoted to the examination and treatment of people who do not require admission to the hospital. This extends hospital services to many more persons in the community than the hospital's beds could accommodate. It saves the patient the expense of full hospital care and allows him to continue a normal life and, often, his employment.

What to Take

Travel light when you go to the hospital. All you need to take from home is:

• Several pairs of pajamas or nightgowns if you do not plan to wear hospital-issue clothing.
• A bathrobe.
• Slippers.
• Comb and brush.
• Cosmetics.
• Shaving equipment (for men).
• Toothbrush and toothpaste.
• Books and, for children, toys.
• Personal items.

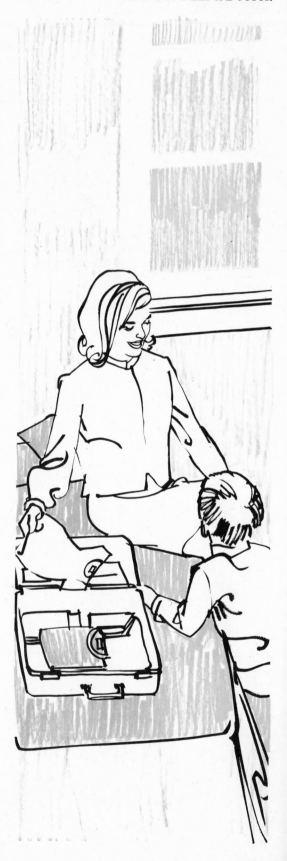

The clothes worn to the hospital will be taken care of by the hospital and be available upon discharge.

Bring only enough money for magazines, newspapers and things of that nature. Valuables, such as jewelry, watches, and the like should not be worn to the hospital. If, however, you arrive at the hospital with valuables, they should be placed for safekeeping in the valuables depository of the hospital. Check with the admitting office in advance regarding bringing a radio or television set. Many hospitals have this equipment available to patients.

Medicines should not be taken to the hospital. During the hospital stay the doctor will prescribe all medications and they will be given by a nurse. Any additional medicines could be harmful.

A word of caution to parents: Be sure to make proper arrangements for the care of children left at home so that they will not be a source of worry. When a mother or other homemaker is hospitalized, the maintenance of the home must be provided for. If no relatives or friends are available, the need may be supplied by the homemaker services which exist in larger communities, often supported by some voluntary agency. Their cost is usually flexible, and may be free if necessary.

Preparing a Child

Hospitalization can be made an interesting, if not always pleasant, experience for a child. By discussing it with him in advance its frightening aspects can be minimized. Inquiries should be made at the hospital to learn what a typical day for the child will be like. This can be done by telephone, but, if possible, a visit to the hospital should be made to see the facilities for children. Most hospitals have very attractive accommodations for children as well as toys, books, and games to keep them entertained when they are well enough to play.

It helps to tell the child some time in advance that he is going to the hospital, and why. It should be explained that doctors and nurses will take good care of him, that he will eat and sleep in the hospital, and be given medicine and care to make him well.

It is very important that adults show no fear. Answer his questions and allay any fears he may have. When going to a hospital or any strange place, a child misses the security of his family. He wants to be assured that parents and other family members will visit him frequently and that they will be on hand when he needs them.

If a child expresses extraordinary anxiety or fear, his doctor should be told about it. With this added knowledge the doctor, nurses, and other hospital personnel can do much to relieve the child's fear and put his mind at ease.

If your child's hospitalization is not planned, if he is rushed to the hospital for emergency care, parents should by all means go with him. They should remain with him, giving him all the comfort he needs until he is ready to return home or until the doctor advises the parents that they may return home.

Be a Good Patient

Many patients complain that hospitals are noisy places where it is difficult to rest. Some activity is necessary in hospitals at all hours, but efforts are made to keep noise down as much as possible. Patients can help by keeping the sound of their radio or television programs low, or by using individual earpieces or under-the-pillow speakers. Visitors can help, too, by coming and going quietly, talking in low tones, and refraining from loud laughter.

Patients and visitors should not smoke unless they have first assured themselves that they will not offend others by doing so.

Patients and relatives often rebel against restrictions on the number of visitors and the length of time they are permitted to stay. These regulations are necessary for the welfare of the patient and to allow hospital personnel time to perform their duties.

Visitors should not bring food to patients without permission from the doctor. Even wholesome foods may be inadvisable for certain patients at certain times.

Most hospitals have informational booklets describing their services. This information will be furnished on request. In addition, a trip through the hospital will reveal the many services available for your care. Hospitals are glad to arrange tours on request, and some regularly schedule them.

Hospital staffs perform many different kinds of services; each is usually the responsibility of a particular group of individuals. Among these, at least in large hospitals, will be found the following, in addition to the attending physicians:

Resident physicians are senior staff members who have finished an internship and in many instances are preparing for a specialty; they are licensed to practice medicine.

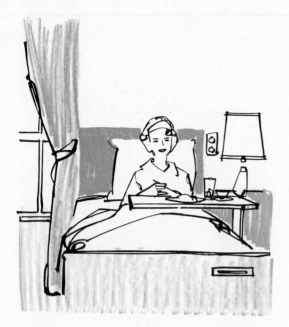

Interns are graduate physicians rounding out their education through hospital experience.

Graduate registered nurses, in charge of floors, operating rooms, or other departments, are responsible—under medical direction—for care of patients, medication, and other nursing procedures.

Practical nurses, trained in performing essential but less exacting services for patients.

Nurses' aides, trained to work with professional personnel in meeting the personal, nonmedical needs of the patients.

"Candy-stripers" are teenage girls who help voluntarily in the hospital by taking many nonmedical responsibilities off the hands of professionally trained personnel.

Orderlies are men who help move patients and perform other heavy duties. Many are male nurses.

Dietitians are specially trained to supervise the hospital menus and to prepare and serve special diets.

Laboratory technicians take blood and other specimens on which they perform various laboratory tests.

X-ray technicians assist physicians in the taking of x-rays and their development, and in giving x-ray treatments.

Physical and occupational therapists help physicians restore patients to normal functioning by their special treatments.

Office staff members attend to admissions, billing, and the keeping of records.

Medical social workers assist patients and families to adjust to circumstances created by illness, and procure assistance for those who require hospitalization and lack the means to pay for it.

Auxiliary and guild members and other volunteers give their time as a public service. They operate gift shops, snack shops, library carts, and countless miscellaneous services to make the hospital stay more pleasant.

Many hospital patients hesitate to ask their doctors the many questions that teem through their minds—about the details of their hospital stay—about the treatment they will receive—even about their illness. Patients often hesitate to ask simply because they do not want to take up their doctor's valuable time. While this attitude is considerate, it is not practical from the standpoint of the doctor, the hospital, or the patient.

The hospital staff, which includes the doctor and all who provide care, is there for one purpose only—to help patients get well. The patient's mental attitude is an important factor in his illness; he should be free from unnecessary concern. Therefore, patients are strongly advised to ignore the tales which "friends" may tell and to seek answers from their doctor and the hospital staff so that they understand to their complete satisfaction the care they will receive. Many have found to their surprise that the hospital is a very interesting and, for the most part, a very pleasant place.

CHAPTER SIX

HOME NURSING CARE

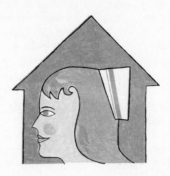

WHEN A PATIENT is sick at home, it makes extra work for the homemaker—usually the mother. The secret of success for her in the role of nurse is organized efficiency, to make each of her moves count, and to avoid all unnecessary walking, lifting, or climbing stairs. The sickroom should be near a bathroom and, if possible, on the same floor with the living rooms and kitchen. It should be light, pleasant, well-heated, and well-ventilated. It should be uncluttered without being forbiddingly bare.

The Patient's Bed

Patients confined to bed are most easily cared for in a high bed such as is used in hospitals. If the illness is likely to be long, such a bed may be purchased; if short, one may be rented. If the patient needs much lifting, a bed that can be mechanically raised, lowered, or tilted, is a great strength-saver to the attendant. For children or helpless old people, the bed should have safety rails. Chairs backed up to the side of the bed are some protection against falling out. Ordinary beds may be raised by removing casters and placing the legs securely on blocks of the desired height; such beds are not easily movable, however.

Patients who can get out of bed to use the bathroom or sit up or move about need a low bed to avoid falls. Such a bed should stand firmly so that it will not slip away from the patient. A footstool is often helpful.

The sickbed mattress should be smooth and soft, but firm. It may be supported by a bed board, which can be cut out of plywood at home or purchased ready-cut.

The principal requirements of a good sickbed are clean, smooth linens, covers of the right warmth for the season, light in weight, and washable. Protective plastic or rubber pads under the hips are needed if the patient is unable to control his bladder or bowels. Disposable waterproof pads are available for this use.

Making the sickbed with a patient in it can also be learned from a visiting nurse or in a nursing course. Essentially it consists in making one half of the bed while the patient lies on the other; then rolling the patient gently to the made-up side and finishing up the other.

Ideally, linens should be fresh daily, but some concessions may have to be made to laundry facilities. The most important feature of the sickbed is to keep it free from wrinkles or crumbs which may irritate the skin and start bedsores.

The very sick patient's position must be changed frequently to avoid continuous pressure on any skin area. In the absence of a mechanical hospital-type bed, backrests may be purchased or made at home. A small chair placed upside down behind the patient will do. Cradles or hoops keep the weight of the bedclothes off the toes. A cardboard carton wrapped in a light blanket may be placed under the covers wherever their weight causes discomfort; a rolled-up blanket or pillow serves the same purpose. To raise one end of the bed higher than the other, blocks may be used. Rubber or plastic rings ("doughnuts") can be purchased for special purposes, such as protection of heels, elbows, and buttocks. Rolled rings of cotton wound with bandages will serve the same purpose, but they tend to flatten out and must be replaced often.

If a regular bed table is not available for serving meals, writing, or other convalescent time-passing, one can be made from a wooden box by knocking out two sides and bracing the ends. If there is a real carpenter in the house, this is a chance for him to show his skills. An ironing board adjustable for height can be placed by the bedside with one end projecting over the bed.

Patients who need help in sitting up or letting themselves back into a lying position often find a strong rope, attached to a post at the foot of the bed, helpful. It should have a loop which is easy to get a grip on.

A bed patient who is not too ill needs help to keep from getting bored. He should have a big bedside table handy, with disposable tissues, drinking water, a clock, a radio, a bell to call for assistance, and room for books, writing materials, puzzles, games, or whatever else he wants. A TV set with remote control is nice if one can afford it. It should be placed where it can be easily seen and where lights and reflections do not interfere with a good picture. An earpiece or under-the-pillow speaker helps to keep sound from disturbing other members of the household.

Planning the Attendant's Day

The usual sickroom attendant is the homemaker, who is compelled to add this duty to her many other responsibilities. Unless she plans her day, she will be likely to suffer under the added strain.

Suggestions for a patient's daily routine are as follows:

"Early morning: Use of toilet, bedside commode or bedpan. Wash hands and face. Brush teeth and hair. Ventilate room. Straightening bedding and patient's clothing.

During the day: Meals and snacks, as permitted in the diet. Bath and linen change. Medications, procedures, and treatments (by homemaker, public health nurse, therapists, etc.) prescribed by doctor. Toileting. Hand and face washing and care of mouth. Back rub and rearrangement of bedding for comfort and support.

During the day: Ventilation of room. Needed articles placed in reach: light, call device, fresh drinking water, bedpan or urinal, if patient can use without assistance.

During the night: Any care the patient requires, or the doctor orders."*

The home nurse should not be too conscientious. The family should insist, for her own sake and that of the patient and the rest of the family, that she get her necessary rest and sleep, except in serious emergencies. She should also get away from the home and the

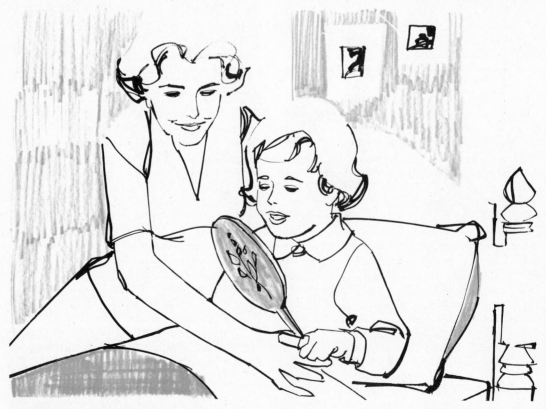

_____
*Home Nursing Handbook, Dorothy White Cotton.
© 1963 Metropolitan Life Insurance Co. Used by permission.

patient from time to time, making arrangements for a substitute to take her place. Relatives who render such service are more useful than those who bring the patient sweets that he cannot have, flowers that he cannot enjoy, or chicken broth which has little nourishment. Even the patient may need to be restricted from becoming too demanding. The last thing the family needs at this time is an exhausted or sick homemaker.

Obviously all routines must be varied to suit circumstances. The important point is that following a system is better than an attempt to do the job in a haphazard manner.

The sickroom attendant should wear simple clothing easily laundered; a coverall apron is desirable, because it can be removed and left in the sickroom after the patient has been cared for. When the patient has a communicable disease, the apron should always be hung inside out when not in use.

Handwashing after caring for the patient is also a necessity, especially when the disease is a communicable one. Disinfectants need not be used on the skin unless the physician gives instructions to do so.

A paper bag fastened to the side of the bed with adhesive tape is convenient for the disposal of handkerchief tissues and prevents contamination from handling used tissues. A wastebasket near the bed is handy for both patient and attendant.

Supplies

The following supplies are helpful to have in the home. Their use and care are briefly outlined:

First Aid Kit. Each family should have a box of supplies that includes finger bandages, adhesive, sterile gauze pads, roller bandage, and a disinfectant. These can be purchased at a minimal price or perhaps put together by a teen-ager who has taken a first-aid course in school.

Thermometer. Normal body temperature is approximately 98.6 F. These are instructions for the use of a mouth or oral thermometer:

1. After washing your hands, rinse the thermometer in cool water.

2. Shake the thermometer with a quick "flip of the wrist" until the mercury goes below at least 95°.

3. Insert the thermometer under the tongue and instruct the patient to hold his mouth closed for at least three minutes.

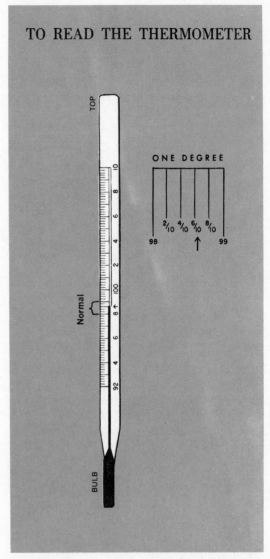

TO READ THE THERMOMETER

Each home medicine chest should have a thermometer.

4. Remove the thermometer and rotate it until the point at which the mercury has settled can be visualized. Each little graduation between the numerals is equal to .2°. Read and note the temperature and the time it was taken.

Use of rectal thermometer:

1. Follow steps 1 and 2 above.

2. Lubricate the thermometer with some petroleum jelly on a piece of tissue.

3. Place the patient on his side, instructing him to breathe deeply through his mouth.

4. Gently separate the buttocks with your left hand and insert the thermometer with your right hand up to the 98.6° mark. The thermometer should remain inserted for at least three to five minutes. It should be held in place for children and elderly patients.

5. Upon removal, wipe the thermometer with the tissue used for lubrication, read, and record.

Wash the thermometer thoroughly with soap and cold water (never hot)—using a piece of cotton, rub vigorously. If the person has a contagious or infectious disease, soak in 70 per cent alcohol or comparable disinfecting agent for a minimum of 30 minutes and preferably overnight.

Hot Water Bottle. The temperature of the water should never exceed 120°. The home nurse usually will have to test the temperature over her wrist if a bath thermometer is not available. The bottle should be checked for leaks. It should never be applied directly to the skin but wrapped first in a turkish towel or piece of flannelette. The condition of the skin should be checked frequently to be certain that the individual is not being burned. A hot water bottle should not be applied without doctor's orders to persons who have difficulties with circulation, who are diabetics, or who are unconscious. Rubber goods can be cleaned with warm soap and water.

Heating Pads. The wiring should be checked carefully. Continuous use is not recommended for small children or older people who may not be aware of the possibility of a burn. The same rules apply as with hot water bottles.

Bedpans, Commodes, Hospital Beds. In the case of a prolonged illness, it is helpful to have this type of equipment in the home. Bedpans are fairly inexpensive to purchase. Commodes and hospital beds may be rented. If the family has inadequate funds, this type of equipment may be borrowed through certain community agencies.

Care of the Bed Patient

No medication should be on a shelf unless it has been specifically ordered for a specific purpose by a doctor. It is a good habit from time to time to clean the medicine shelf and discard old prescriptions *not* into a wastebasket, but into the toilet bowl. Medicines tend to deteriorate or lose their strength and are potentially dangerous to children and older persons. All medicines should be kept out of the reach of children. All bottles should be properly labeled.

The doctor orders medicine on the basis of his diagnosis. He will give directions for dosage and times. It is important to keep enough medicine on hand and not to change or omit dosage unless so instructed by the doctor. Children

occasionally will take pills more easily if they are crushed and put in a teaspoon of corn or maple syrup or jelly. It is not a good idea to use orange juice for this purpose since the child may later associate the bitter taste of a pill with orange juice. Adding medicine to a baby's formula is not recommended since the entire bottle might not be taken.

Some people are sensitive to certain drugs. If reactions appear, the medicine should be discontinued and the doctor called. The following conditions may possibly occur with certain medications as shown below:

1. *Aspirin or Preparations including Aspirin*. Buzzing in the ears, rapid breathing, swelling of lips or other parts of the body.

2. *Sulfa Drugs*. Rash on any part of the body (may look like hives, or may be splotchy or a fine powdery rash), bloody urine.

3. *Penicillin*. Rash (as described above), pains in joints, difficulty in swallowing or breathing.

4. *Digitalis*. Vomiting, diarrhea, irregular or very slow pulse.

Taking the Pulse

Your doctor may ask you to take and record the pulse. If so, do it after the patient has been at rest for a little while. This can be done while taking an oral temperature.

Place two or three fingers (not your thumb) on the palm side of the patient's wrist closest to his thumb. Feel for the beat by pressing down slightly. Once you have located it, count the pulse for one full minute using a watch with a second hand. Record the number of beats per minute and any irregularities you may notice.

Occasionally the doctor will decide that an enema is needed. He will specify the solution; if not, *tepid* tap water is safe. If a soapsuds enema is ordered, swish some mild soap through the water. Never use a detergent. When giving an enema, all of the necessary equipment including protective covering for the bed, a cotton bath blanket, toilet paper, a pitcher, irrigating can or enema bag, with attachment and clamp, lubricant, and rectal tubing should be assembled. Prepare the solution in a pitcher, then transfer it to the enema bag.

Place the patient on his left side in bed. Let some solution run through the tube to remove air bubbles and then close clamp. Lubricate the rectal tube with petroleum jelly and insert no more than three to four inches of its length into the anal opening, and open clamp. The can or

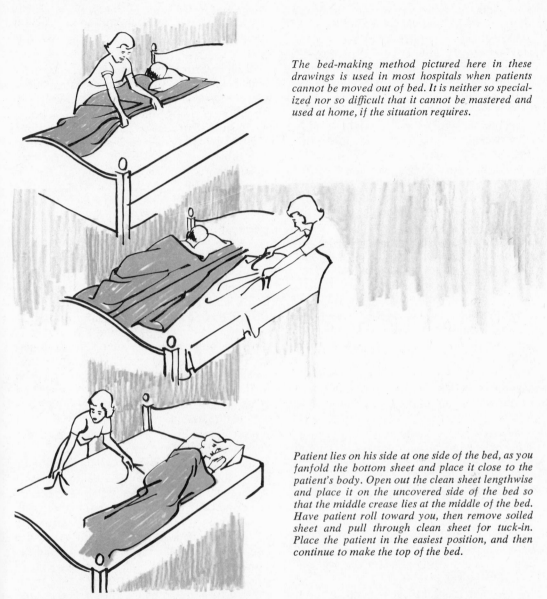

The bed-making method pictured here in these drawings is used in most hospitals when patients cannot be moved out of bed. It is neither so specialized nor so difficult that it cannot be mastered and used at home, if the situation requires.

Patient lies on his side at one side of the bed, as you fanfold the bottom sheet and place it close to the patient's body. Open out the clean sheet lengthwise and place it on the uncovered side of the bed so that the middle crease lies at the middle of the bed. Have patient roll toward you, then remove soiled sheet and pull through clean sheet for tuck-in. Place the patient in the easiest position, and then continue to make the top of the bed.

bag should be held no higher than 18 inches from the surface of the bed. The solution should go in slowly and the patient encouraged to retain it for 5 to 10 minutes. If able, the patient may walk to the bathroom—if not, he can be placed on a bedpan. In some instances a patient either cannot retain the solution or he cannot turn on his side. In such a case, he can be placed on a bedpan for the enema.

Comfort, cleanliness, prevention of bedsores, and nutritious foods are very important in a long illness.

The teenage daughter in the family may volunteer to see that the patient washes his face and hands in the morning and possibly prepare and serve the breakfast. Then later some other person can bathe the patient. All parts of the body from head to foot should be washed, the back massaged, and the skin observed for sore and reddened areas. The bed covers, during the bath, can be folded down and an old cotton blanket used to cover the invalid and keep him warm.

The bath water should be obtained only after the other supplies have been assembled as it cools quickly and chills the patient. Near the end of the bath, the patient's feet should be washed in a tub of water—the bed can be protected with newspaper or a piece of plastic material. If possible, the sheets can be tightened or changed while the patient is out of bed in a chair for a few moments.

If the patient cannot get out of bed, the following procedure can be used:

1. Assemble clean sheets and pillowcases in a convenient place. Pillowcases can be changed first if desired. Remove spread, blankets, and drape over a nearby chair. Loosen top and bottom sheets.

2. Ask patient to lie on his side at one side of bed and place sheets loosely, close to his body. You stand on the opposite side.

3. Fan-fold the bottom sheet and place close to the patient's body. The bed has now been half-stripped and the remaining linen pushed up to patient.

4. Open out clean sheet lengthwise, place on the uncovered side of the bed so that the middle crease lies at the middle of the bed. Tuck the sheet on this side.

5. Have the patient roll toward you protecting him from rolling too far with your body. Then walk around to the other side of the bed.

6. Remove the soiled sheet; pull through the clean sheet and tuck in securely.

7. If necessary, a draw sheet to protect the bed could have been placed on top of the clean bottom sheet and pulled through with it.

8. Place the patient in a comfortable position and make the top of the bed.

If the invalid has no control over his elimination, a plastic mattress cover can be used to protect the mattress, and soft pads can be used to protect the bed linen. Disposable pads can be purchased in a drugstore or made at home from odd pieces of material. It is important that the patient not lie in a wet or wrinkled bed for any length of time since his skin must be kept dry to avoid bedsores and consequent serious difficulties.

It is also important that the patient not lie on his back or in one position for any prolonged length of time. He should be encouraged to move or if necessary turned several times during the day to avoid bedsores and congestion of the lungs. When lying on his side, the patient's back can be supported by a pillow placed lengthwise and folded under once. A plastic covering will protect the pillow from becoming grossly soiled.

Keeping sickroom records is a great help to the physician, the home attendant, or any visiting nurse who may be engaged to come in for special treatments. A simple notebook will do, or a chart may be purchased or drawn for making the records. Any instructions from the doc-

tor should be written down so as to avoid misunderstanding; so also should the questions it is desired to ask the doctor, lest they be forgotten when he arrives.

Such records should include not only pulse and temperature but the patient's complaints, signs of restlessness, pain, or other unusual observation, giving of medicines, time of bowel action, and frequency and amount of urination.

A back rub can be given with hands warmed and lubricated with alcohol or a prescribed lotion. Starting at the neck, the massage is carried with long, slow gentle strokes to the buttocks and back again. It usually follows the back. It is relaxing and comforting and helps to prevent bedsores.

Giving Medicines

Giving medicines exactly as the doctor ordered is best assured by setting an alarm or electric timer for the times when medication is due, or by routinely giving it at the same time the pulse and temperature are taken. Medicines should not be left where the patient can take them. In giving medicine the label should be read before opening the bottle or package and again after the dose has been measured to be sure that there is no mistake. Bottle labels can be protected by covering with transparent plastic tape, and by pouring from the side opposite the label. Medicines which "settle" or grow cloudy should always be shaken.

Those for external use only should be identified by an adhesive strap over the stopper. This signal gives warning immediately when the bottle is handled. Liquid medicine doses are best measured with a medicine glass or a measuring spoon, since household utensils vary in size. Drops should be counted out loud.

Medicines should be given at the exact time ordered by the doctor, since absorption is influenced by food in the stomach; some drugs are less irritating when taken on a full stomach.

Pills or powders are more easily given with a spoon. You should place the medication well back on the tongue and have a glass of water or juice ready.

When giving medication to children, you should treat it as medicine, not as candy. Confusion between candy and medicines accounts for many poisonings in childhood, aside from the fact that honesty is the best policy, especially since the children are not deceived anyway.

Changing dressings may be necessary for a

while after surgery or injury. Here it is important to avoid infecting the wound or carrying infection from the wound to the dresser's hands and so to others. Sterilized dressings can be purchased in packages; but it should be remembered that as soon as the package is opened, it becomes nonsterile. It should therefore not be opened until it is to be used at once.

The hands should be washed thoroughly beforehand, and kitchen forceps sterilized by boiling. These forceps are used to handle the soiled dressings, which are dropped into the disposal bag at the side of the bed. The clean dressing is then applied and held in place with adhesive straps which have been cut beforehand. The hands are washed again, and the forceps sterilized. The disposal bag is then closed and burned. Finally, the dresser's hands are washed again.

Heat applied locally may be prescribed by the physician, who will specify whether it is to be given through the use of a hot water bottle, a heating pad, radiant heat from an electric heater, or a hot wet pack. Heat must be applied with caution to avoid burning the patient, especially if he has been bedridden for a long time. Heat should not be kept on during sleep. Hot water bottles should be wrapped in towels to prevent direct contact; heating pads should be kept at low or moderate heat. All heat applications should be watched closely.

Hot wet packs require careful protection of the bed against wetting by use of rubber or plastic sheets. Cloths should be wrung out of water which has been carefully checked for temperature to avoid burning, and placed over the area to be treated. The wet cloth is then covered with another plastic or rubber sheet to retain heat and moisture. The patient's comfort should be checked constantly, or if the patient is unconscious, the condition of the skin

watched to prevent burning.

Steam inhalations may be given by boiling a kettle on an electric plate so as to fill the entire room with vapor. The steam source can then be safely placed away from the sickbed. If inhalation directly into a steam tent over the patient must be given, great care is necessary to avoid fire or burning the patient with hot steam too close to the body. Such a steam inhalation should always be closely watched by an attendant to prevent accidents caused by the patient's movements in bed. This is particularly important when the patient is a child, or is very ill, very old, or in a state of confusion. Exposure to cold air or drafts should be avoided for at least an hour after a steam treatment.

Very sick patients or weakened convalescents should have as much rest and as little disturbance as possible. They should receive their necessary care quickly and quietly, and various procedures should be grouped to avoid frequent disturbances. Patients who are recovering rapidly may welcome more frequent attention to help them avoid boredom.

The attending physician should be asked for specific instruction about whether a sleeping patient should be awakened for pulse and temperature observations, medications, or other treatments. Sleep may be more important, or vice versa, depending on the circumstances.

Whenever a home-care procedure appears difficult or is not fully understood, a demonstration can be had in most communities by calling a health department or a visiting nurse association and arranging for a nurse to call at the home. The expense is small.

Since few homemakers will escape becoming sickroom attendants, especially where there are old people or children, a course in home nursing offered by the American Red Cross or other community agency is a sensible preparation.

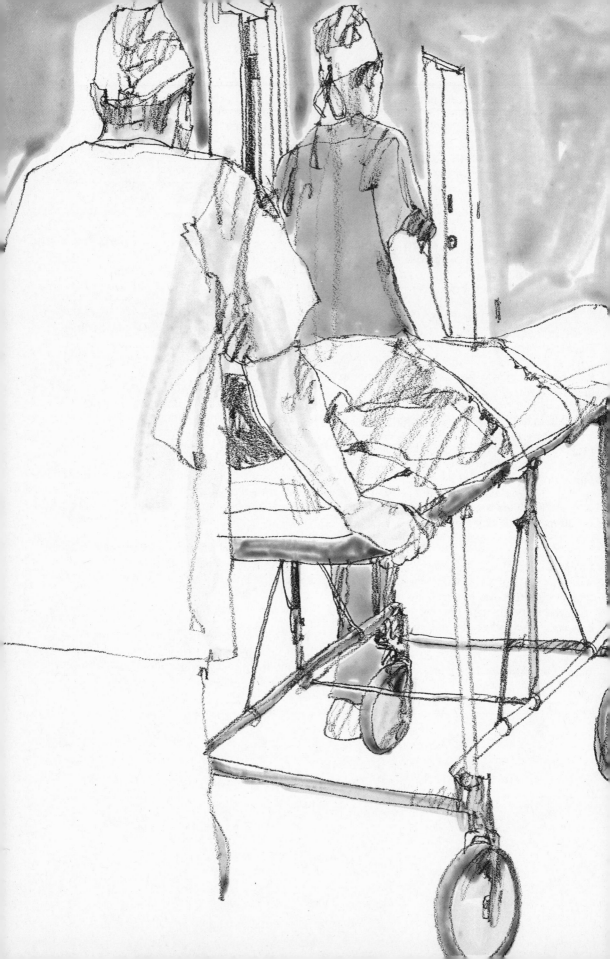

PART X

Dangerous and Disabling Diseases

CHAPTER ONE

THE HEART AND CIRCULATORY SYSTEM

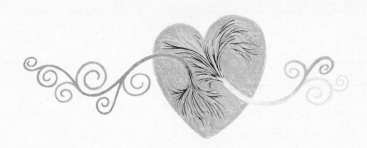

THE TERM HEART DISEASE actually applies to a number of different illnesses that affect the circulatory system—the heart and blood vessels. A more exact name is cardiovascular diseases—cardio (heart) and vascular (blood vessel).

The circulatory system is a complicated mechanism that in most people runs smoothly for a lifetime. The heart itself is the strongest, toughest muscle in the body. Yet, like all machinery, it can sometimes break down. When any part of the circulatory system is impaired, a part of the body does not receive the blood supply it needs and thus is damaged. The damage may occur in the heart itself, in the brain, the lungs, the kidneys, the skin, or the limbs.

More than 10,000,000 Americans of all ages have some form of heart or blood vessel disorder. These diseases are by no means always fatal, but they cause more than half of all the deaths in the United States every year. So many people are affected by just one of the cardiovascular diseases, arterial atherosclerosis, that it has been called "the epidemic of the 20th century."

Great improvements have been made in the treatment and control of some of these diseases. Because of medical advances, thousands of people are living today who 10 or 20 years ago would not have survived their illness. With proper medical care, most people with cardiovascular ailments can work and live useful lives. Rheumatic fever, which may lead to one form of heart trouble, as well as a few other less common heart diseases, can now be prevented. Consequently the incidence of these diseases already is decreasing in frequency.

To make the best use of modern medical knowledge about heart diseases, it is important to visit your family doctor regularly for a physical checkup. If you think you have any symptoms of a heart ailment, don't try to diagnose the condition yourself—see your doctor. If all is well, he will relieve you of your worries. If something is wrong, the earlier it is detected, the better.

Atherosclerosis

Atherosclerosis is a form of arteriosclerosis, or hardening of the arteries. Most heart attacks can be traced to atherosclerosis of the coronary arteries, through which travels the blood which nourishes the heart muscle. Most strokes result from atherosclerosis in the arteries that deliver blood to the brain.

This disease may begin at an early age and go undetected until the middle years or later. Most people have it to some degree without troublesome symptoms and live a normal life span.

In atherosclerosis, the inner walls of the arteries are gradually thickened and roughened by deposits of fatty material. As more layers of deposits are formed, they narrow the channel through the artery, hindering the flow of blood. When the artery wall is considerably roughened, blood clots may form on the roughened areas and block circulation at that point.

Research scientists are seeking the causes of atherosclerosis and ways to prevent and cure it. Changing the fat content of our diet may be one approach, and long-range studies are underway to discover whether a modified fat diet will help to prevent heart attacks and strokes. Other factors being investigated include the role of exercise or its lack, emotional stress, heredity, excessive smoking, and sex hormones.

Excessive smoking, especially of cigarettes, is regarded by many scientists as a contributory cause to heart and blood vessel diseases, because of the constricting effect of smoking on the smaller arteries. In one arterial disease,

Buerger's disease, smoking has a definitely unfavorable influence and perhaps may even be a precipitating cause. (See also Part XII, Chapter Three.)

Heart Attacks

Usually what is meant by a heart attack is what doctors call coronary thrombosis or myocardial infarction. It is a sudden blocking of one of the arteries that supply the heart muscle with blood. A clogged artery may be closed by a blood clot (thrombus), and the part of the heart muscle fed by that artery may deteriorate or die from lack of blood. In such cases, healing begins almost immediately, and scar tissues begin to form in the damaged area of the heart. Treatment and rest give the heart time to heal itself. For some patients, doctors prescribe drugs to prevent new clots from forming.

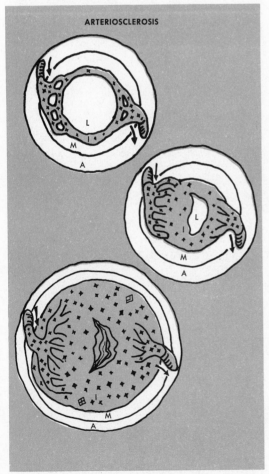

Arteriosclerosis changes normal artery (top) to severe condition (bottom): media (M) is thinned; lumen (L) has blood clot (C) on portion of intima (I).

Heart attack symptoms vary greatly and are not easy to identify. However, when the following symptoms occur, a doctor should be called at once:

● Moderate or severe pain or an uncomfortable sensation of pressure in the front of the chest. This sometimes spreads to the arms, throat, or back, and often lasts for hours, especially when it is accompanied by sweating, shortness of breath, weakness, or occasional loss of consciousness. Often the patient does not experience what he considers to be pain and hence does not think he has a heart attack.

● Nausea and vomiting. These symptoms can be mistaken for acute indigestion; only a physician can tell the difference.

Until the doctor takes charge, the patient should be placed in a position most comfortable for him, either lying or sitting. Tight clothing should be loosened. The patient should be kept from chilling, but he should not be made to perspire by use of too many blankets. He should not be lifted or carried without the doctor's supervision, or given anything to drink without the doctor's advice.

The time needed for a patient to recover depends on the extent of heart damage, the rate of healing, and whether or not complications develop. Most people can return to work after recovery, although some may have to make adjustments in their jobs and manner of living.

Angina Pectoris

Angina pectoris is an uncomfortable sensation of pressure, tightness, or pain usually in the front part of the chest. It is a sign that the heart muscle is not getting enough oxygen through its blood supply. An attack is ordinarily brought on by overexercise, excitement, or overeating. Usually, rest or nitroglycerine tablets will relieve the pain in a few minutes.

Angina pains may occur both in a person who has recovered from a heart attack, or in one who has never had a heart attack and may never have one. Nevertheless, severe chest discomfort should always be reported to a doctor because it could be the forerunner of a heart attack. Chest discomfort, of course, can also have many other causes.

Stroke

A stroke occurs when the blood supply to a part of the brain is reduced or completely cut off. This can be caused by a blood clot or by

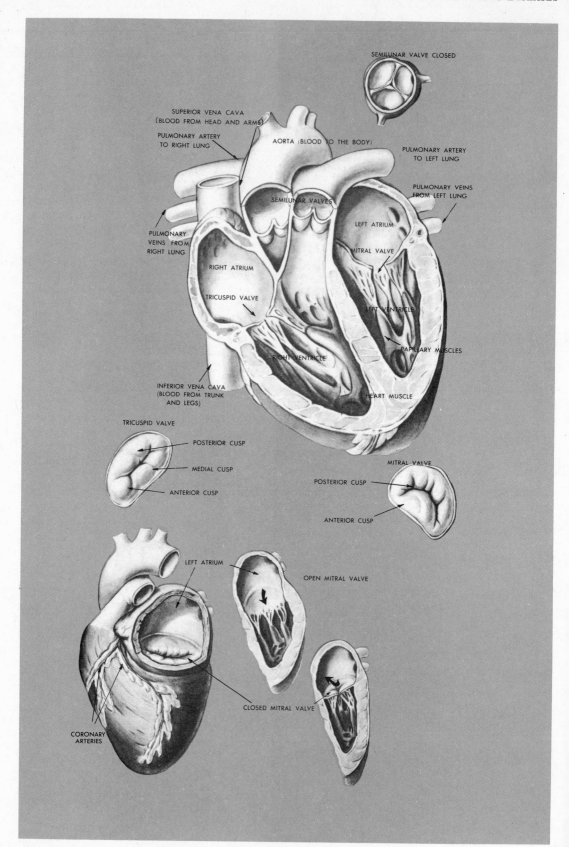

SEMILUNAR VALVE CLOSED

SUPERIOR VENA CAVA
(BLOOD FROM HEAD AND ARMS)

PULMONARY ARTERY
TO RIGHT LUNG

AORTA (BLOOD TO THE BODY)

PULMONARY ARTERY
TO LEFT LUNG

PULMONARY VEINS
FROM LEFT LUNG

SEMILUNAR VALVES

LEFT ATRIUM

MITRAL VALVE

PULMONARY
VEINS FROM
RIGHT LUNG

RIGHT ATRIUM

TRICUSPID VALVE

LEFT VENTRICLE

PAPILIARY MUSCLES

RIGHT VENTRICLE

INFERIOR VENA CAVA
(BLOOD FROM TRUNK
AND LEGS)

HEART MUSCLE

TRICUSPID VALVE

POSTERIOR CUSP

MEDIAL CUSP

ANTERIOR CUSP

MITRAL VALVE

POSTERIOR CUSP

ANTERIOR CUSP

LEFT ATRIUM

OPEN MITRAL VALVE

CLOSED MITRAL VALVE

CORONARY
ARTERIES

hemorrhage—bleeding from an artery in the brain. Medical terms used for various kinds of strokes are cerebral vascular occlusion, cerebral thrombosis, cerebral embolism, and cerebral hemorrhage.

When the nerve cells of a part of the brain are deprived of their blood supply, the part of the body controlled by these nerve centers cannot function normally. The result may be weakness or paralysis, difficulty in speaking, or loss of memory.

Some patients recover quickly, and can resume their normal activities. Others may suffer such serious damage that even a partial recovery will take a long time. Immediate treatment with proper exercises and other forms of therapy can do much toward helping a patient regain the use of muscles and speech. If a stroke is brought on by a narrowed blood vessel or, in some instances, a blood clot, the doctor may use anti-coagulant drugs to prevent another stroke. When neck arteries leading to the brain are involved, a surgical operation can sometimes remove the obstruction to circulation.

Rehabilitation for stroke requires the cooperation of the doctor, the patient, and the family. The patient's own will to avoid invalidism and to become independent is especially important.

Rheumatic Fever

Rheumatic fever usually occurs between the ages of 5 and 15, although adults can also have it. It accounts for most of the heart disease found in children and young adults. Rheumatic fever may affect any part of the body temporarily, but damage to the heart, which can be long lasting, is the greatest danger.

Rheumatic heart disease results from the scarring of the heart muscle and valves by rheumatic fever. This may interfere with the vital work of the heart. Many patients recover from rheumatic fever without permanent injury to the heart valves. However, this disease has a way of repeating itself, and each attack renews the chances of heart damage.

Rheumatic fever is always preceded by a streptococcal infection such as a strep sore throat, scarlet fever, or a strep ear infection. Rheumatic fever can be prevented by treating the strep infection promptly and thoroughly with antibiotics. Because persons who have had rheumatic fever are susceptible rather than immune to repeat attacks, long-term preventive treatment is often prescribed for them. Regular doses of penicillin or sulfa drugs, under the direction of a physician, can prevent further strep infections and thus ward off subsequent attacks of rheumatic fever.

You can protect your own child against rheumatic fever by calling the doctor if he develops a sudden, severe sore throat, or if he has been exposed to someone with scarlet fever or another strep infection.

High Blood Pressure

Blood pressure is the pressure put on the walls of the arteries as the heart pumps blood through them. It is perfectly normal for blood pressure to vary from time to time; it may go up when we are excited and go down when we are at rest. However, in some people blood pressure remains at higher levels than it should. This condition is called hypertension and about 5,000,000 people in the United States have it. Continued high blood pressure overworks the heart and circulatory system and thus reduces their ability to function as well as they should. The kidneys can also be affected.

Hypertension sometimes causes no symptoms and only a doctor can tell when it is present. Treatment can do a great deal to control it. Doctors can choose from an increasing number of drugs and other methods of management, such as diet and changes in living habits.

Low blood pressure occurs in many healthy people, and is usually considered an asset.

Congenital Heart Defects

This kind of heart defect is present at birth, although it may not be discovered until later. In it, the heart or a major blood vessel near the heart fails to mature normally during the period of growth before birth. About 30,000 to 40,000 children are born with heart defects in the United States each year.

Mild inborn defects may never cause trouble; but serious ones may interfere with circulation of the blood, slow the child's growth, and reduce his energy. Because of great progress in heart surgery, most patients with congenital heart defects can be restored to normal or near-normal health.

Congestive Heart Failure

To say that a person has heart failure does not mean that his heart has stopped beating. In congestive heart failure, the heart muscle goes on working, but with less strength than is needed for good health. This condition may follow a severe heart attack or rheumatic fever, or it may occur in connection with a congenital heart defect or with very high blood pressure. It often results, especially in elderly people, from muscle damage due to atherosclerosis of the coronary arteries.

The usual symptoms are swelling of legs and ankles (edema) and extreme shortness of breath. Treatment includes drugs to strengthen the action of the heart; rest to ease its work load; and diet or drugs, especially digitalis and diuretics, to control edema.

Patients who follow their doctor's instructions faithfully find that their heart failure can be controlled. Usually they can carry on their normal activities while guarding their hearts against extra strain.

Other Ailments

Bacterial endocarditis is an infection of the lining of the heart. People with rheumatic heart disease or inborn heart defects are particularly susceptible to it. To protect these patients, doctors prescribe antibiotics to be taken when bacteria have a chance to enter the bloodstream— for example, in conjunction with dental treat-ment that breaks the gums; operations of the mouth, nose, or throat; childbirth; or surgery of the gastrointestinal or urinary tracts.

Peripheral vascular diseases affect blood vessels of the extremities—chiefly the legs and feet, and less often the arms and hands. By interfering with circulation, these diseases cause symptoms ranging from mild discomfort to pain and swelling. If allowed to go untreated, they can result in more serious complications, such as skin ulcers that are difficult to cure. Varicose veins, the bulging veins that usually appear in the legs, are a common peripheral vascular disorder. Atherosclerosis of the extremities is another. In it, arteries in the limbs are affected by the same process of atherosclerosis that takes place in arteries of the heart and brain.

In thrombophlebitis, the inner wall of a vein is inflamed and a blood clot is usually attached to the vein wall. Venous thrombosis is a similar condition but without the inflammation.

These are the most common cardiovascular diseases which, in the majority of people, can be treated successfully by medical or surgical means. The ideal, of course, is to prevent these diseases from occurring altogether. Each year medical science is gaining knowledge that brings us closer to that goal.

CHAPTER TWO

DIABETES

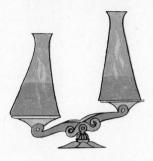

MORE THAN 3,000,000 diabetics in the United States face the prospect of disability from their disease. Their number is increasing rapidly because of the general aging of the population. These patients, their families, and friends should attempt to understand the nature of diabetes. Particularly important are the problems of adjustment of its victims and the principles of therapy involved. With proper education and care, the diabetic can live a nearly normal life.

Diabetes mellitus is a disorder in which the body fails to make proper use of sugar. An excessive amount accumulates in the blood and often passes in the urine. Normally, insulin helps to burn sugar and provide energy. This is a hormone secreted by the pancreas which is a gland situated in the upper abdomen. When the pancreas fails to produce enough insulin, the person cannot utilize sugar, and his body chemistry is upset. He is, in short, a diabetic. Insulin must then be injected in most instances to make up for the patient's deficiency. Oral or tablet treatment is limited to milder cases in older people.

The cause of diabetes is unknown, but it is usually due to an inherited tendency. It is more common over the age of 40, in women, and in obese individuals. In some cases the adrenal, pituitary, or thyroid glands are also involved.

Diabetes is one of the oldest diseases known to man. Records in ancient Egypt describing the condition date back to 3,000 B.C. The word "diabetes" was provided by the Roman physician Aretaeus in A.D. 50. It means "to pass through" and refers to the common symptom of frequent urination. The sweet taste of the urine was noticed by Willis of Oxford in his studies of diabetes conducted during the seventeenth century.

In 1889 Von Mering and Minkowski removed the pancreas from a dog and subsequently noted sugar in the urine. In 1922 Banting and Best discovered insulin in extracts of dog pancreas. This knowledge formed the basis for the modern treatment of diabetics.

Recognizing Diabetes

The typical symptoms of diabetes are absent in early or mild cases. Severe disease may cause copious urination, excessive thirst and hunger, tiredness, weight loss, itching, blurred vision, and skin infection. Older people have fewer symptoms, and they can usually be controlled by diet or by pills. Younger patients have unstable sugar balance, may become ill rapidly, and need insulin injections. The disorder may be suspected by the patient or his physician from the nature of his symptoms, or a routine urine test may reveal sugar and indicate a moderately severe case.

Normally the blood glucose ranges between 80 and 120 mg. per 100 cc. of blood after 12 hours without food. Definite elevation on more than one blood sample to more than 140 mg. establishes the diagnosis. Estimating the value two hours after a meal generous in starch is even more conclusive. When the diagnosis is in question, a glucose tolerance test is performed. The blood sugar is measured before, and hourly for several hours after, taking a large amount of glucose. This test indicates the body's efficiency in disposing of sugar and permits the doctor to determine definitely whether the disease is present or not. Mild diabetes may exist even though the urine test is not positive. Even if sugar is present, the doctor must rule out other possible causes, such as spilling of nonglucose sugars, drug administration, kidney, and nervous diseases. The fact that other members of the family have had diabetes often suggests the diagnosis in the person under consideration.

Managing Diabetes

The object of treatment of diabetes is to control it without interfering unnecessarily with

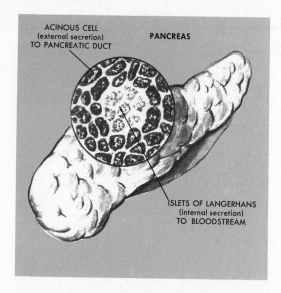

ACINOUS CELL
(external secretion)
TO PANCREATIC DUCT

PANCREAS

ISLETS OF LANGERHANS
(internal secretion)
TO BLOODSTREAM

the patient's daily routine. This is considered to be accomplished when the urine is almost always free of sugar (although it may still be present after a meal), when weight and energy are adequate, and when the blood sugar is reasonably normal. Besides improving the symptoms, good control offers a reduced likelihood of infection, undernutrition, acidosis, and blood vessel disease. Even though the excess sugar and other manifestations may be eliminated by therapy, diabetes cannot be cured because the pancreas still does not produce enough insulin.

Diet: Diabetes may be controlled by diet alone in at least half of those patients who developed the disease after the age of 30. Foods containing large amounts of sugar and starch increase the amount of sugar which the body must burn. Thus their intake must be limited. If the patient is obese, his caloric intake must also be limited because losing weight improves the patient's condition by reducing the demand on the pancreas for insulin.

The important consideration in the diabetic's diet is that he should eat the correct amount of the proper kind of food every day. Starches are limited and fats are increased proportionately. The method used to control intake may be either a system of weighing the food or the ordinary household measuring system. Which method is chosen depends on the severity of the disease, the patient's intelligence, and the physician's opinion. The quantitative program, in which the patient learns to estimate weights of foods accurately, permits delicate balancing of the carbohydrate content of food against the

amount of insulin injected. This program is carried out most rapidly and effectively in the hospital where adequate medical, dietary, and laboratory information is available.

"Free" sugars, such as those found in candy, jelly, syrup, and honey, are omitted, and artificial sweeteners are substituted. Hard or soft drinks containing sugar are prohibited, but carbonated beverages low in sugar and calories may be taken. Substitution lists for the major food groups (milk, vegetable-fruit, bread-cereal, and meat) are provided so that the same amount of carbohydrate, protein, fat, and calories may be eaten daily. This provides variety, and mixed dishes may be prepared when the patient gains understanding of food content. The physician calculates the dietary prescription to provide good nutrition and proper weight and sugar balance with regard to insulin, work and exercise habits, and possible oral medication. Details should be discussed with a dietician if possible.

Testing: Every diabetic should learn to test his urine for sugar and for acid indicators. Not to test is like trying to drive an automobile with your eyes closed. Tests depend upon a chemical reaction which occurs when a copper sulphate solution (Benedict's) is exposed to urine containing sugar (glucose). The standard method is to heat the urine with Benedict's solution, and observe the color changes which occur if glucose is present. These range from green through yellow to orange; the greater the color change, the higher the percentage of sugar.

For convenience, this test can be made on paper tapes, but these are subject to change if they become moist, and it is safest to check with the heat and chemical version. This can be made more convenient with a package containing tablets which furnish both the reacting chemical and the necessary heat. The physician will advise the patient how to procure test materials and how to use them. He will also advise about the acidosis test, which should be made whenever there are indications of sugar in the urine.

Acid substances are formed by the body in severe diabetes when excess sugar is present in the blood and urine because adequate amounts of insulin are lacking. These tests should always be performed when urine sugar is heavy. A positive test is a danger signal and should be reported to the doctor immediately.

Injections: The purpose of insulin is to help the body burn and store sugar. Since the diabetic lacks insulin, sugar accumulates in the blood and tissues. If the diabetic cannot reduce his food intake to the amount which can be burned by the inadequate hormone (insulin) supply from his pancreas, then insulin must be obtained from another source (usually cow or pig pancreas) and injected. Such patients cannot usually get along on oral medication.

In some cases injections are necessary only temporarily, since the disease improves with treatment. In other cases, large amounts must be injected once or even twice every day of the patient's life. This is usually true in young patients and in those with diabetic symptoms or other associated disease. In acute diabetic complications, insulin must be injected every one to six hours in order to control infection, coma due to acidosis, or healing of wounds after surgery or injury.

Three types of insulin are available commercially. Regular or crystalline insulin lowers the blood sugar rapidly but only temporarily (8 to 12 hours). It is used in such emergencies as infection, acidosis, or surgery.

Zinc or protein has been added to some types of insulin so that action is intermediate or prolonged. Greatest effect with their use occurs at 8 to 12 hours; the duration of action is 24 to 36 hours. NPH, Lente, and Globin insulins are the most common types used because their action prevents rise in blood sugar following meals during the day and wears off at night when it is not needed.

Protamine zinc insulin acts slowly but its effect lasts for two or three days. It is useful in controlling mild diabetes in older people.

To make an injection, the skin of the leg or abdomen is cleaned with cotton soaked in alcohol, then it is pinched into a fold, and the needle inserted deeply to the hub. Even if he is not taking insulin, every diabetic should learn to give insulin to himself because of the possibility of urgent need in the future.

If an excessive amount of insulin is taken, the body sugar may drop rapidly to a low level. The lack of sugar supply to the nervous system may cause such symptoms as weakness, shaking, fatigue, drowsiness, extreme hunger, and sweating. As the condition worsens, confusion, poor judgment, hostility, incoordination, and even unconsciousness and convulsions may occur.

In addition to excessive insulin intake, low blood sugar may be caused by improper food intake, diarrhea, or unusual exercise. Or, an improvement in diabetic control with a consequent reduction in need for injected insulin may be another cause.

The standard treatment for a low blood sugar reaction is eating of hard candy or lump sugar which diabetics taking insulin should always carry. The diabetic should also wear an emergency identification symbol and carry an identification card (see Part IX, Chapter One) in case of diabetic coma or insulin shock.

When unconsciousness or difficulty in swallowing is present, the doctor must be called immediately so that sugar may be injected to raise the blood sugar rapidly. The insulin dose is then reduced approximately 10 per cent on the following day. The most important way to prevent reactions is to establish stable sugar balance under the doctor's supervision. Insulin should be injected at the same time each day, meals eaten within a half-hour of schedule, and infections controlled promptly.

Oral Compounds: Until 1954 efforts to replace inconvenient insulin injections with insulin taken by mouth were unsuccessful. In that year a drug was developed in Germany to help control diabetes, and others have been

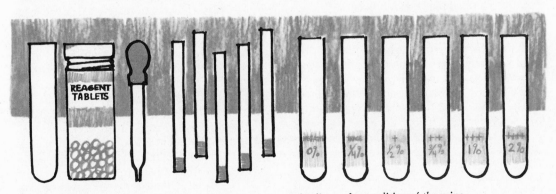

Diabetes test, using materials above, indicates presence of the disease by condition of the urine.
Materials supplied by Diabetes Association

developed since. While these are not true "oral insulins," most mild cases of the disease in patients over 40 which do not respond solely to diet control, may be controlled with these medications. These agents either stimulate the pancreas to produce insulin or increase sugar uptake by the tissues. Thus they may be substituted for small doses of injected insulin. They cannot be employed in severe diabetes or when acute complications are present. They are, however, useful in treating older patients who have difficulty in using an insulin syringe, and also help to control unstable diabetes in persons who use insulin.

Personal Hygiene: The diabetic should indulge in reasonable and regular exercise. It helps to maintain muscle tone and prevent obesity. It may also reduce the insulin dose necessary by using up sugar which otherwise would require insulin. A regular amount of exercise daily will help stabilize the sugar balance. Extra food may be taken if unusual or strenuous exercise is contemplated. Half a sandwich and half a glass of milk may be needed before swimming or playing a set of tennis, full portions before playing 18 holes of golf. Nervous tension and fatigue tend to cause fluctuations in or to elevate blood sugar as a result of the action of other hormones, adrenalin, or cortisone. Changes in the sex hormone balance such as the menstrual cycle, or excessive use of tobacco, alcohol, coffee, or medication may also alter the sugar balance.

An additional reason why many physicians advise their diabetic patients not to smoke is that diabetes is often the cause of arterial deterioration, to which tobacco is believed to contribute in some instances. (See also Part XII, Chapter Three.)

Complications

Failure to maintain a good diabetic balance increases the diabetic's susceptibility to infections. They usually involve the skin, throat, teeth, respiratory system, urinary tract, or feet. Even minor infections should be treated with respect. They tend to recur, as for example, a fungus rash of the skin. Boils may persist and require hot compresses or drainage; wounds may be slow to heal. The diabetic is susceptible to tuberculosis and should have his chest x-rayed annually.

Modern treatment of the diabetic woman has made her chances for fertility normal. With careful control requiring frequent sugar tests and extra insulin, successful delivery is possible in as many as 90 per cent of cases. Diabetic women are more likely than non-diabetic patients to have toxic reactions such as high blood pressure or excessive water retention during pregnancy. Early delivery is usually necessary, about three to four weeks before the anticipated time of birth. A Caesarean section may be performed if normal delivery techniques are not possible or advisable.

When excess sugar accumulates in the blood, fat is burned instead of it for energy. This imbalance, if not corrected, may cause toxic symptoms due to the acid products of fat breakdown. These include abdominal pain, persistent vomiting, dehydration, even coma and death. Acidosis usually results from uncontrolled infection, inadequate insulin dosage, wrong diet, or other factors causing poor diabetic control. Any stress, such as surgery, injury, infection, burns, or severe illness, will contribute to excessive loss of sugar and may lead to acidosis. It is identified by testing the urine. This should be done whenever heavy sugar appears in the usual urine test. If the test indicates that acidosis has occurred, the doctor should be notified immediately. Diabetic acidosis and coma are treated by administering extra insulin and salts and water into the vein.

Changes affecting the heart and blood vessels connected with aging tend to appear somewhat earlier in the diabetic. Coronary artery disease, damage to the small arteries in the eyes, nephritis, and arteriosclerosis of the brain and arteries in the legs may even appear before diabetes is recognized. Symptoms include chest pain, shortness of breath, swollen ankles, dizziness, coldness, and numbness or burning of the legs. Acute ailments, such as heart attacks, visual impairment, uremia, strokes or gangrene, are due to blocking of arteries supplying the affected organs. Normal treatment is to control the sugar balance carefully so as to keep the disease from worsening. Reduction of weight and blood cholesterol is also helpful, and it is probably necessary to increase the ratio of vegetable (unsaturated fatty acid) fat to animal fat in the diet. The doctor must control these treatment factors, but the patient must understand them.

CHAPTER THREE

ARTHRITIS AND RHEUMATISM

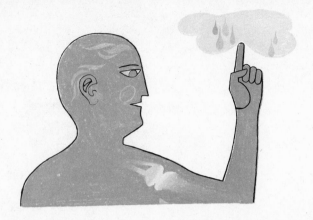

IT IS A RARE ADULT who never experiences some form of arthritis or rheumatism. These diseases are extremely common and are among the oldest known to man. Only in recent years has the magnitude of the health problem of arthritis and rheumatism been appreciated in the United States and throughout the world. As a result, a great deal of new knowledge, understanding, and treatment is available today. Medical scientists have discovered new leads in their search for the causes of various forms of arthritis. Though cure is not yet available, treatment is generally satisfactory, especially if started within the first six months after onset. Very few people today need be crippled by arthritis.

About 12,000,000 Americans have some form of rheumatic disease, that is, about one person out of every 20. Rheumatic diseases are by far the most commonly occurring chronic illnesses in this country—or in the world. In the United States there are twice as many people with rheumatic disease as have the next most common chronic ailment, heart disease. It is estimated that rheumatic disease costs the nation $1,500,000,000 a year. Next to nervous and mental disease, rheumatism causes more days lost from work in our country than any other chronic disease.

Rheumatism is a general term used to describe stiffness and aching pain. Rheumatic diseases are those in which abnormalities are located in the supporting structures of the body, the ligaments, tendons, joints, muscles, and bones—the tough parts of the body.

The body is often regarded as a great aggregation of cells, all of which must be held together and supported by a framework. The framework is called connective tissue, and is mainly made of tough fibrous materials. Con-

nective tissue is an appropriate name for this system since it does, in fact, connect the cells and the parts of the body together. When something goes wrong with the manufacture or the maintenance of the big molecules that make up the tough structures of the body, the result is aching, swelling, pain, stiffness and sometimes heat, redness, and gross inflammation.

Though most rheumatic diseases involve joints, many connective tissues other than joints are also affected. Arthritis really means inflammation of a joint and nothing more specific than that. Thus, though arthritis is a frequent part of most rheumatic diseases, it is certainly not the only part.

There are about 50 different rheumatic diseases. Diagnosis of them is often difficult, requiring considerable study by a physician, many laboratory tests and x-rays. One reason for failure in treatment is that the particular type of rheumatic disease is not identified in the first place. One should not assume one has "arthritis" or "rheumatism" until his doctor has reached a decision regarding diagnosis and appropriate treatment. Some rheumatic diseases require little or no treatment; a few more serious varieties require very extensive and prolonged treatment.

The first step in consideration of any rheumatic disease is accurate diagnosis. The physician usually makes an over-all assessment of the probable outlook and an outline of the treatment program. The treatment is quite individualized. The intensity of the inflammation, the degree of pain and swelling, the patient's age, how long he has had the disease, and his type of work are all factors in determining the best treatment program for any one patient. Drug treatment may be needed in one patient and not in another.

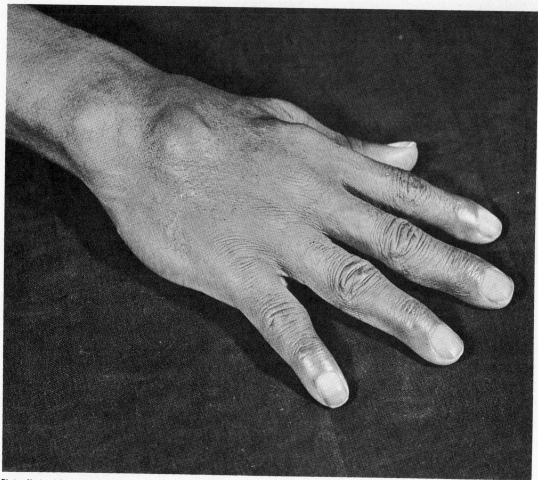

Photo: National Institutes of Health

Rheumatoid arthritis characteristically involves swelling of the knuckles and the finger joints nearest the hand.

The most common rheumatic diseases are rheumatoid arthritis, osteoarthritis, and gout. In addition there are the collagen diseases.

Rheumatoid Arthritis

Rheumatoid arthritis is potentially the most serious of the three chief diseases. However, many victims have only mildly annoying trouble. The disease characteristically occurs in attacks of joint pain and swelling, weakness, fatigue, and stiffness, especially in the morning. The attacks may last for weeks, months, or years, but usually the intensity of the disease fluctuates. The disease varies in severity from time to time, seldom completely disappearing, though a few people have recovered completely. A very small percentage of patients have severe, steadily-worsening arthritis that finally results in crippling and deformity. Rheu-

matoid arthritis is indeed a capricious disease.

The best treatment of rheumatoid arthritis includes a variety of different methods and techniques. When applied in a comprehensive daily program it is very effective. Dependence on any one drug or other single means of treatment is doomed to failure. Rest is a cardinal principle of management and is usually prescribed as a number of hours per day. Details of rest are outlined by the physician or physical therapist. Rheumatoid arthritis is a disease of the whole person, and rest must include the mind and the body as well as the inflamed joints. The bed should be firm; pillows under the knees or back should be avoided. The feet should be supported by a footboard. The bed is easier to get in and out of if blocks six to eight inches in height are placed under the casters. Plaster of Paris splints are used for severely inflamed joints to assure proper rest.

Rest is alternated with exercises and activity. Prescription of the proper balance is the physician's responsibility. Specific exercises are prescribed, among which are muscle strengthening exercises. Joint deformity can be prevented by daily putting the joints, actively or passively, through a full range of motion. The paradox of alternately using exercises and rest puzzles many patients. The arthritic requires both. However, if pain lasts for more than 15 to 20 minutes after exercise, it has been too much.

Rest is necessary to reduce joint inflammation but exercise is required also to retain muscle and joint function and prevent insidious and gradual onset of deformity. Many patients believe they "must keep moving" for fear of "stiffening up." This is not the case; proper balance of rest and exercise is the keynote.

Warm or hot tub baths once or twice daily are helpful. Hot towels wrung out of hot water, applied to the joints and then wrapped in plastic sheets, provide muscle relaxation. Infrared lamps are useful when applied at an 18-inch distance. A towel may be put over the joint being treated. This does not interfere with penetration of the rays, but does avoid skin burn.

Other methods of treatment and aids to the patient include hot paraffin to hands and feet; special splints for specific joints; contrast baths, hot and cold; surgical procedures for certain joints; elevation of the chair the patient sits in, and a special elevated toilet seat. Joint care entails positioning in bed, postural exercises, diet for reduction of body weight, and prescription of certain kinds of work to exercise the joints and muscles.

Education about the characteristic and expected behavior of the disease is very important in order to help the patient anticipate in a general way what his future is to be and to learn how to deal with his problem in a positive and predictable way. A patient who has experienced pain and disability for years will understandably grasp at any straw that promises relief. He should be warned against quackery and the use of expensive and ineffective drugs or appliances. The field of rheumatic disease is and always has been a fertile one for the quack and charlatan. (See Part VIII, Chapter Five.) The family members of the patient with rheumatoid arthritis are his most important allies. They should be trained in home care and instructed in special techniques of treatment. They should understand the nature of the disease, and participate in the overall treatment program.

Drug treatment includes simple aspirin, chloroquin, hydroxychloroquin or plaquenil, gold salts by injection, and the cortisone family of drugs. Each must be prescribed by a physician. Drugs are by no means always used. Dosage varies and requires considerable skill in prescription to gain the best results and to avoid undesirable effects.

Osteoarthritis

Osteoarthritis is the relatively mild and usually non-crippling form of "rheumatism." It is extremely common and usually constitutes little more than a considerable and continuing nuisance. The chance of getting it increases with age. The weight-bearing joints are more commonly involved, but one hereditary form of osteoarthritis involves the end and middle joints of the fingers. The joints, one by one, become painful, tender, and have hard, bony swelling. They pass through a painful phase and end up as painless but knobby fingers. There is deformity, but function is generally quite good. Stiffness in sitting is characteristic of osteoarthritis. Unlike rheumatoid arthritis, osteoarthritis causes pain but very little heat or redness. It also causes a bony type of joint enlargement, not a soft tissue swelling.

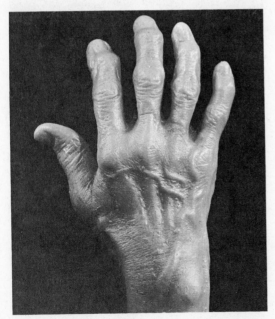

Photo: National Institutes of Health
Osteoarthritis involves the joints nearest the tips of the fingers. In severe cases, other joints are affected.

The treatment of osteoarthritis is simpler than that of the more severe forms of arthritis. This disease is due to a gradual destruction of cartilage. Its precise cause is unknown, but it is no longer regarded as a simple "wear and tear disease." Heredity appears to play a part in its cause. The first step in treatment is to assure the patient that it is not a crippling, deforming disease. This is often a great relief to him since he usually thinks he has a destructive form of arthritis. He may have more of a problem with fear of the future than his disease warrants.

Joint rest is important and special exercises are needed. Postural exercises are important aids in treatment. The body weight should be kept down. Drug therapy is kept to a minimum and the cortisone drugs are not used. The principal drug treatment is aspirin as required.

Gout

Gout is one of the first diseases ever described (by Hippocrates in 500 B.C.). It is characterized by severe acute arthritis, generally affecting one or two joints only. It comes on commonly at night. The pain is extremely severe; heat, redness, and tenderness in and about the joint are noted and a maximum intensity of pain is reached in only a few hours. It lasts from several days to a few weeks. Recovery often seems to be complete. The patient is quite well until the next episode which may come weeks, months, or years later. A more severe form of gout is a chronic continuing kind of arthritis. Gout is related to a hereditary defect in the chemistry of the uric acid in the body. The disease is fairly common and often presents a problem in diagnosis.

Gout as a general disease is treated quite successfully with one of several drugs which speed up the elimination of uric acid. An acute attack can also be treated successfully with a drug. Treatment must be supervised at all times by a physician.

Collagen Diseases

Other types of rheumatic diseases are grouped under the general heading of collagen diseases. Collagen is the term applied to the

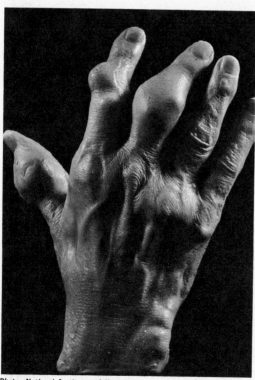
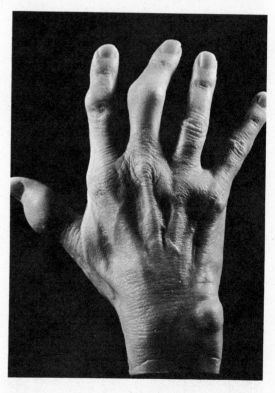

Hand at left is of a person suffering with gout. The large lumps are caused by an accumulation of urate crystals. Right, the same hand after treatment with uricosuric agents. If left untreated, urate crystals destroy the joints.

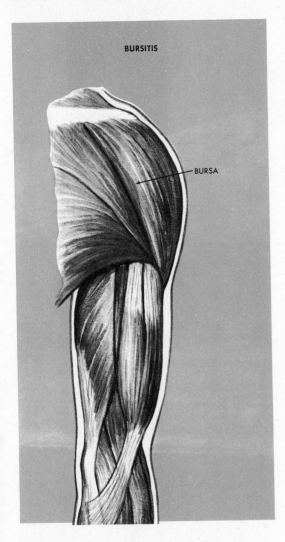

BURSITIS

BURSA

supporting connective tissues of the body.

Bursitis is an inflammation of a bursa or pocket (from the Latin for purse) lined with smooth lubricating membrane. Such bursae are located near joints and where muscles slide over each other. Their purpose is to minimize friction. A commonly inflamed bursa is the one near the shoulder. A formerly common condition, housemaid's knee, was due to an inflammation of the bursa below the knee-joint.

Fibrositis is an inflammation involving the fibrous tissues in tendons, joint-supporting sheaths, or capsules or muscle sheaths. This is variously named tenosynovitis (inflammation of tendons), tenomysositis (inflammation of tendons and muscle) and lumbago. The latter is a form of low-back pain due either to spinal disc injury or to rheumatic inflammation of the mixed muscle-tendon-joint structures at the base of the spine. Because many stresses occur here, the area is frequently subject to rheumatic influences.

The Future

Any arthritic or rheumatic victim should consult with his family doctor. In most instances this is all that need be done to determine the type of rheumatic disease and the appropriate treatment. Hospitalization may be necessary for periods of a few days to a few weeks at the onset. The doctor may request the consultation of an internist (medical specialist in diagnosis and treatment) or a rheumatologist (medical specialist in the rheumatic diseases) if the problem is not clear or is unusually complicated. There are many clinics in the United States where topflight care at little expense can be obtained. The Arthritis and Rheumatism Foundation maintains lists of clinics and doctors specializing in rheumatic diseases.

A nationwide, indeed a worldwide, program is carrying on a vigorous organized attack on this group of diseases. Faith in the results of such a program is justified. Research correlated with education and patient care, when done on a wide enough scale, will surely result in finding the cause of the rheumatic diseases. The several large organizations engaged in research, education, and care of the rheumatic disease patient have splendid coordination of efforts. Before many years all of these organizations will have done themselves out of business by finding a cure for arthritis; this is their hope and goal.

CHAPTER FOUR

HEADACHES

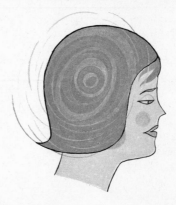

HEADACHE is one of the most common complaints of 20th century man. Since headache is an almost universal complaint, it is a topic that almost everyone can discuss from painful, first-hand experience.

Headache, it should be quickly recognized, is not a disease by itself, but rather a symptom of a disease or a functional disturbance. The causes of many headaches are relatively simple to discover; others may tax the collective brains of topnotch specialists. Thanks to recent research, the diagnosis of headache has become more exact and its treatment more certain than ever before.

In searching for headache causes, a physician will require a detailed history and frequently a complete physical examination of the patient. He will ask many questions about the nature of the headache—where it is located, whether the pain is sharp or dull, at what time of the day it is worse, and whether there is a family history of migraine or high blood pressure. If the patient relates his symptoms accurately, the physician may find significant hints and clues as to where the trouble lies. When headache causes are obscure, to arrive at a diagnosis the doctor may require various tests for the eyes, blood pressure, blood, urine, nerve reflexes, and other functions.

Emotional and Mental Causes

Tension headaches and headaches of emotional origin are extremely common, probably constituting the most usual cause of headache observed by physicians. They occur in so-called normal persons as well as those afflicted by emotional problems, and they differ in the same person on different occasions. In many instances the emotional difficulty is unknown. A considerable time may ensue between a siege of worries, anxieties, and fatigue and the actual appearance of headache. Headache will sometimes persist long after the emotional state subsides. Nor is it necessary for a person to undergo a period of emotional upheaval to bring on headaches. The chronic wear-and-tear of everyday living is enough to tax a person and produce his headache.

Headaches that occur at regular intervals in everyday life are likely to be mental in origin. Overly-conscientious professional men and women, business executives, and white-collar workers are especially vulnerable to such headaches at the end of a trying, demanding day. Since the causes are often deep-seated and difficult to recognize, emotional or mental headaches account for many headaches dismissed casually as being "nervous" in origin. The suffering that follows can sometimes be as real and intense as headaches that are produced by organic disease.

Headache victims with emotional problems are best treated in the doctor's office. One of his main tasks is to understand the origin and development of the complaint in relation to the patient's work, social position, and family attachments. By uncovering the patient's hopes, fears, frustrations, anxieties, and ambitions, the doctor often can match up the onset of headaches with periods of particular emotional stress in the patient's life.

Psychotherapy is an important factor in the treatment of emotional headaches. Patients who are given insight into their own reactions to daily living can be shown how to reduce or avoid tensions. Reassurance, suggestion, and re-education are valuable tools employed by physicians to bring to the surface a patient's underlying emotional conflicts. A huge dose of understanding and compassion on the part of the doctor helps many sufferers from tension headache lead healthier, happier lives.

Physical Causes

In contrast to headaches of emotional origin, a headache can warn that something is fundamentally wrong with the brain. While it has been estimated that brain tumors account for only one of every 200 deaths, early recognition of this condition is imperative. Failure to distinguish the ominous headache from the trivial may subsequently cost life. Thus, no chronic headache should be dismissed without investigating the possibility of its having a serious cause.

Headaches due to eyestrain, for example, can be corrected by using proper glasses. Still others are caused by glaucoma, the condition that produces hardening of the eyeball. Although migraine headaches are never fatal, they cause more discomfort than many other diseases. Many migraine victims could become reasonably comfortable if they would learn how to correct faulty ways of living. Of paramount importance is regularity in living—regular habits, regular meals, and regular hours of sleep. Excesses or overindulgence should be cut down or, better yet, avoided. Each case of migraine has to be studied by a physician to determine its underlying cause. Many migraine victims can be taught to reduce attacks when the actual roots of their difficulty are brought to light.

Diseases of the nerves leading to the head and face, as well as infections of the ear, nose, throat, and sinuses, can also cause headaches. In addition, some headaches are caused by such diseases as influenza, pneumonia, and measles; in these, cure of the headaches depends upon the cure of the underlying infection. Finally, acute infections of the nervous system—inflammation of the brain, meningitis, or polio—are almost always accompanied by severe headaches.

Recurring pain at the back of the head and the upper part of the neck may result from contraction of the neck muscles and scalp or from head injuries. Although headache is often associated with high blood pressure, its severity

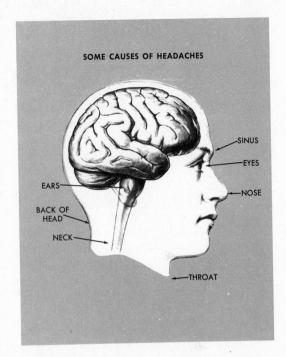

SOME CAUSES OF HEADACHES

is not necessarily related to the height of the blood pressure reading. Happily, a number of excellent drugs will reduce high blood pressure and the accompanying headache.

In general, a person suffering from severe or recurring headaches should consult a competent physician as soon as possible. Prolonged self-treatment with headache pills or powders, which many Americans purchase nonchalantly at the corner drugstore, is unwise, for the promiscuous use of these drugs may give a false sense of security and occasionally lead to serious trouble.

Aspirin is a safe drug to use and probably one of the most effective. For the average person afflicted by an average headache, one or two tablets is all that is required for relief. However, some persons with recurrent types of headache, especially those without benefit of medical attention, will desperately turn from one headache nostrum to another without securing relief.

Do these concluding words on headache make your own head ache? They shouldn't— if you will take intelligent advantage of the strides modern medical science has made in relieving and curing headaches.

CHAPTER FIVE

NEUROMUSCULAR DISEASES

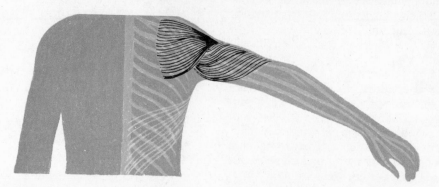

NEUROMUSCULAR DISEASES affect the muscles through disturbing the nerve supply which keeps the muscles healthy. These diseases occur in many different forms, but they are all due to similar underlying causes which center in the brain and the central nervous pathways in the spinal cord.

Many of these diseases have a hereditary basis and most of them are, as yet, poorly understood. However, progress is being made and it is worthwhile for families to have an understanding of these conditions and to know that even when no cure is possible, the physician is often able to make the patient feel a great deal better and help preserve or restore muscular function.

Muscular Dystrophy

Muscular dystrophy is a chronic disease, characterized by gradual wasting away of muscle tissue. It affects both males and females. It more frequently attacks children than adults (about 78 per cent of all victims are children), and is an inherited disease. In most cases where there is no previous family history, the cause of the disease is unexplained. Animals may have this disease, including mice, sheep, hamsters, and chickens.

The most common victim of the disease is the child who develops pseudohypertrophic muscular dystrophy. In this type the muscles of the legs and lower back are first affected. As the muscle tissue disappears, fat takes its place and the legs appear to have greater than normal muscular development. In the adult, the most common types of the disease affect either the muscles of the pelvic girdle (lower back, hips, and thighs) or the shoulder girdle (the muscles controlling movement of the shoulders and neck). In this latter type the muscles of facial expression are also affected so that these pa-

tients gradually lose the ability to smile, scowl, or grimace; their lips protrude somewhat and give the appearance of pouting.

Diagnosis in the majority of these patients may be made by the family physician. Since some of these diseases have a history and physical findings that are not entirely typical, the family doctor may desire consultation to make certain of the diagnosis. This consulting service is available through 57 active Muscular Dystrophy Association, Inc. clinics throughout the United States. At them, specially-trained doctors with specially-designed diagnostic equipment and laboratory facilities are usually able to make a positive diagnosis as to whether the patient has the disease or not.

Treatment of muscular dystrophy consists of careful general as well as specific measures. Since there is no known cure (nearly 300 different medications have been tested in treatment clinics with negative results), the emphasis lies in preventing any complications associated with the progressive loss of muscular activity.

Due to lack of activity and outside interest, most patients tend to eat too much. Adding fat to already failing muscles will inevitably speed up the weakening process. Thus, patients must avoid any excessive weight gain.

The disease affects the muscles of breathing. Patients gradually lose the ability to cough and eliminate secretions from the throat and lungs. As a result, a common cold to the dystrophic is as serious as pneumonia is to normal individuals. Treatment is preventive; influenza vaccine should be given annually. Active treatment with antibiotics can help to prevent infections, especially those of the nose, throat, or lungs.

Psychological problems of the dystrophic vary with his condition. Educational opportunities and recreational outlets must be provided. The dystrophic child must not be pampered. Basically he resents being treated as inadequate and, as a result, often becomes hostile toward his brothers and sisters. Parents not infrequently have a strong guilt feeling about their dystrophic children; unless recognized, evaluated, and guided, this attitude may destroy the value of an otherwise excellent program of treatment for the patient.

Patients benefit by physical therapy. It is more beneficial for them to receive this treatment at home rather than at a clinic since frequent trips to and from the treatment center may unnecessarily tire the already disabled patient. In the clinics, doctors specializing in physical medicine or their trained staffs teach the patient's parents physical therapy methods. They can then carry out the program at home. The goal of the therapy is to keep the walking patient walking and the wheel chair patient sitting up as long as possible.

The dystrophic occasionally needs short leg braces. Rarely does surgery to correct deformity provide any benefit. Time lost in convalescence from surgery can result in irreversible physical disability. A properly prescribed wheel chair is essential to the comfort and security of the patient able to use it. The child's wheel chair will have to be changed progressively to larger sizes as the child grows.

At least once a year, alleged "breakthroughs" in muscular dystrophy provide headlines in newspapers and magazines. The false hope and bitter disappointment following these announcements are heartbreaking. Until reputable, rigid clinical trials have clearly established the usefulness of a drug, the patient must depend upon the physician and/or clinic responsible for his care.

The Muscular Dystrophy Association of America, Inc. has nearly 400 active chapters that are anxious to assist in the diagnosis and treatment of the muscular dystrophy patient. In areas where chapters do not currently operate, wheel chairs and other equipment may be obtained through the Medical Department of the national office on prescription by the family doctor.

Parkinson's Disease

For generations Parkinson's disease was known as "shaking palsy." It first attracted serious medical attention in 1817 when James Parkinson, an English physician, published "An Essay on the Shaking Palsy." Strictly

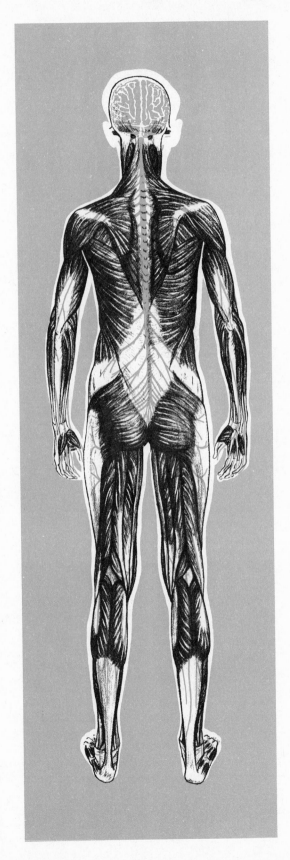

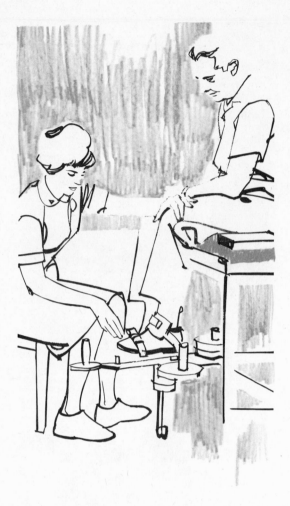

Trained physical therapists, like the girl above, show the disabled and the handicapped how they can build up strength in wasted muscles, and regain capabilities.

speaking, the malady is not a disease but rather a group of symptoms that may or may not be associated with such known diseases as encephalitis. Regardless of cause, the basic disturbance is believed to be some malfunction of centers deep in the brain. What causes the malfunction remains obscure.

One of the first symptoms of the disease is tremor in a particular part of the body, usually one of the limbs. The tremor is rhythmic at first and slight. Gradually, however, it increases in intensity and may become widespread. Along with or soon after the tremors begin, muscular rigidity occurs in tight muscles that cannot be relaxed. The combination of rigidity and loss of autonomic movements produces a peculiar, stooped posture first described by Dr. Parkinson in his essay. More disabling is the

eventual loss of autonomic movements which gives a masked appearance to the face and causes a rapid, shuffling gate.

These three symptoms—tremor, decreased autonomic movement, and rigidity—occur in varying degrees in different patients. They generally increase gradually over the years, more slowly in some cases, more rapidly in others.

A state of helplessness can be postponed, in some cases indefinitely, by the patient who enthusiastically follows a program of medication, special exercises, and healthful habits. In rapidly advancing cases, surgery has been employed with varying degrees of success.

The ideal drug for the treatment of Parkinsonism has not as yet been found. However, about a dozen drugs are widely used. These drugs will reduce the rigidity and tremor of Parkinsonism if used properly under a physician's guidance. Unfortunately, no drugs have yet been discovered that can restore automatic movements and correct weakness.

Physical therapy is one of the most helpful means to relax rigid and frozen muscles. However, since a physical therapist cannot always visit the home regularly, it becomes most important that the patient carry out a regular program of home exercise on his own. Every activity, be it work, walking, visiting, shopping, or playing cards, is exercise and should be engaged in to the fullest in order to keep the muscles alive and in good working condition. Special exercises have been devised and can be readily taught to patients by physical therapists trained in this area.

Neurosurgeons have been attempting operations on the brain in the hope of relieving Parkinsonism. Several such procedures devised recently may relieve tremor and rigidity, sometimes markedly. However, authorities agree that surgery can help only about 10 per cent of Parkinson cases. These are mainly younger patients whose chief disability is tremor or rigidity limited to one side of the body.

More than 90 per cent of all patients with Parkinson's disease live at home with their families. The family's goal should be to make the patient as comfortable and contented as possible in spite of his affliction, to encourage him to take part in outside activities and to exercise regularly, and to increase their own understanding of the disease.

In an attempt to answer the question, "Should the patient be told the nature of his illness," 300 patients were asked their feelings on the subject. Almost all felt they should be told by their doctor when he was certain of the diagnosis. Doing so improves the prospects of immediate and intensive treatment and gives the patient a better outlook. Doctors feel, too, that neighbors and visitors should be told frankly and honestly that the patient has Parkinson's disease.

Since Parkinson's disease makes for awkward movements, the home should be arranged to minimize falls. If possible, all doorsills should be removed, since they are a constant cause of stumbling when a patient goes from one room to another. It is also wise to remove any sharp pointed tables and small pieces of furniture that might cause the patient to stumble. An adequate rail should be installed on both sides of all stairways. As an added measure of safety, a carpenter could install metal or wooden handles on the walls next to all doorknobs to give the patient more security in standing as he opens a door. If a special chair can be set aside for the patient, 2" x 4" blocks can be placed under the back legs to make it easier to get in and out of. Getting in and out of bed can be made easier by tying a sheet to the bedpost and a knot at the other end which the patient can grasp to rise to a sitting position. Special elevated toilet seats are now available in surgical supply stores; bars at the side of the toilet prove helpful to the patient in adjusting his clothes. Bars at the sides of a bathtub or shower are also helpful.

Since the Parkinson patient can do only one motor act at a time, he must learn to adapt himself to a new time schedule. For instance, he cannot reach for his electric shaver while brushing his teeth or he will find that the hand being used to brush his teeth will cease to function. Dressing can be most time-consuming but it is important for the patient to do these chores himself in order to keep his muscles in good condition. To make it easier for the patient, and so that he will continue to do these chores, buttons can be replaced by zippers. Elastic shoelaces can be tied in place permanently. Ordinary neckties can be replaced by clip ties which slip under the collar; sleeves of coats widened two inches permit the patient to get his coat on without help. If room temperatures can be maintained a little above average, the patient can get along with fewer clothes and thus will find it easier to dress and undress. The happy and contented patient is one who is completely independent of the help of others.

Working out a proper time schedule for the patient, so that he will not be under pressure or hurried and yet will do as much as possible for himself, requires understanding and cooperation by both the family and the patient.

Seventy per cent of Parkinson patients show a weight loss during their illness. This weight loss can lead to difficulty in standing and walking and it deprives the body of important vitamins which can weaken the bone structure. The loss is due almost entirely to the patient's inability to consume enough calories for his daily needs. Some of it is caused from his failure to finish meals because of slowness.

To make it easier and more pleasant for the patient at the table, his meat should be cut for him in advance and other difficult foods should either be cut or ground up and served as thick soups or meat loaf. Most important, members of the family should be encouraged to sit around the table and carry on conversation rather than leave the patient to finish his meal alone or to feel rushed.

Sometimes it is better for the patient to eat lightly at breakfast, follow this with a mid-morning snack, a light lunch, something in the mid-afternoon, a moderate meal at supper, and a sixth, light meal before going to bed. In this way he can eat an adequate amount.

Patients with Parkinson's disease usually sleep without too much difficulty and fre-

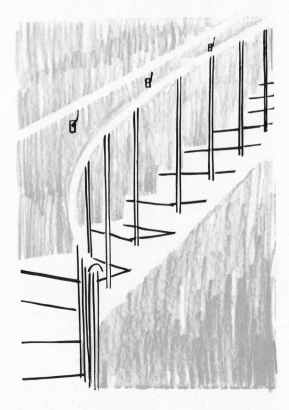

quently may fall asleep in their chairs while watching television or reading. These catnaps should be accepted by the family since they are good for the patient and rarely interfere with his regular night's sleep.

Older patients, either because of their age or a change in medication, may experience nightmares or "hallucinations." Sometimes these can be prevented by keeping a light on at night, leaving a radio playing softly, or keeping the window open so that the patient is not cut off completely from other sounds. Such steps may make it unnecessary to cut down on medication, which sometimes contributes to the problem.

Patients forced to retire find it necessary to develop new hobbies. An occupational therapist can prove helpful in making suggestions and working out interesting activities. Ship model construction, metal and leather work, or light carpentry have their place and appeal. Many patients find new enjoyment in television, radio, records, magazines, and books.

Travel should be encouraged providing the patient has a companion to go along. Automobile rides are particularly good since the movement of the car tends to relieve rigidity. Also, the constantly changing scenery helps to raise the patient's morale. A busy and active patient sleeps and eats well and is generally happy and contented.

From the foregoing, it is obvious that the family plays an important role in Parkinson's disease. The patient's physical and emotional adjustment to his illness depends to a large extent on their support. Many physicians and researchers are confident that investigations now under way will lead to new concepts as to the cause and treatment of Parkinson's disease. Until the proceeds of these studies are realized, much understanding and patience, on the part of the family as well as the patient himself, is necessary to overcome the obstacles involved in this chronic illness.

Multiple Sclerosis

Multiple sclerosis, one of the most common diseases of the nervous system, afflicts between 200,000 and 300,000 people in the United States. It almost invariably affects young people. While rarely fatal in its early stages, its symptoms may get worse and cause prolonged disability.

Multiple sclerosis has no one infallable sign. Indications include loss of muscular coordina-

tion or strength, difficulty in maintaining balance, paralysis, tremblings, numbness, tingling, visual disturbances or abnormal eye movement, speech difficulties, or impaired bowel or bladder control. Such symptoms require medical examination, and each has possible causes other than multiple sclerosis.

Many multiple sclerosis patients seem unusually cheerful and remain hopeful and optimistic despite their increasing disability. Others are severely depressed. Mental symptoms are not common but mental disease is rare.

First symptoms appear most often in adults between the ages of 20 and 40, rarely before 18 or after 45. Typically, symptoms come and go in the beginning, occasionally disappearing completely. As the disease goes on, however, recovery may be less and less complete. Some cases pursue a relentless course with no periods of improvement. In others, symptoms appear suddenly and persist without either improving or worsening.

The disease usually differs markedly from patient to patient and shows so much variation that it is difficult to foretell its course. While some victims are completely paralyzed or incapacitated, many are able to carry on normal or near-normal activity.

The structural change that takes place in the brain and spinal cord as a result of the disease consists of patches of scar tissue scattered throughout the nervous system.

Nerve fibers in the brain and spinal cord are normally covered with a fatty sheath called myelin, which is believed to act as insulation. In multiple sclerosis the myelin in scattered areas dissolves or disintegrates. This is later replaced by scar (sclerotic) tissue, from which the disease gets its name.

Early in the disease only the sheath is affected; the nerve fibers which it surrounds are not destroyed until later. If only the protecting covering is diseased, some nerve impulses can still be transmitted, although not with full strength. Improvement in the sheath's condition may explain periods of improvement in the symptoms.

Patients and relatives must not be influenced by dire rumors or tales about other patients. Actually, the average life expectancy of a patient after the onset of the disease is more than 25 years. Many patients with mild or even moderately severe multiple sclerosis make an excellent adjustment and have continued their careers.

Unfortunately, the cause of the disease has thus far eluded medical science. Many theories about its cause have been proposed: constitutional peculiarity or congenital predisposition; heredity; injury; exposure to heat or cold; a germ or a virus; toxins; vitamin deficiencies; abnormalities of blood clotting; spasm of blood vessels; allergy; even psychological factors. None has been proved.

Of interest is the fact that the disease is most common in cold, damp climates. In Europe it is found most frequently in Scandinavia and the low countries, northern Germany and Great Britain. It is rare in the Mediterranean countries. In the United States it is more common in the northern Atlantic states, the Great Lakes region, and the Pacific Northwest. It is found more frequently in Canada than in the southern United States. However, the disease cannot be cured by moving from a cold to a warmer climate.

Certain factors seem to bring on relapses. These include general poor health, generalized infection, illness with fever, too much exertion or undue fatigue, injuries, allergic diseases, and emotional upsets. The effect of pregnancy in these flare-ups is still a disputed point.

Once nerve fibers themselves are replaced by scar tissue, impulses can no longer be carried along them and there can be no recovery of function. Consequently, with severe or prolonged impairment, return of function is not expected.

Many treatments have been tried and each year new theories of cause and treatment appear. But no single cause, no scientific or absolute treatment, has been discovered. Antibiotics, vitamins, medicines that dilate the blood vessels, corticosteroids, and many other treatments have been used. None is of proved value. The fact that patients often improve spontaneously with no treatment makes it especially difficult to judge the usefulness of any single approach.

The best treatment at present seems to be that of building general resistance, avoiding fatigue and exposure to extremes of hot and cold, elimination of exposure to infection (with vigorous and adequate treatment when infection does occur), and avoidance of the other factors that may bring on relapses. Rest is important and nutritious meals are essential, but there is no real proof that any special diet is of value.

Each patient should be under the care of a physician to prevent infection and control any distressing symptoms which may arise.

Myasthenia Gravis

Myasthenia gravis, which means literally, severe muscular weakness, is a rare type of muscle disease. It affects principally the muscles of the eyes, lips, and tongue. Chewing and swallowing may be difficult. It generally begins during the first half of life, and is often accompanied by an enlargement of the thymus gland. This gland lies under the breastbone and normally disappears at or just before birth. Thymus tumors may accompany the disease. It is more prevalent among women than among men.

The general body muscles of victims of the disease become tired very rapidly upon exertion, but recover quickly. The condition may be limited to the eye muscles or may involve the entire body. The eye symptoms are the most common—inability to keep the eyes open for long, especially late in the day. There is a lack of facial expression and interference with clear speech. Double vision may occur.

The explanation for the muscular symptoms lies in a chemical disturbance at the point where the controlling nerve enters the muscle fiber. Here a substance known as acetylcholine is normally set free in the system; in myasthenia gravis it is either not liberated or is destroyed immediately afterward.

All the symptoms are lessened by rest, but tend to return very quickly upon exertion. Drug treatment is effective in some cases, but must be continued. Good results have followed surgery in some instances. Many patients live a long time, but their lives are full of restrictions.

CHAPTER SIX

POLIOMYELITIS

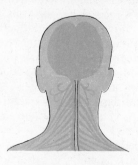

POLIOMYELITIS has been put to rout as a major crippling disease in the United States and most other parts of the world. But so long as people remain who have not been immunized against polio, it remains a threat.

The first known recording of the effects of poliomyelitis is found on a plaque which dates from about 1300 B.C. It depicts an offering to the Phoenician goddess Astarte. The plaque pictures a man standing, using the support of a long wooden pole. His right leg shows the effects of polio. The muscles of the entire limb are wasted; the Achilles (heel) tendon is pulled upward and thus the foot points downward instead of being parallel with the ground; the hamstring tendons at the back of the knee are keeping the knee bent.

However, there is little historical evidence of outbreaks of the disease until the late 19th century when it began to appear in European countries. From then until the Salk and Sabin vaccines were developed, polio epidemics became an increasingly common problem in nations with relatively high standards of sanitation. Although children were the chief sufferers, adults too became victims.

A sizeable number of polio victims in the United States who have survived the disease in recent years still depends upon iron lungs, rocking beds, portable chest and abdominal belt respirators, braces, crutches, wheelchairs, and other aids. In 1964 the National Foundation-March of Dimes reported that more than 1,600 patients living at home were dependent for breathing upon some kind of mechanical aid. The total number of similar patients in hospitals or nursing homes was unknown.

Poliomyelitis is caused by a tiny virus, a disease-producing agent that must get inside a living cell in order to reproduce. The virus generally enters the body through the mouth either in food, by hand-to-mouth contact, or by inhalation. The virus grows freely in the cells lining the intestinal tract.

There are three specific types of polio virus. Each can cause the same disease, but immunity to one type does not provide immunity to either of the other two. If the virus gets into the nerve cells of the spinal cord or brain, it also grows and multiplies there, feeding on the nerve cells themselves. It directly destroys some of the cells and indirectly injures others. The nerve cells that are killed are lost forever, because the body cannot grow new nerve cells to replace those which are totally destroyed. The nerve cells that are temporarily damaged—but not destroyed—in time are able to resume their normal functions.

Not all patients infected with polio virus become paralyzed. On the contrary, for every known case of polio, perhaps 100 to 1,000 persons have the virus in their systems for a limited time without becoming paralyzed or without even showing any serious signs of the disease. Such persons can pass the virus on to others. In many cases, the body's natural defenses combat the virus and prevent it from reaching the central nervous system. Polio vaccination stimulates the body to do this quickly and effectively.

Paralysis of a particular muscle occurs when a majority of the motor cells (the nerve cells that control motion) which relate to that particular muscle are affected. Weakness results when a small percentage of the cells are attacked. Weakness or paralysis may be only temporary if the nerve cells are damaged but not destroyed.

Signs and Symptoms

The usual symptoms of polio are headache (especially important in children), fever, nausea, listlessness, upset stomach, and sore throat. In adults, symptoms are likely to be more vague, without fever, but with pain in the back, stiffness of muscles, and extreme restlessness. In some cases, children as well as adults are highly irritable and restless during the first stages of the illness.

Because the symptoms resemble many common illnesses of children, the presence of polio may be unnoticed or receive only slight attention. Sometimes the early symptoms disappear for several days only to recur with the addition of stiffness of the neck and back, plus extreme muscle soreness. Higher temperature and paralysis may occur. The occurrence of paralysis indicates that the central nervous system has been invaded.

If the facial muscles, vocal cords, swallowing muscles, and the brain centers which control respiration and blood supply are affected, the patient has bulbar-type polio. If the muscles of the arms and/or legs, back or abdomen, and the muscles of respiration are affected, the patient has spinal-type polio. A combination of these two types is known as spino-bulbar type.

Because the progression of the disease may be very rapid, it is extremely important that any symptoms resembling those described above be reported to a physician at once, particularly if the patient has not had polio vaccine. Close and constant observation of a patient suspected of having polio is vitally important, so that life-saving care may be begun and his needs be met at every turn.

Approximately one fourth of all reported polio cases cause no paralysis. About a third of those with paralysis recover with little or no disability. The more severely paralyzed require long-term care. For them, there are special treatment centers where patients receive the benefit of every advance in care and research.

Treatment

Immediate medical attention, bed rest, and good nursing are still the most important first steps in the care of polio victims. Hospitalization may or may not be necessary, depending on the severity of the illness. Some parents wonder if it is better to have their children treated at home or in the hospital. This is not a simple question, nor can it be given a simple answer. A great many factors are involved: the severity of the patient's illness; the availability of help to care for him; the number of other persons in the home and their daily care needs. The physician alone can determine where the most effective treatment and best care can be given.

The physician has a corps of assistants to help in polio care: these include nurses, phys-

ical and occupational therapists, medical social workers, laboratory technicians, and a number of other physician-specialists. Polio treatment will call for any or all of the following procedures, depending on the individual patient.

1. Prompt diagnosis, which involves a physician's skills and judgment plus laboratory and clinical tests and findings.

2. Good nursing care. The nurse through close observation helps the doctor find out how sick the patient is. She isolates the patient to keep him from giving his disease to others or contracting other diseases. She reports changes in the patient's condition, checks his pulse, temperature, and respiration. She watches to be sure the patient takes the right amount of food and fluids each day and keeps him in the correct bed position to prevent deformity.

3. As soon as muscle soreness and spasm have been relieved, the physical therapist, working with the physician, joins the team helping the patient to combat the after-effects of polio. First, tests of muscle weakness and range of motion of joints are performed to give information helpful in planning a treatment program. Then the physical therapist works with the patient using heat and exercises to improve circulation, strengthen weakened muscles, maintain joint motion, and prevent deformities. If the patient needs to wear braces or use crutches or a wheelchair, the physical therapist helps him learn how to use the equipment.

4. The occupational therapist, under the guidance of the physician, uses creative, educational, and recreational activities and human ingenuity to help patients get well. Physical and mental recovery is the main objective of occupational therapy, but a second goal is almost equally important—that of helping the handicapped acquire a job skill. Occupational therapists use a number of methods to help the patient increase his ability to feed, bathe, and dress himself and to perform other actions that he will need in daily living.

5. Medical social work is a professional service to patients, physicians, treatment institutions, and the community. Acute poliomyelitis presents special problems such as greater than usual anxiety and confusion about diagnosis, fear of death in the early stages of the illness and of permanent disability later, distress over disfiguring and physically limiting handicaps, and loss of function as a wage earner or mother in the household. After the acute period, crippling and prolonged treatment present other problems. The social

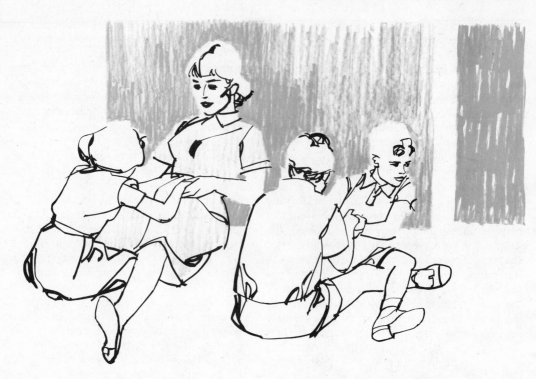

worker is helpful in aiding the patient and his family meet those problems. He can also help in the practical planning required to meet physical, vocational, and financial needs and adjustments.

During the acute phase of polio, supports and splints may be used to help keep the patient's body, arms, and legs in good alignment so that deformities will not occur. When the patient begins his exercise and activity program, splints and braces are used to protect weakened muscles, to keep body parts in good alignment, and to help improve the functional ability of arm, leg, and other muscles. Some patients with severe paralysis will need braces, slings, wheelchairs, and the like for the rest of their lives to perform daily activities and to have the endurance needed to help care for themselves.

A respirator is used when the polio virus has attacked the nervous system in such a way that the normal movement of the muscles of breathing are interfered with. In about 15 per cent of paralytic polio patients, an iron lung or other respiratory device may be needed. If a patient is placed in the tank respirator (iron lung), he is usually "weaned" from it with use of the rocking bed, chest respirator, or abdominal belt respirator. Comparatively few patients require this type of treatment permanently. About 7 out of every 10 patients whose breath-

ing is affected can eventually learn to live without mechanical breathing aids. A high percentage of the respiratory patients eventually return to their homes, and often to their jobs.

Certain patients will benefit in the later stages of their recovery, or children after certain stages of growth, from surgery. The orthopedic surgeon's concern is to eliminate deformities or prevent them; to restore useful function or to assist in its restoration; and to eliminate the need for appliances.

The entire rehabilitation team of medical and other specialists plans a program of home care for the patient, with him and his family taking part, so that the patient's life may be as comfortable and enjoyable as possible. His family is taught how to care for him, allowing him to do what he can for himself. His doctor and other health professionals visit him periodically to make changes in his program as they are indicated. Community resources are called upon to assure that all of his needs are being met—emotional, social, educational, vocational, and physical.

Immunization

There are now two vaccines to protect against paralysis from polio. Both vaccines are effective and are being used at the discretion of individual physicians and public health officials. Your doctor or your local health department can advise you on this question.

Polio vaccine prevents paralytic polio by stimulating the production of antibodies. These antibodies combat the polio virus as it enters the blood stream and thus prevent the virus from reaching and destroying or damaging nerve cells.

The Salk vaccine, in use since 1955, is given by injection. It contains killed polio virus of all three types. Each dose, therefore, provides some protection against each of the three virus types that cause polio. Four doses of the available commercial product are necessary to protect most persons.

The Sabin polio vaccine is taken by mouth. It contains selected live but weakened polio virus. A separate vaccine is used against each of three polio viruses. Each dose, therefore, provides protection only against the type of virus it contains. For full protection, each of the three types is usually taken separately and a

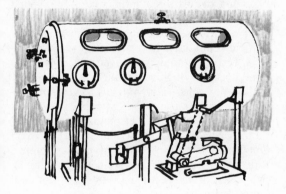

booster dose containing all three types is recommended, especially for infants.

The oral polio vaccine when swallowed must multiply in the lining of the intestinal tract. It then stimulates the body to produce antibodies in much the same way as does the killed polio virus vaccine or natural infection.

The year 1963 marked the virtual disappearance of epidemic poliomyelitis from the United States. Provisional year-end figures released by the Public Health Service showed a total of 121 new cases in 1964, a reduction of 99 per cent from the average for the period 1951-1954. While both paralytic and nonparalytic cases registered further declines in 1964, these were not as dramatic as the reductions achieved in 1957, 1960, or 1961. No cases were reported in 10 states during 1963. Only 94 paralytic cases were reported in 1964.

The devastating effects of paralytic polio on its victims are still very real. The one protection parents can offer their children is to take advantage of the Salk or Sabin vaccine. If a child shows symptoms which resemble those caused by a polio virus, a physician should be seen promptly.

The goal for those physically disabled by polio is to live a normal life in the environment in which they belong. It is natural that physical suffering should be accompanied by emotional distress in the face of crippling. Yet, polio patients frequently seem to make a good psychological adjustment if other emotional factors are not involved, and if there is wise and helpful guidance along the way.

CHAPTER SEVEN

STROKE

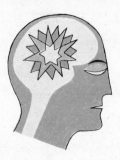

STROKE HAS COME TO MEAN a variety of things, but in general the term refers to sudden brain damage caused by a hemorrhage of a blood vessel in the brain, a thrombosis or clot formed by hardening of the vessel walls, or an embolus, a clot that gets into the blood stream from another diseased or injured part and blocks a brain artery. The brain area affected stops functioning and causes the symptoms related to this loss of function.

Stroke affects not only older people; a high percentage of the death and disability it causes hits people between the ages of 30 and 64.

In ancient times, victims of a stroke were thought to have been "struck down by God." Today, one eminent scientist says that the affliction is often only a stroke of bad luck. If treated successfully during the acute stage, the patient may live a useful life for many years. Perhaps the term stroke persists because the illness it causes is so dramatic in its abruptness.

Estimates are that more than 1,800,000 people in the United States have been crippled by strokes caused by the blood vessels supplying the brain alone. Strokes take more than 170,000 lives a year. Hardening of the arteries in the brain which is related to stroke, is the second leading cause of first admissions to state mental hospitals.

The seriousness of brain damage from strokes can be realized by comparing strokes in the brain with those in other parts of the body. For example, if a small clot lodges in the lung, the lung is not severely handicapped because all its parts perform the same function and can enlarge if necessary to make up for the injured portion. In the brain, a small closure in an artery that relates to such a specialized function as speech or movement of limbs can destroy that particular function. Victims of heart attacks often survive because auxiliary blood vessels quickly appear to send life-giving blood to the injured part. However, extensive research has been able to show little, if any, recovery capacity of the brain, which is our most delicate and our most prized possession.

"Little Strokes"

An often unsuspected cause of mental and physical incapacity is a series of "little strokes." These may start when a person is in the 30's or 40's striking silently at night or passing almost unnoticed as a sudden dizzy spell, a momentary blackout, or just a few moments of confusion. The stroke itself is not severe enough to compel the patient to seek medical aid, but some permanent brain damage remains just the same.

A formerly kind, gentle person may suddenly become highly impatient and irritable with little cause. His judgment is often impaired, and a strong man may become weak and be prone to tears. Suspiciousness is common. A person who has had a tendency toward emotional instability, held in check heretofore by will power, may suddenly develop a psychosis. Some become sloppy in dress and befuddled in thought, others lose their moral sense and become involved in sexual indiscretions. Sometimes the victim merely loses interest in his family and friends and lives secretively, constantly hiding things that through forgetfulness he cannot later find.

When symptoms are mild, as they often are, the person may get along very well, provided he doesn't live in a city. Surveys show that a sufferer of cerebral vascular disease can get along better in the slower-going farm and small-town areas. Fast city living, with its dashing cars, hustling pedestrians, and tight time schedules, serves only to confuse a tired, slowed-up mind and body. The situation is complicated even more because city dwellers are reluctant to admit they want to slow down.

Our lack of natural defenses for the brain makes the problem of a series of small strokes one of the most difficult ever tackled, but medical authorities believe that it can be solved.

The most popular experimental approach is that of finding ways to prevent strokes. Tentative results show that scientists may be on the right track in recognizing early symptoms and treating them so that disastrous effects can be avoided for many years.

Research into Stroke

The dimmest view has been taken of brain hemorrhage, which because of its abruptness, may cause death in a short time. But experts feel that if a patient can be treated quickly, he may survive and enjoy a long, useful life. In studies made, 80 per cent of stroke victims had had high blood pressure. This would seem to indicate that a vital artery breaks after long pounding by too much pressure. Though often claimed in recent years, no real cure for high blood pressure has been found. However, several new drugs do lower blood pressure and much has been learned about how a calm way of life will lessen both tension and hypertension. Recently it has been shown to be of great value for people with a family record of hypertension and cerebral hemorrhage to take precautionary measures long before their blood pressure climbs to the danger mark.

Among such precautions should be regular medical supervision, diet and weight control, carefully considered activities, and moderation in all phases of living. The use of tobacco in the presence of arterial disease should be governed by medical advice. (See also Part XII, Chapter Three.)

The other fairly common cause of massive brain hemorrhage is a ruptured aneurysm or break in the wall of an artery which was not properly formed before birth. In a study of 143 ruptured aneurysms, the ages of the patients ranged from 18 to 89, but almost half were between 40 and 59 years. Only one third died within the first 48 hours after their stroke.

Since none of the breaks occurred in persons under 10 years of age and their number rises with age, these doctors suspect that it often takes hypertension and arteriosclerosis to batter down the weakened vessel. Otherwise, the accident would have occurred much earlier. With modern x-ray techniques giving knowledge of blood vessels and lymphatics, the aneurysms can now be detected when they first cause trouble, and measures can be taken to prevent their recurrence.

Once a hemorrhage has occurred, it presents a problem similar to that of any foreign body

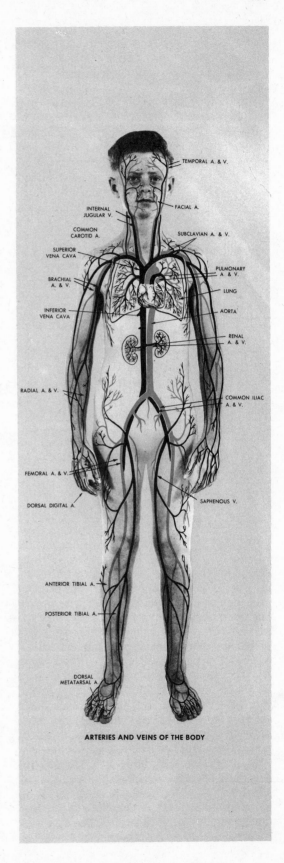

ARTERIES AND VEINS OF THE BODY

and can sometimes be treated surgically. Since certain heart, lung, and other conditions are known to throw off clots that may lodge in the brain, they can often be anticipated and prepared for.

A thrombosis or closing of a cerebral artery by a clot caused by arteriosclerosis comes comparatively slowly, incapacitating the patient gradually over a period of a day or two, in contrast to the instant striking of a hemorrhage.

Little strokes may have occurred when people over 38 have mental or nervous symptoms that seem too severe for the slight abdominal discomfort they feel, when nervous symptoms occur suddenly with no background of instability, or when there are changes in character and performance after a fall or dizzy spell. Since these small episodes may start at an early age, they often progressively incapacitate the victim for 20 or 30 years.

The stroke problem is almost overwhelming because of its many facets and its conflict with our modern, urban way of life. Only a beginning has been made in the recognition of types of cerebral disease, in treatment, and in application of rehabilitation measures. But with the great strides that have been made with coronary disease—which in some ways is similar—the full weight of scientific effort and knowledge is behind the research against one of man's oldest and most feared afflictions.

The Stroke Victim

In carefully considering all aspects of the disrupted living pattern among stroke victims, it becomes obvious that the entire household can be affected. The time sequence for recovery may be long and laborious for each member of the family group. All of a sudden the patient has an extremely short memory and marked difficulty in understanding and expressing both oral and written language, combined with a degree of paralysis. When we consider these facts, it seems reasonable to assume that there will be some drastic difficulties in adjustment. When such patients are subjected to a whole series of unreasonable demands, they may have no choice but to voluntarily withdraw from contact with other people.

Many people with brain damage may reacquire useful and satisfying life patterns. A significant number of stroke patients have been as young as 20 years of age. Such individuals most certainly are not of an age when their contributions to society have been completed. The rehabilitation program will be hampered if the well members of the patient's family are not thoroughly informed and assisted in aiding the recovery process. All problems involving speech disturbances seem to have an undeniably negative effect upon personality adjustments. These, in turn, often markedly interfere with language recovery.

If such patients are to be helped, the entire family must be aware of its own relation to the problem. Many people strongly resist advice and especially criticism or what they regard as nagging. It is easy to condemn such persons, without realizing that we ourselves may be at fault in the manner in which we approach the patient. It is difficult for a normal member of the family, who may have many problems of his own, to understand that the brain-damaged relative has many more problems than the normal person can possibly imagine. Success in helping the patient to adjust can be expected only when relatives thoroughly comprehend the personality changes which result from damage to the brain tissues.

Effects of Brain Damage

When a stroke patient first returns to his home after hospitalization, he may appear to be extremely happy and unconcerned about his condition. It is difficult for both the patient and his family to recognize immediately the numerous deficiencies that have resulted from damage to the nervous system.

Once the patient begins to recognize his own physical, emotional, and communication deficiencies, he may begin to show despair. At this point, the family must be careful not to be discouraged. Professional guidance to hasten their understanding of the patient's over-all condition will help. Unrealistically high goals, continually forced upon such a patient, most often result in his refusal to try, accompanied by a complete rejection of the household. The growth of his anxieties drastically interferes with retraining.

It is necessary for the family to carefully regulate conversations with the patient. Abstract ideas may be extremely difficult to talk about because of the patient's reduced ability to express and understand spoken language. A simple vocabulary must be used, along with frequent references to the topic being discussed. A short memory complicates the patient's language abilities.

The patient's persistence in frequently re-

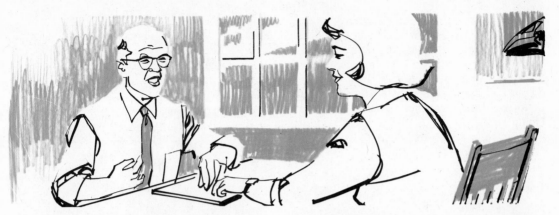

peating the same conversation is involuntary and should not be interpreted as purposeful nagging. He may, for example, be concerned with the fact that fuel for heating the home is extremely low and repeatedly instruct the household members to order more fuel. Even though he may have heard repeated explanations that fuel had been ordered the day before, it is possible that within a matter of two or three hours he may again make the same request. Many times such patients eventually come to understand their own memory inadequacies when the family has had the patience to accept such behavior.

It is important to keep in mind that the patient may be disgusted with himself as he begins to recognize his memory failures. Certainly, he condemns himself enough without having his frustrations increased through unkind comments from those about him. When he is repeatedly blamed for his unavoidable forgetfulness, he has no choice but to develop deep and morbid depressions. The family may need professional counseling to assist them to accept unusual behavior in an unruffled manner, thus providing an opportunity for the patient to improve his insight into his own behavior.

Disrupting factors in our daily lives bring on feelings of helplessness, hopelessness, and exhaustion even in normal persons. The stroke patient, as may be readily understood, frequently develops such feelings. This is apt to occur as he acquires longer memory spans for they may tend to increase his consciousness of his failures in physical and social activities.

Many of our basic attitudes toward our husbands or wives depend upon our ability to express maximum affection toward them. The reestablishment of a stable relationship between a stroke victim and his or her husband or wife may depend upon their achieving an adequate sexual relationship. A short memory span may

handicap the patient in doing this. A vast number of patients, both male and female, have described difficulties in concentrating upon even this basic drive. Such failures can create marked emotional problems for both partners.

Unless the normal sex partner has a good understanding of the recovery that is likely to come, it is possible that he or she will develop a frigid attitude toward such relationships. This reaction can have a severe effect upon the patient's total recovery.

Many stroke patients object to visits by friends and relatives. They often withdraw immediately from the living room upon the arrival of visitors. This reaction may be due to their inability to control emotional outbursts, toilet problems, or conversation. If at all possible, friends and relatives should have careful guidance concerning their conversation. They should especially be warned to avoid negative comments about the patient's condition and welfare. Often they will begin a conversation with the patient and then find that his responses are unrelated to the topic being discussed. When this occurs, visitors should then direct their conversation toward other family members.

If at all possible, the family should prepare their friends and relatives for contact with the patient. They must advise them to allow the patient time to respond, to avoid topics that may upset him, and to do their utmost to allow the patient to take part in the conversation. The better the visitors understand the situation, the less will they fear the patient. As a result, they will assist in improving the patient's social relationships and in building his self-confidence. Everyone should treat the patient with as much courtesy and consideration as they would have before his illness.

The well members of the immediate family must be aware of the patient's reactions to what he may hear and see regarding himself. The family must keep in mind that the patient needs frequent periods of emotional "ventilation." Such outbursts are often his chief means of gaining emotional relief. If the patient has no one to listen to him, his only alternative may be to withdraw completely from all activities. Doing so will, in the long run, greatly reduce the degree of his recovery.

Language Recovery

The ability to use and understand language is the key to successful social adjustment. Communication is far more than precise articulation of speech sounds. Improvements in clear articulation are most likely to develop after the patient has had an opportunity to re-acquire a meaningful vocabulary for expressing himself and understanding others. This involves the patient's recall of words and phrases which he formerly knew, rather than learning new ones.

Communication can exist only when we have a need to express and understand ideas. Too often, families of stroke patients tend to overprotect them, to give them too much help. Many people have the habit of completing the spoken sentences of even well people. We are much more likely to do so with a family member who has suffered a marked reduction in his ability to speak with normal speed. Because we often guess wrong as to what he means to say, we thus often complicate his problem. When we persist in this practice, most patients have no choice but to withdraw completely from any attempt to converse with others.

We should calmly await the patient's completion of his communication unless he indicates a need for assistance. When the patient does forget a key word, he is completely thwarted in finishing his expression. While it is true that he may say that he knows the words but can't get them out, he quite likely means that he is mentally picturing an activity, rather than specific words to describe such thoughts. When a list of words is presented, he often recognizes an appropriate word for which he has been searching; then he can finish what he started to say. To help him best, his family should patiently await his request for help and then be ready to give it to him.

Unless the patient must be confined to his bedroom, he should be, as much as possible, in an environment that encourages him to use language. If this is done in an easy and casual manner, it is quite likely that, with time, he will demonstrate a gradual and even sometimes dramatic recovery in his conversational abilities. When we help an adult patient as much as we do our children to start to use language, the entire household will be far more relaxed.

To help the patient relearn emotional control, he should be allowed to complain. If he has no one to listen to him, his only alternative may be to develop deep depression. This will greatly slow down his recovery.

Finally, and most important, the family must be provided with continued professional counseling. The better we understand the circumstances of any situation, the less we fear what is to come. Consequently, we may effectively provide realistic guidance for the patient.

CHAPTER EIGHT

CANCER

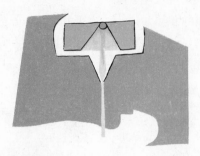

CANCER is perhaps the most feared of all diseases, yet among doctors or researchers it does not inspire fear so much as respect and appreciation of the need for aggressive treatment. Cancer is, if untreated, fatal; but it is curable if treated promptly and properly.

One third of all cases of cancer in the United States are being cured today. In 1963, there were 1,200,000 Americans alive who had been cured of cancer. That is, they had survived, free of the disease, for at least five years since treatment. Another 700,000 American men, women, and children who have been treated for cancer during the past five years will live to join the ranks of those cured.

Nevertheless, the full possibilities of cancer treatment are far from being realized. At least 88,000 people in this country will die of cancer this year. The gap between potential cure and real cure is not solely a medical problem; it is also a communication problem. Not enough people know cancer's Seven Danger Signals or heed them promptly. Not enough people have annual health examinations. Too many resist going to the doctor when they think they might have cancer, usually out of fear caused by lack of information.

Cancer is a disease characterized by an unrestrained growth of abnormal cells which, if untreated and unchecked, eventually destroy the patient. There have been only 103 known and proved cases of cancers that have cured themselves. This is such an extremely small number, fewer than 1 in 100,000 cases, that if offers no alternative to anyone who hopes to be cured.

Since cancer attacks all living things, a wide variety of creatures has aided human science in its pursuit of cancer's causes and cures. Bumblebees, bread mold, the fruit flies, whales, snails, and monkeys have all been "guinea pigs" in testing the use of hormones and chemicals or reactions to viruses, x-rays. The ugly toadfish is a cancer hero, for it is the toadfish's simple kidney and insulin-producing mechanism that has made it possible for researchers to observe blood sugar changes caused by an anti-cancer drug. Even trees, ferns, clams, and salamanders are helping researchers run down cancer clues. Ultimately, of course, the treatments must be tried on man himself. And in this field numberless anonymous volunteers have written an heroic chapter in medical research.

Types of Cancer

There are two main types of cancer. That which arises in muscles, bones, tendons, cartilage, fat, blood vessels, or lymphoid and connective tissue is called sarcoma. A cancer originating from surface cells of the skin or cells which line the internal organs is called carcinoma.

Cancers cause death by spreading. First they invade surrounding tissue; then, in the process called metastasis, they travel through the lymphatic (tissue-fluid circulation) or blood-vessel systems to other parts of the body where they take root and destroy normal tissue.

There is no race of man or any species of life that is free of cancer; nor is any part of man's body immune to the disease. However, more American men than women die of cancer; the ratio is 56:44. Some cancers are extremely fast growing, doubling in size in as few as 30 days, while others grow slowly, taking many months or years to begin to travel beyond their starting point.

Cancers are most readily curable when they are treated while still confined to their original sites. They are less easily curable when they have invaded nearby tissue and least curable when they have traveled farther, or metastasized. Thus, the key to cancer cure is early detection and treatment. As might be expected, this is easiest with the most visible cancers.

Skin cancer, except for melanoma, is the most curable form of cancer because it is so readily detected and accessible to treatment. The cure rate of skin cancer in the U.S. is 93 per cent.

Causes of Cancers

Many causes of cancers are known. For example, it is now accepted by many medical authorities, and denied by some, that excessive cigarette smoking is the major cause of lung cancer. The death rate from this disease, which was extremely rare in 1900, has increased more than 90 per cent since about 1930. Other countries in which cigarette smoking is widespread have had an equal or even a greater increase in lung cancer deaths. Excessive smoking is also believed to be implicated in cancers of the bladder, mouth, throat, and larynx. (See also Part XII, Chapter Three.)

Other cancers are caused by certain dyes and other chemicals, heavy metals, and overexposure to x-rays and sunlight.

The first environmental cause of cancer was discovered by a British doctor in the 19th century. He found that cancer of the scrotum in London's chimney sweeps was caused by the soot that lodged in the skin of the scrotum.

Ever since 1940, when Dr. Francisco Duran-Reynals of Yale University stated his belief that some human cancers were caused by viruses, an increasing amount of work in this

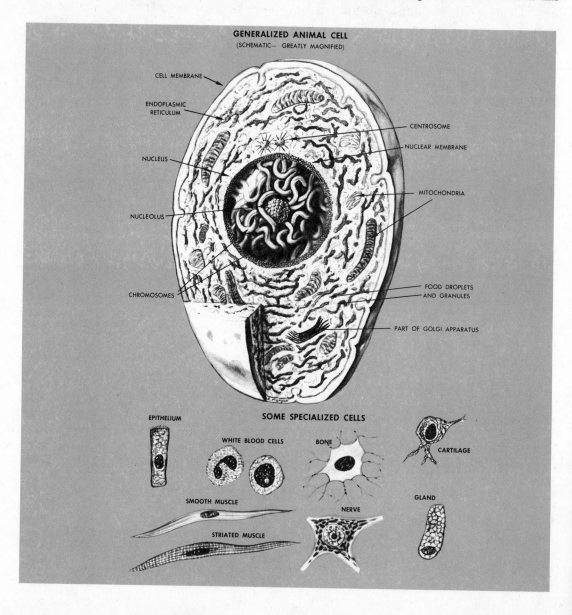

GENERALIZED ANIMAL CELL
(SCHEMATIC— GREATLY MAGNIFIED)

CELL MEMBRANE
ENDOPLASMIC RETICULUM
CENTROSOME
NUCLEAR MEMBRANE
NUCLEUS
MITOCHONDRIA
NUCLEOLUS
CHROMOSOMES
FOOD DROPLETS AND GRANULES
PART OF GOLGI APPARATUS

SOME SPECIALIZED CELLS

EPITHELIUM
WHITE BLOOD CELLS
BONE
CARTILAGE
SMOOTH MUSCLE
NERVE
GLAND
STRIATED MUSCLE

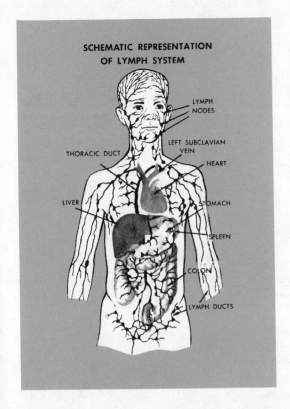

SCHEMATIC REPRESENTATION
OF LYMPH SYSTEM

LYMPH NODES

LEFT SUBCLAVIAN VEIN

THORACIC DUCT

HEART

LIVER

STOMACH

SPLEEN

COLON

LYMPH DUCTS

field has tended to lend weight to this theory. Although no human cancer viruses have yet been isolated, viruses that cause different cancers in mice, hamsters, chickens, and rabbits have been found.

Dr. Charlotte Friend of the Sloan-Kettering Institute in New York City has discovered a virus that causes leukemia in mice. Using this virus, mice have been immunized against leukemia, or cancer of the blood, with some degree of success. This limited success in the field of animal experimentation holds real hope for human beings. The electron microscope has shown Dr. Leon Dmochowski and Dr. John A. Sykes of the University of Texas Medical School virus-like particles in leukemic cells of mice, chickens, and men—particles that appear to be strikingly similar. Thus, if a mouse can be inoculated with a virus against leukemia, it may be possible to do the same for man —providing that the human leukemia virus can be found and a vaccine created. To this end, much experimentation on leukemia viruses is being carried on. Other scientists have been experimenting with limited success with vaccines made from cancer patient's own tumors.

The common occurrence of cancers in the same family has led to much thought about the part heredity might play as a cause. Biologists have been able, though with difficulty, to breed a cancer-susceptible strain of mice. However, most authorities at the present time agree that there is no real evidence to call heredity a cause of cancer. The fact that several cases occur in a family is regarded as a coincidence due to the increasing frequency of the disease in an aging population.

Common Sites of Cancers

Breast Cancer: The leading cause of death from cancer among women in the United States is breast cancer. An estimated 64,000 new cases occur each year, of which about 25,000 are fatal. One out of every 17 women will have the disease in her lifetime. The common type of breast cancer affects a gland. It is most curable when found while still small in size and confined to the breast. Hence, detecting it early is extremely important.

This can be done by monthly self-examination which any woman can easily learn. The American Cancer Society has a film available for free showing on this subject. Also, regular visits to the family doctor—particularly if any suspicious lump is felt—are vital. Ninety-five per cent of women with breast lumps wait too long to see their doctors. In a Scotland study of several thousand women on whom breast cancer surgery was performed, the average size of the tumor was a little over an inch, three times the size of the smallest lump that can be felt.

Lung Cancer: The leading cause of cancer deaths in American men is lung cancer. About 40,000 deaths are recorded in the United States each year from this disease. Yet, a large portion of these deaths could be prevented if there were no cigarette smoking. The more cigarettes smoked and the longer they are smoked, the greater the risk to the smoker. On the other hand, studies show that in those who stop smoking, the risk of lung cancer decreases directly with the length of time they have stopped smoking. Pipe and cigar smokers who do not inhale run little risk of lung cancer, but they are more prone to cancers of the lip, tongue, and mouth than are non-smokers.

Lung cancer is cured in only about 5 per cent of cases even though the potential cure rate is as high as 50 per cent if operated upon in time. Unfortunately, it often gives no clue to its presence until it is too advanced for cure. Prevention by not smoking is the best protection. (See Part XII, Chapter Three.)

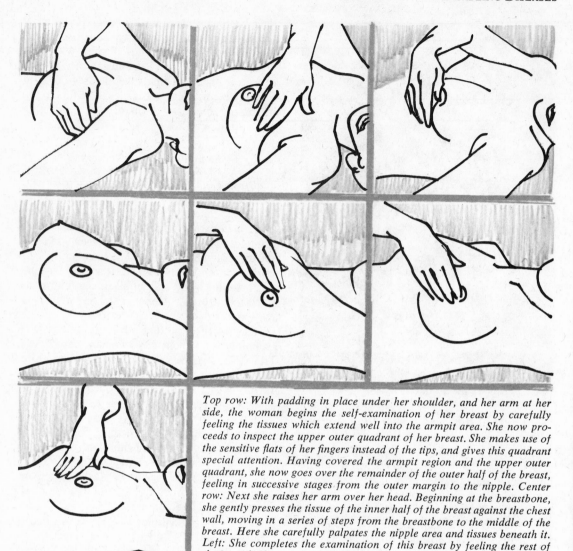

Top row: With padding in place under her shoulder, and her arm at her side, the woman begins the self-examination of her breast by carefully feeling the tissues which extend well into the armpit area. She now proceeds to inspect the upper outer quadrant of her breast. She makes use of the sensitive flats of her fingers instead of the tips, and gives this quadrant special attention. Having covered the armpit region and the upper outer quadrant, she now goes over the remainder of the outer half of the breast, feeling in successive stages from the outer margin to the nipple. Center row: Next she raises her arm over her head. Beginning at the breastbone, she gently presses the tissue of the inner half of the breast against the chest wall, moving in a series of steps from the breastbone to the middle of the breast. Here she carefully palpates the nipple area and tissues beneath it. Left: She completes the examination of this breast by feeling the rest of the inner half systematically. Along the lower margin she will find a ridge of firm tissue; this is normal, and should not alarm her.

Colon and Rectal Cancers: More than 73,000 Americans get colon or rectal cancer each year; the deaths from the disease number approximately 40,000. Regular annual physical examinations which include internal inspection with a lighted instrument (proctoscopy) could detect 75 per cent of these cancers soon enough for cure. The death rate could be cut by more than half if adults would get proper colon and rectal examinations, easily performed in a doctor's office, once a year.

Cancer of the Uterus: A sharp and dramatic decline in cancer deaths has taken place in cancer of the uterine cervix (neck of the womb). Formerly the number one cancer-killer of women, the uterine cancer death rate has dropped more than 50 per cent in 25 years. However, there will be 55,000 new cases of this cancer in any year and 14,000 deaths. The reason for the drop in the death rate is twofold:

1. More and more American women see their doctors for regular pelvic examinations.

2. More and more are getting the "Pap" (Papanicolaou) smear test as part of these examinations.

The "Pap" smear test is painless, extremely reliable, and inexpensive. It costs no more than a hair set or a theatre ticket. The test can detect uterine or cervical cancer when there are no symptoms and while the disease is still curable, often by x-ray therapy. The lives of thousands of women have been saved through the "Pap" smear test. If every woman took it once a year, deaths from uterine and cervical cancer could be nearly eliminated.

Leukemia and Lymphoma: Leukemia kills more children under the age of 15 than any other cancer, and cancer as a whole kills more children under 15 than any other disease. Acute leukemia, the form most often found in children, was once a fast killer. But since World War II, a number of chemical and hormone drugs have been developed to treat both leukemia (a cancer of the blood-forming organs, principally bone marrow) and lymphoma (a cancer of the lymph glands). The drugs slow down the disease for an average of nearly 13 months in acute cases and much longer in chronic cases. Antibiotics and blood transfusions are also useful in leukemia.

Chronic leukemia occurs most often in adults. There will be about 13,800 deaths from leukemia in an average year, of which about 2,400 will be children; and about 14,600 deaths from various lymphomas. There are no cures for these diseases, but patients can now live under treatment for months or years, free of pain and disability, carrying on their usual activities.

Cancer of the Stomach: The number of stomach cancer deaths has declined in the U.S. about 40 per cent in 25 years. The cause of the decline is not known, but some scientists believe that improved nutrition may be one of the reasons. The symptoms of stomach cancer are lack of appetite, persistent indigestion, nausea, and vomiting. As in other forms of cancer, delay or self-treatment can be fatal. It is the patient's responsibility to bring symptoms which may mean cancer to the attention of a physician within two weeks. If stomach cancer is diagnosed when it is still small, and before it has invaded surrounding tissue, about 50 per cent of the patients can be cured by surgery.

Cancer of the Bladder: Occurring three times more frequently in men than in women, cancer of the bladder makes itself known first by a change in bladder habits or by blood in the urine. Blood in the urine is a warning to see a doctor immediately. He can examine the bladder with a cystoscope and determine what course of treatment is required. This may be x-ray therapy, the application of radioactive isotopes, or surgery. Cancer of the bladder is caused by certain dyes, a parasitic infection

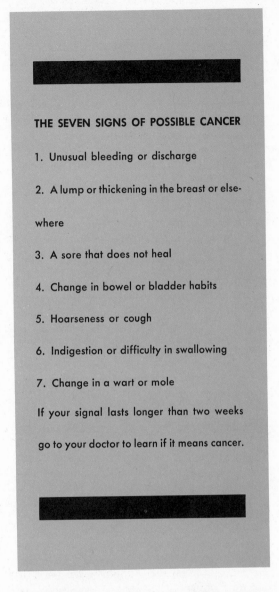

THE SEVEN SIGNS OF POSSIBLE CANCER

1. Unusual bleeding or discharge

2. A lump or thickening in the breast or else-

where

3. A sore that does not heal

4. Change in bowel or bladder habits

5. Hoarseness or cough

6. Indigestion or difficulty in swallowing

7. Change in a wart or mole

If your signal lasts longer than two weeks

go to your doctor to learn if it means cancer.

found mainly in Egypt, and, possibly, bladder stones existing for many years and causing chronic irritation.

Cancer of the Larynx: Persistent hoarseness is the early sign of cancer of the larynx. It can have other causes, but any hoarseness that lasts longer than two weeks calls for a prompt visit to the doctor for examination of the vocal cords. If there is a tumor and if it is small and confined to one cord, it may be treated successfully by x-ray or surgery with little damage to the speech mechanism. However, if the cancer is large or involves both vocal cords, the larynx may have to be removed.

This need not, however, condemn the patient to a speechless existence. He may learn to speak with mechanical devices developed for this purpose or, preferably, through the technique of esophageal speech which consists of swallowing air and forcing it out. With this technique, people without larynxes can learn to speak clearly in a matter of weeks; they can use the telephone, talk with friends, and even make speeches in public. The International Association of Laryngectomees sponsored by the American Cancer Society is an organization of people who have lost their larynxes to cancer. They offer rehabilitation advice and assistance to new laryngectomees.

Melanoma: Melanoma or "black cancer" forms in some moles that are subject to chronic irritation, such as the shaving area of the face, and in special locations such as the feet and sex organs. Such moles should be removed as precancerous lesions. Any change in a mole—ulceration, crusting, or itching—is a warning sign of melanoma and the patient should waste no time in consulting a doctor. While melanoma grows very rapidly, it can be cured with surgery if it is diagnosed early and treated promptly.

Medical Progress

Medical science has made tremendous progress against cancer. Surgery is now much more effective than ever. Radiation treatment offers many promising new techniques such as supervoltage x-ray and other forms of radiation or the use of radioactive isotopes of gold, iodine, cobalt, and other substances. In drug treatment, at least 20 chemicals have been found to be effective against cancer. Recently, one of them (methotrexate) has caused complete disappearance of widespread choriocarcinoma, a rare form of cancer found in women following pregnancy. Some patients so treated have remained cancer-free for more than five years.

The chemical attack on cancer has been aided by the development of ways to use powerful anti-cancer drugs in quantities and for periods of time which add to their potency without endangering normal tissues or the patient's life. The basic technique is known as perfusion.

It consists of isolating the circulation in a cancerous limb, organ, or entire section of the body and injecting into these vessels a chemical which attacks the cancer. Thus, the cancer can be hit hard with dangerous chemicals without damaging the rest of the body. A new technique in this area is the abdominal tourniquet which

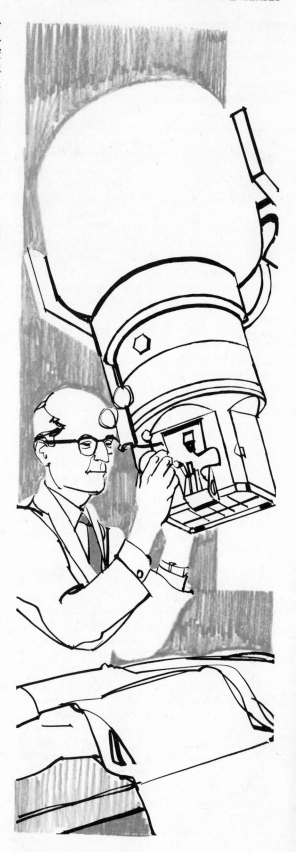

allows the entire pelvic cavity to be perfused with cancer-killing chemicals. D. S. Martin, of the University of Miami, has been working with his colleagues on the development of a combined heart-lung and kidney machine which will allow pelvic perfusion for a period of three to four hours.

Even an inoperable cancer can be treated. The new arsenal of chemicals and hormones can help the physician make life livable for the inoperable cancer patient. Many people have lived for years, even decades, with incurable cancers—and lived full, active lives—under proper treatment.

Cancer Quacks

Radiation and surgery are presently the only proved methods of curing cancer; yet many Americans do not go to physicians and hospitals where they can get effective treatment for cancer. Instead, they go to quacks. An estimated $100,000,000 is spent in the U.S. annually by the public on unproved remedies peddled by quacks. They rely on such "healers" who peddle unproved and invariably worthless remedies, which include anything from corrosive chemicals to fad diets, and who scoff at established methods of treatment. Thus, sufferers often forfeit their chances for cure through failure to receive proper treatment. (See also Part VIII, Chapter Five.)

The following is a list by the American Cancer Society of six helpful ways to identify a cancer quack:

1. If a "doctor" offers a cancer treatment that he claims is available only from himself - beware!

2. If his treatment bears his own name, or is offered in the name of his research organization whose other members, if any, are not listed - beware!

3. If he claims he is being persecuted by the "medical trusts" - beware!

4. If he says that his "cure" is being sabotaged by the medical profession - beware!

5. If his "cured" patients and greatest supporters have only his word for it that they had cancer when they came to him - beware!

6. If he refuses or discourages consultations with specialists in the medical profession - beware!

There are now approximately 800 cancer clinics, approved by the American College of Surgeons, in the United States and Canada, where proper treatment of cancers can be obtained. These are within reach of all cancer patients, and there is no geographical reason why proper cancer treatment should be denied to anyone. Nor is there any financial barrier to proper therapy that cannot be overcome with the help of various private and governmental agencies. Thus, anyone in the U.S. or Canada who avoids or refuses proper treatment for cancer is doing so through personal choice, not through the force of circumstance.

CHAPTER NINE

TUBERCULOSIS

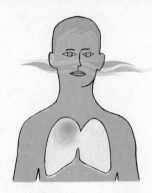

TUBERCULOSIS is a disease that people catch from one another. It has been one of the greatest killers in the history of the world. In the United States alone, five times as many Americans died of tuberculosis between 1900 and 1960 as had been killed in all the wars in U.S. history.

Not so many years ago tuberculosis was primarily a matter of death; today it is first of all a problem of the living.

Until relatively recently there was no specific treatment for tuberculosis. The vast majority of people who contracted the disease died of it. In the survivors, the disease was arrested only after months or even years of rest and possibly such measures as collapsing the diseased portion of a lung.

Today the picture is different. Specific treatment is available. Drugs have been discovered that are remarkably effective against tuberculosis. These, together with improved living conditions, have greatly changed the outlook for tuberculosis.

Although this outlook is brighter than it was only 15 years ago, the advances have brought their own complications. Lessening death rates are a dramatic story. Less dramatic, however, is the story of long months of illness, of the passing of the disease from one member of a family or other close associate to another, of recovery followed by breakdown. Yet this is the story behind the more than 50,000 new cases of tuberculosis reported in the United States each year.

The total number of active cases throughout the United States is estimated at 250,000, while between 30,000,000 and 35,000,000 people have been infected with the tuberculosis germ. Possibly 2,000,000 of these will break down with active tuberculosis during their lifetime. The real tuberculosis problem in the United States today is to prevent those already ill with tuberculosis from passing on their disease to others. This is a problem in preventive medicine that calls for constructive public health action. But because such measures are not so dramatic as curing the seriously ill, their importance is often overlooked.

The Disease

Tuberculosis is an infectious disease that primarily attacks the lung, although almost all organs can be involved. The specific cause of tuberculosis is the tubercle bacillus. Poor social and economic conditions are major contributing factors.

Tubercle bacilli are coughed up by people with active lung tuberculosis. The microorganisms are carried through the air on droplets expelled in coughing or sneezing. They may remain suspended in the air for long periods after the droplet itself evaporates. The bacilli are breathed in and, under conditions favorable to the microorganism, multiply in the lung. Bacilli may also gain entrance into the body through the digestive tract, but this is rare today in the United States because of the testing of cattle for tuberculosis and the pasteurization of milk.

Once infection occurs, the body's defense system is set in motion. Unless there is a massive invasion of bacilli, the system keeps the infection under control and active disease is prevented, for the time being at least. Later, if resistance is lowered or there is a new invasion of bacilli, active disease may develop. Most commonly in infants, but also in some adults, the initial infection may lead to a type of the disease that is scattered throughout the body. This is known as miliary tuberculosis. In other cases the infection spreads to the covering of the brain, causing tuberculous meningitis. Both are serious forms of the disease.

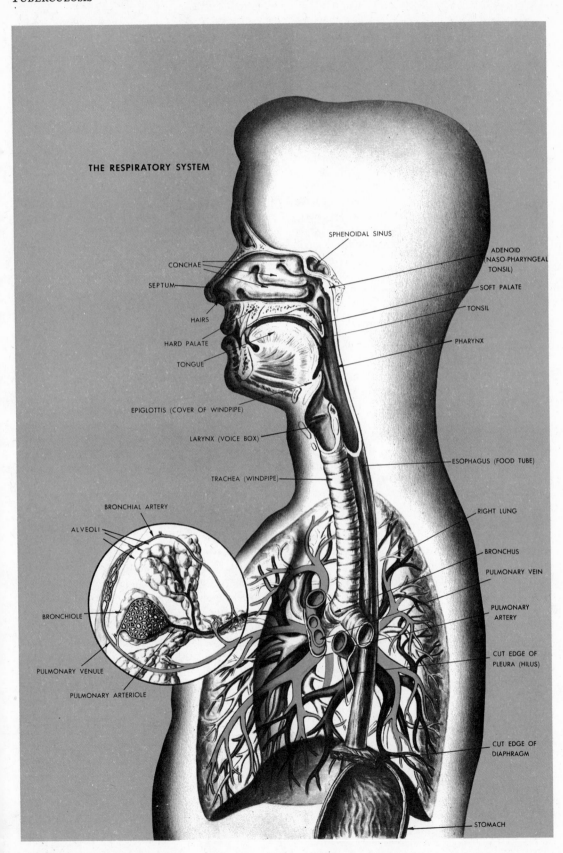

THE RESPIRATORY SYSTEM

SPHENOIDAL SINUS

CONCHAE

SEPTUM

HAIRS

HARD PALATE

TONGUE

EPIGLOTTIS (COVER OF WINDPIPE)

LARYNX (VOICE BOX)

TRACHEA (WINDPIPE)

BRONCHIAL ARTERY

ALVEOLI

BRONCHIOLE

PULMONARY VENULE

PULMONARY ARTERIOLE

ADENOID
(NASO-PHARYNGEAL
TONSIL)

SOFT PALATE

TONSIL

PHARYNX

ESOPHAGUS (FOOD TUBE)

RIGHT LUNG

BRONCHUS

PULMONARY VEIN

PULMONARY
ARTERY

CUT EDGE OF
PLEURA (HILUS)

CUT EDGE OF
DIAPHRAGM

STOMACH

After the first infection, the body's cells become sensitized to the particular proteins of the tubercle bacilli. Thus, when an infected person is given a skin test with a substance containing these proteins, he has an allergic reaction. This is the tuberculin test, a useful tool in the hands of tuberculosis specialists.

In the test a small amount of tuberculin is injected between the layers of the skin, usually on the forearm. If the individual being tested has been infected with tubercle bacilli, within 48 to 72 hours a hard, raised spot will appear at the site of the injection. The uninfected have no reaction. It must be emphasized, however, that the test makes no distinction between *infected* and *diseased* persons. Other steps must be taken to find out if the infected person actually has an active case of the disease.

There are several alternate techniques for the tuberculin test. The choice is made by the physician. The principle is the same in all methods, namely, the reaction of the tuberculin protein upon the tissues of the patient.

Discovery of the infected through the tuberculin test frequently leads to the discovery of a hidden active case. And since most future active cases will come from the infected of today, locating them is essential to starting treatment to prevent the development of active disease. Another important use of the tuberculin test is to distinguish tuberculosis from other diseases which appear similar to it.

Diagnosis

In its early stages, tuberculosis has no outward symptom. Thus, the disease may be quietly making inroads while its victim is unaware of his infection. Later, he may have fatigue, late afternoon fever, night sweats, and cough. These symptoms may send the individual to the doctor in whose office the vast majority of tuberculosis cases is diagnosed. Meanwhile, however, the disease may have reached an advanced stage, which is more difficult to cure than the early stage.

Tuberculosis can occur at any age. Tuberculosis in children has been known to occur as early as five or six weeks after birth. This period is considered the normal incubation time for the disease after exposure to an open case.

Primary tuberculosis occurs in children under the age of puberty. The secondary disease or reinfection, occurs after the age of puberty and chiefly involves the lungs.

The early signs of tuberculosis in children are deviations from the normal curve of growth and development of the child. Children with primary disease usually develop tuberculosis of the glands, miliary tuberculosis (blood stream infection), tuberculous meningitis, tuberculosis of the bone, tuberculosis of the intestines and, in some areas of the world, tuberculosis of the skin and eyes. The latter two types are quite rare in the United States.

A child with any of these types of tuberculosis is a sick child. He does not eat, rest, or grow normally. He may have a feeding problem, he may be exceedingly cross and unsociable, and he may have trouble sleeping. He also may have a low-grade temperature late in the day and the early evening, but a normal or subnormal one in the morning.

Any child deviating from his normal pattern of growth should be seen by a physician. Pediatricians may make a tuberculin test on the first visit to the office. If this test is positive but there are no other signs of the disease, a chest x-ray will be taken. If glands of the neck are swollen, this may aid in the early diagnosis of glandular tuberculosis. Many times the x-ray will reveal enlarged glands in the lungs.

A child with miliary tuberculosis is acutely ill with a high temperature. A child with tuberculous meningitis may be in a coma after several days of illness; a spinal puncture is required to confirm presence of disease. Every case of a positive tuberculin test in a child should be followed by not only medical treatment of the child, but also tests and x-rays of every person who has been in contact with him.

Children who do not appear to be ill are not normally given routine chest x-ray because tuberculosis of the lungs is not found in children before the age of puberty. Children are routinely given tuberculin skin tests to determine whether or not they have been exposed to an active case of disease.

Adults are routinely checked by chest x-rays to discover tuberculosis infection. Many times the x-ray will indicate early signs of disease months before such symptoms as fatigue, night sweats, low-grade temperatures, and the like appear.

The doctor who suspects tuberculosis in his patient will, of course, want to x-ray the patient's chest. He will not, however, base his diagnosis on the x-ray film alone. If the shadows on x-ray film suggest tuberculosis, he will examine the sputum for tubercle bacilli. He may also give the patient a tuberculin test, for a negative test will almost certainly rule out tuberculosis while a positive one, together with a positive x-ray film, is strong evidence of TB.

A new development in the United States, use of the tuberculin test and the chest x-ray at the same time, permits entire communities to identify all positive reactors and to treat everyone who is in danger of developing the disease. To find the unknown cases and see that the affected individuals are adequately treated is a public health measure of greatest importance in the control of tuberculosis.

It must be emphasized that the amount of radiation received from a single chest x-ray from a machine kept in good condition is very slight, especially in comparison with the danger of undiscovered tuberculosis.

As a safeguard, everyone in the household should cultivate good general health habits— proper food, sufficient rest and recreation, and a well-ventilated home.

Treatment

Drugs are the basis of treatment of the tuberculous patient today. The discovery of drugs effective in treating tuberculosis constitutes one of the great medical advances of the century. None of the drugs appears to kill the germs, but several stop the bacilli from multiplying and permit the body's natural healing processes to carry on without interference.

The principal drugs used in the treatment of tuberculosis are streptomycin, an antibiotic that came into use around 1945; para-aminosalicylic acid (PAS), a synthetic chemical compound that has been in use since 1948;

and isoniazid (INH), also a synthetic chemical compound that was first used in 1952.

Of the three, isoniazid is recognized as the most useful. Happily, in addition to its healing value, it has other virtues. It is easy to administer (by mouth), it has few side reactions and these, on the whole, are mild, and it is inexpensive. PAS is also taken by mouth, but it must be taken in large doses and causes stomach upsets in some patients. It has the least value against tuberculosis of the three major drugs. Streptomycin must be injected, and in some it causes dizziness or loss of hearing.

Usually, two of these three drugs are given at the same time. Doing so has been found to delay or prevent the bacilli from learning to live with the drugs.

Because of the chronic nature of tuberculosis, drugs must be taken for a long period; at least two years is recommended by the American Thoracic Society, the chest specialists' section of the National Tuberculosis Association. The American Thoracic Society also strongly recommends that most patients with active tuberculosis have their first period of treatment in a hospital. This serves a twofold purpose. It is a good public health practice because it cuts down the chances that the infectious patient may pass his disease on to others. It is also an advantage in treating the patient to have laboratory testing facilities available at all times and to have the patient under constant observation so that treatment can be changed if he does not respond properly. When infectiousness is under control, the patient may be permitted to go home but must continue to take

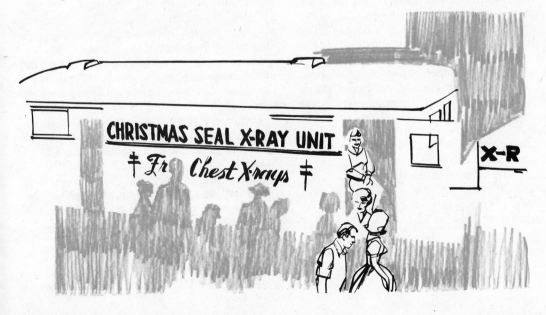

his drugs regularly and to report to his doctor, clinic, or hospital for regular check-ups.

Bed rest does not play a major role in the treatment of tuberculosis today. At one time it was almost the only measure available, but the proper use of drugs makes prolonged periods of complete rest in bed unnecessary. However, bed rest is still recommended for the very ill patient or one who may be running a high temperature.

In addition to drugs, surgery may be used in treatment. Lung surgery today carries no greater risks than the normal removal of an appendix. Lung surgery has been made more effective by advanced methods of giving anesthesia, and by the drugs which control infection, as well as by the use of blood for transfusions. With these advantages and the aid of skilled nursing care, it is possible to perform virtual miracles for tuberculosis patients. Surgery is more often used to remove parts of the lung than to collapse it. The amount of lung tissue removed depends upon the extent of the disease. The aim is to interfere as little as possible with the lung's function while removing diseased tissue.

When, for various reasons, none of the three major drugs can be used in treating a particular patient, certain "second-line" drugs may be of help for limited periods. They are at times lifesaving in keeping the infection under control until surgery can be performed, but they must be used carefully and only in a hospital.

Prevention

The discovery of isoniazid has not only helped in the treatment of tuberculosis, but it can also be used to prevent the disease. Trials undertaken in the Tuberculosis Program of the United States Public Health Service have shown that during one year of administration, isoniazid is approximately 80 per cent effective in preventing tuberculosis among groups that have greater than ordinary exposure to the disease.

The vaccine most widely used to prevent tuberculosis is BCG. This is a vaccine made from a live, weakened strain of the tubercle bacillus named Bacillus of Calmette and Guerin, after the two French scientists who developed it. The vaccine is recommended only in areas where the disease is common, not for widespread use. One of its disadvantages is that everyone on whom it is used reacts positively to the tuberculin test. Thus, this test loses its value as an indicator of infection.

Tuberculosis has been one of the most costly of all man's diseases in terms of personal disability, economic loss, and costs for care and control. Today many lives are being saved and patients do not have to languish for years in hospitals, but often can return to work while taking drugs at home. Even so, the cost of the disease is estimated at more than $725,000,000 a year in the United States alone.

The bulk of the money spent comes from state, county, or city funds since the control of tuberculosis, as of other communicable diseases, is the responsibility of official health agencies. Added to these funds is the money spent by the voluntary agencies, particularly those affiliated with the National Tuberculosis Association, which work with the official agencies in control and research programs.

Not so many years ago tuberculosis was considered a hopeless disease. Today there is hope not only for the individual patient who is ill with tuberculosis, but even for its disappearance in the United States. The outlook in many other parts of the world is not so bright. Tuberculosis is still the most serious health problem in many parts of Asia, Africa, and South America.

The progress made against tuberculosis is due in part to such general factors as improved economic conditions, which have resulted in less crowded housing, better diets, and better ventilation and sanitation. It is due in part also to scientific triumphs such as the discovery of drugs effective in treating the disease. It is also due to broadened ideas about public responsibility for health measures, such as the maintenance of public hospitals and clinics for the diagnosis, supervision, and treatment of tuberculosis patients.

Unless effort slackens, there is reason to anticipate a day when tuberculosis will no longer be a threat to anyone in the United States. When that day comes it will be because the public has insisted that efforts be stepped up to find and treat every person with active tuberculosis. Only in this way can the chain of infection-to-disease-to-infection be broken.

ALLERGY

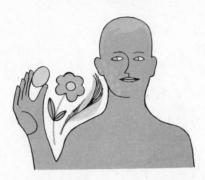

PEOPLE HAVE AN ALLERGY when their bodies are sensitive to substances most other people's bodies are not. The allergic person may have distressing symptoms from what he breathes, eats, or touches, while the nonallergic person is not troubled by them. The normal individual enjoys a bright summer day unaware of the tiny, microscopic pollen grains in the air. To the allergic person this same summer day with its pollen grains means hay fever or asthma. The nonallergic person enjoys his food. The person allergic to a particular food may have, if he eats it, stomach pain, hives, eczema, or other skin rashes, asthma, or migraine headaches. The normal woman can enjoy a beautifully dyed dress. The person allergic to the dye used may develop an intense itching rash on the slightest contact with it.

Whatever it is that produces an allergic reaction is called an allergen or an antigen.

Our Defense Mechanism

The cells of the body of both allergic and nonallergic persons can distinguish between "self" and "nonself." In other words, they recognize substances which are identical in composition with them and accept them as harmless, while they recognize those that differ in composition as foreign and potentially harmful. The latter must be prevented entry.

Entry of such foreign substances as bacteria and foreign proteins is prevented by the surface covers which separate the body cells from the outside world. These include the skin and the linings of the breathing, digestive, and reproductive tracts. These coverings actually form one continuous sheath. It differs in appearance and structure in the different areas, but it is alike in separating our internal cells from the outside world.

These surfaces protect the inner cells from both dryness and too much moisture, from a loss of our own fluids, from cold, heat, bacteria, chemicals, and other harmful influences.

The first barrier may, however, be breached. Skin broken by injury may be invaded by bacteria or the skin may be punctured for injection of vaccines, antibiotics, or other medicines.

Most substances which find entry past the outer barriers are foreign to the person's cells. Usually these can be expelled through the kidneys, the intestines, or the lungs without trouble. Some substances, such as bacteria or proteins (for example antitoxins), cannot be eliminated without being broken down into smaller units. The cells of the body are prepared to do this.

Certain body cells can manufacture substances called antibodies which can combine with specific invading foreign material. Moreover, after such antibodies are first formed, they can be manufactured much more rapidly with the next invasion of the same or a similar material. These antibodies combine with the foreign protein and release ferments. These split the foreign chemical units into smaller units which can be eliminated from the body more easily.

The action of such antibodies is defensive and does not harm the body cells. In combining with bacteria and viruses, antibodies protect the body against harm. However, when antibodies combine with proteins, the body cells themselves are injured in the process of splitting and getting rid of the foreign materials. The combination of antibodies with proteins results not only in a release of ferments, but also of histamine and other related substances which injure the body cells and cause illnesses. Such illnesses are called "allergies."

Everyone's body cells form antibodies which react with foreign protein. The same processes occur in most lower animals as well. Therefore, it can be truly said that all people and most animals can become allergic if a large enough

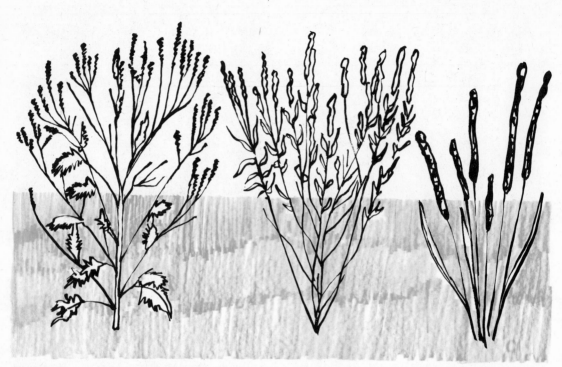

Typical allergy-producing plants include (from left): short or common ragweed; southern ragweed; and timothy.

amount of foreign protein gets past one of the body's defensive barriers. The nonallergic as well as the allergic person can thus become sensitive to any protein.

The difference between the allergic people who make up 10 to 20 per cent or more of the population and the remaining 80 to 90 per cent, is that they are sensitive to materials which come in contact only with the skin and other outer coverings of the body. For the allergic individual to react, these materials need not be injected past the barriers. The allergic individual is capable of producing special antibodies called "skin-sensitizing" antibodies which combine with such foreign material as pollen or food protein. When this happens, histamine and similar substances are released and allergy symptoms occur every time there is contact with the offending material.

Allergic people inherit the tendency to become allergic. Most of them have allergic parents, grandparents, uncles, or aunts. However, they need not be sensitive to the same substances or have the same symptoms as their allergic relatives. Only the tendency to become allergic runs in their families. If people from two allergic families marry, the chances are three to one that their children will become allergic. If only one of the parents is from an al-

lergic family, the chance for allergy in the children is reduced to two to one.

The symptoms of allergy involve primarily the surface linings of the body. Other deeper tissues are affected, but most of the symptoms that the patient complains about are due to changes in the surface coverings. In hay fever, the nasal and eye linings are involved; in asthma, the lining of the bronchial tubes; in eczema, the surface of the skin; in allergy to foods, the surface of the stomach, gall bladder, and intestines. However, when the substances causing the allergy manage to pass the surface barriers they can also cause allergic symptoms in other organs, such as the deeper layers of the skin, the joints, liver, brain, or blood.

The Respiratory System

The linings of the nose, the windpipe, and the bronchial tubes separate the deeper cells of the breathing system from the outside world. These linings are affected in hay fever and asthma, the two allergies of the respiratory system.

To most people hay fever means nasal allergy to pollens, most commonly to the ragweed pollens of August and September. Most people think of hay fever as a seasonal condition, affecting the patient regularly during cer-

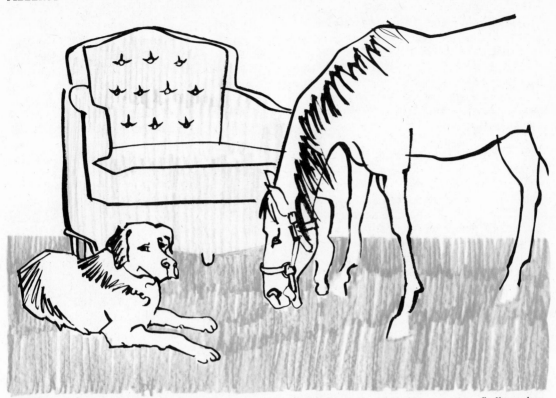

Animal-related allergies include those caused by dog and horse hair. Hair-stuffed chair may give off allergy dust.

tain months of the year. This concept tells only parts of the story. There are other types of nasal allergy which are also common and as important as August-September hay fever due to ragweed—June-July hay fever due to grass pollens, and spring hay fever due to tree pollens. People in grain-growing areas often get seasonal hay fever and asthma during the warmer months from the small spores of molds which commonly grow on vegetation. The dusts created by disintegrated insects can also cause seasonal symptoms.

Nasal allergies may be caused by many other allergens besides pollens. House dusts or the dust particles from feathers or animals can cause the same symptoms all year around. Hay fever symptoms, therefore, may be present not only during a certain season, but also throughout the entire year.

Smokers may have allergies to tobacco which may be overlooked in the belief that they are merely irritations from too much smoking. Such allergies may be particularly important where the patient's allergy is expressed as asthma or emphysema, both of which are discussed later in this chapter. (See also Part XII, Chapter Three.)

The symptoms of hay fever are familiar to most people. They include sneezing attacks and itching or running nose or eyes. These are the familiar symptoms of nasal allergy, but many patients have less typical complaints. They may complain of a blocked nose because of the swelling of the nasal membrane, but have no sneezing or itching. If the sensitivity has come on gradually and has been present the year round for many years the patient may have become so accustomed to the blocked nose that he accepts it as "normal." These patients frequently awaken with a dry mouth because they have breathed through their mouths during the night. They may have headaches and temporary or permanent loss of smell, due to swelling of the nasal lining.

Such patients frequently, but incorrectly, think that they have a "sinus condition." And their allergy may at times be associated with a sinus infection because the swelling of their nasal lining may lead to more frequent colds along with sinus infection.

But sinus infections are secondary and in addition to their nasal allergy. At such times the clear watery secretion typical of nasal allergy changes to a thick yellow or green secretion characteristic of infection. Chronic nasal allergy may cause polyps to grow in the nose, and may cause mouth breathing that can deform the dental arch.

Before nasal allergy can be satisfactorily treated, the cause or causes of the allergy must be found. It is not enough simply to recognize that a person has nasal allergy. The allergic person is seldom sensitive to only one thing; he is almost always sensitive to many things. He may be sensitive to a dog, a cat, feathers, molds, pollens—to several or all these things. Unless all the causes are determined, the patient can be helped only partially or not at all.

The patient's story will frequently reveal to the experienced doctor the causes for the symptoms. Sneezing attacks or a blocked nose present only during certain summer months are attributable to the pollens present during this period. Symptoms present during the entire summer may be due to pollens, molds, or insects or to a combination of these. Symptoms present all year around require a more careful search for causes to be found in the patient's home or at his work.

Skin tests with suspected materials, if properly interpreted, may help establish the causes. Skin tests without a careful history, however, are worthless or misleading. A reaction obtained to dog dander may not be related to the patient's present allergy. The dog that first caused the sensitivity may have been disposed of years ago and there is no longer a dog around to cause trouble. It should be remembered that allergic patients are inclined to become sensitive to new things. One must sort out the former from the present causes of trouble.

Let us assume that through a careful history, confirmed by skin tests, the doctor finds that a patient's nasal trouble is due to ragweed pollen in August and September and to feathers and dog dander the rest of the year. How does he treat the patient?

First, he can give him some relief by prescribing one of the many antihistamine drugs. It will be recalled that allergic symptoms are caused by the release of histamine in the system. Antihistamine drugs act in just the way their name signifies, against histamines. These drugs prevent histamine from injuring cells. Unfortunately, antihistamines can help only to a limited degree. They are not effective when a large amount of histamine is liberated and when symptoms are more than mild. The physician, therefore, takes other measures in addition to prescribing these relief drugs.

Two procedures are open to him: First, he advises that offending materials be removed from the home if possible. A patient sensitive to feathers, dogs, cats, or other substances should not be exposed to them. Rubber or synthetic filled pillows can be substituted for feathers. Even a small bird can shed enough feather dust in a room to make the susceptible person miserable. Disposal of pets is occasionally a trying emotional experience for children or even for some adults. Sometimes a patient may choose to endure his allergy rather than give up a beloved pet.

Frequently, the patient who is allergic to pollens can go away during his hay fever season to a place which is free from the offending pollen. If he can't do this, he can remove the pollen from his environment. Home or room air filters may help, as may nose or face masks during temporary exposures.

Second, when the causes of allergy cannot be removed or the patient cannot remove himself from them, the doctor may try to reduce the patient's sensitivity by careful injections of the offending material. Unfortunately, the procedure is not curative, even though it helps a large proportion of patients. While the injections usually must be continued for many years, the large number of patients who accept this treatment speaks for its usefulness. Severe, acute attacks can be controlled with some of the new steroid drugs.

Asthma

The lining of the nose continues into the bronchial tubes. Asthma in most cases is an extension of nasal allergy into them. About 40 per cent of patients who have nasal allergy develop asthma. The same substances that cause swelling and increased secretion in the lining of the nose produce similar results in the lining of the bronchial tubes. The bronchial tube passages become narrower because of swelling of their linings, contraction of the muscle tissue in the bronchial walls, or from plugging with thick mucus. These cause difficulty in breathing and induce coughing attacks, the major symptoms of asthma.

As in hay fever, the physician must do more than recognize the condition as asthma; he must discover its causes. And again, like hay fever, the causes may produce seasonal asthma due to pollens or all-year-around asthma due to many other causes. It should be noted that the term "asthma," which means "breathless," is a general term used to describe symptoms due to causes other than allergy. For example, "cardiac asthma" is breathlessness due to impaired heart action.

Asthma is a much more serious and much more complicated condition than hay fever. Years of asthma can produce a variety of abnormal changes and responses. The patient's bronchial tubes become so sensitive to irritation that strong odors, cold air, and the common infectious cold will produce asthma. Emotional tension may aggravate the condition and make the patient more prone to asthma attacks. Emotional tension, alone, is rarely the major cause of the patient's trouble. Instead, like cold air or the odor of fresh paint, emotional tension can produce attacks in the patient whose symptoms have been present for many years and whose bronchial tubes have thus become easily irritable. The most feared complication of asthma is emphysema, a stretching of the lungs which makes the person short-winded.

Because asthma tends to become more severe and more complicated as it persists, it should be taken care of as early as possible. The same principles of treatment used for hay fever must be pursued even more thoroughly in treating asthma. Those causes for the attacks that can be removed from the home must be. If diet studies and skin tests determine that certain foods cause trouble they should also be eliminated. When a patient is sensitive to substances like pollens and molds that cannot be eliminated, his resistance to them may be increased by careful injections as for hay fever.

Numerous drugs have been developed for the relief of asthma. Great relief can be obtained by the injection of epinephrine (adrenalin) solution. This is a potent drug that should be used only under a physician's guidance. Ephedrin preparations help mild cases. In the past 15 years hormones (ACTH) and cortisone-like preparations have given the physician valuable relief measures. Hormone treatment for asthma should be used cautiously and only for as limited a time as possible.

The question most frequently asked by the asthmatic patient is whether a change of climate will benefit his condition. Frequently, without seeking advice, parents will sell their home and leave their work in the hope that a warm dry climate will cure a child's asthma. Asthma in children is rarely helped by change of climate. Sometimes a child is relieved by an escape from pollens or molds to which he is sensitive. But often in such cases the patient develops sensitivity in two to three years to the pollens of his new environment.

The patients who are helped by warm, dry equable climate are those whose asthma is due primarily to chronic bronchial infection or those who have had asthma for many years and are affected by cold air. These patients are usually older people whose asthma occurs primarily in winter.

The allergic conditions of the respiratory tract have been discussed in detail because of their importance. Three other surface coverings are left to be considered: those of the urinary tract, the skin, and the digestive tract.

The urinary tract is not frequently affected by allergy, but the other two are.

The Skin

The skin is the site of two types of allergic symptoms, eczema and hives. Eczema is properly used to describe all types of itching skin rashes which are allergic. When the material (antigen) causing the rash comes from outside sources the eczema is called "contact dermatitis." Contact dermatitis is usually limited to the skin areas actually touched by the offending material, but in acute attacks it may spread beyond these areas.

Some materials are such strong sensitizers that almost everyone can become allergic to them. Poison ivy and poison oak or sumac are outstanding examples of strong sensitizing materials which can produce allergic rashes in any person following adequate exposure. Because of their strong effect, these substances often produce severe, blistering rashes.

Many other substances produce less severe rashes which cause itching and redness in the affected areas. Among the most important are dyes (used to color clothes or to dye hair), chemicals in cosmetics, shampoos, and creams, lacquers, plastics, mercury and nickel compounds, furniture polishes, detergents, and a host of other substances.

A diagnosis of the cause is essential in treating contact dermatitis. Keen detective work and experience are required. Skin tests by applying the suspected material to a normal skin area for 24 to 48 hours may be tried. Caution must be used not to apply materials which can harm the normal skin. When the cause of contact dermatitis is discovered, its care consists of avoiding contact with the material.

Allergic eczema may be caused by substances taken internally. In severe cases the rash may cover the entire skin. When milder, the face, neck, back of the knees, or folds of the elbow are the areas most often involved. Ex-

428

tremely severe itching results in scratching and this in turn leads to rawness, thickening, and scaling of the skin. The condition is most common in infancy and tends to clear up in some cases by the end of the fourth year of life. Not infrequently, however, this type of eczema lasts for many years.

The discovery of the cause or causes of this form of eczema is often very difficult since substances that are inhaled as well as those that are eaten or drunk may cause eruption. In many instances no cause can be found. Emotional disturbances and nervous tension can make an attack much worse. Because such dermatitis makes the affected areas very sensitive, contact with other substances that normally are only mildly irritating can cause marked flare-ups.

Relief of itching requires the use of a variety of local medicines as well as internally administered drugs. Colloid (oatmeal or starch) baths are frequently prescribed. Hormones may be used under strict medical supervision.

Hives (urticaria) are temporary swellings starting below skin surface. They may be caused by a variety of allergy-producing substances, but often no cause can be discovered. They resemble mosquito bites. The most common causes of hives are drugs and foods, but they may have a number of other causes.

As the use of drugs for relief of many conditions has increased, sensitivity to them has correspondingly increased. A typical example is offered by antibiotics, especially penicillin. While these drugs can save lives, they also can produce sensitivity. The injection of a drug like penicillin or of an antitoxin in a person sensitive to the material may produce not only hives, but sometimes more serious and even fatal symptoms. A person who has once had hives following the use of any drug should be aware of the greater danger if the same drug is given again, especially if it is injected. He and his physician must be aware of his sensitivity to any drug. Such persons should wear a medical identification tag, carry a warning card, or both. (See Part IX, Chapter One.)

Commonly used drugs such as aspirin, sleeping medicines, and laxatives can produce hives. This is in no way due to the fault of the drug, but to the sensitivity of the person.

Any food may be the cause of hives and it is wrong to think of one food as a more likely cause than another. In searching for the cause, it should be remembered that frequently a substance like onion, garlic, or other food flavoring may be the cause rather than the food it is used to season.

The Digestive Tract

While foods are the most common cause of allergic symptoms in the gullet, stomach, or intestines, drugs may also cause allergy. The gall bladder as well as the gastrointestinal tract may be the site of symptoms.

The symptoms of gastrointestinal allergy vary from mild discomfort (bloating and constipation or diarrhea) to severe abdominal pain. Abdominal allergy may resemble one of many diseases of the abdominal organs, for example, stomach ulcers, appendicitis, or gall bladder disease. It should be emphasized that allergy cannot cause any of the conditions it resembles. Pain in the gall bladder is much more frequently caused by gallstones than by allergy to foods. But when the lining of the gall bladder becomes swollen because of allergy, the resulting pain may closely resemble that from gallstones.

To treat abdominal allergy requires finding its causes. A very careful diet study is necessary with tests in which suspected foods are eliminated or purposely tried to observe their effect. Intelligent observation, in which the physician's skill and the patient's patience play important roles, is essential. The only effective treatment is to avoid the substances causing the condition.

KIDNEY DISEASE

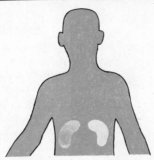

THE STRUCTURE OF THE KIDNEYS and how they work is dealt with in Part III. Here we consider the important diseases of the kidneys and what may be done to keep their consequences to a minimum.

Nephritis

A great deal of nonsense appears in popular literature on nephritis, the disease that is more properly called glomerulonephritis and is popularly known as Bright's disease. Backache, general weakness, "debility," and getting up at night to urinate are all suggested as being caused by "kidney disease." All sorts of peculiar remedies are offered for sale in newspaper and magazine advertising, ranging from mineral waters to "magnetized" belts.

The plain facts are that nephritis is a serious disease and its diagnosis can be made only by a physician. Its onset is often associated with infection of the throat, ear, or skin. There may be fever, sore throat, puffiness of the eyes, and swollen ankles. The urine may be scant and bloody. But nephritis may also begin insidiously with less obvious symptoms. The first signs may be swollen ankles, a pasty complexion, and vague signs of illness. The examining physician may also note a rise in blood pressure. He will find albumin, a protein substance which forms part of the blood serum, and very small amounts of blood in the urine in this type of nephritis. The patient may be anemic.

Curiously, those with the worst initial symptoms often do better in the long run than those with a gradual or slow onset. But in either case, it is of great importance that the patient go to bed and stay there until the infection subsides and sometimes even until the albumin all but disappears.

After the disease has subsided, the patient should lead a normal life, but try to avoid infection and chilling. He can take no special precautions except to have regular consultations with a doctor once the acute phase of nephritis is past. But if any operation—even a tooth extraction—is to be performed, he should warn his physician about having had nephritis so that he can take all necessary precautions against infection.

Much has recently been written about so-called "artificial kidneys" and kidney transplants. The machine known as an "artificial kidney" performs the kidney function of excretion and may replace this normal function for periods up to several years in length. But it is a time-consuming, expensive treatment and can be used only in a few highly selective cases. It is not something the average patient should count on.

Transplantation of one kidney between identical twins has been very successful. Few people, however, are identical twins. In all other cases, the body recognizes a foreign kidney, even though it may come from a member of our family, and rejects it. This "rejection phenomenon" is the major reason for transplant failure. Much work is now in progress to overcome it, and some of it has had modest success.

Transplantation is in its early stage and the hope that the problems will be solved in the not too distant future seems justified. If it is, then patients with the terminal uremia (kidney failure) of nephritis may well have a second chance to live.

Can nephritis be avoided? The answer is probably no. Every effort should be made, however, to clear up infections wherever they may be as quickly as possible, especially if the patient is "run down." But there is no specific way which guarantees that nephritis can be wholly avoided. By knowing the kind of disease it is, one may suspect its occurrence and avoid neglect or the pitfalls of quack treatment.

Nephrosis

Nephrosis is a disease closely allied to nephritis. It is confusing in that there are some people who seem to have a "pure" form of it

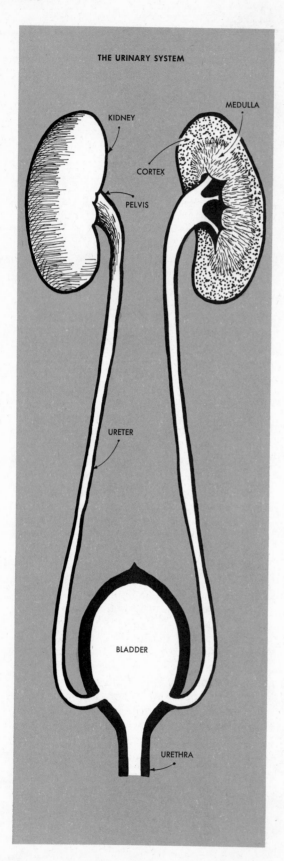

THE URINARY SYSTEM

KIDNEY

MEDULLA

CORTEX

PELVIS

URETER

BLADDER

URETHRA

while most people have it as a stage of nephritis itself. In the latter it is referred to as the "nephrotic phase" or the "nephrotic syndrome." In any case, it is a kidney disease characterized chiefly by a large loss of albumin through the urine and by marked swelling or "dropsy" of the tissues. The face, abdomen, and ankles may be greatly swollen with water.

Some treatments for nephrosis have been quite successful but the remedies require skillful use. The patient himself can help the treatment by avoiding as much salt as possible and including a goodly amount of meat or other protein in his diet. The outlook for nephrosis depends entirely on the particular circumstances of the disease in the individual patient.

Kidney-Caused High Blood Pressure

One of the most spectacular recent developments in the field of kidney diseases has been the demonstration that the kidneys can cause high blood pressure. This condition can often be cured surgically by removing the obstruction that blocks the free flow of blood in the main artery of the kidney. There is no way an individual can recognize the presence of such an obstruction in his own kidneys, but when physicians find a person's blood pressure to be abnormally high, they will make a careful search for such an obstruction.

Not all patients with this kind of high blood pressure need be operated upon for repair of the artery to the kidney. Treatment with drugs often will cure the condition. People who are effectively treated can usually live quite normal lives.

Cystitis and Pyelonephritis

Infections of the bladder and kidneys are not uncommon, especially in girls and women. Usually so-called cystitis (inflammation of the bladder) comes and goes but does not result in serious infection of the kidneys.

Bladder symptoms may occur as a result of cancer. These may also be due to irritations from stones, to chemicals in the urine, to excessive smoking, or to changes in the bladder lining for which specific causes are not always identifiable.

On the other hand, much that masquerades as "cystitis" is in reality an infection of the kidneys known technically as pyelonephritis. It is for these reasons that cystitis should always be carefully investigated and any necessary corrective measures be taken by a competent surgeon or kidney specialist.

Medical treatment for cystitis and pyelonephritis usually has to be carried on regularly or from time to time during the life of the patient. Many physicians believe that only in this way can the serious consequences of pyelonephritis be avoided.

Pyelonephritis itself is a form of Bright's disease. Usually the urine is cloudy with pus cells and there will be albumin. The blood pressure may rise. The patient is often listless and tires easily. In many cases, the condition is difficult to distinguish from nephritis. Pyelonephritis, if unchecked, tends to reduce the patient's chances for a long and full life and must, therefore, be taken seriously.

Polycystic Kidneys

Some people are born with kidneys in which there are little lakes of fluid called cysts. These cysts take up space that should be occupied by normal kidney tissue. If cysts become infected, they further reduce healthy kidney tissue.

There is no known way to prevent the formation of these cysts, and about the most that can be done is to treat infection when it appears. Attempts have been made to remove or wipe out the cysts by surgery, but this kind of operation so far has not appeared to aid the patient significantly.

The kidneys, the heart, and the blood vessels function closely together. The condition of one organ affects that of the other two. Thus, kidney disease can cause high blood pressure and this in turn can injure the blood vessels and the heart. It works the other way, too. Blood vessel disease can injure the heart and kidneys, and heart disease injures the blood vessels and kidneys by impairing the nutrition of all the tissues. That is why the combination problems of heart, blood vessels, and kidneys are often called medically cardio (heart)-vascular (blood vessels)-renal (kidney) disease.

The frequently hidden nature of diseases of these vital systems emphasizes the importance of the periodic health examination. Small changes from the normal may be detected and prevented from growing into big ones.

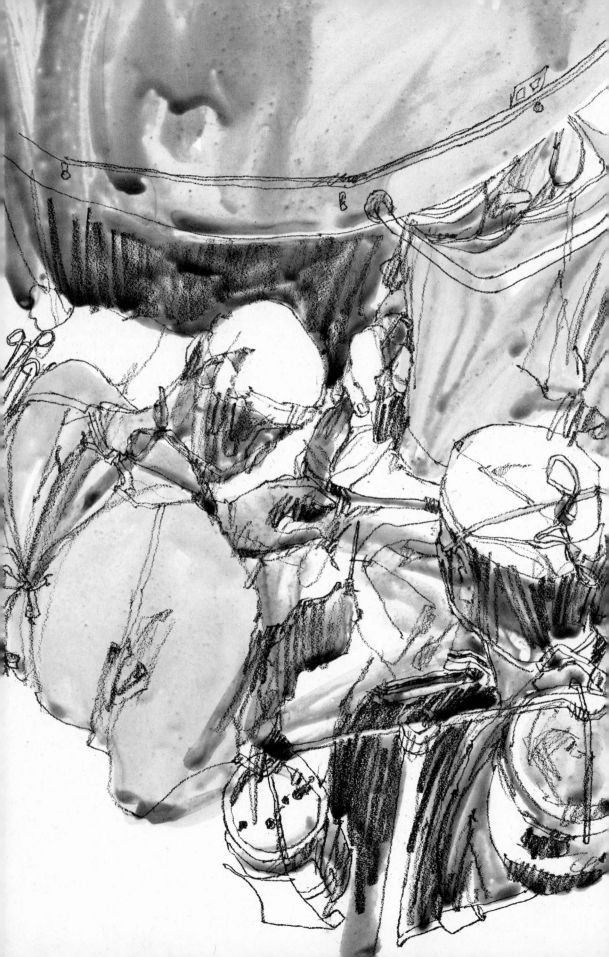

PART XI

Surgery Today

WHEN SURGERY IS NEEDED

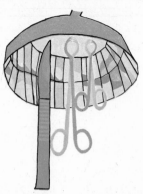

THE NEED FOR SURGERY, especially emergency surgery, almost always comes as a shock to the patient and his family. Despite modern advances, most people still have an instinctive fear of hospitals and anesthesia. Many people doubt that immediate surgery is really essential. Few people know how to select a surgeon. These and other problems related to surgery can best be solved with the aid of your family physician.

In the early years of this century there was little specialization in surgery. A good surgeon was good at performing almost every operation that had been devised. Today the situation is different. Operations are now being done that had not even been dreamed of 50 years ago. The heart can be safely opened and its valves repaired. Clogged blood vessels can be cleaned out or broken ones mended or replaced. Lungs, whole stomachs, pancreases, and parts of the brain can be removed and still permit the patient to live a comfortable and satisfactory life.

But not every surgeon wants to or is qualified to do these operations. It is not realistic to expect any one surgeon to be expert in all the complex branches of surgery. The fact that you got along so well after your appendectomy does not imply that the surgeon who operated on you would be equally well qualified to operate on your heart. This is where your family doctor enters the picture. It is his job to know the qualifications of various surgeons in various fields and to help you select the one whose skills best suit your case.

If there are alternative methods of treatment or if there are differences of opinion between the various physicians who have seen you, there is no reason why you should not ask your family physician to refer you to a specialist in your disease. Often such a consultation will resolve your doubts and reassure you in the choice of the surgeon you first consulted.

The scope of surgery has increased remarkably in this century. Its safety has increased too; deaths from most operations are about 20 per cent of what they were in 1910. Surgery has been extended in many directions, for example, to the treatment of certain types of birth defects in newborn babies and to life-saving operations for the aging. The hospital stay after surgery has been shortened to as little as a week for most major operations. Many patients are out of bed on the day after an operation and may be back at work in two or three weeks.

Many developments in modern surgery are almost incredible. They include the replacement of damaged blood vessels with artificial ones made of plastic, the replacement of the valves of the heart with plastic valves, transplanting of tissues such as the cornea of the eye, the development of the artificial kidney to clean the blood of poisons, and the development of artificial hearts and lungs. All these miracles open a hopeful vista into the future of surgery. It even seems that we are on our way toward breaking the greatest barrier to the surgical conquest of disease—the barrier of individual differences.

Organ Transplants

Every person, except identical twins, is unique to himself; no one else is like him; he has his own unique fingerprints and his unique body tissues. Hitherto no person, (except, again, identical twins) has been able to accept into his body the tissues of another person without reacting against them and eventually killing them.

Recently, as a result of long experimentation, it has been found that, after x-raying the entire body or treating it with drugs whose effects mimic irradiation, it is possible to graft

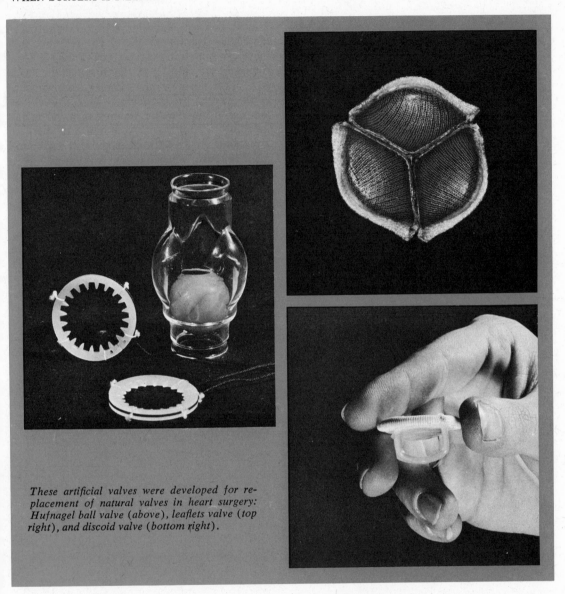

These artificial valves were developed for replacement of natural valves in heart surgery: Hufnagel ball valve (above), leaflets valve (top right), and discoid valve (bottom right).

tissues from one person to another which will survive for periods of a year or more. Kidneys have been successfully transplanted in a few instances when the donor and the patient were twins. Attempts, as yet unsuccessful, are being made to transplant livers. Lungs have been transplanted in animals.

If at some time in the future it becomes feasible to transplant organs, you might quite possibly go to the hospital and have your worn out organs replaced by new ones. But this is a dream of the future. Surgery, to date, cannot accomplish such miracles. We must be content with the miracles it can and is accomplishing. You can be happy if your surgeon says to you, "Yes, I can operate."

Even the most competent surgeons may disagree as to whether or not an operation should be done. Some specialists advise surgery for all patients with gallstones whether they are producing symptoms or not. Others recommend operations only when symptoms make the patient uncomfortable. Even in cases of rectal cancer there may be disagreement, this time not as to whether treatment should be given, but as to what type of treatment is best. Some surgeons believe that the most curative type of operation is removal of the entire rectum while others believe equally sincerely that in many patients part of the rectum can be saved. Usually when specialists disagree on treatment, there is not much difference in the results of the types of treatment that each favors. Rather, each one simply prefers a method with which he has been successful.

The patient cannot hope to read and understand all of the medical literature on his ailment. For him to go from specialist to specialist seeking an ideal answer to his dilemma becomes confusing and frustrating. It is better for him to discuss the question frankly with his family physician, ask him to explain the possible alternatives, and accept his advice as to what surgeon he should consult. When a patient tries to decide for himself whether he should have an operation or what operation he should have, he may do himself serious harm.

If you have an agonizing pain in the abdomen and a gallbladder full of stones, it doesn't take much persuasion by the surgeon to convince you that you need an operation to remove the gall bladder. If you know enough to recognize the possible significance of a lump in your breast, you will unhesitatingly go to a surgeon and have it removed. But if you feel fine and have no symptoms except occasionally a little blood in the stool, you may find it difficult to accept the need for operation for rectal cancer. You may find it particularly hard if such an operation involves the making of an artificial opening in your body. Acceptance of such an operation may require deep thought and complete investigation of all the possibilities.

It has been said that "you are lucky if they can operate." This is true. An inoperable cancer of the rectum means that the cancer is incurable. If an operation could not be advised to treat the gallstone colic that was giving you abdominal pain, it would be because your general condition was so poor that you could not stand an operation. In general, surgery is advised for diseases that are in favorable stages for treatment. Thus, in this respect, you are lucky if you can be operated on.

CHAPTER TWO

ANESTHESIA

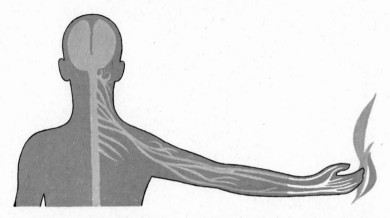

ANESTHESIA is a state of insensibility or "not feeling." It may be produced in part of the body by a local anesthetic drug, or it may be produced in the whole body by a general anesthetic. The general anesthetics, such as ether and so-called laughing-gas (nitrous oxide), also produce sleep. To many people anesthesia means being put to sleep with ether so that a surgical operation may be carried out without pain. Ether was first used for anesthesia in 1842 and is still used in many operations today.

Before the advent of modern anesthesia, attempts were made to relieve the pain of operation or to produce unconsciousness by giving such substances as henbane, poppy, mandragora, and hemp. Opium, made from the poppy, was used in various forms to relieve pain many centuries before Christ. It is said that Aesculapius, the Roman god of medicine, used nepenthe to make his surgical patients unconscious, and Hippocrates produced the same effect by giving inhalations of the vapor of bhang (an East Indian plant).

By 1900 ether, nitrous oxide, or laughing gas (1844), chloroform (1847), and ethyl chloride (1894) were the only drugs available to provide general anesthesia. Since that time many new drugs have been discovered which make anesthesia more pleasant and safer for the patient.

Although anesthesia is well known to cause a state resembling sleep and to render the person insensitive to pain, it has another effect which is very important—relaxation of the muscles. This is needed to make it easier for the surgeon to operate inside the abdomen or chest or to set broken bones and dislocated joints.

Most general anesthetic agents produce some degree of relaxation and the local anesthetics produce deep relaxation. In addition, certain substances such as curare (a poison used by South American Indians on their darts), when purified and used in small doses, provide excellent muscular relaxation.

Research on new drugs and methods of anesthesia is being carried out in many universities, clinics, and hospitals. New anesthetic drugs are tested carefully over long periods in the laboratory before they are used on human patients. The results of these research programs are published in many medical journals so that all anesthetists have an opportunity to use the safest and most effective treatment possible.

It is not usually difficult to produce anesthesia in most patients with the potent drugs available today. But the highly developed skill of the anesthesiologist is necessary to maintain careful control of the essential body functions (blood pressure, pulse, and respiration) and to keep them as nearly normal as possible during anesthesia and surgery.

In a normal person not under the influence of anesthetics or other drugs, his many control mechanisms work to preserve a normal condition throughout his body. Several of these mechanisms are concerned with the action of the heart and lungs. For example, if during vigorous exercise the muscles need more blood, the pumping action of the heart is stimulated to supply it. The muscles' activity produces substances which are carried in the blood. When they reach the brain and a sensitive organ on the carotid artery in the neck, these organs signal the lungs to increase breathing. The lungs then provide more oxygen to the blood and remove more carbon dioxide from the body. These reflexes do not operate well when the anesthetized patient is "asleep," and for this reason the anesthesiologist must take over the responsibility of assuring satisfactory blood circulation and breathing.

The anesthesiologist of today not only administers the anesthetic drugs but also does the following:

• Estimates the safety of anesthesia for the individual patient;

• Gives certain medicines to prepare the patient for anesthesia and operation;

• Observes carefully the blood pressure, pulse, color, and respiration of the patient while anesthetized;

• Administers drugs other than anesthetics when necessary during this period; and

• Supervises the care of the patient while he is recovering from anesthesia.

Before the Operation

The decision as to how much risk is involved in producing anesthesia is very important. The history of the patient's former and present diseases is carefully discussed to determine if there are any effects of such diseases that will make anesthesia more difficult or dangerous. Diseases of the heart, blood vessels, and lungs have special importance, but conditions affecting the brain, liver, and kidneys must also be considered. A physical examination adds much valuable information about the patient's ability to tolerate anesthesia. Routine laboratory tests of the blood and urine are carried out on all patients.

With older patients or those with complicated conditions, additional laboratory examinations are made to test the functioning of various organs and body systems. The sum total of the knowledge gathered by all these methods helps to determine the best way to prepare a patient for anesthesia and surgery. This may involve a delay of one or more days to improve certain body functions or restore them to normal, to administer certain medicines, or to give blood transfusions. The information obtained before operation is also needed to determine the most suitable form of anesthesia and the amount and character of operating which can safely be done.

The medicine given before anesthesia often consists of three drugs: a barbiturate, a narcotic (morphine or a similar preparation), and atropine. A barbiturate is given either by mouth or injection an hour and a half or two hours before surgery, and morphine and atropine are given by hypodermic injection one hour before the schedule time of surgery. The barbiturate and morphine act as tranquilizers to quiet the fears of the patient. The morphine also helps to make him less sensitive to pain. The atropine decreases the secretion of saliva and counteracts some of the undesirable reactions to anesthesia.

During the Operation

After the patient has been placed on the operating table, a blood pressure cuff is applied to one arm above the elbow and, in most cases, an intravenous infusion of a solution of dextrose, a special sugar, is begun in the other arm. This infusion supplies necessary fluid and also provides a way to put anesthetics and other drugs into the blood stream where they will have an immediate effect upon the body.

When general anesthesia is to be used, sleep is usually first induced by injecting a barbiturate solution through the infusion needle carrying the dextrose solution into the vein. The patient loses consciousness within a few seconds and the anesthetist then gives oxygen with a mask attached by long tubes to the anesthesia machine. Anesthetic gases or vapors are added to the oxygen to produce anesthesia.

While the operation is in progress the anesthesiologist keeps a chart on which he records the patient's blood pressure, pulse, and breathing rate. In operations upon the heart or in patients with serious heart disease, an electrocardiograph may be attached to the patient during anesthesia so that it is possible to see any changes which occur in the electrical impulses produced by the heart. If there is bleeding with a severe fall in blood pressure during the operation, the anesthesiologist may elect to give blood, or may be requested to do so by the surgeon. Under other circumstances blood pressure may be raised by giving various drugs or by changing the patient's position.

At the end of the operation, the anesthesia is discontinued and the anesthesiologist keeps the patient under observation either in the operating room or recovery room until the anesthesia has lightened to such an extent that the patient can safely be returned to his own room in the hospital.

The patient and his family can help considerably during the operative period. It is important that the patient have complete confidence in both his surgeon and his anesthesiologist. Each is a trained specialist in his own field. Their decisions as to what type of anesthesia is

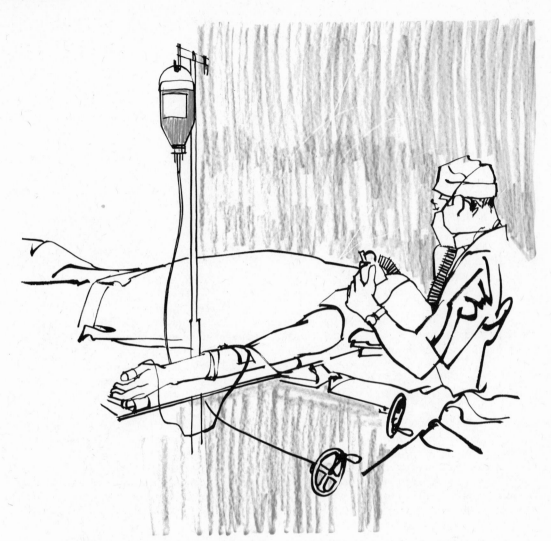

safest for the patient should be accepted without question. The patient must have a sensible attitude toward anesthesia—one free from fear. He should understand that anesthesia is many times safer today than it was in the early part of this century. It is especially important to discuss anesthesia with children before they go to a hospital for an operation. Any child who has been taught the facts about anesthesia should be able to cooperate well with the anesthetist.

Anesthesia service provides unconsciousness, absence of pain, and relaxation of the muscles. It includes care of the patient before, during, and after the operation and a careful supervision of all the important body functions during this time. The knowledge of anesthesia has been growing for many centuries and today provides the safest, most efficient conditions during which complicated and extended surgery can be accomplished.

CHAPTER THREE

THE ROLE OF BLOOD

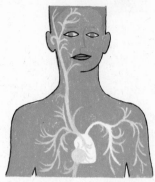

MAN HAS ALWAYS been fascinated by his blood. Blood has played an interesting role in history, from the battlefield to the altar of worship. Blood looms large in the religious philosophies of both pagans and Christians. Peace treaties have been sealed and friendships pledged in blood. It has been used in black magic. Now it is one of the most important modern medicaments. Modern science confirms that life is in the blood. So, sometimes, is death.

Long before man understood the nature and function of blood, he tried to use it medically, through bloodletting and the application of leeches. Both of these procedures probably did much more harm than good. Men also sought to control bleeding when injured. In the course of the centuries, bandages, ligatures, hot oil, and cautery were used to control loss of blood. Although attempts to transfuse blood between animals and from animals to man were made as early as the 17th century, blood lost was not replaceable until this century.

Today it is possible to replace lost blood with blood from another human being, a donor. The word "donor" is perhaps the most crucial one in the whole story of blood. There is no other source of blood for use in modern medicine than a human donor. This fact lays an obligation upon every healthy young person to give blood for others, to maintain a supply in case one should need it for himself or a member of his family. Money is needed to gather, process, and store the blood, but the blood itself must always be a gift of compassion. Blood has been taken from dead bodies in some parts of the world, particularly in Russia, but this practice has not become established in the United States.

The procurement of human blood, its preservation, selection, and transfusion are medical procedures which require the direction and supervision of a physician. The ultimate objective of this procedure is the welfare of patients who require blood or blood derivatives.

The most spectacular use of blood is in surgery. It is a striking and dramatic event when a transfusion saves the life of a person who has suffered a severe injury. Transfusions are commonly used in surgery when blood loss is expected, to prevent the development of an emergency due to bleeding. In many cases, transfusions before an operation can greatly reduce its risk.

The first known transfusion took place in 1654 when a Florentine monk tried to transfer blood from one animal to another; the recipient died. During the 17th century blood from calves was used for transfusing to human beings, but this practice soon stopped because bad results followed more often than not. Modern success in transfusion resulted upon the discovery in the early 1900's of the variations in blood types and ways to type and match blood before using it in transfusions.

Blood Types

The details of blood grouping or typing are technical, but the principles are simple, and everyone should understand them. Each person's blood is individual as are all the cells of his body. If the donor's blood is of differing type, it will be destroyed by the recipient's blood if injected into his veins. Occasionally the recipient's blood may also be destroyed in the process.

Blood groups are classified in four categories. The letters A, B, and O refer to substances present in the red blood cells. The words "anti-A" and "anti-B" refer to substances in the plasma able to react with and destroy the red cells containing the substances A or B.

Group O. This blood has no substance A or B, but it has in its plasma anti-B and anti-A; it exists in 46 per cent of the population.

Group A. This blood has anti-B; it exists in 42 per cent of the population.

Group B. This blood has anti-A; it is found in only 9 per cent of the population.

Group AB. This blood has no anti-A or anti-B; it is found in only 3 per cent of the population.

Some persons with blood of the O group may under certain circumstances be used as donors for persons of other blood groups, and those with group AB blood may under certain circumstances receive blood of other blood groups, but only in emergencies. The tests for blood groups which should always precede transfusion are not enough in themselves. Additional cross-matching tests with the donor's blood cells and recipient's serum, and vice versa, are required to assure that neither person's blood contains antagonistic or incompatible blood mixtures.

Aside from the use of whole blood in transfusions, the so-called blood fractions are useful in surgery. The liquid or plasma, separated from the cells, can be frozen and stored for long periods of time. This can be used on the battlefield or in disaster areas without concern for blood grouping. It is an important emergency measure to restore lost blood volume, but it furnishes no cells. The element in the blood that is responsible for clotting is also useful in surgery, and red blood cell suspensions have been used to heal wounds, especially burns. A plasma foam is used in the abdomen to help prevent adhesions.

Until recently, it has been impossible to keep whole blood or blood cells for more than 21 days. As a result, blood which was not used within the time limit was wasted. Now blood cells can be frozen, making it possible to keep them for years. Plasma products, including the important gamma globulin, can also be stored for long periods.

Blood and Childbirth

Use of blood has added to the safety of pregnancy and childbirth. Transfusions restore blood lost in excessive bleeding from a miscarriage or following labor. Another principal service which evolved from modern research on blood is the saving of infant lives through the discovery of the Rh factor. This is a blood discrepancy between parents which causes the mother's blood to destroy that of the infant. The complicated mechanism of this process may be explained by the following steps:

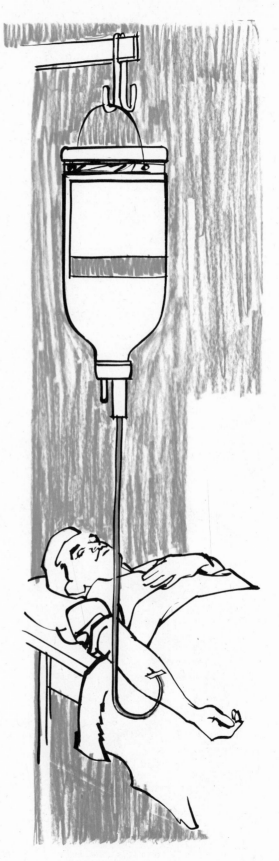

1. About 85 per cent of the white population has a blood factor known as the Rh factor; this occurrence is governed by heredity. Persons who have it are called Rh positive.

2. If both prospective parents are Rh positive, which is most often the case, the matter can be ignored. If both are Rh negative, there is no problem.

3. If the father is Rh negative and the mother Rh positive, there is no effect on the baby.

4. If the mother is Rh negative and the father Rh positive, difficulties may arise, usually in pregnancies after the first one, for the following reasons:

5. The blood of the mother defends itself against the Rh positive blood of the baby by developing antibodies.

7. These antibodies pass from the mother into the blood of the baby, destroying the baby's red blood cells. This results in miscarriage, still birth, or early infant death, unless. . .

7. The Rh status of father and mother are learned before the pregnancy and steps are taken before delivery to replace the baby's blood with blood which does not contain the anti-Rh factor of his mother and the Rh factor

of his father. This is done by transfusion immediately after birth, replacing all the baby's blood. This is a highly successful procedure.

8. There are occasionally differences even between Rh positive persons, which may lead to complications in pregnancy, but they are rare and complex and need not be considered here. Physicians are aware of them, and know ways to protect babies against ill effects resulting from them.

Because of the Rh factor, it is necessary to determine Rh factor compatibility as well as blood type when giving any transfusion to a woman of childbearing age. Only in this way can the creation of Rh problems in future pregnancies be avoided.

Treating Disease

Aside from surgery, transfusions are useful in cases in which the blood is changed through diseases. These include leukemia, chronic infections, nutritional disorders, such wasting diseases as cancer, chronic poisonings with blood-destroying chemicals like lead, diseases of the blood-forming organs (bone marrow), and continuous small blood losses as from ulcers or cancers. Transfusion of plasma fractions may also be helpful in a condition known as purpura, in which there is bleeding under the skin, into the tissues and joints and sometimes into the body cavities or hollow organs such as the stomach, intestines, or bladder.

Before the development of vaccines such as those for measles, gamma globulin, a blood plasma fraction was often used to give temporary immunity against diseases—especially for pregnant women and other people for whom the disease was a dangerous risk. Whole blood was sometimes injected in order to stimulate the immunity mechanism of the body as a whole. Human serum from persons recovering from a disease was also used to combat certain infectious diseases. More modern vaccines have largely taken the place of these uses of blood in medicine.

Blood as a Diagnostic Aid

When the doctor pricks the finger or the ear or draws blood from a vein, he has a large number of tests at his command. Ordinarily he wants to know how many red and white blood cells and blood platelets the specimen contains; how healthy the cells are, and how much hemoglobin pigment is present to carry oxygen to

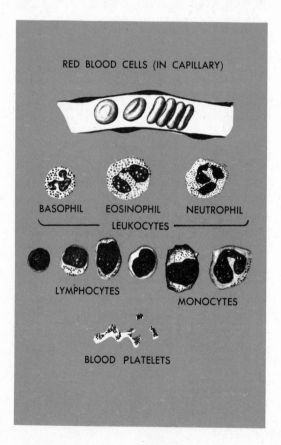

RED BLOOD CELLS (IN CAPILLARY)

BASOPHIL   EOSINOPHIL   NEUTROPHIL
└──────── LEUKOCYTES ────────┘

LYMPHOCYTES

MONOCYTES

BLOOD PLATELETS

the tissues. He wants to know the proportion of various types of white cells. Chemically, he is interested in blood sugar, cholesterol, and many other substances which give information about the body. Immunity reactions performed on the blood plasma can tell him about past diseases or the state of protection against currently common diseases. The rate at which the red blood cells settle into a sediment gives the doctor useful clues about tissue injury and the progress of chronic disease processes. There is a world of useful diagnostic information in just a few cubic centimeters of blood.

Giving Blood

The importance of blood in modern medicine emphasizes the importance of keeping a constant supply on hand. It is needed both for ordinary daily use and for the unpredictable demands likely in case of floods, earthquakes, fires, explosions, or war. Every healthy person between the ages of 21 and 60 should seriously consider giving blood in advance of an emergency. Any large hospital is likely to have a blood bank where the donation can be made. In many communities, small as well as large, national agencies or local groups operate blood banks. By making such blood donations, persons can assure themselves as well as others of a supply of blood in case of need.

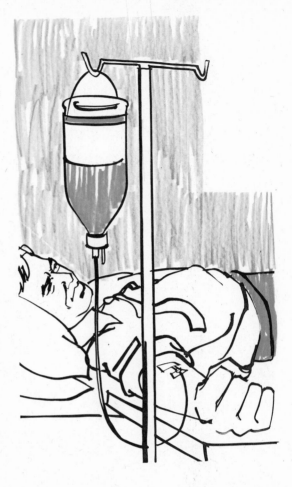

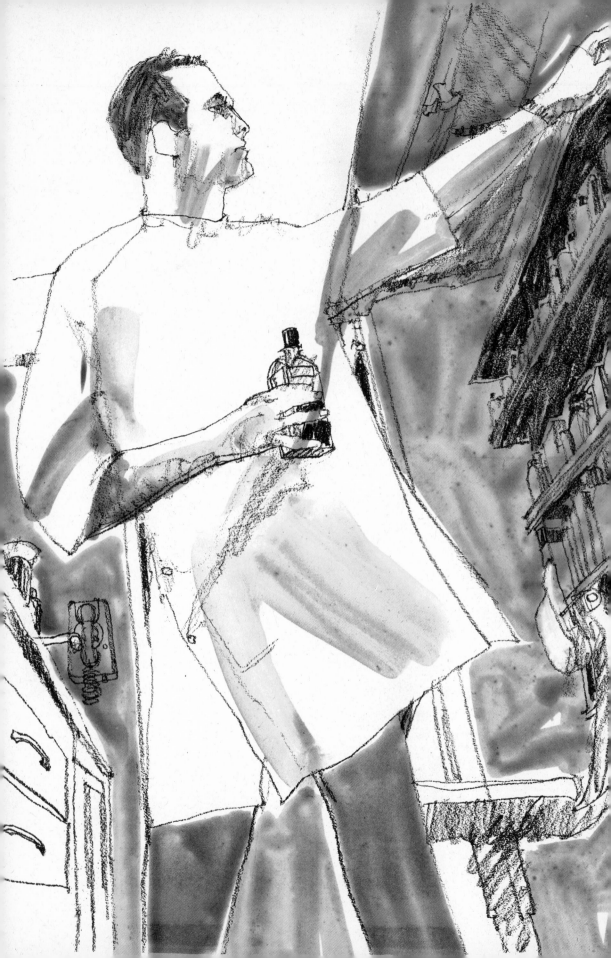

PART XII

The Proper
Use of Drugs

THE DRUGS YOU USE

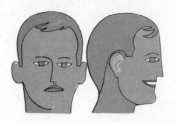

A DRUG IS DEFINED as a substance used to treat illness, protect against disease, or promote better health.

Between 800 and 900 different drugs are in fairly extensive use currently in the United States and new ones appear at the rate of about 30 to 40 each year. Some of the older drugs disappear as more effective new ones take their place. Generally, the newer drugs are more powerful and much more effective than those used 10, 20, or 30 years ago, and they must be used with greater care, often only under a doctor's prescription. This chapter describes some drugs widely used for the more common ailments. It advises on the intelligent use of drugs so that your health, or the health of your loved ones, can be restored or preserved.

Non-Prescription Drugs

Drugs for the relief of pain are used by hundreds of thousands of people with little or no harmful side effects. A few people are sensitive to certain drugs and have skin and other reactions that may be serious and occasionally need prompt professional attention. This allergic reaction to drugs is similar to the reaction some people have to hair, house dust, or molds.

In addition, some drugs can be directly harmful because of their potency. Such medicaments obviously should be given only under close medical supervision by someone who can judge if the risk, whether slight or grave, is outweighed by the possible benefits for the patient. This is where professional skill and judgment based on training, experience, and general ability are important as the patient is guided from illness back to health.

Laxatives are widely used and with more safety than in earlier years, because they contain less dramatically effective and therefore less harmful ingredients. In general they are much more gentle than 20 or 30 years ago. Nevertheless, they can cause serious harm if

unnecessarily and persistently used and when the patient has appendicitis or an intestinal obstruction. Long-term or chronic constipation can be a symptom of serious disease. Therefore, instead of using laxatives, a physician should be consulted in all cases of long lasting constipation.

Sedatives and sleep producers should be used only for occasional relief and not as a perpetual crutch. Physicians seldom prescribe such agents over long periods of time except in cases of persistent disease. Prolonged, unsupervised use of those agents is not wise. This is particularly true for prescription drugs used by victims of insomnia who prefer to suffer in silence rather than seek out the cause of their problems. As in other situations, abuse causes more problems than use.

Very often compounds which relieve pain or dull one's perception of pain mask the severity of an illness, and adequate medical care is delayed. Everyone should realize that the earlier a serious illness receives attention, the greater are the chances for complete recovery. In addition, some drugs that physicians prescribe for their beneficial effects unavoidably do other things, for example, slow down reactions to unexpected dangers. Obviously, patients using such drugs should heed the warnings of the prescribing physician.

Stimulants or "pep pills" enjoy a wide and promiscuous use in some age groups. Any such drugs that truly have the ability to stimulate the body may cause excessive fatigue or collapse. Their use without consulting a physician can be dangerous. Weight-reducing compounds with powerful ingredients may also be dangerous to use on one's own initiative because of possible harmful effects. In most instances, it is unwise to take several drugs at once or to mix drugs with alcohol.

The effectiveness of ointments and lotions for skin afflictions varies with the percentage of the drug used and the cause of the skin condition. One type of condition may require a skin-stimulating agent. Another may be harmed by application of such a medicament. Sometimes it is necessary to apply a dry powder, or sometimes an ointment or a lotion. If one is used when the other is needed, the condition may be aggravated. The treatment of severe skin ailments is best left in the hands of physicians. But many minor skin ailments can be treated to obtain relief with remedies obtainable through the pharmacy without a prescription.

There are also many kinds of skin and wound antiseptics on the market. Some have limited usefulness, others are quite effective. Those which are specific and effective for severe infections are usually obtainable only on a doctor's prescription and should be applied under medical supervision only.

Often the physician may wish to treat the condition by applying drugs internally, even by injection. For such treatment, it is obvious that home medication is out of the question.

Prescription Drugs

The most effective medicines today are those obtainable only on prescription. Because of their effectiveness, such drugs are likely to be exceptionally potent and require use only under certain conditions and only as directed. That is why this medicine is available only through a prescription—to guard your health.

The most widely publicized types of prescription drugs are the lifesaving "sulfa" drugs and antibiotics. The first of these was sulfanilamide, which opened the way to a variety of sulfa drugs. Some sulfa drugs are still available today, but their use for a serious ailment, like that of the antibiotics, must be regulated by a physician. His choice of treatment will depend on the kind of infection being treated, the dose necessary for the severity of the illness, the specific drug used, perhaps the weight of the patient, and a knowledge of the patient's expected—and sometimes unexpected—response to drugs. Only a physician can weigh all these factors.

Penicillin is generally effective against bacteria causing bone infection, boils, and carbuncles, against blood poisoning, and against bacteria normally responsible for pneumonia and venereal diseases. Occasionally, however, some persons have an allergic reaction to penicillin. This is usually a skin rash, although it may be more serious. To avoid such reactions the physician may test the patient for sensitivity

to this antibiotic or he may be prepared to use a drug to combat any unwanted reaction.

The family of "mycin" drugs, for example streptomycin and chloramphenicol, attack bacteria against which penicillin or other antibiotics may be ineffective. Many other antibiotics are also available and most are needed because of the variation on the part of patients in response to drugs and because of the resistance that bacteria sometimes develop to drugs after prolonged use. The research laboratories are constantly seeking new and better drugs in this field as in others.

Another entirely different class of drugs are those for the heart and circulatory system. Digitalis is primarily used to prevent or treat heart failures. It increases the working capacity of the heart by strengthening the contraction of the cardiac muscle. Diuretics aid in getting rid of excess fluids from the body, thus taking the strain off the heart and the circulatory system. The effect of such action is dramatically evident in reducing swelling, such as around the ankles, in the presence of certain kinds of heart disease. Another class of drugs often used after a so-called heart attack, includes the anti-

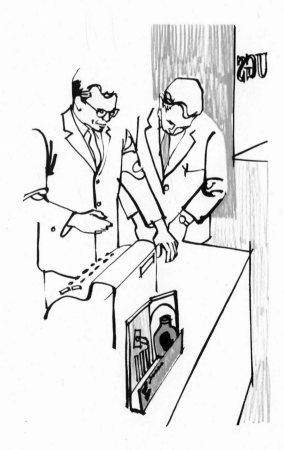

coagulants which help to keep the blood in a proper fluid state and thus help prevent further clot formation. A number of drugs also have been developed which lower blood pressure almost at the doctor's bidding. Needless to say these drugs are very potent and should be employed only under the doctor's orders.

Acute and severe pain can be relieved by a number of substances of which morphine and codeine, both of which are alkaloids derived from opium, are perhaps best known. It is easy to become addicted to such drugs, however, and they should be used only on a doctor's prescription. Morphine substitutes to reduce the risk of addiction are available, but scientists are still searching for the ideal one. Furthermore, the cause of the pain must be attacked as well as the pain itself, which is only a symptom of some underlying cause. Thus, arthritis is attacked by the corticosteroids as well as by other agents. In the same way, a brain tumor causing headache would have to be removed before the pain could be expected to disappear. And a diseased gall bladder would have to be removed before the symptoms of gall bladder disease would be gone.

Insulin has been used since 1922 for the treatment of diabetes, but it must be taken by injection. There are also chemical substances that can be taken in pill form by many, but not all, older patients for controlling the body chemistry that is upset by this disease. Many other diseases that involve the endocrine or hormone-producing glands of the body can be similarly treated.

For inducing sleep, many compounds are available under a variety of names. A proper dose of a drug can bring sleep in 20 minutes to an hour. This sleep may last for a short time or for a longer period depending on the drug used and how it is administered. Unfortunately, some of these drugs become habit-forming in some people and an overdose can be fatal. It goes without saying that use of the prescription drugs in this class of remedies must be carefully regulated and controlled.

Spectacular progress in drug discovery in recent years has been made in the area of tranquilizers and drugs that affect a person's mood. The first of such drugs was reserpine, derived from the ancient rauwolfia serpentina, the Indian snakeroot. Chlorpromazine and meprobamate followed in short order. Then came the drugs that relieve mental depression—phenelzine, nialamide, and imipramine, among others. These drugs have emptied many wards in men-

tal hospitals, and enable many persons to live a relatively normal life through self-treatment, under a doctor's supervision, at home.

Scores of antihistamines are in use against various allergies. Griseofulvin taken internally has proved effective against certain fungus infections, such as athlete's foot. A score of substances are now used in the treatment of cancer, but none of these are cures. They may prolong the lives of cancer victims and even cause significant easing of the symptoms of certain forms of the disease.

This is only a brief reference to the many drugs that today are available. They probably have done more to revolutionize the practice of medicine than any other single element. But their effectiveness depends on knowledge of the value of other measures such as surgery, good nursing care, and proper nutrition, and on an awareness of the limitations as well as values of such dramatic tools.

How to Use Drugs

From the foregoing discussion it should be evident that today's drugs should be handled with great respect. They are capable of doing a great deal of good, but used indiscriminately they are capable of producing harm.

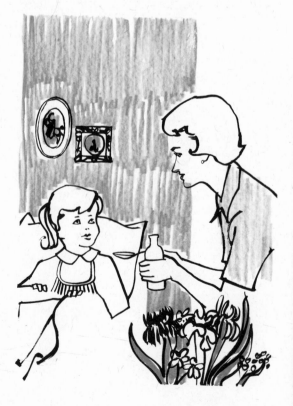

It is important, first of all, to use a prescription drug exactly as the doctor directs. An overdose or underdose, or failure to take the medicine at the prescribed intervals, can lessen the drug's effectiveness in restoring you to good health.

A common mistake is for someone to give medicine prescribed by a physician to another complaining of similar distress. A physician writes a prescription for a definite purpose, the treatment of a specific disease, or the relief of a specific symptom in a specific person. It cannot be used for a variety of diseases, nor should it ever be used by other persons. The proper dosage is often determined by individual factors such as the age, body weight, and sex of the patient. A drug which is highly effective for one person can actually be dangerous to another.

It follows, then, that when a prescription is no longer of use to the patient for whom it was prescribed, it should be discarded. There is nothing to be gained by keeping a bottle of medicine that was compounded some years ago. The active ingredients of that prescription, especially if in liquid or ointment form, may have lost their therapeutic value. Futhermore, any new condition, even if similar-appearing, may require a different medicine. The progress of drug discovery is so rapid that much more effective medicines may be in use.

Keeping old drugs beyond their period of usefulness may lead to accidents and poisoning. Time after time we hear of mistakes made in choosing poorly marked or mislabeled bottles. Children, too, can get hold of the drug and take a fatal dose.

All bottles should be labeled so that there can be no mistaking their contents or their purpose. A dangerous drug should be kept on the highest shelf and not mixed with personal care and hygienic items which several family members may use. A flashlight kept in the medicine chest is useful to distinguish labels during an electrical failure. Poisons should preferably be kept, not in the medicine cabinet, but in a separate, locked cupboard, and in containers plainly marked "poison."

The medicine cabinet should be out of reach of small children. Too often they find they can easily reach their goal by climbing upon the bathtub or washbasin. If the cabinet cannot be kept out of their reach, it should be fastened securely by lock, and the key kept in a nearby place accessible only to adults.

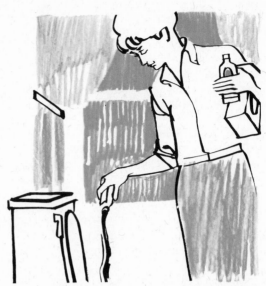

In buying drugs it is usually better to rely on well-known manufacturers than to take a chance with lesser-known but cheaper brands. Drugs have many important properties besides their chemical formulae that can make the difference between an effective and ineffective medicine of the same basic name. In such cases it is usually false economy to buy the cheaper brand.

Recent years have seen unparalleled progress in medicine and drug therapy. Deaths from many diseases have been drastically reduced. For example, acute poliomyelitis has been cut 75 per cent; acute rheumatic fever, 83 per cent; syphilis, 89 per cent; influenza, 90 per cent; tuberculosis, 91 per cent; measles, 94 per cent; whooping cough, 96 per cent; and diphtheria, 99 per cent.

A quarter of a century ago, 1 out of every 157 mothers died at childbirth. This number had been slashed by 1960 to 1 out of every 2,778. Infant and child mortality is down 63 per cent for babies under 1 year, 80 per cent for children 1-4, and 71.5 per cent for children 5-14. During the past 25 years, a decade has been added to the life expectancy of the newborn child.

Reduction in mortality between 1935 and 1960 accounted for a 1960 contribution in earnings to the gross national product of $10,400,000,000. Of this total, almost half is due to the decline in death rates from four diseases: tuberculosis, pneumonia, influenza, and syphilis. These are diseases for which the availability of drugs is critical to the treatment and cure.

Thirty years ago, a patient entering a mental hospital could expect to remain there for up to 30 years, or for the rest of his life. Today about two thirds of those now being admitted to mental institutions are discharged during their first year there. Increasingly effective psychiatric care, partially through drug therapy, has saved more than $2,000,000,000 in hospital construction costs alone since 1957.

Almost half the beds used for care of tuberculosis patients in 1956 are now available for other purposes, and many tuberculosis facilities have been shut down entirely or have been converted to other uses.

Cancer survival rates have improved from 1937's rate of one in seven to today's one in three. Early diagnosis and better surgical, radiological, and drug techniques are responsible.

The average cost for a prescription in 1939 was $.91. To pay for it, the average wage earner had to work 1 hour and 41 minutes. Today the average (and much more effective) prescription costs about $3.26. But to pay for it, the wage earner works only 1 hour and 23 minutes. Thus today's better drugs actually take less of the medical-care dollar than the inferior drugs of 25 years ago. Furthermore, the wholesale price of prescription drugs has actually declined 10 per cent since 1949 while the wholesale price for all commodities has risen 26 per cent.

The price of individual new drugs may seem high when they are first introduced. However, as production and distribution methods are improved and as some of the research investment is recovered, the price of new drugs invariably goes down, often dramatically if research opens the door to more efficient and productive ways to manufacture them. For example, in 1943 one manufacturer sold penicillin for $100 per 100,000 units. By 1956 the price was only 22.2 cents for the same quantity. One company's initial price for cortisone was $200 per gram. By 1957, it was only $2 per gram. Likewise, the price of terramycin has gone down 25 per cent; polio vaccine, 43 per cent; and streptomycin and cortisone, 99 per cent.

Each year the drug industry tests more than 100,000 substances, of which only about 40 turn out to have enough value to be marketed. In fact, in 1962 more than 160,000 substances were isolated but probably fewer than 40 will eventually reach the doctor for prescribing. It requires five to six years, as an average, from the time an idea is born in a test tube until it appears in medicine as a usable product. And from $5,000,000 to $8,000,000, or more, may have been spent on perfecting it and making it useful. This does not include the cost of building any new production plants that may be necessary or opening channels of distribution to ensure it is available when it is needed.

This means that for every useful drug product that reaches the public, more than 2,500 compounds are studied and discarded. Even when a successful drug is developed, newer and better products may make it obsolete within a very short time. The life of many so-called miracle drugs often is comparatively short as research discovers new and even more effective drugs.

CHAPTER TWO

THE DANGER IN SELF-MEDICATION

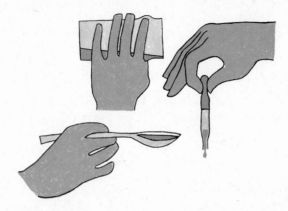

MANY PEOPLE THINK that doctors lean over backwards in advising against self-medication. What's wrong with it, they ask? Why shouldn't I take an aspirin when I have pain, or a sleeping pill? Or vitamins? Or a laxative? Or nose drops for a cold? Or something for an upset stomach? I can't dash to the doctor's office for every little thing, can I? What's wrong with self-medication?

Many, if not most, of the ills that afflict modern man are minor in the sense that they do not produce profound or lasting changes in body tissues. We cannot always know what is or will remain a minor ailment, but most people assume that they need not worry about something which is not severe or long lasting or which they have previously treated satisfactorily with self-medication. With some relief measures, they believe time and nature will cause the discomfort to disappear.

As a matter of fact, nature is an especially good friend, and the body, unaided except perhaps by sleep and rest, can take care of most ailments, although medications ease their distress. Furthermore, some of the more reliable home remedies can assist or speed up the process of healing. But when there is doubt, it is always wiser and often more economical in the long run to seek the advice of a physician.

The conditions most commonly subject to self-medication are some skin afflictions, temporary headaches, occasional sleeplessness, muscular aches, allergic symptoms, and colds. The agents used for such self-treatment include aspirin and other pain relieving drugs, sedatives, skin lotions, and ointments. Of course remedies that can be sold only on prescription cannot, or should not, be purchased by those without proper medical training, nor should they be used simply because some pills are left over from someone else's prescription. Federal laws limits what drugs can be sold without a prescription.

Obviously, one cannot run to the doctor for every trifling discomfort. If everybody did, the doctors would be swamped with unimportant chores, the way they are in countries where medical care is supposedly "free." It is to be expected that certain everyday discomforts can be cared for by simple home methods, such as rest, a hot water bottle or an ice-cap, and perhaps an aspirin tablet to relieve pain.

The trouble is that self-medication doesn't stop there, and that many times mistakes are made in judging what is trifling and what is the beginning of real trouble. For example, in Part IX, Chapter Three, you will find a list of common symptoms which are trivial if they happen once, or once in a long time. They cease being unimportant when they keep coming back again and again, or when they are present all or most of the time, or when they are extremely severe, or when they are the source of worry and apprehension.

Self-medication means using powerful drugs for the self-treatment of symptoms, without having a medical diagnosis of what those symptoms mean or how they are caused, and without medical advice about the drug being taken, its dosage, and its possible dangers. Even such commonly used drugs as pain-relievers, antacids, and laxatives should not be used often or for long periods of time, because of the danger of overlooking serious advancing disease.

Dangers of Self-Medication

Self-medication, except for minor and temporary conditions, doesn't make sense for the following reasons:

- Symptoms are confusingly similar and deceptive because the same symptom can arise from many causes. It is not logical or effective to be treating oneself for something when one does not know what it is.

- Reactions to drugs differ with different people, and in the same person at different times and under different conditions; therefore all but the most simple drugs must be given with care and subject to medical judgment. Among such "simple" drugs are pain-relievers, antiacid agents, laxatives, cold tablets, nose drops, nose and throat sprays, and external applications. Sleeping pills, "pep" pills, and tranquilizers are not included in this group.

- Covering up pain with a pain killer, insomnia with a sleeping pill, anxiety with a tranquilizer, or fatigue with a stimulant fails to get at the basic causes of these conditions and may permit serious disease to progress to a point of danger.

- Using a left-over drug from a previous illness under what seem to be similar circumstances, a common practice among people who dose themselves, is unlikely to be helpful. It may be useless or even dangerous. It may waste valuable time in getting proper treatment.

- Using a drug prescribed for someone else, another common practice, is likely to be useless, detrimental, or even dangerous because individual circumstances, needs, and reactions are likely to be different or dosage unsuitable.

Nonmedical persons do not understand how complicated modern drugs are, the dangers of side effects, and the importance of keeping close watch on the effects of a drug—both those reactions which are desired and those that are not.

Only a physician is prepared to evaluate the results of using a drug. Such evaluation is so difficult that when experiments with drugs are made, the danger that personal reactions will interfere with judgment is counteracted by the double blind system. This consists of using two preparations with code numbers. Neither physician nor patient knows whether what the subject gets is the drug under investigation or a so-called placebo, a substance without medical action. Sometimes a third or fourth coded preparation may be used when comparisons between several drugs are wanted. The double blind eliminates the psychological element in evaluation. The self-medicator obviously cannot be sure whether any benefits that *follow* the taking of a drug are necessarily *due to* taking that drug.

Many minor conditions improve with or without treatment. With few exceptions, it is reasonable to assume that if relief through drugs is necessary on a continuing basis, there is need for much more than self-prescribed drugs. Medicine has long gone beyond the era of the coated tongue and the universal faith in a good "physic."

Drugs may have unexpected effects. Most people are astonished when they are told that laxatives are the principal cause of constipation in many persons. How can that be, they ask? Aren't laxatives supposed to overcome constipation? The answer, believe it or not, is no. They simply make the bowels move, which is a very different thing from overcoming con-

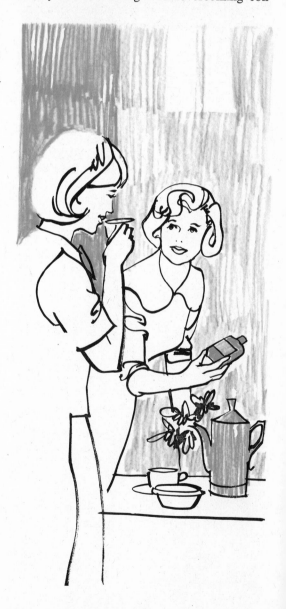

stipation. Habitually used in the false belief that the bowels must be cleaned out daily, laxatives set a vicious circle in motion. The bowels do not act because they have nothing to act upon, and the victim, thinking he is constipated, takes more laxatives, making a bad matter worse. In the end he may really become constipated because of his indiscriminate use of laxatives.

Many symptoms are not what they seem, for example, "acid stomach" as the announcers say on TV. What to do? Why, take an alkalizer, stupid! What else? What else, indeed! First, the stomach is normally acid, and if it gets too much alkali it starts producing more acid. If the over-acidity is due to an ulcer or to a rebellious gallbladder, no amount of alkali is going to solve the problem. If the trouble is due to a stomach cancer, serious danger lies ahead. Even an inflamed appendix can give trouble in the region of the stomach. So can emotional disturbances for which no amount of "coating" the stomach with alkali will do any good. Another kind of stomach symptom is due to a special form of anemia in which the stomach produces too little of the right kind of acid, food ferments, and the wrong kind of acid develops.

These are some of the reasons why self-medication does not make sense. They add up to the fact that it is illogical and inefficient to try treating a condition which has not been diagnosed with a drug whose effects you do not understand. It is like searching in a dark cellar for a black cat that isn't there.

Besides being dangerous and ordinarily useless, self-medication is expensive. The unnecessary use of laxatives and vitamins runs into millions of dollars annually, to say nothing of the alkalizers, cold tablets, and pain-killers. All of them give no permanent relief but merely cover up symptoms, postpone proper treatment, and in many instances, allow serious disease to progress. The annual waste of money on self-medication would go far toward paying for the medical diagnosis and care which is really needed.

Recognizing the dangers in self-medication, the Federal government has laid down requirements to the effect that certain drugs may be sold only on prescription. This is intended to protect the patient who might try to use, without supervision and without knowledge of the dangers, a highly potent drug. Unfortunately, many persons get around this law. With the best of intentions, they give their partially used prescription to others who have "exactly the same thing I had"—which is often something entirely different. Even if the condition were the same, the same drugs might not be used, or the dosage might be different.

Of all "neighborly" acts, the most unneighborly is the loaning or giving away of left-over prescriptions. The results are often bad. Occasionally they are fatal.

CHAPTER THREE

SMOKING: FACTS YOU SHOULD KNOW

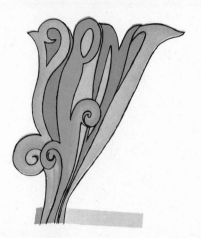

AMERICANS SMOKE about 500,000,000,000 cigarettes, the equivalent of about 2,777 cigarettes a year for every man, woman, and child in the country or over seven cigarettes per day.

The smoking habit usually begins in the early teens. By the 12th grade from 40 to 55 per cent of all children are found to be smokers, according to one study. Another survey in American secondary schools indicates that about one of every four boys smokes cigarettes, and one of every eight girls. The boys also are heavier smokers. This ratio follows through in adult life. Figures fluctuate, but it has been estimated that 60 per cent of American men smoke compared to 30 per cent of American women.

Since 1939, numerous scientific studies have been conducted to determine whether smoking is a health hazard. The trend of the evidence has been consistent and has permitted sound evaluation of the health risk. Based on evidence derived from human population studies, clinical and autopsy studies, and animal experimentation, the smoking of cigarettes does constitute a definite risk to health. Skilled research personnel have conducted studies that prove tobacco smoking, particularly cigarette smoking, is associated with a shortened life expectancy. Cigarette smoking is regarded as an important factor in the development of cancer of the lungs, and cancer of the larynx, and is believed to be related to cancer of the bladder, esophagus, and oral cavity. Male cigarette smokers have a higher death rate from coronary heart disease than nonsmoking males. Cigarette smoking is regarded as the most important of the causes of chronic bronchitis in the United States, and is also a significant factor in laryngeal cancer. A relationship does exist between pulmonary emphysema and cig-

arette smoking, but it is not established that this relationship is causal. The majority of physicians and researchers believe these observations to be correct and say, "Don't smoke! If you don't smoke, don't start."

Some competent physicians and research personnel are less sure of the effect of cigarette smoking on health, although their number is dwindling. They believe the increase in these diseases may be explained by other factors in our complex environment, although evidence to support this view has not been forthcoming. Nevertheless they advise: "Be moderate if you must smoke."

An individual may try to reach a solution about his own smoking by studying the evidence, making a rational decision, and acting on it. Accordingly, let us review some of the evidence that has accumulated from the research of many investigators during the last decades.

Physiological Effects

What is smoke? Smoke, a product of combustion, is a mixture of gases, various vaporized chemicals, and millions of minute particles of ash and other solids. These are drawn into the nose and throat during smoking and into the lungs by inhalation. The smoke includes some vaporized nicotine, a toxic substance found in tobacco, although much of it is changed by heat. It contains tars and other products from the partial burning and distillation of the tobacco.

A smoker gets more nicotine and tar if he smokes a cigarette to the end. A significant amount of carbon monoxide is also produced which is quickly picked up by the oxygen-carrying hemoglobin of the blood and reduces its oxygen-carrying ability.

Effect on the Respiratory System

As smoke is drawn into the breathing passages and the air sacs of the lungs, the gases and particles in the smoke settle onto the surrounding membranes. One point of great concentration is where a large tube (bronchus) divides into two smaller ones. Interestingly, this point is where most lung cancer begins.

Pathologists—physicians skilled in the microscopic anatomy of disease—consistently find that the lining membranes of the air passages of smokers are thickened and abnormal. The hairlike cilia on these membranes become damaged and are less effective in removing the toxic and irritating chemicals introduced by the inhalation of smoke.

Pathologists also have found that smoking not only thickens the lining membranes of the air passages and obstructs them with secretions, but also stimulates a contraction of the muscles in the air passage walls which narrows them and further reduces air flow. There is considerable evidence that a single cigarette will markedly reduce the air flow of even an experienced smoker. Potentially harmful particles are deposited into the air sacs, the point where emphysema develops. Recent pathological studies in humans suggest an association of these changes found in smokers and development of this disabling lung disease.

Smoke also affects the membranes lining the larynx or voice box. A pathologist identifies a smoker's larynx by the thicker, often swollen vocal cords. The changes in the voice box are similar to those that occur in the air passages and in the lungs. These irritations cause swelling and increased secretion and result in "smoker's cough."

Effect on the Circulatory System

Smoking affects the heart and blood vessels. Nicotine, if injected or taken in tobacco smoke, stimulates that part of the nervous system that controls the heart, blood vessels, and other internal organs that function almost automatically. For years, smoking has been known to be related to Buerger's disease, a constriction of the small arteries in the hands and feet that can lead to gangrene and necessitate amputation. Smokers also die more often from coronary heart disease.

Among other effects of smoking are those of an apparent tobacco allergy in some sensitive persons and aggravation of peptic gastric ulcers. Patients with these conditions are generally advised not to smoke.

While all tobacco smoking affects health and life expectancy, cigarette smoking appears to have a much greater effect than cigar or pipe smoking. Among the possible explanations are that cigar and pipe smokers often do not inhale and the temperature at which the tobacco burns is different.

Filters and denicotinization of tobacco or cigarettes are alleged to reduce the hazards. However, denicotinization has no effect on the kind or amount of tar in the smoke, and filters can only reduce, not eliminate the hazards.

Psychological and Social Aspects

That smoking is related to psychological and social situations is well known not only in the reasons people give for smoking, but also in other obvious reasons which they do not give. Young people often start smoking in imitation of older people who smoke or as an expression of a subconscious wish to be like them. Older children and youth want to be accepted by their friends and associates. Often friends dress alike, talk alike, and have other behavior in common. Smoking may be part of this attempt to conform. Not smoking could also be part of a group pattern.

As a means of relaxation, the mechanical aspects of smoking are recognized. Under tension or during an awkward lull in activity, smokers probably do relax by taking out a package of cigarettes, choosing one, getting matches, lighting the cigarette, and handling it.

Some authorities suggest that a cigarette represents a reward that a smoker can offer himself whenever he wishes, or that the act of smoking represents a means of self-expression. In young people, it may represent freedom to do as one pleases, or be a reaction against adult authority. Others believe that people smoke because of the need for oral activity to fulfill an unsatisfied sucking reflex.

Recent studies have shown that youngsters whose parents smoke will also tend to smoke. If older brothers and sisters smoke, the younger ones are more likely to become smokers.

Much research remains to be done before an understanding is reached regarding the factors in smoking that produce satisfaction and often lead to habituation.

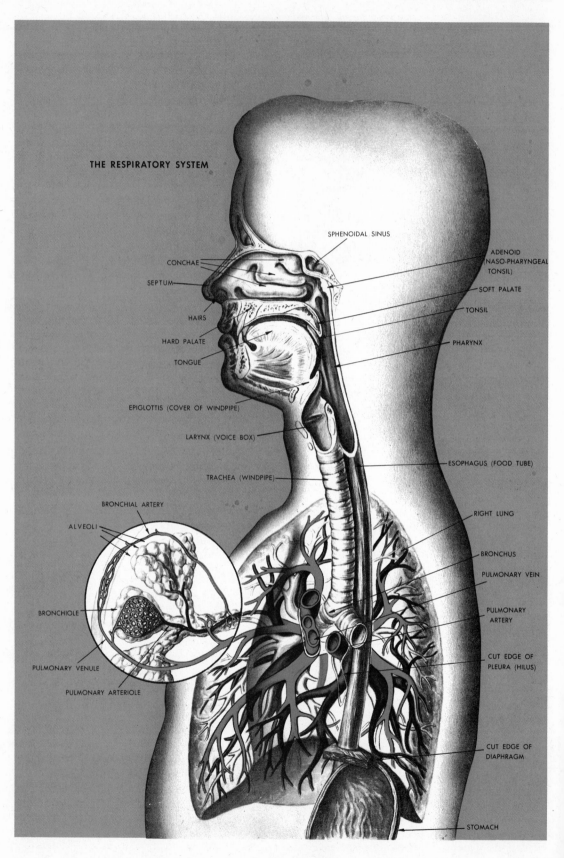

THE RESPIRATORY SYSTEM

SPHENOIDAL SINUS

ADENOID (NASO-PHARYNGEAL TONSIL)

CONCHAE

SEPTUM

SOFT PALATE

TONSIL

HAIRS

PHARYNX

HARD PALATE

TONGUE

EPIGLOTTIS (COVER OF WINDPIPE)

LARYNX (VOICE BOX)

ESOPHAGUS (FOOD TUBE)

TRACHEA (WINDPIPE)

BRONCHIAL ARTERY

RIGHT LUNG

ALVEOLI

BRONCHUS

PULMONARY VEIN

BRONCHIOLE

PULMONARY ARTERY

CUT EDGE OF PLEURA (HILUS)

PULMONARY VENULE

PULMONARY ARTERIOLE

CUT EDGE OF DIAPHRAGM

STOMACH

Physicians, other scientists, and many health agencies have studied the relationship of smoking to health and most are in general accord.

The most extensive examination of smoking was published in January, 1964, by the Advisory Committee to the Surgeon General of the U. S. Public Health Service. The committee reported that "cigarette smoking is causally related to lung cancer in men; the magnitude of the effect of cigarette smoking far outweighs all other factors. The data for women, though less extensive, point in the same direction."

The dangers in smoking, especially heavy smoking of cigarettes, are recognized all over the world. Statements on the subject have been issued not only by the United States Public Health Service, but also by the Royal College of Physicians in Great Britain and a special committee of the World Health Organization.

The American Medical Association stated officially at its Annual Convention in 1964:

"The American Medical Association is on record and does recognize a significant relationship between cigarette smoking and the incidence of lung cancer and certain other diseases, and that cigarette smoking is a serious health hazard."

The House of Delegates of the American Medical Association has officially endorsed the actions of the Joint Committee on Health Problems in Education of the National Education Association and the American Medical Association. This Committee, recognizing that "the specific components of tobacco exerting harmful effects on the human organism have not yet been defined and the exact pathological and physiological actions of these components have not been determined, nor the psychology of smoking fully understood, recommended authoritative research. . .in smoking such as that being conducted by the AMA and others."

The Joint Committee also resolved "that schools, physicians, health departments, and other community agencies cooperate in an aggressive program designed to discourage children from starting the smoking habit and to influence youth who are smoking to discontinue the habit."

The American Medical Association has not confined itself to mere endorsement. It has never allowed tobacco advertising in its health magazine, *Today's Health,* since publication began in 1923, and it banned tobacco advertising from its Journal for physicians and its exhibits at scientific meetings in 1954, long before the hazards of smoking became scientifically apparent. It is sponsoring clinical and scientific research, as well as an educational program on a continuing basis to call to the attention of the public, particularly young people, the known evidence against smoking.

Manufacturers are trying to reduce the hazards of smoking by modifying tobacco, reducing nicotine content, and filtering tars. The long-range effects of these efforts are not known.

Research has been initiated to find and isolate or refine harmful substances so that those who smoke may continue to smoke safely. Thus far, the results have been discouraging. As part of its concern with this problem, the American Medical Association is sponsoring a large-scale study to determine mechanisms by which human ailments may be caused or aggravated by smoking, in order to define more accurately the role of tobacco in disease.

While to smoke or not to smoke is a matter of individual choice, most authorities now agree that never to smoke is preferable. Further, they would agree that significant evidence is accumulating which indicates the desirability for the heavy smoker to stop smoking or cut down to the point of moderation.

The longer one smokes, and the more one smokes, the greater the risk of developing lung cancer. In those who quit smoking, the risk is diminished. Pipe smokers run more of a risk than nonsmokers, but far less risk than cigarette smokers.

Medications are being sold which are intended to keep the smoker from smoking. Unfortunately, these have not been successful. Antismoking clinics are being continually developed and may help many smokers. Persons who contend that smoking helps them control their weight by decreasing their appetites can find more healthful controls.

Whether to smoke or not to smoke is a major decision for anyone to make. A person who has not started the habit should carefully consider all the facts before doing so.

For those who really wish to discontinue smoking, the following suggestions are offered, out of the experience of a physician who successfully stopped smoking cigarettes, and has not resumed after 13 years. It takes doing, but it can be done.

How to Quit Smoking

To quit smoking is not easy. It makes no difference whether the daily consumption is three cigarettes or three packs, or any number of cigars or pipes, to quit smoking is a difficult task. Success depends on wanting to quit, willpower, and the use of various gimmicks to break the habit pattern.

One who is not sold on quitting may stop for a few days or even a few weeks, but always reinstates his habit. Wanting to quit involves both a rational reason (based on facts which are now well documented) and a motivation that leads to positive action, the actual act of stopping.

There are two schools of thought on the process of stopping. One advocates gradual withdrawal, the cutting of smoking in half each day till elimination of the last smoke makes one an abstainer. The other recommends the sudden cutoff. Now you smoke—now you don't. For most people gradual withdrawal is more likely to fail, since the presence of tobacco and the knowledge that it can be smoked dilutes the resolve to quit. Sudden cutoff may become uncomfortable, both physically and emotionally, but has a certain finality that helps. This is an "either—or" situation where one knows whether one is smoking or not smoking. There is no confusion about how much is smoked, or whether one has used his quota for the day.

The habit patterns of smoking have become a part of the social and business life of the smoker. Most smokers crave a cigarette after each meal. Knowing this, special effort must be made to do something after meals, not previously associated with smoking. Students who cannot smoke in class do so during their socializing between classes. In a similar way office workers smoke during their coffee breaks. In such cases, the desire to associate smoking with these periodic opportunities must be recognized and one's behavior at these times changed as much as possible.

It is easier to quit smoking when the whole living pattern to which one is accustomed can be changed. The most common of these is a vacation. With the timing of events different from the routine of office or shop, the signal for another smoke is met less often.

Hospitalization for treatment of an illness or for surgery is another such opportunity. Though not pleasant in many cases, it does provide a change of pace and habit and several days of forced abstinence on which to build.

Smoking is a gregarious habit. Usually when one person lights up, other smokers will. The person who has quit is tempted. He must state his position. It is therefore a wise precaution, after being sure that to quit smoking is the desired end, to announce that you have quit smoking. It may cause some good natured joking, but it will reduce the offers of smoking materials. It will also establish a social pattern in which the person quitting doesn't dare smoke, and this has a very healthy influence.

When the typical smoker quits he can expect a certain pattern of experiences. The first day is not bad, his enthusiasm is at high pitch. The next few days—up to a week or more—are uncomfortable. Part of the discomfort is the pain of breaking a habit, part is the elimination of the chemicals absorbed from tobacco smoke. By the end of two weeks the craving is nearly gone, though it returns on viewing others smoking or on smelling smoke. By now the senses of taste and smell have improved and with them appetite. Food tastes so much better that great care must be taken not to overeat. But even though the smoking habit is weakened, it is not broken. One cigarette or one cigar can return the backslider to the ranks of confirmed smokers. At this stage, unfortunately, the ones who return may smoke as much or more than they did before trying to quit.

Success comes in three to six months, when a former smoker can go through his daily routine and associate with smokers while having no desire to smoke himself. The acme is reached when at the end of a year of abstinence the former smoker overreacts, and an effort is made to avoid places where people smoke— and there may even be a tendency to be critical of the people themselves.

Where does one's physician fit into this picture? There are two circumstances in which he should be consulted. Medical supervision during the first few weeks of abstinence could so support one during this change that troublesome reactions would be less likely.

The other circumstance is the case where "the spirit is willing but the flesh is weak"— the resolve is made but the willpower to carry through is lacking. Here your doctor can prescribe drugs that may help some, although this is not always indicated. For some people such drugs can make the nervous tensions associated with breaking the habit less annoying.

"Secret" drugs which can be put into the smoker's food or drink without his knowledge have no value.

CHAPTER FOUR

ALCOHOLISM

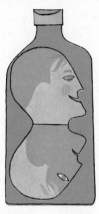

ALCOHOLISM is both a major chronic disease and a major social problem. The illness afflicts between 5,000,000 and 6,000,000 persons in the United States alone. Because of the peculiar nature of the illness and because most of its victims are adults with families, three or four times that many people are directly affected by it. In addition, the alcoholic's friends and employers share the brunt of his affliction.

The economic and social costs of alcoholism are tremendous. Alcoholics cost their employers millions of lost man hours each year and they cost their families many millions of dollars in lost pay, in money spent (or lost) in drinking bouts, in accidental injuries and damages, in crimes and misdemeanors, in hospitalization and treatment. Society as a whole must expend huge sums in maintaining institutions for alcoholics—hospitals, sanatoria and clinics, and jails—where alcoholics form a substantial proportion of the inmates. Alcoholism is believed to be one of the major causes of the nation's traffic accidents, costing several thousands of lives and several million dollars worth of property damage each year.

Until fairly recent times, alcoholism was considered by most persons to be a social problem. The alcoholic was thought to have a "weak character." It is now universally recognized that alcoholism is first and foremost a disease. As a disease, it is defined in several ways. In its active phase, it is simply the habitual consumption of too much alcohol. In addition, alcoholism is an addiction, an allergy. The alcoholic is almost never "cured" in the sense that he becomes able to drink moderate amounts of alcohol without disastrous effects.

Because the nature of alcoholism has become generally understood, it is now being faced more squarely as both a medical and social problem. It is being attacked by various approaches. Relatives and close friends of the alcoholic have become interested in the effects of alcohol on the body, how the habit begins, and how the alcoholic can be restored to health. The public in general also has gained insight into the problem and has developed a desire to find a solution to it. As a result, there are encouraging prospects that alcoholism, like many other chronic diseases, can come to be controlled. There is new hope that the disease will become far less of a problem for the alcoholic, his family, his employer and fellow workers, his community, and professional persons in the fields of medicine, health, and social service.

Effects of Alcoholism

The consumption of alcoholic beverages has for too long been associated with ideas of merriment and good cheer. This is indicated by the slang terms applied to their effect, such as "high" or "happy." Alcohol is not a stimulant in any sense. Instead, it is an anesthetic, acting on the body in the same way as ether or similar anesthetics. It is worth noting that when ether was first introduced, medical students and others who had access to this anesthetic used it at "sniffing parties" to produce the same effect as liquor.

One of the first parts of the body to show the depressing effects of alcohol is the front portion of the brain. In that area are the centers that govern self-control, finer judgments, conscience, inhibitions, and moral sense. As these are dulled, the drinker begins to talk and act with reckless abandon, and is easily led into all sorts of antisocial conduct. The "good cheer" is actually a response to the deadening, brake-releasing effects of alcohol.

As more alcohol is consumed its level in the blood rises and coordination diminishes. Ordinary movements like walking or driving a car become difficult or clumsy. Speech becomes slurred, and the eyes may not focus properly. Studies have shown that sometimes the eyes jerk from side to side rapidly. This probably accounts for the sensation that the room is turning around.

Because inhibitions and caution have been cast to the winds, the impulse to continue drinking becomes stronger. Finally, as the alcohol level in the blood goes still higher, vital centers in other parts of the brain are affected. These are responsible for such life-sustaining functions as breathing and other reflex actions. If breathing should become too slow or should stop, death will occur.

It is believed that some individuals apparently develop a certain amount of tolerance to alcohol if they are habitual drinkers. This means that they must drink more liquor to produce the effects described above. Thus, a vicious circle is set up, and there probably occurs

a change in the basal metabolism of the brain cells, so that they become dependent on alcohol in order to function. It has been suggested that this is responsible for some of the frightening withdrawal symptoms that occur when an alcoholic stops drinking. These include the "shakes," nervousness, delirium, and hallucinations observed by the drunkard who is sobering up. They probably explain his frantic craving for more alcohol at this time.

Because alcohol is a strong chemical, it may damage other delicate body tissues if constantly present in the blood and body fluids. Actually, alcohol is used in the pathologist's laboratory to "fix" or harden tissues that are being prepared for microscopic examination. Because the liver must "break down" alcohol, exposure of its cells to this fixing action can produce permanent changes that eventually impair the normal functions and structure of that organ.

Alcohol is as addicting as narcotics. That it can be obtained legally and without difficulty by any adult, in no way alters the seriousness of

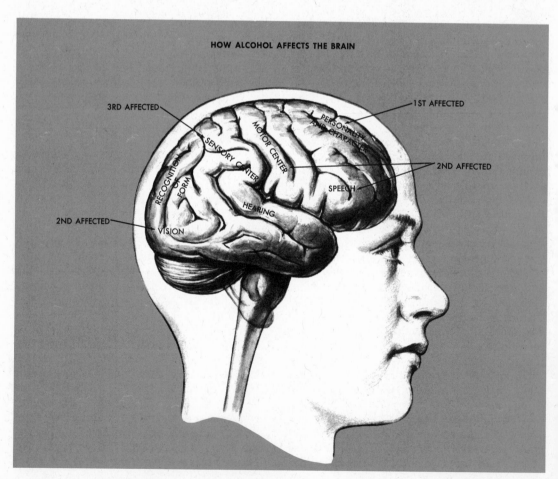

its effects. This important fact must be kept in mind constantly, because in almost all localities there are no other reminders—no laws forbidding its use by others than minors.

Among the harmful effects of alcohol must be included the annual death toll attributed to the drinking driver, who is not necessarily a full-blown alcoholic. Each year, about half of the deaths resulting from automobile accidents—and these come close to 50,000—involve a drinking driver.

Finally, but of importance, are effects of alcoholism on the individual's personality and, in turn, on his social status and family relationships. Because all his pride has gone, the excessive drinker pays no attention to the way he looks. Unshaven, unkempt, unwashed, wearing dirty, unpressed clothing, he arouses repugnance and distaste in all with whom he has contacts. This reaction turns easily to anger and rejection on the part of business associates, friends, and relatives. And because of this, the alcoholic continues along his same course, seeking even more eagerly the oblivion provided by alcohol. It is not surprising that family discord develops, with all its shattering effects on morals and the feeling of pride and security in the home.

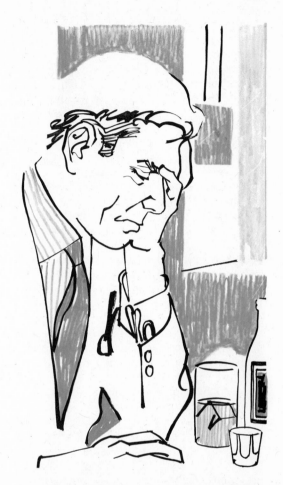

Causes of Alcoholism

Even without all the convincing evidence that has been produced in the last 15 or 20 years to indict alcoholism as a pernicious, life-threatening disease, its destructive end-results have been known to mankind for centuries. Why, then, has addiction to the use of alcohol continued to increase? The answer must be sought in aspects of man's reactions to his environment other than merely the desire to have a "good time," for no sensible person would take such risks for the brief pleasure expected.

Because alcoholism can be such a serious threat to health, social status, and home and community security, it is vitally important to detect the cause at the earliest possible moment. It has been estimated that about six per cent of people who drink are candidates for addiction. Unfortunately, early discovery is not always easy. There are no clear-cut signs that enable a relative or even a physician to say, "This person is a potential alcoholic." However, individual reactions at relatively early stages of drinking are often helpful. For example, a person whose character or personality changes after only a drink or two, who

becomes unusually aggressive or argumentative or perhaps blatantly boisterous, will be well advised to take stock of himself. He should decide then and there that abstinence is the best course. Often "blacking out" after only a few drinks is a significant sign.

Much evidence suggests that many alcoholics have common characteristics that incline them to addiction. Those whose background, home training, and emotional makeup have failed to help them face the realities of living are likely candidates for this escape from reality. Detection of such persons is not always easy. Many are borderline cases, able to meet average social, family, and occupational responsibilities, but always close to the edge of retreat from demands that to them appear excessive. As they discover how the anesthetic effect of alcohol dulls their fears and feelings of inadequacy, they tend to turn more and more to this easy way out. And since their problems melt into oblivion when they are in a stuporous alcoholic state, they tend to resort to alcohol all the more frequently. Because an alcoholic "binge" in itself demeans the addict and emphasizes his inadequacies, he is encouraged to further excesses.

On the other hand, some observers interpret these same facts to indicate that the alcoholism is the cause of the deterioration which may occur, rather than the effect of a pre-existing weakness.

Whether or not alcoholism should be called a mental disorder is not easily decided. Definite evidence of psychiatric imbalance, if not actual psychiatric disease, will be found in some alcoholic victims. It is considered desirable for all alcoholics to have psychiatric evaluation as part of their general treatment program. Those in need of specific treatment in this area can be helped greatly if the need is uncovered.

In other alcoholics, psychiatric and psychological tests indicate they have no basic problem in facing the realities of living. Instead, it has been their drinking which has created the inadequacy. Physicians who have studied this problem extensively report that more than half of their patients gave no indication of having previous neurotic tendencies, and that when the drinking habit was broken, they were able to live on a normal basis.

Undoubtedly the basic problem is the invariable tendency of the potential alcoholic to drink more and more as time goes on. Strangely enough, this often occurs without the alcoholic's recognizing that he is increasing his intake. Not until he has become seriously habituated may he become aware of this. And by this time, he has progressed to the point where he cannot get along without his drink. Cutting down then becomes much more difficult, and in many cases impossible without outside help.

Many other theories and concepts regarding the cause of alcoholism have been set forth. For example, some biochemists believe there may be a deviation from normal body chemistry in persons who are vulnerable to alcoholism. And, as has been indicated earlier, social scientists have held that cultural and environmental factors have a tremendous bearing on the cause of alcoholism.

Diagnosing Alcoholism

In its full-blown state, alcoholism is of course easily diagnosed by relatives and friends of the alcoholic. The state of chronic semi-intoxication, with its detachment from reality, imperviousness to reasoning or persuasion, and general body deterioration, requires no scientific evaluation or pronouncement. But there are somewhat earlier signs that will serve to alert the family and associates of the potential victim to the need for prompt, constructive action. These include:

● Drinking excessively and frequently.

● Getting drunk without really intending to.

● Needing a drink at odd times, with no "party" excuse.

● Going on "sprees" that are practically disabling.

● Constantly thinking about drinking.

● Drinking alone.

● Letting drink become the only important thing in life.

● Losing time from work because of the effects of drinking.

● Making elaborate excuses for drinking.

● Rationalizing the amount taken and reason for drinking.

Sometimes alcoholism may not come to general attention until, through some unexpected change in his daily routine, the alcoholic loses access to his usual supply of liquor. This calls to mind the classic story about the wife who discovered her husband's illness only because he happened to come home sober one night. Alcoholics develop unusual cunning in covering up their use of intoxicating beverages, and are often able to maintain a "normal" front in contacts with friends, business associates, and even members of their family. Of course, as the habit becomes more solidly entrenched, such caution is usually abandoned, the drinker's only interest in life being alcohol. He becomes indifferent to what others think or say.

Treatment of Alcoholism

Many treatment approaches are now available for effective conquest of alcoholic addiction. Two important facts that are basic to any and all treatments are:

1. The patient must recognize his problem and ask for help to correct it.

2. The condition must always be thought of by family and friends as a disease, not as a "sin" or perversion that can be cured by punishment.

If alcoholism has been long-standing and severe, a program of physical rehabilitation may be required before specific treatment can be given. Many chronic alcoholics are undernourished, weak, nervous, and without appetite. Some may even be suffering from marked vitamin deficiencies. Some time may be required to restore such patients to a reasonably normal physical condition. Unless this is done, active treatment programs are likely to prove much less effective.

In the medical area, in addition to the often important assistance provided by psychiatric treatment, certain drugs may be employed. Two that have received considerable attention are products that, when given, cause serious body reactions if any alcoholic drink should be taken. Although these symptoms, which include nausea, vomiting, and marked prostration, are impressive to the patient, they are not life-threatening. Usually no more than one or two demonstrations of the cause-and-effect sequence will be required to convince the alcoholic that if he continues the treatment program he must abandon further drinking. The decision to use these substances must depend on the doctor's evaluation of the patient's general health.

Other medical ways to set up a "conditioned" reaction in the patient are available. With one, a preparation that causes vomiting may be injected by the physician after one or more drinks have been taken. After several such trials, weaning the patient away from alcohol will be considerably simplified.

Drugs that are often employed effectively, especially during the acute withdrawal period, include tranquilizers and sedatives. They will help the patient keep calm and refreshed as well as provide him the restful sleep that he so often needs. However, the physician will not put the patient on prolonged use of any of these products, since to do so might simply transfer him to another addiction, perhaps not so serious but nevertheless as undesirable and unnecessary as alcoholism itself.

Hypnotism may be tried in properly selected cases. This measure is not something that can be used casually or in a parlorgame type of setting. Only specially trained psychiatrists are considered competent to apply hypnotism and, as has been indicated, careful patient selection is essential.

Counseling has always been recognized as having an important place in the therapy of alcoholism. In appropriate situations, the physician can do much to reconstruct the alcoholic's thinking and his attitude toward his problem and its underlying causes. So can a clergyman who has the modern concept of alcoholism as a disease, rather than a sin or a weakness.

Probably one of the most important forms of counseling that has been developed is the aid provided by the organization known as Alcoholics Anonymous. This group, which is now world-wide in its operation, bases its services on complete, personal understanding of the alcoholic's problem, derived through personal experience. Each A.A. member is himself a convincing demonstration that it is possible, no matter how extreme a person's former drinking habits, to live productively without alcohol.

Giving of aid by an Alcoholic Anonymous member is always on the personal or "buddy" level. There are no lectures, no dwelling on the horrors of alcoholism, no reproaches. Instead the alcoholic receives sympathetic understanding and encouragement.

Early in its operation, A.A. developed a set of steps that its members believed summed up the essentials of a comeback from alcoholism. These were based on the experiences of members themselves, rather than being obtained from non-alcoholic counselors, physicians, ministers, or others who, despite their sincere desire to help, had never gone through the personal torture of having descended into the depth of alcoholism and then climbed back up. Only an A.A. member knew, they believed, what should be done. Nevertheless, the steps, 12 in number, are never presented as dogma, but as suggestions to be tried out. They are:

1. We admit we are powerless over alcohol —that our lives have become unmanageable.

2. We have come to believe that a Power greater than ourselves can restore us to sanity.

3. We have made a decision to turn our will and our lives over to the care of God as we understand Him.

4. We have made a searching and fearless moral inventory of ourselves.

5. We have admitted to God, to ourselves, and to another human being the exact nature of our wrongs.

6. We are entirely ready to have God remove all these defects of character.

7. We humbly ask Him to remove our shortcomings.

8. We have made a list of all persons we have harmed, and have become willing to make amends to them all.

9. We have made direct amends to such people wherever possible, except when to do so would injure them or others.

10. We have continued to take personal inventory and when we are wrong promptly admit it.

11. We have sought through prayer and meditation to improve our conscious contact

with God as we understand Him, praying only for knowledge of His will for us and the power to carry that out.

12. Having had a spiritual awakening as the result of these steps, we have tried to carry this message to other alcoholics and to practice these principles in all our affairs.

As the recovery of thousands of alcoholics has demonstrated, A.A. can be helpful in many seemingly hopeless situations. Obviously, both the alcoholic and his family must try to understand the organization's program.

Contact with A.A. can be made virtually anywhere in the United States. In larger cities, the local groups are listed in the telephone directory. In less populous areas, information about A.A. groups probably can be obtained from health or welfare departments. Even casual inquiry among friends or neighbors will very probably reveal a contact. Like alcoholism, A.A. is everywhere.

At regular A.A. meetings, personal experiences are exchanged and helpful attitudes developed. Both open and closed meetings are held. At the latter, family members can be helped to gain more insight into the alcoholic's problems and how home situations can be developed to help him. In some larger cities, there are special family meetings, and there is even an organization known as the Alateens. Its members are teenage sons and daughters of alcoholics who meet together to gain understanding of the problems that are involved and how they can make the home and family relationship easier for the alcoholic, and thus speed his recovery.

Prevention of Alcoholism

Alcoholism is more likely to occur in children when the disease has afflicted one or both of their parents. However, there is no evidence that it is actually inherited as diabetes tends to be, or like the color of hair and eyes or specific blood types. In looking further for possible causes, one realizes that certain personal characteristics, which may be acquired or inherited, can perhaps represent predisposing factors. As has already been pointed out, a person who is nervous, easily upset, tends to be withdrawn, and has difficulty in adjusting to life situations is a more likely candidate for alcoholism.

Agreement is general that the environment is of vital importance in considering the causes of alcoholism. If the child has been brought up in a home where there is peace and harmony, where each member of the family recognizes and accepts his or her responsibilities, and where there is a feeling of security and satisfactory adjustment to the demands of society, there will be little chance of alcoholism developing. The high incidence of alcoholism among those who give a history of family discord, of irresponsible parents, of separation or divorce provides eloquent testimony to this fact.

It is obvious that prevention of alcoholism begins at an early age. Its effectiveness will be directly proportional to the level of family living and adjustment that has been reached.

Knowledge is another important deterrent to alcoholism. Young people should be told in simple, straightforward terms what alcohol does to the body. Emphasis should be placed on the permanent effects that can be produced by unwise use of this poisonous anesthetic that causes "good cheer" only through its deadening effect on the brain.

In good family surroundings, most young people will automatically acquire the ability to adjust readily to life's demands. They quickly recognize that life will not always be easy, that there will be frustrations, and that everyone has certain physical and mental limitations. Accepting these realities, they will know that one cannot run away from life's problems, but must face them squarely and do the best one can. Unfortunately, all too many alcoholics are inadequate in this aspect of living. They have "run away" into the temporary oblivion provided by alcohol, not realizing that this simply compounds their problems.

Important also in the family atmosphere is the example set by parents. Too much value must not be placed on drinking. Insistence on a routine of one, two, or perhaps more highballs or cocktails before dinner may establish an undesirable pattern for the children in the family. The giving of "make-believe" drinks or diluted alcoholic beverages to young children tends to establish wrong values in their minds. Often, young people drink only because they want to be considered "grown-up," and because that is what the grown-ups they know do regularly. It hardly needs to be pointed out that the example set by a parent who is an alcoholic can have a tremendous influence on children exposed to such a home situation. Youngsters, because of insecurity engendered by alcoholism in the home, may use the same method of escape from their problems as they have seen a parent use.

Prevention of alcoholism at its onset, before the pattern has become firmly established, is equally important. In addition to attention to the personal characteristics that suggest the possibility of beginning alcoholism, other helpful reminders are available. It must always be borne in mind that early detection and prevention must rely heavily upon the honesty and good sense of the individual involved, as well as upon the alertness and judgment of those about him. Because alcoholism is such an insidious disease, its victim rarely recognizes it in its early stages. That is why he will deny there is any possibility that he is drinking excessively, and why it is necessary for friends and relatives to insist that the potential patient face the matter honestly and make a sensible analysis of it.

All too often, social customs operate to make prevention of alcoholism difficult. It has been stated, with reasonable justification, that alcohol occupies too great a part of our culture. Social pressures to drink are often tremendous. But refusal to drink alcoholic beverages, with or without reason, is a personal privilege that should always be respected.

Fortunately, the feeling is becoming more widespread that critical or joking comments about an abstainer are impolite and out of place. Also, the term alcoholism no longer carries the stigma it once had before the condition was recognized as a disease. Therefore, persons with this problem are no longer as likely to be embarrassed by having public attention called to it when they refuse liquor.

Casual, understanding acceptance of such refusal will help reinforce the patient's determination not to drink, and help to prevent his becoming self-conscious and uncomfortable. The host and hostess who are alert to all possible desires of their guests will have available, without question or challenge, soft drinks, fruit juices, coffee, and tea to meet every preference.

Public tolerance of drunken behavior is unfortunately still widespread. Drunkenness is a matter for laughing and joking, and the comedian who presents a drunkard skit on the stage or television is enthusiastically applauded. This attitude must change. Everyone must recognize and accept the obvious fact that there is no acceptable reason for voluntarily drinking excessively. Where drunken behavior is not tolerated, there we find little alcoholism. For example, among the Chinese, where drinking is frowned on, there is almost no alcoholism.

The simple fact with which all alcoholics must learn to live is that once the disease is halted, alcohol can never be taken again. There is no half-way measure. Like diabetes, alcoholism is never cured. Eternal vigilance and avoidance are necessary. It is as dangerous to take "just a glass of beer" as it is to drink a pint of whiskey. As time passes, as the alcoholic gets better and better adjusted to normal living and realizes that he can function happily and productively in such an atmosphere, the temptation to drink will lessen. But still the alcoholic must always keep his guard up.

CHAPTER FIVE

NARCOTIC ADDICTION

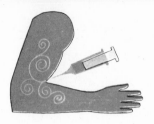

THOUSANDS OF AMERICANS awakened this morning with one driving need—to obtain enough illegal drugs to see them through the day. They are victims of a habit so powerful and so expensive that many will commit crimes before the day is done in order to pay for their drugs.

The drug addiction problem is centuries old. In this country it dates back at least to the Civil War period. Recognition by the American public of addiction as a public health problem, however, is relatively new. Such awareness has developed only during the past few decades.

The term "dope fiend" brings to mind images of wild-eyed derelicts given to violence and crime. It is true that addiction is linked to crime, but usually in an indirect way. The addict's crimes are most often the result of his urgent need for money to buy more drugs. Seldom does the use of drugs in itself lead the addict to commit a crime. A substantial number of younger addicts have a preaddiction record of antisocial activity, but no relation between these acts and the use of drugs has been shown. Despite these facts, it is difficult to supplant the image of an addict with the truth about addiction.

Narcotics addiction is a complex human problem which has benefited little from the remarkable advances in knowledge in related fields. Partial explanation for this fact lies, perhaps, in the very nature of the problem. Addiction is often a solitary affair—a quiet, unobtrusive habit. The addict associates chiefly with other addicts. Unlike the alcoholic, he is not likely to be obnoxious or to bother other people. His problem is easily kept in a dark corner because, for the most part, it develops in society's shadowy corners. It is only when he is driven to crime to finance his habit that the addict attracts public attention.

Addiction is a serious illness, with frequently tragic consequences. It is also linked in the public mind with the underworld, which today in the United States is the source of narcotics. As a result most people are concerned with addiction as a crime rather than with addiction as a disease. Such is the nature of addiction that the public has felt justified over the years in considering it more of a problem of morality than as a psychiatric and public health problem.

In numerical terms, the addiction problem seems small and insignificant when compared with alcoholism or with the venereal disease problem. The truth is that no one can say, with complete certainty, how many people are addicted to drugs. Addicts are hardly eager to be counted in a census, knowing that their behavior is illegal and considered immoral.

In addition, the size and significance of the addiction problem must be measured in terms of human suffering, disrupted lives, and the financial cost to society. The effect on the addict's family is often devastating. The family is often in the position of longing for help but not knowing where to turn for it, and at the same time, fearful lest its secret be discovered.

The typical narcotics addict requires $10 to $30 daily for drugs. Male addicts usually turn to stealing in one form or another to obtain the necessary money. Since stolen merchandise brings the thief only a small proportion of its original cost, addicts must steal items worth far more than the cash they need for drugs. It can safely be said that the typical male addict may steal in a year's time merchandise valued at from $30,000 to $90,000. The figure of $350,000,000 has been suggested by the Federal Bureau of Narcotics as the amount spent annually for illegal drugs.

The typical female addict usually resorts to prostitution to obtain the money she needs. It is likely that more than half the women in the prisons of our large cities are both prostitutes and narcotic addicts.

It is clear that society is paying an exorbitant price, in a variety of ways, for continuing to let this problem go unsolved.

Drugs Used by the Addict

True addiction occurs only with sedative drugs and is associated with the continued use of barbiturates and opiates. Addiction has three separate but related phases: tolerance, habituation, and physical dependence. Tolerance is the diminishing effect of the same dose of a drug, or the need to increase the size of the dose in order to get an effect similar to the earlier ones. Habituation is the emotional or psychological need which is met by the drug. Dependence is the body's need to get the drug.

Opiates that have been used by addicts in the United States are opium, morphine, heroin, and the synthetic drugs that are manmade but have an effect similar to that of an opium derivative. In the early 1930's, opium ceased to be the drug of choice among American addicts, giving way to morphine. A few years later heroin, a morphine derivative, became their preferred drug. Heroin is nearly twice as powerful as morphine and is used by most of today's opiate addicts. Heroin is illegal in the United States, and anyone possessing it is violating the law, for either the heroin itself, or the opium from which it is made, must have been smuggled into the country.

Although not an addicting drug, cocaine is habituating and is used by some opiate addicts. It gives an almost instantaneous "charge" which is very concentrated and intense but of short duration. It stimulates, whereas opiates depress. Addicts seldom use cocaine by itself consistently because it is extremely highpriced on the illegal market and because its effects are so short-lived. Some experienced addicts like to mix heroin and cocaine into a "speed ball" which combines the immediate "kick" of cocaine with the extended afterglow of heroin. Addicts also call this mixture a "love affair," because heroin is often referred to as "boy" and cocaine as "girl."

Other drugs which are under federal regulation, even though they are not opiates and not addicting, are marijuana and peyote. They, too, are stimulants—not depressants.

The barbiturates, or sleeping pills, are regarded as genuinely addicting drugs when used to excess. Evidence gathered in the past few years strongly suggests that overuse of barbiturates may lead to an addiction as serious, if not more so, than the opiates. Some narcotic users take barbiturates if their regular drug is not available, and some take both.

Many people still believe that an addict can be identified by his appearance. He cannot. As a matter of fact, members of an addict's immediate family may not observe any changes in his appearance due to his use of drugs. It is true, however, that heroin users may have scars or sores on their arms resulting from repeated injections of the drug into the veins.

Identifying the Addict

It is extremely difficult to recognize an opiate user who is receiving a regular supply of his drug. If the drug is withdrawn for one or two days, however, the addict is easily identified by a series of definite involuntary reactions called the withdrawal or abstinence syndrome. The severity of the addiction can be measured by the severity of this reaction pattern. A mild abstinence syndrome involves sneezing, yawning, perspiring, watering of the eyes, and a running nose. A moderate response includes tremors of the body, goose flesh, loss of appetite, and dilation of the pupils.

A severe syndrome often involves fever, increased blood pressure, rapid breathing, insomnia, and acute restlessness. In its most intense form, the response takes the form of vomiting, diarrhea, weight loss, and spasms of the limbs. The reaction pattern begins when the effect of the last "shot" starts to wear off. For the typical heroin addict, this period is nearly 6 hours; for the morphine addict, it is 12 hours; for the opium addict, 24 hours.

Contrary to a widely held belief, drug addicts are not necessarily members of society's lowest class—economically, socially, or mentally. Through history, a few highly intelligent, talented, well-known figures have been addicted to narcotics. This is true today as well. But the addict group that attracts the greatest attention and elicits the deepest public concern today is made up of teenagers. The bulk of them come from the slums of our large cities and from the underprivileged minority groups living in these slums. Some of these young addicts are members of gangs and have been involved in delinquent and even criminal activities prior to their development of the drug habit. Their use of drugs represents simply one more phase of the antisocial pattern of their lives. In this respect, today's young addict differs from the drug user of the 1930's who usually had a clean record until his need for narcotics drove him to criminal activity.

How Addiction Starts

Most addicts begin using drugs as a result of associating with those already using drugs. It must be pointed out, however, that many, if not

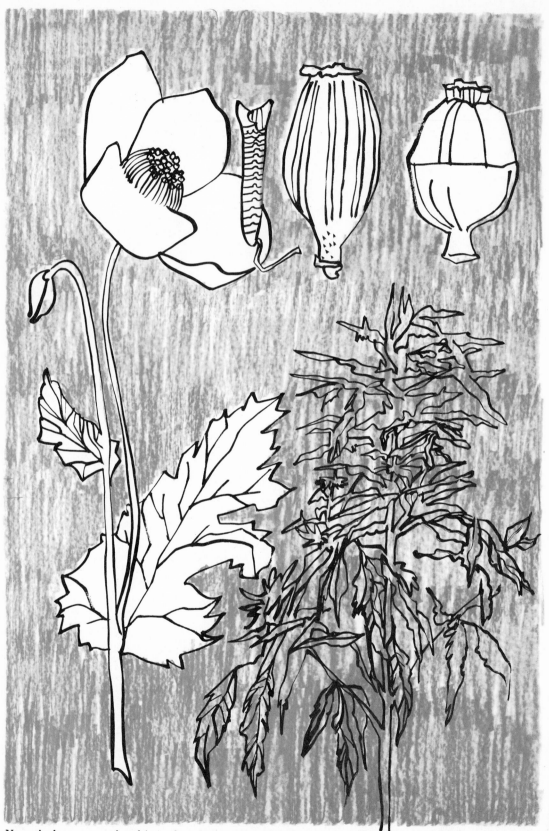

Narcotic drugs are produced from the opium poppy and pods (top); *marijuana from the weed at bottom, right.*

most, persons who try drugs out of curiosity do not use them a second time and certainly do not become addicted. It is likely that only those persons who feel that drugs help them cope with their serious personal problems continue to use narcotics and ultimately become addicts. It is not possible to make generalizations about the reasons for drug use because it appears that drugs meet different needs for different persons. For example, some addicts may begin using drugs to be like the members of a group they admire, while others may develop the habit to accent their individuality and to set them apart from a group that does not take drugs.

A substantial number of addicts in large cities begins using narcotic drugs at approximately the age of 16, the age when adolescents are likely to be faced by the new challenges of maturity. Many of these teenagers suffer from a personality disturbance so severe that they seek to "tune out" reality and its commitments and decisions. Different kinds of inadequate persons may begin and continue to use drugs. There is no general agreement about the type of personality make-up that is most likely to be found in addicts, although many seem to have a schizoid, or split, personality. There is urgent need for more research in this field to determine the common denominators of the addict personality, if there be such.

Treating the Addict

The two largest facilities providing treatment for narcotic addicts are federal hospitals —one at Lexington, Kentucky, and the other at Fort Worth, Texas—with a total of 1,800 beds. The Lexington hospital is devoted exclusively to addicts, while the Fort Worth facility is a general psychiatric hospital with a section for addict patients.

The number of beds in these two facilities is greater than the combined total of beds available for treatment of addicts in all the other state, city, and private hospitals in the United States. Only one community (New York City) has a hospital exclusively for drug addicts and it admits only addicts under 21 years of age. California is planning a large hospital for the treatment of addict patients.

Treatment in the federal hospitals consists of giving the addict a continually smaller dosage of a synthetic opiate until his habit is broken. It is a fairly routine medical procedure, often followed by psychiatric treatment. If it were as

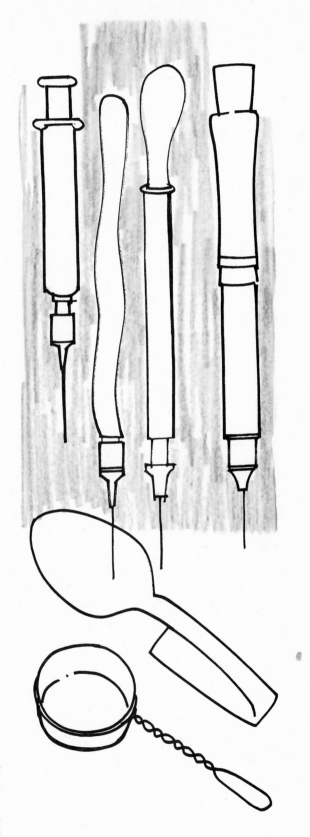

easy for the addict to remain off drugs as it is for him to be withdrawn from them, the problem would be comparatively simple.

Much of the difficulty in treating addicts stems from the public's lack of information about and understanding of drug addiction. Many people are repelled, even while fascinated, by the addict, viewing him as a demonaic "dope fiend." This is unfortunate, for a necessary part of any effective treatment program is an attitude which accepts the addict as a sick person who suffers from a serious disease.

The ex-addict returns to his home from a federal hospital under extremely difficult circumstances. He is back in the environment which helped to make him an addict, and people are likely to know he is a former addict. Usually, he returns with no money and when he goes looking for work, he finds that employers are very wary about hiring ex-addicts.

The chances are that his relations with his family have been strained by his long absence and by the community's obvious disapproval of addiction. His non-addict friends may be suspicious of him, and his addict friends may be far too available. Social agencies often are reluctant to help the former addict because they feel the chances of his successful adjustment are too slight to warrant the necessary expenditure of time and counseling talent.

In view of the lack of support the former addict receives, it is not surprising that he often goes back to drug use as a way of expressing his disenchantment with his community. He does so even though he may have been eager to break his habit and return to normal living. It is heartening to note that a number of voluntary, non-governmental groups have been working in some areas to provide neighborhood facilities for such returnees.

On the other hand, there is evidence to support the belief that some—perhaps many—addicts go through a process of "maturing out" of their habit. They stop taking drugs, often without much treatment. The very passage of time is a major factor in this process.

The Causes of Addiction

The sociologist sees addiction as a problem that develops in certain geographical areas, in specific environments. He points to the underprivileged groups in a few big city neighborhoods who form a large segment of the addict population. He equates addiction with economic depression, cultural deprivation,

and a high rate of juvenile delinquency. The psychologist, on the other hand, interprets addiction among minority groups as an expression of the frustration and hostility they feel but cannot express outwardly. The psychoanalyst sees the addict developing in and responding to a specific kind of family situation.

Many people hold fast to the idea of addiction being strictly a problem of law enforcement. They feel that if the smuggling rings are smashed and the "pushers" thrown in jail, drug addiction will disappear because there will be no illegal drugs available.

Another group holds the opposite view. They insist that addiction is an illness and that law enforcement cannot cure an illness. They point out that prohibition did not eliminate alcoholism. Drug use, they point out, is a symptom of other serious problems, and any treatment for addiction must take these problems into consideration.

This group also argues that making addiction a crime may actually increase the number of addicts. Because drugs are illegal, they are expensive; because much money can be made from their sale, the underworld and the "pushers" try to make as many addicts as possible. This group points to the low number of addicts in Great Britain. There addicts may register with the police, without penalty, and receive drugs at low cost while undergoing medical treatment.

Formidable barriers stand in the way of progress in the narcotics addiction field, but the situation is far from hopeless. As this is written, there is a new stirring of interest in the drug problem, there is encouraging action on a number of fronts, there are many hopeful signs.

Special efforts have been made by several state probation and parole departments to test the usefulness of intensive casework by parole officers to help the addict make a satisfactory social adjustment.

A number of church-sponsored groups have pioneered in providing services to support addicts trying to break their drug habit. A few voluntary agencies are developing experimental casework services tailored to the needs of the addict struggling with the problem of readjustment.

The mass media are focusing the public's attention on the problem of narcotics addiction. It is not uncommon these days to pick up a popular magazine and find an article dealing with some facet of drug addiction. More and more television panel programs present discussions of various aspects of the problem. Many motion pictures dealing with addiction have been produced.

Narcotics Anonymous, patterned after Alcoholics Anonymous, was founded in 1949 by Daniel Carlson, a former addict. It now has branches in a number of cities and is gaining experience in providing effective resources for addicts. NA accepts only members who are off drugs, and offers the ex-addict the opportunity to discuss his problems with others who are facing similar difficulties. The group gives many ex-addicts the kind of support they need.

While addiction can be treated successfully in some instances, it is a long and hard fight, and relapses are common. It cannot be emphasized too often or too earnestly that the only way to be safe against drug addiction is to avoid any practice that might lead to it. Trying marijuana just for kicks often leads to heroin addiction. Glue-sniffing by adolescents, using airplane model glue, can lead to serious physical results, and the effects it produces may cause a desire for bigger and stronger "kicks." Other dangerous drugs include peyote (mescaline), Mexican mushroom, jimson weed, and LSD-25. These drugs are known as hallucinogens; they create a temporary illusion of well-being, but their ultimate effect is trouble.

Temptation to experiment with drugs accompanies the idleness forced upon young people unable to find jobs. This will be greater if they associate with groups whose morals are lax, and whose leadership is perverted.

Another form of drug use which leads to habituation rather than addiction is the use of stimulants or "pep pills," such as amphetamine, commonly employed by students and others who wish to keep awake under difficult conditions. Often sleeping pills are alternated with stimulants. These create first artificial sedation and then stimulation, an undesirable substitute for normal rest and sleep.

While drug addiction has been decreasing in the United States, it remains a serious problem in areas where minority groups are numerous, and where social and economic conditions are unfavorable. Young people should be warned in a factual, unemotional, but emphatic manner of the dangers involved in trying a drug "kick" just once.

The only safe way to use any kind of drugs, except possibly a few common household remedies, is under medical supervision.

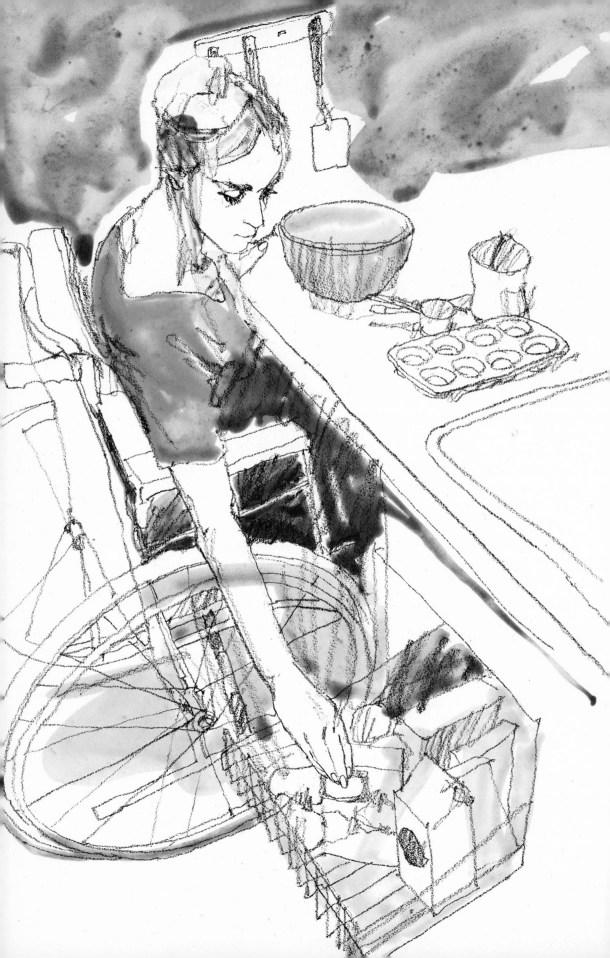

PART XIII

Physical
Handicaps

CHAPTER ONE

THE HANDICAPPED ADULT

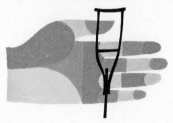

THE PACE of modern living has impressed every individual with the need for saving money, time, and energy. Efficiency is seen in short-order restaurants, drive-in banks, movies, and motels, frozen and prepackaged foods, industrial production lines, and jet transportation As the pace increases for the non-disabled, it is particularly important that the disabled make the most of their capabilities.

Actually, labor-saving methods and devices are made to order for those with physical limitations, allowing them to take their place in society side by side with their non-disabled neighbors. However, not all devices are usable without some individual modification, and only some of these modified devices are at present available commercially. The following is presented to help disabled individuals and their families become acquainted with what does exist. And it may inspire the creative to invent other devices.

Problem Areas

Some of the activities that are apt to be the most frustrating are the simple, everyday acts which most of us do without particular thought but which, because they must be done regularly, cannot be ignored. Eating is necessary to sustain life, and it usually is done three times a day. To be dressed—and comfortably so— is a physical need, while to be attractively dressed is almost a psychological necessity.

Have you ever tried cutting meat with only one hand? Getting into a bathtub with stiff, painful, and paralyzed legs? Or zipping up the back of your dress, even with two good hands and arms?

Other basic problems may range from inability to hold a pencil or telephone to opening a can of food, from reaching objects on high shelves to reaching and turning on water faucets, from threading a needle to manipulating a slide rule.

The approaches and devices which are described herein are not intended to be set forth as the only answers that exist, nor will all be of equal value to all. But it is hoped that this discussion will help make your efforts more fruitful. Much time may be saved by not duplicating work already done and avoiding common pitfalls and disappointments.

Hints for the Family

It is understandable and quite normal that you should wish to *do for* the disabled member of your family, but it may be more helpful to allow him to do for himself.

To make sure that you are really being helpful, it is wise to check with the patient's physician and have him outline the patient's real capabilities and limitations. It may seem incredible that the miracles of modern medicine do not include a cure-all for all our ills. However, there are some facts that we must accept. We know that the aging process, for one, often brings with it less than 20-20 vision and joints that are not as limber and flexible as those of youth. Certain illnesses may also cause irreversible damage—some arthritis, for instance, or spinal cord injury—and activity may thenceforth be restricted or modified.

It is sometimes possible that the patient is not interested in minimizing his physical problem. There may be many reasons for such an attitude and they may or may not be changeable. Real psychological problems are best handled by a competent psychologist or psychiatrist, but the following list may serve as an illustration of various kinds of problems.

• The dependent nature of some people, which their disability tends to accentuate.

• The lack of intellectual ability or educational background.

• Plain laziness.

• The need to let others do the work after having spent a lifetime of "doing for others." (The parents who now feel that the children should take care of them.)

• The aesthetic type who may object to equipment or to certain techniques (such as use of mouthstick, wearing of splints, etc.) because they are not cosmetic or graceful in use.

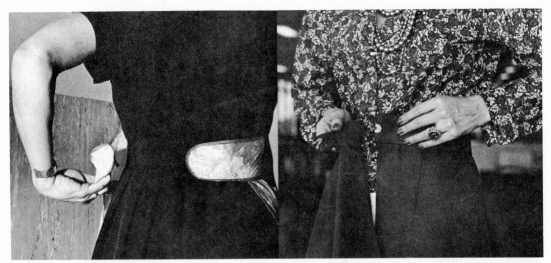

Dressing aids for handicapped women include non-tie apron (left) and easy-opening hooks in place of buttons.

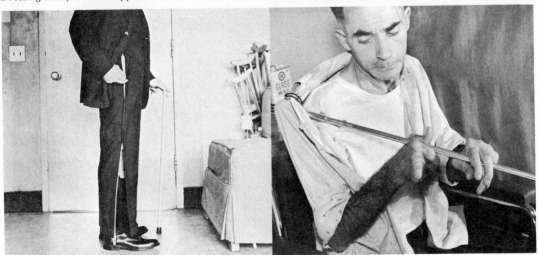

Three-piece suit has special side-seam trousers with two-way zippers. Dressing stick (right) helps in many ways.

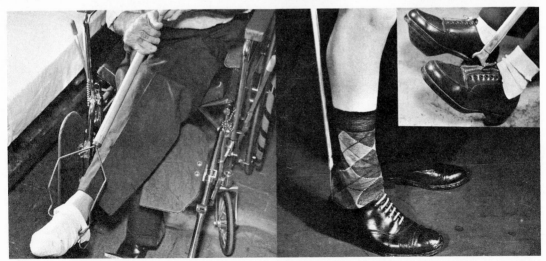

Modified dressing stick (left) used in putting on socks, even shoes. Shoe horn on stick helps with step-in shoes.

● The expectation of complete recovery, so that devices are not seen as a necessity.

Once you know what can realistically be expected of the handicapped individual, and you know that he is desirous of receiving help, then your help can prove invaluable. Even here, though, a few cardinal points of procedure may prove useful to you.

1. Offer help, but don't try to force it upon someone.

2. Find out what activity is most important to the individual and start with that—be it eating, putting on make-up, reading, or playing cards.

3. Seek the patient's ideas. If he has some, it will be more rewarding for you both to pool your efforts. Otherwise you may be only gratifying your own desires.

4. If possible, seek the guidance or consultation of a physician or therapist. There may be some techniques that they can recommend as more helpful than others.

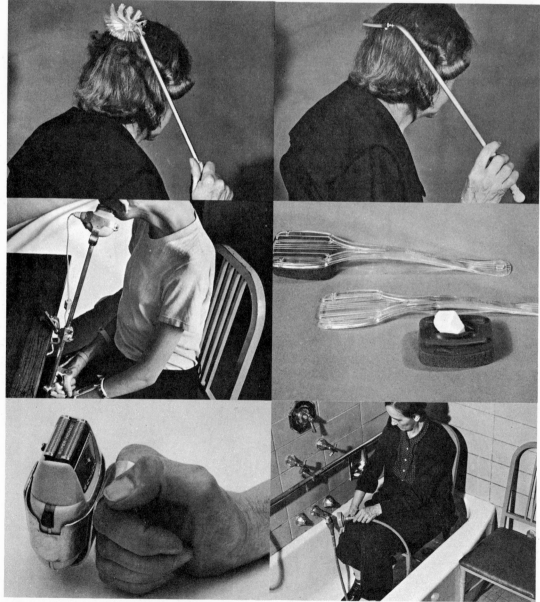

Occupational Therapy Service, N. Y. U. — Bellevue Medical Center

Personal grooming aids for the handicapped person include special, long-handled brushes, combs, and electric razors, and chair baths. Good personal appearance is especially important to the morale of the handicapped.

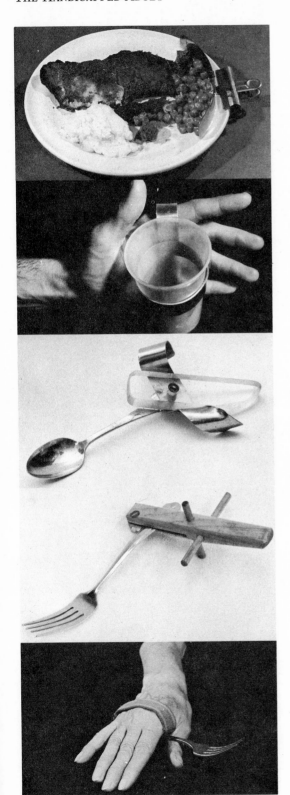

Those with hand or muscular-coordination handicaps can eat without great difficulty or fear of embarrassment with specially-designed utensils and table aids.

5. Keep an open and receptive mind to ideas of others. It is instinctive to try to "better" someone else's creation. But be sure you understand it before altering or rejecting it.

6. Keep devices simple. The "Rube Goldberg" may be an interesting conversation piece, but not necessarily a useful piece of equipment.

Hints for the Disabled

A few more hints, these for the disabled person himself, are:

• Accomplishment is more important than how it is done (except at the expense of energy or of medical danger).

• Give it your best try. A tie or a shoe lace can be tied with one hand. A glass or an electric razor can be held with two hands if your grasp is weak. Put the emphasis on what you can do.

• Don't be afraid to experiment a little and make a few mistakes. And remember that the first attempt may not be perfect. One does not learn to drive a car or play the piano or bake a cake without some practice.

• Remember that anyone forced by necessity to stay in bed for a while must learn to walk again. The athlete who does not keep in practice becomes "rusty" very quickly.

• Accept help graciously when it is offered. Just as service is the hallmark of a good restaurant, some "waiting on" is ordinary courtesy extended from one person to another.

Finding Solutions

Every activity that we perform is managed with certain kinds of motions, most of which are commonly used by all of us. Even though some of us do hold a pencil or a spoon in a slightly different manner, two things dictate the procedures. One is custom—and this may vary in different localities and countries—and the other is structure and anatomy of the human body. Each person, for example, has approximately 57 muscles with which to manipulate his one hand and arm, and these muscles perform designated movements. The devices shown in this chapter offer assistance to or a substitute for certain motions that are no longer possible.

Homemaking Hints

The disabled homemaker has been long neglected. Many of her problems can be solved by providing assistance to permit her to carry out her activities of cooking, cleaning, ironing, bed-making, and sewing.

In the kitchen, where a large portion of the homemaker's time may be spent, there are many ways to simplify tasks. Sometimes special equipment may help, but more important is the arrangement and placing of standard equipment and tools already in use.

Few non-disabled housewives would admit to being inefficient. But many—and they include the community's most respected cooks or housekeepers—accomplish their tasks through unnecessary work energy expenditure. Modern equipment has helped to make more time available for everyone, but even this is not the real secret of energy saving.

The increased production of industry is based largely on time and motion studies of the various jobs involved. Much that has been learned is applicable to the homemaker and her job. Some of the cardinal rules for her to follow are:

1. Most trips are made between sink and stove. Locate them as close together as possible to save steps.

2. The refrigerator is best located next to the sink, as items are usually used there first.

3. A work space between the refrigerator and sink and between the sink and stove reduces the carrying of utensils and may make sliding of some items possible.

4. Work heights should be convenient for you. Slightly lower than elbow level is most usable, although a lower surface is indicated for heavier tasks such as beating and chopping.

5. Tools and supplies should be stored at their place of first use (sometimes a duplicate item is helpful).

These general principles of work are worth keeping in mind and should be checked against your present method of doing things regularly. It may be difficult to accept a change, but if you are the adventurous type of person, you may find it rather stimulating as well as helpful to alter your old procedures.

While many answers to the problems of the handicapped have already been found, there are many more to be invented. And simplification and improvement of those in existence is to be anticipated, inasmuch as this is a relatively young endeavor. It is the right of every disabled person to seek independence through the use of whatever tools or devices will assist him in his efforts to make use of his inherent skills and abilities and to become a productive and useful member of society.

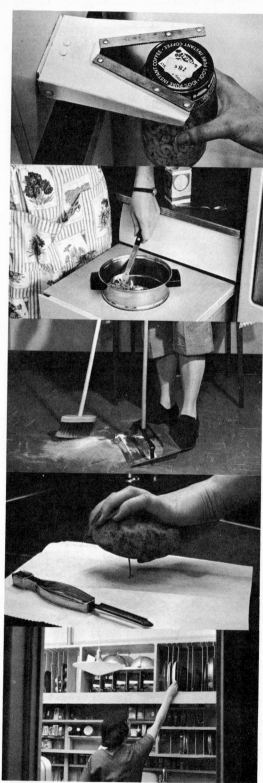

Photos on this page present special devices—from jar opener (top) to special storage area (bottom)—which allow the handicapped to do routine jobs in the kitchen.

CHAPTER TWO

BIRTH DEFECTS

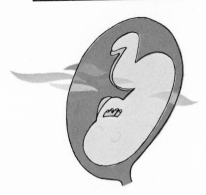

BIRTH DEFECTS constitute today's greatest unsolved childhood medical problem. More than 250,000 babies are born in the United States each year with serious birth defects. Such malformations also cause more than 30,000 deaths and stillbirths annually.

As the population increases, and as more infants are protected from childhood infections, the number of those with disabling birth defects who live to adulthood increases. A single victim who must be institutionalized yet who lives a normal life span, as many do, may cost his family or the state more than $100,000.

What do we know about preventing birth defects, a problem as old as time? Are there any specific rules to prevent such defects that we can give a pregnant woman? What do we know that we did not know before? Fortunately, recent research has been most productive, as can be seen from this progress report of March of Dimes-financed projects:

Test for galactosemia: Development of an accurate blood test helps to detect both victims and symptom-free carriers of an inherited disease called galactosemia. Galactosemia is a chemical birth defect which causes mental retardation in babies when they drink milk. This test is an important new weapon for early detection of this inherited disease.

Test for maple sugar urine disease: Development of a simple blood test helps to identify infants with a rare condition termed maple syrup urine disease, so-called because of a sugar-like odor to the urine of its victims. This inherited condition involves abnormalities in body chemistry which generally result in mental retardation and death by the age of two.

Homograft barrier: Apparent cracking of the "homograft barrier" is a notable achievement in efforts to make adult animals permanently tolerant to organ transplants and skin grafts, which may open the way to solving the

problem in man. Success in this area may make it possible to repair many birth defects by transplants.

Clues to how cells specialize: Evidence has been found, in experiments with combination "chicken-duck eyes," that chemical messengers between living cells instruct cells of one kind to change their specific job. Some birth defects may be caused by errors, occurring during pregnancy, in this messenger system.

New kind of gene discovered: Studies of inner workings of cells reveal a new kind of gene (unit of heredity) which controls the assembling of living protein matter into its proper structure. This gives us useful clues as to how birth defects come about.

Viruses and birth defects: Tentative identification has been made of several viruses as causing birth defects when mothers-to-be are infected during pregnancy. Preliminary and inconclusive figures from a four-year study indict ECHO 9 virus, three Coxsackie type viruses, and influenza virus, the latter in connection with miscarriages only.

Synthesis of biologically active DNA: For the first time the master code-of-life chemical DNA (deoxyribonucleic acid) has been synthesized in the laboratory in a form that is biologically active. This is as close as anyone has come to creating life in the test tube.

New clue to birth defect cause: New leads point to causes of certain birth defects produced in studies of fluid inbalance in chick embryos. Several factors, such as too little oxygen, too much salt, and foreign substances, resulted in salt imbalance in the blood, followed by excess accumulation of body fluids and the development of major defects and often death of the chick.

Outbreaks of spinal birth defects: Three reports have appeared of unusual outbreaks of a serious birth defect involving the spine. An in-

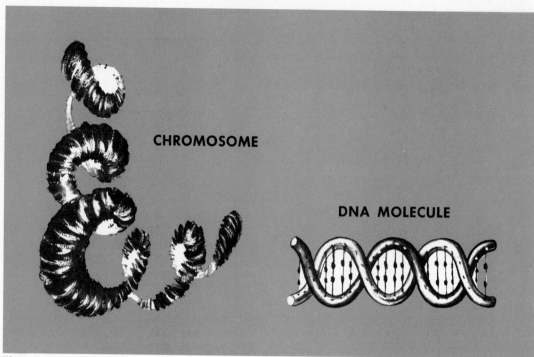

CHROMOSOME

DNA MOLECULE

These diagrams of the DNA molecule and chromosome were developed from research in cellular composition.

creased number of referral centers for birth defect patients and vastly increased concern about the problem are considered responsible for spotting these "epidemics." However, the outbreaks remain unexplained.

Arthritis clues in twin study: Strong evidence which indicates that emotional stress can bring on rheumatoid arthritis was produced in a study of five sets of identical twins in which only one of each pair was found to have the disease. Significant data minimized the influence of inherited factors and pointed to the role of upsetting experiences in development of this puzzling and crippling disease.

To this record of achievement should be added the test for PKU—or phenylketonuria —a defect in the body chemistry that prevents the body's assimilation of an amino acid found in most protein foods. This defect eventually causes mental retardation. By a newly developed blood test for the disease, involving only one drop of blood from a newborn baby's heel, PKU babies can be diagnosed before they leave the hospital, and a protective diet designed to prevent mental retardation can be prescribed for the babies. Thus it is now entirely possible that a child with PKU can grow up as healthy and as mentally alert as any child.

As you can see from this partial list, we do know more than we ever knew before about birth defects and their prevention. While there still is much we don't know, we can nonetheless give a pregnant woman some rules to follow. Ever since 1958, when the National Foundation-March of Dimes turned its attention from polio to birth defects, the development of a child within its mother has been a subject for special study.

Advice to Pregnant Women

At the Second International Conference on Congenital Malformations sponsored by The National Foundation in 1963, one of the most interesting speakers was Dr. Widukind Lenz, a West German geneticist on the staff of Hamburg University. Dr. Lenz published the first article connecting the serious outbreak of birth defects to the sedative, thalidomide.

According to Dr. Lenz, "Formerly, many human biologists, taking a normal uterine environment for granted, used to attribute almost every malformation to heredity."

There is, he said, a need for a change in this type of thinking, because "the chemical environment of man has greatly changed in recent decades due to the introduction of many chemicals. Some of these have been devised with the special purpose to block chemical reactions in man, animals, plants, or unicellular organisms."

This new medical trend warrants this advice to a pregnant woman: At present, any woman who is in the first few months of pregnancy, or is uncertain as to whether or not she is pregnant, should not use a drug unless it is necessary to save a life. Take a drug for a headache? Better not. Why? Because, according to Dr. Lenz, "almost nothing is known of the role of chemicals in the production of human malformations."

This then, would be the first rule for a pregnant woman: Do not take any medication at all—no matter whether you got it with a prescription or without a prescription—unless it is specifically prescribed to you by your doctor *for use at this time*. Never, during a pregnancy, take pills which your doctor gave you before you became pregnant. Never take pills prescribed for anyone else. At least one thalidomide tragedy in the United States occurred when the woman took pills prescribed for her husband, and not intended for her.

Here are other rules for a woman about to become a mother:

● See your doctor—or a prenatal clinic—as soon as you think you are pregnant. Only recently, we have found that the first few months of pregnancy are most important, and that good care at this time is vital for the baby.

● Cut down on your smoking and follow the diet your doctor prescribes. Don't take extra vitamin pills or other vitamin supplements without checking with your doctor.

● Know your Rh factor blood type, and your husband's. Tell your doctor.

● Inform any other doctor whom you have reason to see that you are pregnant, or that you think you are pregnant. This information is vital in the case of x-rays or fluoroscopy, which, during the early months of pregnancy, might harm the unborn child. If these procedures can be postponed until after the first three months of pregnancy, your doctor will certainly do so.

● Never knowingly expose yourself to German measles or to any other infectious disease when pregnant.

CHAPTER THREE

UNDERSTANDING PARENTS' FEELINGS

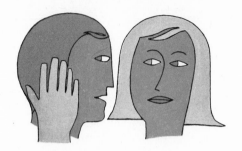

THE OBSERVATION that handicapped children generally make handicapped families is almost a cliche today. More and more parents are seeking help for their own problems. Professional workers with handicapped children are recognizing that attention must be given not only to the child, but also to the child as a part of a family. There is much evidence that parental reactions to the handicapped child's condition often result in the development of psychological problems. These must be given attention if the family unit is to be fully rehabilitated.

These problems of psychological adjustment have their beginnings in very common attitudes and feelings. Since the birth of a child is anticipated for several months, the parents, during this time, usually look forward eagerly to its arrival and have bright dreams of its future. It never occurs to many parents that their child will be anything but perfect.

Others, while aware of the possibilities of having a handicapped child, hope and pray that this will not happen to them. Few parents are prepared to have a handicapped child; many parents report being shocked and confused upon learning of their child's condition.

Professional workers have observed that the most painful period in the lives of parents of handicapped children is the period between the moment they learn that their child has a handicap and the time when they learn what they can do about it. Confusion follows naturally from a lack of information about the child's problem and the absence of a positive treatment program. If not redirected, these feelings of confusion sometimes lead to the parents' feeling defeated and frustrated.

We should not consider it abnormal, therefore, for parents who have been expecting or hoping for a "perfect" child to feel deeply disappointed upon learning that their child is handicapped. A mother of a cerebral palsied daughter expressed this feeling when she said,

"Ann will never be able to wear the pretty clothes I wanted to make for her." A father did so when he said, "I just can't do any boasting about my boy." Sometimes these feelings of disappointment are so deep that the parents fail to develop warm, loving feelings toward their child. Without understanding why, or perhaps without being aware of their feelings, disappointed parents may find it increasingly difficult to play with their handicapped child, to take him visiting, or in other ways show the affection which children need in order to feel wanted and accepted.

Deep concern about the handicapped child's welfare is also an early parental reaction. Not only do parents worry about their child's physical pains, but they worry about his future social and economic adjustments. Our culture places a premium on such skills as walking, talking, and writing. Even the simplest social relations require the participants to move about and talk. The parents of a child whose handicap might interfere with the development of these skills have reason to be concerned about their child's social future. In our culture, parents always hope that their children will "do better than Dad and Mom."

It is very natural for them to ask such questions as, "Will my child be able to take care of himself? If not, who will take care of him after we're gone?" Anxieties develop when parents are not helped to find answers to these questions. If not properly directed, these sometimes result in too much concern and protection of the child. This robs the child of any chance to develop independence.

Embarrassment is one of the most common emotional problems of parents of the handicapped. Many have reported being embarrassed, and often angered, by their friends' expressions of sympathy or pity, or the way people look at their handicapped child. Unless the causes of such feelings are recognized, they may lead to hostility toward other people including those who are trying to help the child. Often, during early conferences, the physician will find parents displaying hostile feelings which have grown from such small beginnings.

Guilt Feelings

Parents often report that they feel they are to blame for what has happened to their child. One of the major causes of such guilt feelings is the lack of accurate information about the nature of the child's condition and its causes. In the absence of reliable information, parents often feel that the handicapped child is their punishment for having committed some sin.

Guilt feelings sometimes arise, too, from the parents' feeling that they have not done enough for the child or have not done the right thing. This attitude was illustrated by a mother when she said, "I'm a poor mother. John would probably be able to walk today if only I'd taken him to a doctor sooner." A father kept blaming himself repeating, "I just can't understand now why we kept thinking everything was going to be all right. We should have started his treatment three years ago."

These attitudes often lead the parents to be overaffectionate to their children. They cannot be firm with the handicapped child and they try to protect him from experiences which might be painful or difficult. As a result, their children often fail to make the physical and social development of which they are capable.

There is another natural outgrowth of guilt feelings which it would be helpful for parents to recognize. Just as our bodies try to develop defenses against diseases, our personalities attempt to develop protective mechanisms to keep us from being hurt emotionally. It is not unusual, then, for parents who feel that they are in some way to blame for their child's condition to become very defensive. Therapists and counselors often find it difficult to break through these defenses to provide the family with the kind of help which is most needed.

Another reaction which sometimes results from a lack of information about the child's difficulty is that one parent becomes suspicious of the other. Being unable to recognize anything in his life for which punishment has been meted out, the parent assumes that the mate is at fault. One mother confided, "I guess I just didn't know my husband well enough before we were married. His past sounds all right, but how can I be sure?" Sometimes a parent assumes that the child's condition is hereditary and, finding no history of abnormality in his family, feels sure that there is a skeleton in the closet of the other's family. In our natural desire to protect ourselves it is easy to permit such wonderings and suspicions to grow until they affect all family relations.

Family problems often develop because the handicapped child makes unusual demands on finances, time, and energy. Mothers, for example, often become hostile toward fathers because they do not do their share in caring for the child. Fathers become hostile because the mothers devote most of their time and energies to caring for the child and then have little time or energy left for normal family activities. As one father complained, "She just doesn't seem to think of me any more. Doesn't she realize that I still need some affection and attention?" His wife had earlier remarked, "I'm completely worn out after I get the children to bed. If John would only help more it would be so much easier."

The expenses of medical care, therapy, and the other special attentions which handicapped children need may strain family finances. Financial worries make a fertile ground for the growth of tensions which further aggravate family problems. Though these feelings start from very simple beginnings they can come to pervade all relations between a husband and wife.

These are not, of course, all the problems which might develop in a family where there is a handicapped child. Like those described, though, other problems will have simple beginnings in the natural feelings and reactions of parents and, unless understood, they may become so complex as to affect the behavior and adjustment of every member of the family. Many families are finding the following program helpful in working out their problems:

1. Become informed about the child and his problems. Parents should recognize that shopping around from one specialist to another can be only an ineffective approach to their problems. Instead of looking for someone to perform a miracle or to tell them the optimistic things they naturally want to hear, they should have a detailed study made of their child under the guidance of one specialist. He can coordinate the work of other specialists and then put all their findings together for a better understanding of the child's problems. Included in this study should be a thorough medical and psychological evaluation.

The results of this study should be discussed

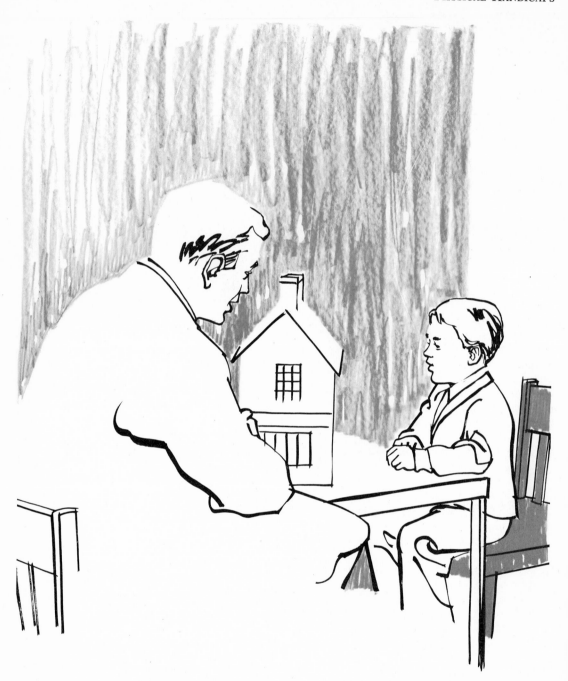

with the parents by a qualified professional worker so that they will understand the present nature of the child's condition, what might have caused it, and the child's potentialities and limitations. It is not necessary for parents to understand all the details of the medical findings. It is important, however, for them to have misconceptions cleared up and to learn enough to enable them to carry out their role as parents effectively.

The parents should become familiar with the patterns of growth and development in children. Unfortunately, parents do not always take the proper approach to this subject. While they expect to have to learn to drive a car or to sew, they do not usually realize that they must also learn how to direct the growth and development of their children. Consequently, parents who recognize that their young child is physically not mature enough to carry a sack of potatoes and would not expect such a feat from him, become disturbed because he can't play without fighting or doesn't know the difference between "right and wrong." Learning that emotional and intellectual development—like physical development—follow certain patterns, will not only make child rearing a more pleasant experience but will also prevent the development of many psychological problems in both the child and the parents.

Because parents have not had an opportunity to observe the development of a large number of children from infancy to maturity, they have no basis of comparison with which to judge the behavior of children. They very naturally tend, therefore, to react to each emotional outburst or each breaking of the rules or each violation as an isolated bit of behavior. Parents have spoken disparagingly about books dealing with child psychology because these books have not given specific answers on how to handle these disturbing episodes. If a father and mother will take the time to read and discuss a good book on child growth and development, they will gain the perspective that is necessary to interpret these episodes as part of an unfolding pattern. With this knowledge, much of the previously disturbing behavior will no longer seem so alarming, and more effective techniques can be worked out to manage those episodes which really require attention.

Parents should also become familiar with the broader aspects of their child's problem. Knowing something about the number of other children in the country who are similarly handicapped and about the facilities available for their care and treatment will help parents see their problems in a better light. Many parents have reported feeling better able to carry on when they realize that they are not alone, that many other parents face the same difficulties. The awareness that specialists have been studying these problems and have accumulated knowledge and skills which can be applied to the treatment of handicapped children is in itself encouraging.

2. Develop a positive action program. Probably nothing is more effective in helping parents adjust than the feeling that they are doing things which will help their child develop and improve his welfare. The first action step should be to see that the child receives all the medical attention which has been advised by the specialist who is coordinating their program. Second, parents should make those arrangements which are necessary to obtain the special therapies which have been recommended. Next, through conferences with the therapists, determine exactly what part home training should play in the child's program and carry this out conscientiously. Finally, identify with the cause.

This does not mean that parents should become missionaries or gadflies to prod their communities into action. Rather they should join organizations which have competent professional advisors and should contribute both time and money to worthwhile programs for handicapped children.

3. Talk out all problems. When problems are kept bottled-up they often grow more serious. Talking about them will not only make them seem less important, but may also lead to solutions. Several types of discussions are important. First, husbands and wives should realize that only by their mutual understanding and cooperation can the handicapped child be best helped. Together they should become informed and together they should plan and carry out the positive action program. Against this background of information and action they should discuss all problems as they develop.

Second, opportunities should be sought to discuss problems with other parents. Parent counseling groups in which parents meet to work out their problems with the help of understanding professional workers have proved very effective. Many parents are helped just by talking with another parent of a handicapped child.

Third, parents should not hesitate to consult a professional worker who specializes in dealing with emotional problems if some disturbing feelings or attitudes persist after these discussions.

Psychological terms, such as "anxiety" or "rejection," sometimes make parents feel afraid or ashamed and they are reluctant to discuss their feelings with anyone because they are afraid of being stigmatized. As has been described, these feelings have very natural beginnings. It is only when they are not understood and properly directed that these natural reactions develop into more serious adjustment problems. Talking with other parents or professional workers is one of the first steps in learning to understand these feelings and to direct them into wholesome channels.

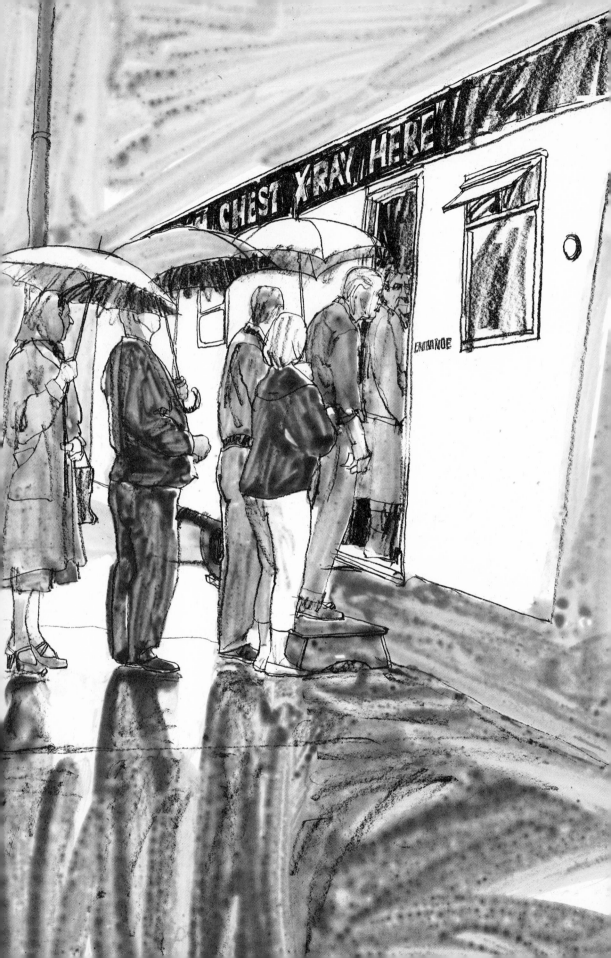

PART XIV

Community
Health

CHAPTER ONE

COMMUNITY HEALTH RESOURCES

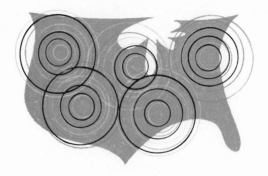

HEALTH IS ESSENTIALLY a matter of personal responsibility and most health problems can be solved by the individual person under the guidance of his family physician.

There are, however, some health problems, or problems in which health and medicine play a significant role, that people cannot ordinarily solve by themselves. These are health problems which may demand long-term or exceptionally expensive or complex care, or which require highly skilled personnel and elaborate facilities not available in the average community. Or they may be problems dealing with health conditions in a person's neighborhood, such as water supply, waste disposal, air pollution, or the sanitation of milk and food supplies.

When faced with such problems, each person must supplement his own resources by calling upon his community for assistance. Even the most rugged individualist should not try to "go it alone" when he comes up against a problem which he can not reasonably be expected to solve with his own resources. That's what the community's health and social service agencies are for—to help in time of need.

While communities vary in the number and type of their health and social service agencies, every community has, or should have, certain basic public health services to support and protect the health and well-being of its citizens.

Approximately 2,500 of the 3,073 counties in the nation are served by a health department, or other type of health unit. Of these, over 900 counties have a county health unit of their own and more are being developed all the time. In addition, there are more than 300 city health departments, and each state in the union has a state health department which stands ready, within the limits of its facilities, to be of assistance to its state's citizens. Similarly, while

every area may not have a full complement of voluntary health organizations or social service agencies, the services such agencies perform can usually be obtained from district, regional, or state organizations.

With the aid of his physician or by calling upon the appropriate state agency for the name and address of the nearest local organization concerned with his problem, the person who lives in a small community or even a rural area can find help when he needs it.

This chapter discusses a number of problems which most often require the assistance of some community health or social service agency for solution. The list is by no means complete, but it includes those problems which experience suggests are either common or likely to cause the individual the greatest difficulty. Where reference is made to a particular agency not present in the community, it is suggested that contact be made with a district, regional, or state unit for assistance. For ease of reference, the topics are listed alphabetically.

Air Pollution

The contamination of the air about us has been of increasing concern in recent years. As a nation, we have become even more urbanized, increasingly mechanized and industrialized, and our industrial processes have become exceedingly complex. The result has been a mounting stream of pollutants released into the atmosphere. Home heating plants, apartment house incinerators, burning fallen leaves, smoldering garbage dumps, burning car bodies, exhaust fumes, and many other urban sources of smoke and fumes add to the pollution from factory chimneys.

Increasing concern with the problems of air

pollution has resulted in more and more communities enacting air pollution control ordinances. These give the local health department or other agency the authority to control air pollution. These local agencies are backed by a number of state air pollution control agencies and by the U.S. Public Health Service.

Every citizen can aid in the work of control agencies by reporting promptly any instances of air pollution that come to his attention and by insisting that the plans for any new industries, large buildings, incinerators, or other potential air polluters be checked by qualified engineers to eliminate or minimize the risk of pollution. If the community or state lacks adequate laws against air pollution, each citizen can make his voice heard through community action programs insisting that such laws be adopted and enforced.

Alcoholism

There is increasing recognition that the alcoholic is a sick person in need of help. Unfortunately there are still far too few facilities to which the alcoholic or his family may turn. However, some communities, and their number is growing, have recognized the need to help this unfortunate group.

Hospitalization is often needed for the alcoholic in the acute stage of this disease and the patient's family physician should be consulted. After the acute stage is over and the alcoholic is "dried out," he must learn to live in a world free of the alcohol which he can not handle. Community clinics or other facilities may provide the help needed for this rehabilitation. The local chapter of Alcoholics Anonymous has much to offer many alcoholics. A clergyman's counsel may be of aid. The sympathetic understanding and support of the family physician has been of help to many alcoholics. A skilled social worker from one of the local social agencies may help by counseling on home or financial problems.

To find out what help is available in the community, consult your family physician or minister or check with the local health department, mental health agency, Community Chest, or Council of Social Agencies. (See also Part XII, Chapter Four.)

Blindness

While nothing can, of course, ever completely replace the blessing that is sight, much can be done to help the blind or the partially-seeing to become self-supporting and to enjoy life. The federal government, every state, and many local communities provide various types of assistance for the blind. These range from vocational training to enable the visually handicapped to earn a livelihood to "talking books" from the Library of Congress. The latter permit the blind to enjoy good literature and to be kept up-to-date on contemporary happenings through the recording of books and current magazines.

The family physician or the eye specialist can usually put the blind person or his family in touch with the proper community or state agency. There are also voluntary agencies for the blind in many communities. These can be located through the local Council of Social Agencies or the Community Chest. The local welfare department, the local health department, or a local family service agency are also sources of information and assistance. In rural areas, inquiries may be addressed to the State Commission for the Blind or the State Health Department for information and advice. (See also Part IV, Chapter Seven.)

Cancer

Any person who feels that he has one of the "Seven Cancer Danger Signals" (See Part X, Chapter Eight) should go promptly to a physician. Often the problem will turn out not to be cancer. However, if it should prove to be cancer, and involved treatment ensues, many community services are available to aid the cancer patient. Some of these, such as "loan closets," are operated by local chapters of the American Cancer Society.

The loan closet provides on a loan basis, without cost or at most a small fee, such items as wheel chairs, hospital-type beds, commodes, bed-pans, and other sick-room equipment. Many loan closets also make available pads and other types of dressings. Local health departments or visiting nurse associations can provide home nursing service. In some communities "homemaker" or part-time housekeeper services are available to keep the home going during the illness of the wife or mother. Where this is not advisable, the possibility of convalescent-home or nursing-home care may be explored.

For information about these or other services that may be available, call the local chapter of the American Cancer Society, the local health department, or the local Council of Social Agencies. The family physician is usually familiar with the community's resources and can often help guide the patient or his family to the proper local agency. (See also Part X, Chapter Eight.)

Drug Addiction

Addiction to a drug is not in itself a disease. Rather it is a symptom of an underlying emotional problem. There are a considerable number of drugs to which susceptible persons may become addicted. However, in this country the most common are the barbiturates, the amphetamines, and the narcotic group of drugs of which heroin is the most addictive. It is the latter drug which is chiefly involved in the addiction problem in our large cities. The treatment of drug addiction, particularly heroin addiction, is difficult because of the patient's tendency to relapse and return to using the drug. This does not mean that the addict should be denied treatment. On the contrary, when addiction is suspected, prompt medical attention should be secured.

The first step involves the withdrawal of the drug in an environment such as a hospital, where conditions ensuring a drug-free environment can be provided. Following withdrawal, a program of rehabilitation is necessary to help the addict learn to adjust to life without the drug upon which he has come to depend.

The first step when addiction is suspected is to consult the family physician. He may institute treatment or refer the addict to one of the specialized facilities maintained by the U.S. Public Health Service, or to one of the narcotic treatment facilities operated by the state or local government. Private sanatoria also offer treatment for drug addiction. (See also Part XII, Chapter Five.)

Handicapped Children

No effort is more deserving of universal support than that directed toward rehabilitating the handicapped child. The effort is supported wholeheartedly with research scientists, the medical profession, social agencies, and government all joining together. Their common goal is a simple one: to ensure that no American child is denied the benefits of modern rehabilitation techniques because of race, creed, color, or the ability of his parents to pay for the needed care.

The effectiveness of this united effort has been matched by the scientific advances which have continually pushed back the limits of what can be accomplished. Open-heart surgery, the

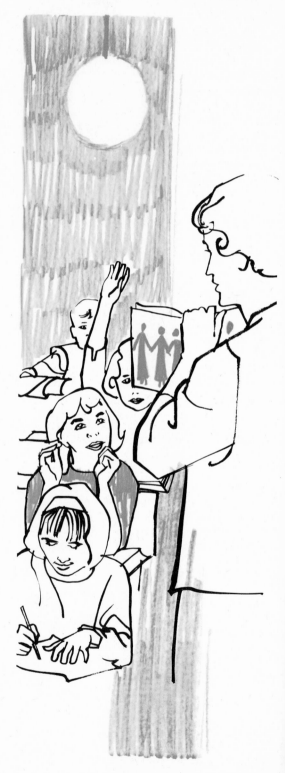

skilled use of antibiotics and other new drugs, the phenomenal growth and development of the specialty of "physical" medicine, and many other advances have all made possible the restoration of countless children to useful, productive lives.

So that children may derive the maximum benefit from all that modern medical science has to offer, parents are urged to seek medical attention promptly for any observed defect or suspicion of abnormality. The physician can then advise remedial procedures should such be necessary. If financing the cost of the needed care will pose problems, parents should check with the local health department, the local welfare department, the local Council of Social Agencies, the State Health Department, or the State Commission or Board for Crippled Children where such an agency exists. No child need go without care because his parents are financially unable to pay. (See also Part XIII, Chapters Two and Three.)

Health Education

Do you want a pamphlet on sex education or one on hay fever or a booklet on baby care or information about septic tanks, or an exhibit on health for the county fair, or a health film or a speaker on a health subject for your club or church group? All of these and other health education services and materials are available simply for the asking, or at most, for a nominal charge. Where do you go to get them? The sources are many and include the local (county, city, and district) health department or local chapter of the voluntary health organization with an interest in the particular topic; the county medical society; the state health department; the American Medical Association; the U.S. Public Health Service; and the national headquarters of the national voluntary health organization in the particular field, e.g. the American Cancer Society, National Foundation, National Tuberculosis Association, etc.

Health education was never more important than it is today when everyone needs the knowledge that will enable him to take prompt advantage of the many protective health measures being developed through medical research. (See also Part XV, Chapter Two.)

Mental Illness

In recent years there has been an increasing awareness of the problem of mental illness, a problem which affects some 17,000,000 Americans to some degree. There has also been an increasing public acceptance of mental illness as another form of sickness and not a subject for shame and rejection. While this acceptance has by no means reached the point to be desired, it has brought about growing public concern about the nature of the facilities for the treatment of the mentally ill.

This concern has been hastened by the almost revolutionary advances in the treatment of mental illness brought about by new drugs and techniques. The previous picture of mental illness as a hopeless oblivion from which there could be no return has been altered by the thousands of mentally ill who have been treated and returned to their families and to useful, rewarding lives.

The revolution in treatment is by no means over. For example, there is growing support for the concept that many forms of mental illness are best treated in specialized facilities of general hospitals right in the patient's home town and that such treatment may be more desirable in some cases than that provided in some distant hospital, good though it may be. Along with advances in treatment, have come efforts to modernize laws pertaining to the handling of the mentally ill, some of which are as out of date as the chains used in Bedlam. While much remains to be done, it is already easier in most states for the mentally ill to undergo voluntary treatment without complicated legal entanglements, but with adequate safeguards for the patient's civil rights.

When faced with a problem of mental illness, the first step is to seek the advice and counsel of the family physician. He can arrange for psychiatric consultation when needed, and for institutional treatment if indicated. He can also advise regarding local laws or regulations in an emergency situation where an acutely ill person may be dangerous to himself or others. (See also Part V.)

Nursing Care

A new baby in the home, an elderly family member with a chronic illness, the presence of someone in the home with tuberculosis, a child with a contagious disease, an expectant mother . . .all of these have one thing in common. They represent occasions when a public health nurse is likely to visit a home in many communities. The list is by no means complete, but it does give an idea of the valuable service

rendered by public health nurses (or the Visiting Nurses Association in some communities).

Most often it is the physician who asks the
nurse to call in order to teach the new mother
how to care for the baby, how to give the grandmother a bed-bath or an insulin injection, to
give some needed treatment to a member of the
family, or to aid in countless other ways. Unless their conditions demand the specialized
skills of the hospital, most people are better off
at home when they are sick. They are happier,
they often do better medically, and it is less of
a strain on family finances, particularly when
the illness lasts a long time.

The services of a public health (or visiting)
nurse can be obtained through the family physician or a call may be made directly to
the local health department or local visiting
nurse association. Services are provided without charge or at a nominal cost. Public health
nursing service should be available in every
community. If your community lacks it, join
with your neighbors in urging that it be established. (See also Part VIII, Chapter Two.)

Poison Control

The home safety section of this guide (Part
VII) contains information regarding precautions against poisoning from substances in the
home. However, there are times when the physician who has been called in a case of poisoning, or the parents or whoever may be on the
scene in an emergency when no physician is
available, need information quickly about the
possible toxic effects of a particular household
product.

To meet this need, a nationwide network of
poison control centers has been established.
These centers, supported by state and local
health departments and by the U.S. Public
Health Service with the cooperation of other
local agencies, are manned 24 hours a day and
stand ready at all times to provide information
and advice. The centers, with the cooperation
of manufacturers, maintain up-to-date information regarding the contents of thousands
of household products from cleansers to insecticides, and can provide on a moment's notice
this information together with an estimate of
the poisoning hazard presented by a particular
product or substance. Your physician will know
the location of the nearest poison control center. However, in the absence of a physician,
check with the local health department or drug-
gist for the name of the local center. In most

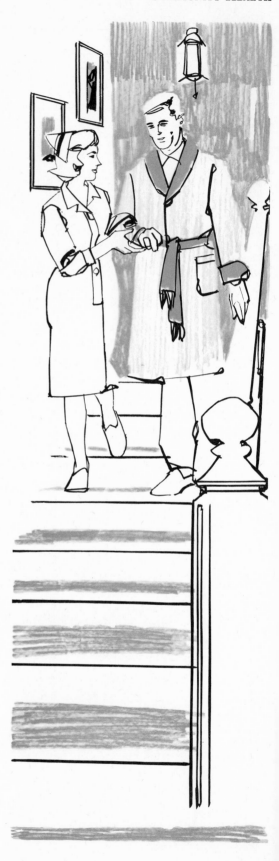

instances these are located in the local hospital. (See also Part IX, Chapter Two.)

Pre-Marital Examinations

Many states now have some requirement regarding pre-marital examination of the groom or both the bride and groom. In some instances all that is required is a blood test for syphilis, while other states have various requirements including, for example, a physical examination by a physician.

In many areas there is a mandatory delay between the issuance of the license and the performance of the marriage ceremony. Such requirements are intended to be a protection to those to be married and they usually pose no problems when the principals are being married in their home community and both are available for an examination by a local physician familiar with the state's regulations. This is not always the case, however, and there are many instances when one of the "intended" is away in the Armed Forces, at college, or at work in a distant place. Problems also arise when the wedding is to take place in another state. Then complications can and do sometimes arise.

A call to the local health department, or a call or a letter to the Bureau of Vital Statistics at the State Health Department will bring information regarding the specific requirements of the state in which the wedding ceremony is to be performed. This will include information on procedures when the principals will not be available for examination locally—what the state's requirements are regarding physicians' certificates and the qualifications of laboratories acceptable for the blood test, and other details.

Rabies

The bite of a dog, cat, or other animal is not only a painful experience, but it also carries with it the risk of rabies, a uniformly fatal disease. Because of this, most communities have some type of local ordinance requiring that bites of dogs or other animals be promptly reported to the health department or other appropriate local agency. Regulations regarding such bites usually require that where possible the dog or other animal be confined and observed by a veterinarian for a period of 10 days. The animal should not be killed if at all possible. Vaccinations should be begun at once if circumstances suggest the likelihood of rabies

in the animal, or if the animal cannot be found for observation.

The basis for such regulations lies in the fact that rabies is a fatal disease in domestic animals. Thus, if the animal survives the 10-day period with no suspicious symptoms, the bite victim can be assured that there is no risk of rabies. If the dog or other animal develops symptoms of rabies, prompt action must be taken in providing the "Pasteur treatment" or vaccination against the disease. Vaccine is usually available from the health department for administration by the family physician (one injection a day for 14 days, or 21 days in severe or multiple bites).

Rabies is a fatal disease, and protection lies solely in prevention. A difficult problem is presented by the bites of stray or wild animals (including bats and foxes) where it is not possible to capture and confine the animal. A decision as to whether to administer the vaccine must be made by the physician, usually after consultation with the health department. This office keeps up to date as to whether rabies has been found recently in dogs or other animals in the area. Since there is also the risk of other types of infection from all animal bites, a physician should be consulted promptly in all cases of animal bites so that he may provide whatever immediate treatment is necessary.

Retarded Children

The family of the mentally retarded child must face many questions for which unfortunately there are no easy answers. First comes the hardest of all, "Is little Johnny or little Mary really different from other children?" Acceptance of the answer if it is "yes" is not easy. Once there is acceptance and the realization that the little one is an "exceptional child," the question arises of what is best for the retarded child and the entire family, including the other children.

In the past, many parents were advised that institutional care provided the best answer. Recently, however, has come the realization that for many of these children and their families it is better for the child to remain in the home, with the community providing support in the way of special classes and vocational training. The decision in each case depends upon many factors, such as home conditions, the family's financial and other resources, the attitude of the parents and other children, the availability of special classes or other educational facilities in the community, and, of course, the condition of the child. The problems of home care are made much more difficult when the retardation is extreme or when the child has another physical defect requiring continual medical or skilled nursing care.

The advice of the family physician should be sought. He in turn may wish to consult with appropriate specialists before making a recommendation to the parents. Local social agencies, such as one of the family service agencies or the local welfare department, may be helpful if there are financial or other special problems. The local health department may also provide public health nursing service in teaching those in the family the techniques of caring for the child. Parents of retarded children may also find support through joining with others in local chapters of the National Society for the Aid of Retarded Children. Such groups have accomplished much in persuading communities to provide educational and other services for the mentally retarded. (See also Part XIII.)

Sewage Disposal

The best way to dispose of sewage from the home is by connection to a municipal sewer system that provides safe and adequate treatment of the community's sewage.

In rural areas and in many rapidly growing suburban areas where sewer systems have not kept pace with the population growth, the only practical approach is that of a home sewage treatment plant such as a cesspool or septic tank, the latter usually being more satisfactory. A well-designed septic tank—one of adequate size with a properly laid tile drainage field of sufficient length—can provide satisfactory sewage disposal for many years. It is most important, however, to be certain of the suitability of soil conditions—heavy clay soils will usually not absorb the liquid flow from the septic tank—and of the design and installation of the tank and tile pipes which carry off the liquid portion of the sewage to be absorbed underground by the soil.

Any prospective homeowner planning to build or buy a home equipped with a septic tank should check with the local health department to see whether soil conditions make a septic tank feasible in the area. He should also get the department's recommendations regarding size of the tank, length of the tile field, and suggestions concerning installation. In many areas, approval of the health department is re-

quired before land can be subdivided and department inspectors must certify the adequacy of the septic tank installation before an occupancy permit can be issued for the house. Zoning regulations should also be checked.

If you are purchasing a new home in an area which can be expected to have sewers in the not too distant future, you will save a great deal of money and later inconvenience if the developer lays the necessary sewer pipes in the street before it is paved and the builder lays service pipes in the yard before the lawn is planted and also "stubs in" piping connections within the house. In this way, extensive alterations will not be necessary to connect to the sewer when service becomes available.

Tuberculosis

The decline in the death rate from tuberculosis (Part X, Chapter Nine), a 64 per cent drop between 1952 and 1961, is most dramatic. While the 37 per cent decline in reported active cases of the disease during the same period is not so great, the two figures together do reflect the tremendous strides that have been made in the fight against tuberculosis. These advances have been satisfying but they by no means suggest that tuberculosis has been conquered. Thousands of cases still occur every year and for each of them the disease is still a problem. With the changes in the prevalence of the disease, there have also been changes in the nature of the group most affected.

Whereas tuberculosis once most frequently attacked the young adult, it is now found in an increasing proportion among the elderly, particularly in older men. This means that community efforts to locate persons with the disease must be directed toward older persons, those in occupation groups involving dusty atmospheres, and toward certain other groups such as jail populations and "Skid Row" tenants where a higher incidence of the disease may be expected. While these groups are more likely to have tuberculosis, the disease can affect anyone, and a chronic cough or other symptom should be the signal for getting a chest x-ray. Fortunately, in a high percentage of cases the disease yields to careful treatment employing new drugs and techniques.

It is generally agreed that most tuberculosis patients benefit from a several-month stay in a hospital especially devoted to the treatment of the disease. After the initial period of hospitalization, the treatment can usually be carried out safely on an outpatient basis. Of importance is the checking for tuberculosis among the members of the patient's family and all of his contacts. The local health department will assist the physician in tracing all of the contacts and notifying them of the need to be examined.

Unwed Mothers

The plight of the unmarried expectant mother demands the full support of health and welfare services so that she may be helped through the trying period of her pregnancy and aided in the adjustment that must come after the birth of her baby. Equally important, her baby must be assured the care that will provide it with a start in life with the minimum of handicaps. The unmarried pregnant girl and her family need the assistance that social agencies can provide and these services should be made available as early in pregnancy as possible.

The agencies can help solve such problems as medical care during pregnancy, a proper place for the birth of the baby, financial support particularly during the latter part of pregnancy, and the placement or care of the baby. Since many people are not directly familiar with the services of social agencies, or lack the knowledge of what particular agency to contact, the first step is for the expectant mother or her family to ask the family physician or priest, minister, or rabbi for advice or counsel.

In larger communities a direct approach may be made to a family service agency, to the local welfare department, or to the local Council of Social Agencies for information or referral to the proper community agency. The important point is for the unwed expectant mother, beset by countless anxieties, to know that there are skilled, kind, and helpful people who are ready to help her and that she should seek their aid promptly without fear of embarrassment.

Venereal Disease

At any suspicion of a venereal infection, a physician should be consulted promptly. This will ensure that the person will be given the necessary tests and receive such treatment as is needed. It will not in itself, however, ensure that the chain of infection which led to the particular victim of the disease will be broken. This will require cooperation with the physician and with the health department to whom he will often turn for assistance.

Venereal diseases are usually contracted through sexual contact with infected individuals, rarely in other ways. Infected individuals may be completely unaware of their infection and may, unless treated, pass their disease on to others who in turn may infect still others. Every person who contracts a venereal disease has an obligation to cooperate fully in the important task of breaking the chain of infection along which venereal diseases spread. This means providing the physician, or the representative of the health department who may assist him, with the names of *all* sexual contacts. The health department, without revealing the source of the information, will contact the individuals named and see that they are referred for tests and for treatment if they are found to be infected. No false sense of modesty or foolish fear of causing trouble for others should prevent anyone from cooperating fully with the physician and the health department.

Water Pollution

No country was ever more blessed with an abundant supply of clear, sparkling streams and lakes or possessed of more beautiful sea coasts and inviting beaches than America. Yet as we have become more urbanized and industrialized, we have seen one after another of these beautiful resources polluted by the by-products of our urban industrial civilization.

We are finally beginning to realize the seriousness of the problem and to make efforts to prevent further pollution and abating insofar as possible that which now exists. To be successful, these efforts must have the wholehearted support of every citizen, support that is not only local, but is also backed up by a willingness to spend the money to build the treatment facilities needed to prevent or correct pollution.

The place to start is in each community by asking if the sewage treatment plant is adequate in size and properly designed to treat the community's sewage. A similar question may be asked regarding local industries: Are they "good citizens" that adequately treat their wastes or are they grossly polluting the waters at the community's door? Each citizen can also join with others to see that legislation which will deal adequately with the pollution problem is enacted at local, state, and national levels and that the legislation is backed up by sufficient appropriations to make it work. Only when pollution is licked, can we make full use of the nation's God-given water resources.

Other Community Health Resources

Aside from health resources furnished through municipal or state health departments, there are a number of health services provided through other local, state, and federal governmental agencies.

In many communities, police and fire departments provide emergency services which include ambulance service, oxygen applied by mask or tent, rescue teams for disaster situations, and sometimes litters or crutches and other first aid equipment. In a serious emergency, a telephone call to the police or fire department may often make such services available. In some communities, civil defense departments may likewise distribute such information or services.

All states in the United States now have workmen's compensation laws which require employers to furnish medical care to employees whose injuries or occupational illnesses occur from and in the course of their employment. Most industries usually employ industrial physicians for this purpose. These physicians may be in plant medical departments or available on call to care for patients with occupationally-related disabilities.

In many of the states, the workmen's compensation laws also provide for rehabilitation of injured employees through the use of consulting physicians or rehabilitation centers. These rehabilitation centers may be departments of general hospitals or they may be independently organized centers set up either by state agencies or by voluntary health organizations. Their function is to provide medical care designed to restore an injured or ill patient to full employment on a job adapted to the remaining physical capabilities of the patient after recovery from his injury. Most states have a Governor's Committee for the Employment of the Handicapped which further aids disabled patients to become restored to self-sufficient employment.

Health and medical resources are also available to certain groups in the community as a result of their participation in the military services. Many communities have a Veterans' Committee, one of whose functions is to administer the medical care of war veterans for disabilities sustained during their military service or for non-service connected disabilities if they cannot afford to pay for care themselves. Medical care for such veterans is available through the United States Veterans Administration either at a regional veterans hospital or by physicians in the community designated by the Veterans Administration.

Similarly, servicemen in any of the armed services and their dependents receive medical care at federal expense. Servicemen themselves—except in emergency—must receive such care at the nearest available military hospital. Members of their families may receive their care either at a military installation or through civilian physicians and hospitals at government expense.

CHAPTER TWO

VOLUNTARY HEALTH AGENCIES

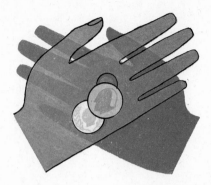

ALMOST EVERYONE is interested in good health and the prevention of disease. Evidence of this fact is shown by the widespread growth of voluntary health agencies at the national, state, and local levels. Through gifts of time and money, millions of Americans show their desire to help combat illness and disease.

Voluntary health agencies make important contributions to the public health resources of a community. They can be classified into two general types:

1. National agencies concerned with a single disease, which use their funds primarily for health education, professional education, research, and in some instances, medical care. Three examples of such agencies are the National Tuberculosis Association, The American Cancer Society, and the American Heart Association.

2. Agencies concerned with people who have common problems resulting from a variety of related diseases. Examples of such agencies are the National Foundation, the National Society for Crippled Children and Adults, and the National Association for Mental Health.

The voluntary health agency as such is an American institution, developed within the past half century. Health and welfare efforts abroad have been largely governmental in nature. To date, there are about 100 national voluntary health agencies which are devoted to the laudable purposes of aiding the unfortunate; disseminating knowledge—both medical and lay—concerning the disease or diseases in question; promoting research; framing and promoting legislation required to combat the disease or diseases effectively; and serving as consultants, advisors, and watchdogs to official agencies at all levels.

A clear picture of just what a voluntary health agency is can be obtained by tracing the history of one specific agency. The organizational activity and financial structure of the National Tuberculosis Association are described because it was the first such agency and because its experiences have helped the organizers of other similar agencies.

In 1904, when the National Tuberculosis Association was formed, tuberculosis was the chief cause of disease and death. Robert Koch's discovery of the tubercle bacillus in 1882 had been hailed as opening the way to solving the tuberculosis problem. However, actual progress in controlling the disease proceeded at such a slow pace that physicians and other particularly interested persons were moved to form associations to encourage more rapid progress.

Edward Livingston Trudeau, himself a victim of tuberculosis, formed the first semi-charitable sanatorium in the United States in 1884 at Saranac Lake, New York. He worked steadily to encourage both medical men and laymen to support his institution and to organize to combat the disease. Trudeau recognized that tuberculosis was transmitted from one person to another and that the way to combat it was to isolate those who were sick. In this way, it would be possible to prevent the transmission of the disease to those who were well.

Lawrence F. Flick of Philadelphia, who had also had tuberculosis and who specialized in the treatment of the disease, attempted with little success to organize a crusade in the 1880's. By 1892, however, he had founded the Pennsylvania Society for the Prevention of Tuberculosis, apparently the first voluntary health agency in the United States composed of both medical and non-medical persons. Although it was difficult for him to obtain enough funds, he did persuade Henry Phipps to donate money to establish the Henry Phipps Institute.

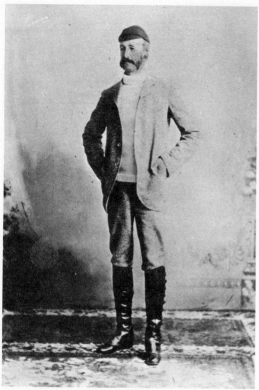

Dr. Edward Trudeau, the founder of the National Tuberculosis Association.

Flick became the Institute's first director and began a research program which was to continue with productive results for many years.

The National Association for the Study and Prevention of Tuberculosis, later to be known as the National Tuberculosis Association or NTA, was formed in 1904. At that time the death rate from tuberculosis was approximately 200 per 100,000 population. One can only guess as to how much effect the formation of the National Tuberculosis Association had in reducing the death rate to approximately 6 per 100,000 population at the present time. But it was certainly a major influence in bringing about modern control measures throughout the United States and the debt owed to the early pioneers in tuberculosis control is hardly measureable.

Trudeau was a powerful instrument in developing the early vigor of the association. He was elected president at the first annual meeting, where he said prophetically: "The first and greatest need is education, and education of the people and through them education of the state. It is evident that if every man and woman in the United States were familiar with the main facts related to the manner in which tuberculosis is communicated and the simple measures for their protection, the people would soon demand and easily obtain effective legislation for its control."

Fund raising was a serious matter for the young Association. Fortunately the group stumbled upon a veritable gold mine—the Christmas Seal. This was suggested by Emily P. Bissell, who adapted the Danish idea of a Christmas stamp which she proposed should be sold before Christmas to raise funds. Originally, Emily Bissell raised money by this means for the care of some tuberculosis patients in Delaware. Somehow it caught the imagination of the American public, coming as it did near Christmas. It was too good a method of fund raising to remain local. In 1908, 33 state branches of the American Red Cross sold the seals which then bore the emblem of the International Red Cross. They raised $135,000 which was then turned over to tuberculosis institutions.

By 1910 the directors of the National Tuberculosis Association realized that here was a method which would solve the financial problems of the Association. In 1920 the Red Cross, which had pioneered the sale, turned over the seal sale to the National Tuberculosis

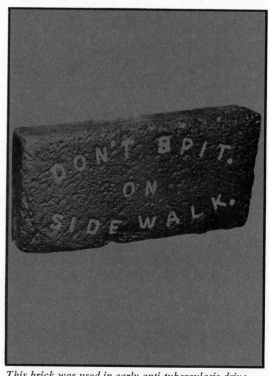

This brick was used in early anti-tuberculosis drive.

Association, and the double-barred Lorraine cross became the official emblem. Since then the National Tuberculosis Association and all its affiliates have depended on the sale of Christmas seals for the major part of their financing.

As noted before, it is difficult to say how much the efforts of the Association have contributed to the decline of the tuberculosis death rate. During the first 15 years of the Association's existence, the death rate declined from 200 to 125 per 100,000. Further impetus to tuberculosis control came when the Metropolitan Life Insurance Company became interested in a demonstration—later to be known as the Framingham Demonstration because of its location in Framingham, Massachusetts—which showed what could be done in a typical American community when all available knowledge and techniques were applied to the discovery and control of tuberculosis. The intent was to examine everyone in the community periodically and to isolate and care for all tuberculous patients as soon as possible.

When the demonstration began, the town's death rate was apparently 121 per 100,000, according to official records. After the project was under way, however, it was discovered that the death rate was really much higher. Inadequate reporting had failed to show that there were many more active cases of tuberculosis in the community than had been known. In the six years of the demonstration, the tuberculosis death rate dropped 68 per cent in contrast to a 32 per cent drop in neighboring communities where lack of control still ruled. This was proof that the National Tuberculosis Association's efforts were sound and that its program could be fruitful if support were forthcoming.

After the Framingham Demonstration, the sanatorium movement, both public and private, developed rapidly. As an offshoot of the National Tuberculosis Association, the American Sanatorium Association was formed. This suborganization later became known as the American Trudeau Society and after 1960, as the American Thoracic Society. Its members comprise more than 5,000 of the leading chest specialists of the United States. It directs the research activities of the National Tuberculosis Association and publishes a well-known scientific journal.

Closely related but independent of the National Tuberculosis Association is the National Conference of Tuberculosis Workers. This is composed of full-time employees of the various

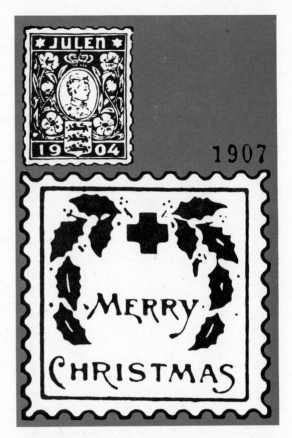

affiliated and local organizations. Thus the National Tuberculosis Association now consists of the parent organization and two subsidiary organizations, plus more than 2,400 tuberculosis associations throughout the country. All of them rely on the Christmas seal sale for financial support.

Voluntary health agencies vary in their organizational structure. The practice of having laymen and physicians on their boards of directors varies. As in most organizations of this type, much of the work of the NTA is carried out by committees. An effort is made in committee formation to include representatives from both the American Thoracic Society and the National Conference of Tuberculosis Workers. Medical guidance is obtained through the American Thoracic Society, particularly through its governing council, and its own committees on medical research, medical education, and therapy.

Since the National Tuberculosis Association was the first voluntary health agency, we can credit it with giving impetus to the voluntary health movement. The agencies organized after the NTA developed various types of programs and their structures differ, but basically they are all alike in following the American principle of helping one's neighbor in time of need. The American public caught on quickly to the idea of banding together and directing their efforts toward alleviating sickness and promoting good health. Today the national voluntary health agencies receive generous support from the public.

National Health Council

The National Health Council was established in 1921 by a group of national voluntary and professional health agencies to help them work together and with others in the cause of health improvement. The Council has three major functions:

1. To help member agencies work together more effectively in the common interest.

2. To help identify, call attention to, and promote solutions of national health problems.

3. To promote better state and local health services, whether governmental of voluntary.

The Councils' member agencies, all national in scope, include voluntary health agencies, professional associations, governmental agencies, and civic and business groups having a major interest in health. Financial support of the Council comes principally from membership contributions and special grants.

The Public's Role

All voluntary health agencies depend on the contributed time of volunteer workers interested in promoting the agency's objectives, as well as on voluntary contributions. It is estimated that between 45,000,000 and 50,000,000 volunteers aid these agencies in one way or another. These health agencies are truly an instrument of public policy, for their very existence depends on the public's time and money.

Citizens have expressed their interest in good health and disease prevention by giving overwhelming support to the voluntary health movement. Total gifts for all health purposes in 1961 were conservatively estimated at $1,000,000,000.

All voluntary health agencies make an annual accounting of their finances to the public. This is done mostly through annual reports and campaign literature. The citizen can obtain a copy by writing to the national office of the agency in which he is interested or by phoning the local unit of that agency. A volunteer or contributor should learn about the stated purpose, organizational pattern, and program of those agencies he supports.

A citizen who wishes to check on the legitimacy of a voluntary health agency should call his local Better Business Bureau, Chamber of Commerce, or medical society. National groups and organizations which supply informational reports on voluntary agencies to their members are the National Information Bureau, National Social Welfare Assembly, National Health Council, Better Business Bureau, and National Industrial Conference Board.

Fund Raising

Voluntary health agencies conduct fund raising campaigns throughout the year. They use two basic methods: the independent drive and the federated drive.

Independent drives are conducted by health agencies who feel that the health education aspect of campaigns for funds is vitally important. When they ask the citizen to give, they educate him on the disease or disability with which they are concerned. These health agen-

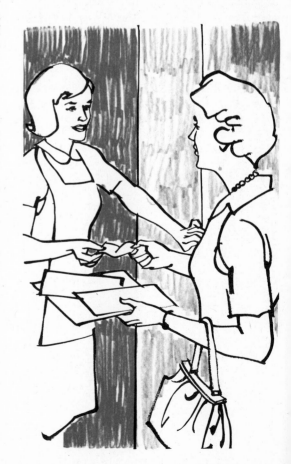

cies campaign during specified months. Some examples are:

> *December:* Christmas Seal Sale—
> National Tuberculosis Association.
> *January:* March of Dimes—
> The National Foundation.
> *February:* Heart Month—
> American Heart Association.
> *April:* Cancer Month—
> American Cancer Society.

The federated drives are conducted once a year in October. The United Community Fund and Council of America is the national organization which oversees local federated campaign drives. UCFCA gives out technical materials, furnishes advice on organization, public relations, and fund raising to local campaigns. The community merges the campaigns of local and national health, welfare, and recreational agencies in one big drive. The funds collected are disbursed by committees of community civic leaders.

Much controversy has taken place over the relative merits of independent vs. federated campaigns. The individual voluntary health agencies have taken a firm stand on the method they wish to use to gather funds from the public. Therefore, the citizen who wishes to give money to a particular health cause should know those health agencies included in his community fund campaign and those who conduct independent campaigns.

Principal Voluntary Health Agencies

The following are brief descriptions of the purpose of the principal national voluntary health agencies. Local addresses are omitted from these listings because they tend to change. Since most of the agencies have local chapters in the larger cities, and many have them in small communities, there should be no difficulty in making contact with any of the organizations. The local health department or medical society can usually furnish local or national addresses.

The National Council on Alcoholism, organized in 1944, is a voluntary agency devoted to the control and prevention of alcoholism through education, research, and community services. It is the only agency in the field that provides inclusive services for a broad public health program on a national and international level.

The Allergy Foundation of America (formerly the American Foundation for Allergic Diseases) was established in 1953 by the American Academy of Allergy and the American College of Allergists to interpret the scope and true nature of allergic diseases and to provide funds for leadership, technical training, and facilities for the correction or prevention of allergic diseases.

The Arthritis and Rheumatism Foundation was established in 1948 by a group of doctors and laymen concerned with the medical, social, and economic problems of arthritis. It works with the American Rheumatism Association. It has these primary objectives: to find the cause and cure for arthritis and other rheumatic diseases; to foster and finance research for better treatment methods, as well as the final cure; to increase and improve local treatment facilities; to provide training in rheumatic diseases to more doctors, therapists, medical students, and nurses; to extend public knowledge and understanding of arthritis and protect its victims from exploitation by those who deal in worthless or misrepresented treatments; to raise funds to finance the expansion of these programs of research, patient care, and public education.

The National Society for the Prevention of Blindness was organized in 1908 to find causes of blindness or impaired vision and to carry on activities for their prevention and the conservation of vision through research, education, and demonstration and community programs.

Fight for Sight—the National Council to Combat Blindness, Inc.—was organized in 1946. Its primary purpose is to stimulate and finance research in ophthalmology and its related sciences. The objective of this program is to restore and preserve sight by determining the causes, means of detection, prevention, treatment, and cure of visual disorders, impaired sight, incipient blindness, and blindness. This objective is pursued through the financing of grants-in-aid, post-doctoral research fellowships, student fellowships, and, from time to time, support of clinical service projects.

The Eye-Bank for Sight Restoration was established in 1944 to make available to qualified hospitals and surgeons a supply of fresh or preserved corneal tissue for the corneal graft operation. In brief, its objectives are:

To establish sources of supply of salvaged eyes and corneal tissue, and to provide the means for their collection, preparation, storage, and redistribution.

To encourage and extend, by teaching and research, the knowledge and skill required to perform corneal graft operations.

To stimulate interest in research work on blindness with special emphasis on blindness from corneal damage. To undertake complete pathological studies of all eyes sent to it.

The Brain Research Foundation was organized in 1953 to arouse public interest in the need for more research and better research facilities in the field of brain disorders. The Foundation is negotiating to establish a Brain Research Center in the Chicago area.

The American Cancer Society was founded in 1913 and reorganized in 1945. The Society's medical and lay volunteers seek to wage a total, nationwide attack on cancer and to utilize present knowledge to save lives by public and professional education and service. It devotes about a third of its funds to research aimed at the eradication of the disease.

The Leukemia Society was established in 1949 to fight leukemia by stimulating new research efforts all over the world and to aid those afflicted through patient services.

The Damon Runyon Memorial Fund for Cancer Research, Inc., founded in 1946, devotes its entire resources to supporting research into the cause and control of cancer. It does not support any treatment facilities other than a limited number of hospital beds for cancer research programs.

The United Cerebral Palsy Associations was founded in 1949 to promote research in cerebral palsy, the treatment, education, and rehabilitation of persons with cerebral palsy, and to subsidize professional training programs of all types related to the problem of cerebral palsy. It seeks to spread information concerning all aspects of the problems of cerebral palsy by professional and public education; to promote better and more adequate techniques and facilities for the diagnosis and treatment of persons with cerebral palsy; to promote the employment of persons with cerebral palsy; to cooperate with governmental and private agencies concerned with the welfare of the handicapped; to solicit, collect, and otherwise raise funds and other property for the above purposes.

The National Cystic Fibrosis Research Foundation was organized in 1955 as a charitable organization for the benefit of, and in aid

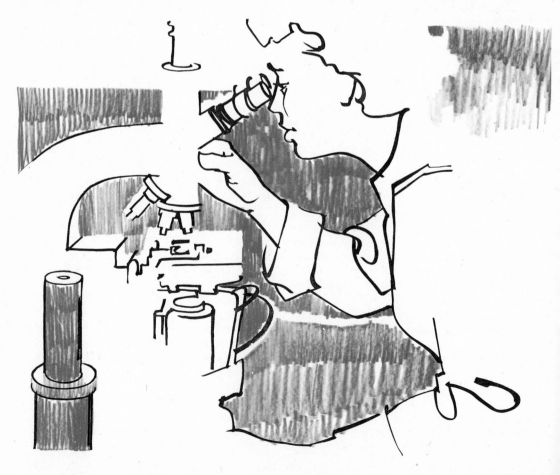

of, scientific research, study, and training and dissemination of information in respect to cystic fibrosis and related diseases, and to provide indirect services to victims of cystic fibrosis.

The National Epilepsy League, Inc. was founded in 1939, as the "Laymen's League Against Epilepsy." It later changed its name to the American Epilepsy League and, in 1949, to the above name. Its purposes are to encourage research in epilepsy, assist epileptics by making information about such illness available to them, and by informing them of the resources for medical care and employment. It also seeks to increase the public's knowledge about and understanding of epilepsy and to widen the opportunities to epileptics for both education and employment.

The United Epilepsy Association was founded in 1941 as the "Association to Control Epilepsy." After two other changes in name, reflecting varying emphasis in program, the organization adopted its present name in 1954. Its purposes are to provide funds for research in the causes and treatment of epilepsy; to encourage medical treatment facilities in epilepsy; to create and assist the development of voluntary health organizations carrying on community service programs for persons with epilepsy; to assist persons with epilepsy by making up-to-date information about this disorder available, and by informing them of resources for medical care, rehabilitation and employment; and to increase the public's understanding of epilepsy.

The National Society for Crippled Children and Adults founded in 1921, incorporated in 1939 as the National Society for Crippled Children of the U.S.A., changed its name in 1944 to the above. Its purposes are to extend and develop the rehabilitation services which can alleviate the physical, psychological, social, and vocational effects of crippling disease or injury; to conduct educational programs for the public, professional personnel, parents of crippled children, and employers, to create greater understanding and greater acceptance of the crippled; to conduct research into the causes of crippling and its prevention, and to improve methods of care, treatment, and education of crippled children and adults.

The American Hearing Society exists to provide information and consultative services to individuals and communities relative to hearing and speech problems; to educate the public concerning the identification, conservation, prevention, and rehabilitation of persons in all age groups with hearing and speech impairments; to stimulate scientific efforts in these areas.

The American Heart Association was incorporated in 1924. Until its reorganization in 1948 as a national voluntary health agency, it was primarily concerned with furthering professional education. Since then, its efforts have been directed to the integration of research, professional and public education, and community services for control and ultimate conquest of diseases of the heart and blood vessels.

The National Hemophilia Foundation was organized in 1948 to make grants and donations for research and clinical study of hemophilia, abnormal blood conditions, and similar ailments; to publish information and knowledge relating to the treatment of these diseases; to provide medical scholarships; and to grant funds to or for persons suffering from hemophilia and kindred ailments.

The Sister Elizabeth Kenny Foundation, an organization of international scope, was founded in 1943 and reorganized in 1960. It stresses training, education, and research in the broad field of rehabilitation of neuromuscular and skeletal disabilities and disorders.

The National Kidney Disease Foundation was incorporated in 1950 to direct, unify, stimulate, coordinate, and further the knowledge of and work done on any and all phases of kidney disease, including nephrosis and nephritis.

The Leonard Wood Memorial for the Eradication of Leprosy was organized in 1928 to carry on, maintain, and support laboratory investigation, clinical observation, and all manner of research with respect to the disease of leprosy; to disseminate information concerning the source, diagnosis, treatment, and prevention of leprosy; to voluntarily aid, establish, maintain, and support leper colonies, receiving stations, clinics, hospitals, and laboratories with proper staffs and equipment for diagnosis and treatment; and to aid and cooperate with organizations and agencies, public or private, having a similar or related purpose.

The National Association for Mental Health was incorporated in 1950 to consolidate the three principal national voluntary agencies working at that time in the field of mental health. Its purposes are to develop a coordinated citizens' voluntary movement to work toward the improved care and treatment of the mentally ill and handicapped; for improved methods and services in research, prevention,

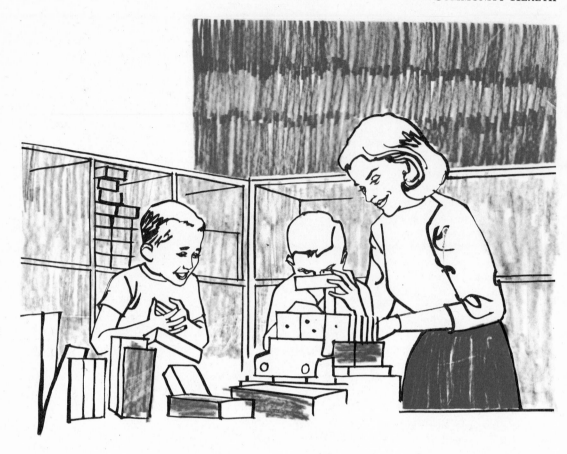

detection, diagnosis, and treatment of mental illness and handicaps; and for the promotion of mental health.

The National Multiple Sclerosis Society was organized in 1946. Its aim and purposes are to stimulate, coordinate, and support research in multiple sclerosis and related diseases; to encourage and assist in establishing chapters, branches, and units of the National Society; to aid in establishing MS clinics and centers; to aid individuals disabled as a result of multiple sclerosis and related diseases, and their families; and to make grants of money for the prevention, diagnosis, treatment, alleviation, or cure of multiple sclerosis and related diseases.

Muscular Dystrophy Associations of America, Inc., was founded in 1950. It is dedicated to the scientific conquest of neuromuscular diseases through basic and applied research into nerves, muscles, and metabolism.

The Myasthenia Gravis Foundation was organized in 1952 to support research into the cause, prevention, alleviation, and cure of myasthenia gravis, and to disseminate information

about the disease to the medical profession and to the general public.

The National Foundation for Neuromuscular Diseases, Inc. was founded in 1953 as the National Foundation for Muscular Dystrophy, Inc. Its name was changed in 1960 to define more precisely the scope of its purposes and objectives. These include: monetary support of intensive, long-range research in leading medical teaching institutions to promote basic understanding, to improve the treatment, and ultimately to cure or prevent crippling neuromuscular diseases; an education program to inform the public about these diseases, and to make available to the medical profession current scientific knowledge; and the provision, through its local chapters, of adequate patient care services.

The National Association for Retarded Children is a non-profit association incorporated in 1953 to improve the welfare of retarded persons and promote a united attack on mental retardation problems.

The American Social Health Association was organized in 1914 "to promote those conditions of living, environment, and personal conduct which best protect the family as a social institution." Its specific programs are in the fields of venereal disease, prostitution, narcotic addiction, and family life education.

The National Tuberculosis Association was founded in 1904. Its purposes are to study, to disseminate knowledge concerning, and to encourage the prevention and scientific treatment of tuberculosis and other respiratory diseases; to coordinate and stimulate the work of the more than 2,400 tuberculosis associations throughout the country; to cooperate with medical societies and with other non-official and offical organizations interested in tuberculosis and related problems; and to promote international relations in connection with control of tuberculosis and other respiratory diseases.

The National Foundation was organized in 1938, to lead, direct, and unify the fight against poliomyelitis by promoting study and research into the cause, nature, and prevention of poliomyelitis and prevention of its harmful sequelae, as well as to provide medical care for patients afflicted with the disease. In 1958 the name of the organization was shortened to The National Foundation and its objectives were expanded to become ". . . an organized force for medical research, patient care, and professional education (with specific goals initially), flexible enough to meet new health problems as they arise." Its initial programs cover arthritis, birth defects (congenital malformations), virus diseases, and disorders of the central nervous system, as well as poliomyelitis.

Other Agencies of Medical Interest

The American Foundation for the Blind was established in 1921 by action of the agencies serving blind persons and by their friends to promote higher standards of service throughout the United States on behalf of all blind and deaf-blind persons.

The American Diabetes Association was established in 1940 as a national medical organization. The association is a nonprofit membership organization and the only non-governmental voluntary group in the field of diabetes in the United States. The association's major interests are professional education, patient education, public education and case finding, and research.

The National Rehabilitation Association was established in 1925 to advance the rehabilitation of all physically and mentally handicapped persons by research, professional services, and public education.

The American Rehabilitation Committee was established in 1924 as a voluntary nongovernmental association. Its aim is to prepare the disabled person physically, mentally, and vocationally for employment as quickly, effectively, and efficiently as possible. The major portion of its operating cost is derived from voluntary contributions.

The Association for the Aid of Crippled Children supports research in this and other countries on the nature, causes, and consequences of handicapping among children and youth. In addition to giving grants for both medical and social research, conferences of various types are held to stimulate communication and collaboration among scientists and to explore areas of investigation which are now receiving little attention. The Association conducts a publishing program, primarily for professional audiences.

The Maternity Center Association, in its program of education for childbirth, is broad in scope. In addition to its local programs of expectant parent education, the Association publishes books, leaflets, film strips, charts, and posters designed for use in biology and family living courses in high school and college, in classes for expectant parents, and in medical and nursing schools.

The American Association for Maternal and Infant Health. Although the role of the obstetrician remains paramount in the medical care of the maternity patient, her total care may include the services of the anesthesiologist, nurse, nurse anesthetist, pediatrician, hospital administrator, nutritionist and dietician, social worker, public health nurse, and others. The purpose of the American Association for Maternal and Infant Health is to provide a close integration of all of these disciplines. The Association serves as a forum for their mutual problems, providing guidance, educational needs, and a common meeting ground for everyone interested in maternal and infant care. A program for the participation of the lay public is in the process of development. It will emphasize the establishment of local educational facilities for the instruction of mothers and fathers in preparation for pregnancy, delivery, and the care of the newborn.

The Planned Parenthood Federation of America was incorporated in 1922 as the American Birth Control League. In 1949 its name was changed to the above, and its program was broadened to include education for marriage and medical treatment of infertility.

The purpose of the Federation is to provide leadership for the universal acceptance of family planning as an essential element of responsible parenthood, stable family life, and social harmony; the provision of the necessary medical services; and the promotion of research in the field of human reproduction including treatment and development of improved contraceptive methods.

The Margaret Sanger Research Bureau, named for its founder, is a center for research, education, and service in family planning, infertility, and marriage education.

The National Society for Medical Research was founded to deal with a symptom of public ignorance and misunderstanding of medical and biological science—the antivivisection movement. It is primarily an association of research agencies.

The People-to-People Health Foundation was initiated in 1958 by the President of the United States as part of a program to promote world peace through increased understanding between the people of the United States and the people of other nations. This program has several committees, one of which is the Committee on Medicine and Health Professions which has a corporate entity, the People-to-People Health Foundation, or Project HOPE (Health Opportunity for People Everywhere).

The purpose of Project HOPE is to bring the skills and techniques developed by the American medical professions to the people of other nations in their own environment, adapted specifically to their needs and their way of life. Initially, the chief vehicle of the project is a fully equipped and staffed hospital ship. Staffed by 15 full-time and a rotating group of 70 volunteer physicians, the ship serves as a training and treatment clinic, a medical school, a base for medical, nursing, and sanitation teams, and the logistic center for medical aid and health and exchange programs carried out in the interiors of the countries it visits.

The American National Red Cross was founded in 1881 and received its first congressional charter in 1900. A new charter in 1905, with its subsequent amendments, outlines the present obligations of the organization. It is charged with furnishing volunteer aid to the

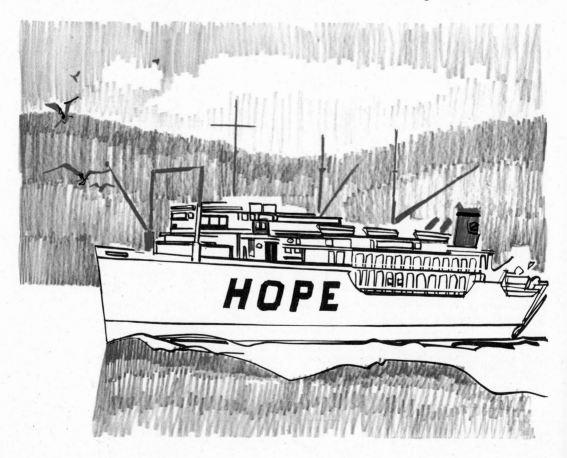

sick and wounded of the armed forces in time of war and to act in matters of voluntary relief and as a medium of communication between the people of the United States and their armed forces. It is further charged with providing a system of national and international relief to mitigate the sufferings caused by pestilence, famine, fire, floods, and other great calamities, and to devise and carry out measures for their prevention.

The American Epilepsy Federation is a national health agency representing 35 lay societies in 16 states and Canada. The purpose of the Federation is to unite all lay groups so that epilepsy can have a national voice. The Federation also assists affiliates to develop effective local programs, encourages the development of lay societies in areas of the country where none exists, and cooperates in a nationwide attack on the problems of the epileptic.

The National Medical Foundation for Eye Care was established in 1956 by a group of leading American ophthalmologists. It is incorporated in New Jersey as a non-profit association.

Its purpose is to study social and medical factors affecting eye care; to disseminate information to the profession and the public relating to scientific eye care; to promote the conservation of vision and prevention of blindness through more effective utilization of this knowledge; to represent the professional interests of ophthalmology in matters of general or interprofessional concern; and to provide an organizational mechanism through which ophthalmologists can study problems and formulate policies affecting their profession and service to the public.

The Deafness Research Foundation was established in 1958 as the only national voluntary laymen's organization devoted to support of investigation into the causes, prevention, and cure of impaired hearing. The principal objectives of the Foundation are threefold: to make available for research documented temporal bones; to stimulate the study of these inner ear structures by qualified investigators in established laboratories throughout the country; and to develop a nationwide program of public education concerning the serious psychological, social, and economic effects of impaired hearing.

CHAPTER THREE

HOME, SCHOOL, AND HEALTH

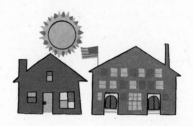

PARENTS HAVE A RESPONSIBILITY, as well as an opportunity, to teach their young children about healthful living. The child's development of sound health behavior patterns and attitudes should get a good start in the home before he starts to school. During this period he should learn at home basic facts about body growth and development, body structure and function, and health and safety practices.

What Parents Can Do

Parents' responsibilities for their child's basic health needs include providing him with adequate, comfortable sleeping quarters, a well chosen diet, good habits of hygiene, and the correction of remediable defects with the aid of their family physician and dentist. Thus provided for, the child can better perform his school tasks.

The fundamentals of learning to live effectively in a complicated, fast-moving social order should begin in the home. The child can learn at first hand what it means to respect the rights of others and to share in their pleasures and responsibilities.

When, however, parents cannot provide adequate care or help the child develop good habits of social living, they should seek help at the community level. In the rare cases when parents are unwilling to meet their responsibilities and where neglect can be demonstrated, the case may be referred to a child welfare agency or other community organization.

Children differ greatly in their physical and mental capacities. They vary in their abilities to adjust socially and emotionally. For a child to perform to his best ability, he must have the highest possible degree of health attainable. He must be free from communicable disease and from defects which can be corrected. For example, hearing or vision loss and problems of

weight control or undernourishment can be treated, and undesirable personality traits or habits may yield to understanding and care. It is the responsibility of the home to take care of such problems.

A child with impaired vision or hearing, or a shy, selfish, or overaggressive nature will have problems in making friends or taking part in group activities as well as keeping up in his studies. Any of these problems may prove to be handicaps to learning.

Behavior problems may be studied jointly by parents and counselors. Teachers and parents alike must be led to realize the need for early identification of such problems and their subsequent correction.

An ill child should remain at home for his own sake and that of his classmates. Parents should realize the importance of complying with this policy. Parents of school children who ride school buses need to be especially careful not to let their children go to school when they are ill. Once on the bus, the ill child may infect other children because of the close quarters. Most schools no longer strive for 100 per cent attendance.

Another phase of parent-school cooperation usually includes insistence upon regular attendance in physical education classes—unless there are valid reasons for not attending. These classes afford the child an opportunity to develop physical skills and an appreciation of the value of exercise and recreation. They also help establish attitudes of good sportsmanship. These programs are entirely in keeping with our national interest in physical fitness.

Some children, of course, cannot keep up with their schoolmates in the regular classes in physical education. The child's physician can arrange for his enrollment in a modified activity. Prescription of individual programs based on specific needs should replace blanket excuses. Better understanding between parents, family and school physicians, and other school personnel may result through their joint representation on a school or community health council, or by informal conferences. Where physical education programs adapted to children's varying needs are available, this problem is seldom troublesome.

Parents and Teachers

For about 180 days each year, children spend from five to six hours a day in school under the supervision of a professional staff who observe them closely both as individuals, and in their relations with other children in the class. For the teacher to be able to do an effective job, he must know as much as possible about the children in his class, including their background and home life. It is unwise and unfair to a child for parents to withhold pertinent information concerning his health status or history which might help a teacher develop a better understanding of the child.

No child can face alone all of the influences which our complicated way of living imposes upon him. He needs adult support from his home, his school, and his community. If these fail him, he may seek help through unsupervised and often undesirable association with others who need the same kind of help. It is in this way that many gangs of juvenile delinquents develop.

A child's happiness has its roots in a happy home life. Children coming from homes where strife and discord replace love and understanding have little chance to achieve satisfying social and emotional relationships with other children. Often, too, they fail to get along with other adults because their home life makes them hesitant to trust adults. Through parent-teacher conferences, some degree of understanding of the child's problem may be achieved.

In some cases not much can be accomplished to correct an unfavorable situation. When economic and competitive pressures are so great as to warp the real meaning of family living and the home becomes merely a place in which to eat, sleep, worry, and quarrel, children often feel insecure and unimportant.

While family counseling is not primarily the job of school personnel, a conference between parents and a teacher or nurse may bring home problems into sharper focus and reveal the need for professional help for the child's sake.

Illness in the family, sudden financial reverses, and moving too often—or any circumstance which results in loss of childhood friendships and frequent change in home and school environment—foster feelings of insecurity in the child. These leave their mark on the child's school attendance and his ability to concentrate on school work. The impact is greater in the lower elementary grades where home dependence is still a large factor in the child's life.

Teachers have a real opportunity to help a child adjust to disappointing and sometimes crushing circumstances. Guidance in learning to live with others may come from a teacher who has an understanding of people and a mature insight into the child's problems.

Every child needs a home where his longing for encouragement is understood and his accomplishments are appreciated. He needs enough time for study and a good place to do it. Every child has a right to some time of his own when he does not have to do chores, babysit, or engage in afterschool activities which parents dream up to keep him occupied and to contribute to his cultural life. Time budgeting is as important a learning skill as typing or playing a musical instrument.

Every child has an obligation to contribute to his family as one of its members; he has duties as well as rights. As the child matures, he will need to learn more about how to share responsibility in the home. The school can help lay the foundation for improved family relations by means of class discussion, acting out imaginary situations, the use of visual aids, and assigned readings in the studies of family living. By stressing the importance of getting along well with others and the need to attain emotional maturity and stability, the school may be able to help the child develop a better understanding regarding his responsibilities toward his home and family.

What Schools Should Do

Children differ greatly in their physical, mental, social, and emotional characteristics. They also vary in their capacity to achieve, which cannot always be judged by their mental ability. The desire to learn and the opportunity to do so rank high in importance along with the ability to learn.

The school can lend its support to the home through opportunities for parent education and for parent conferences with teachers and other school personnel. These include health special-

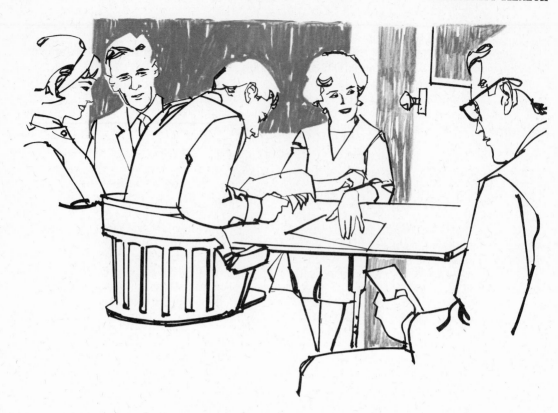

ists responsible for medical, dental, nursing, psychological, or psychiatric counseling.

A school health program has a better chance to succeed when there is mutual respect and understanding between parents and school personnel, and between the family physician and school health personnel.

In building functional and adequate school health programs, most schools have formulated school health policies in cooperation with parents and other people in the community interested in child health and education. Such school health policies should be explained to all parents of school children.

The school has a threefold responsibility for child health: First of all, it must educate for safe and healthful living. Second, it must create and maintain a safe and healthful environment. Third, it must offer an adequate health service program including emergency care in case of accident or sudden illness.

In a health education program, the school aims to provide factual information about health in such a way that the child may develop acceptable health attitudes and practices. He should be given the opportunity to learn the basic facts of healthful living and be introduced to recent health discoveries.

Major topics which should be included are elementary first aid, home safety, and safety at school and on the way there. At the proper age, every child should be taught bicycle safety and driver training. In many of these phases of health education, parents have the major responsibility.

The basic facts of consumer health should also be presented to the pupil. For example, he should learn how to choose a doctor, how to call one in an emergency, and how to obtain hospitalization. He should learn the dangers of self-diagnosis and self-medication. He should have a chance to learn how to tell fact from fancy in advertising of health services and related products.

The child should learn the basic facts of communicable disease control and how to protect himself and others as much as possible from infection. He should assume some responsibility for maintaining his own health by keeping records of his immunizations and his medical and dental appointments. As soon as he is mature enough, he may learn to make his own appointments and be responsible for keeping them.

Home nursing as well as the basic facts of education for family living, the use and abuse of stimulants and depressants, and community responsibility for personal health maintenance are usually emphasized in the upper elementary and junior high school grades, although some phases of these topics may be introduced at the intermediate grade level.

The health curriculum should be tailored to fit the special health needs of each particular grade and should use community resources whenever possible to supplement formal teaching. For example, a unit on communicable disease control can be more stimulating if it is related to a particular community drive for immunization against poliomyelitis or measles. Such a community program would involve parental acceptance and consent, pupil education by the teacher, program coordination between the school nurse and doctor, and public health agencies and the child's personal physician. Such a program may point up the importance of maintaining an adequate immunization status and become a basis for building good attitudes toward future immunizations.

Dynamic health teaching will carry over into the home, resulting in the improvement of family and home hygiene, together with a better understanding and fuller use of community health resources.

Parent-teacher organizations may become aware of important community needs and, under the school's leadership, bring about community health improvements. The raising of housing standards, removal of safety hazards, or improvement of food sanitation in restaurants and markets are examples of improvements that may result.

Communicable disease control can be effective only to the degree in which it becomes a total community project. Sanitation standards must be kept at a high level in the home and in the community in order to support the school efforts.

School responsibility to the home includes notifying the family in case of emergency or sudden illness. Also, there must be a plan for emergency first aid in case of disaster. There should also be a way to inform parents if a disease epidemic threatens to develop in the community.

Insistence on periodic medical and dental examinations for each school child points up to parents the importance of this procedure. By indicating the need for early correction of remediable defects, the school performs a vital service in laying the foundation for continued attention to health preservation throughout adulthood.

Teachers may point out the significance of health examination results or of the child's special health problems, and encourage parents to obtain necessary care. Both parents and children may be motivated through personal conferences to accept the need for treatment.

During such conferences, parents also have the right to be listened to with respect and to be guided in the ways in which they may best understand and meet the health problems of their children. In such conferences, too, children can be taught to evaluate their own health assets and liabilities and to adjust to them. For example when participation in certain athletic events is prohibited, other compensations must be offered. A skilled teacher can offer guidance in this direction.

Classes in home economics and mechanics provide information and practice in skills for the promotion of better family living. The establishment and maintenance of adequate school lunch programs find support through the joint concern of home and school for improving the child's nutrition.

Through the use of the "Lighted School House" program with evening classes for adults and recreation for all, schools can do much to raise their contribution to wholesome community living.

CHAPTER FOUR

COMMUNICABLE DISEASES

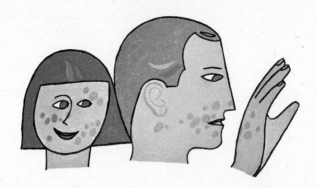

EVERY MAN, WOMAN, AND CHILD at some time in life suffers illnesses caused by infection. Infections which can be passed from person to person, or from animals to persons, are called communicable diseases. These diseases are caused by germs (primarily bacteria or viruses) which gain entrance to the body and multiply at particular sites. Depending on where the germs multiply, different types of illnesses develop. If a germ enters the body through the nose or mouth and multiplies in that region, a sore throat, tonsillitis, sinusitis, ear ache, cough (bronchitis), or even pneumonia will result. If the germs are swallowed with food, milk, or water, gastrointestinal symptoms such as nausea, vomiting, cramps, and diarrhea frequently result. If the germs enter through broken or cut skin, infections such as boils, skin ulcers, or other inflammations may occur.

The severity of infection results from such factors as the inherent properties of the specific germ, the number of germs, and the ability of the body to fight them. The same type of germ may vary in its ability to invade the body. This ability depends upon a large number of factors, only some of which are completely understood. The most important factor in determining the severity of infection is the number of germs actually entering the body. If all other conditions remain the same, the larger the number of germs invading the body, the more severe will be the illness. Of prime importance in the course of an illness is the ability of the body to fight infection.

The ability of the body to resist infection is termed immunity. It may be natural or acquired. Natural immunity is the sum total of the defenses in all normal people which enable the body to resist infection under ordinary conditions. These defenses include, among many others, intact skin and mucous membranes which act to bar the entrance of germs; the tissue fluids and blood, which contain cells and other substances which engulf and destroy foreign objects; and the ordinarily harmless population of bacteria and viruses found in the body which prevent or interfere with the growth of harmful bacteria or viruses. All of these processes of natural immunity are based on an individual's physical characteristics. These depend upon proper nutrition, physical fitness, rest, age, sex, and environmental influences such as humidity and temperature. Throughout one's lifetime, many germs may actually enter the body, but natural immunity prevents infection. When this natural immunity is depressed by illness, inadequate nutrition, lack of adequate rest, or other conditions, a person may develop infections which healthy persons ordinarily would not.

Acquired immunity is that defense against infection which an individual develops through exposure to germs or their products. Each germ acts as a specific antigen. An antigen is a substance foreign to the body which stimulates the body to form antibodies. Antibodies are protective proteins which the body forms in response to an antigen. For instance, when measles viruses enter the body, they cause the body to form antibodies because the measles virus is a foreign substance. These antibodies are for specific use against the measles virus, and help the body fight and kill the virus. They do not help to fight other viruses such as the poliomyelitis virus, however. The body forms antibodies against each germ that invades it. Until the body has had at least one encounter with the germ, no antibodies can be formed against it.

Immunity may be acquired naturally, that is, by actually developing the disease. In the course of an illness, antibodies appear and the patient begins to recover. These antibodies then persist in the blood stream and protect the individual from developing the same illness again. Not many years ago, this was the only way people could develop immunity. Today, however, modern medicine has developed vaccines by which we can develop immunity artificially. Vaccines are antigens which cause the body to build antibodies against a particular disease without becoming ill.

Some vaccines contain living germs, such as the smallpox, yellow fever, and oral polio vaccines. These living vaccines have been rendered harmless in the laboratory, so that they do not cause the harmful effects of the disease. But they still provoke the formation of antibodies. Some vaccines contain killed germs, such as typhoid and the Salk polio vaccines. These vaccines contain germs which have been killed in the laboratory so that they cannot cause disease, but will still cause the body to form antibodies against the specific disease.

Other antigens are made from the products of germs which cause disease, such as the tetanus and diphtheria vaccines. Tetanus and diphtheria are diseases caused by a toxin poison released by the germs. Tetanus and diphtheria preventives, therefore, contain a modified toxin called a toxoid which has been rendered harmless in the laboratory but will cause the body to build antibodies. In this instance, the antibody formed is called antitoxin.

Artificially acquired immunity protects the individual from developing the disease the first time. As a result, hundreds of thousands of people are spared the suffering from these diseases, and many thousands of lives are saved. Artificial immunity, however, does not last so long as naturally acquired immunity. As a result, a booster shot of vaccine is periodically needed to stimulate the production of more antibodies. In developing artificial immunity, the body makes its own antibodies in response to a given antigen. This is known as active immunization.

There are occasions, however, when we cannot wait for the body to make its own antibodies or where we do not have an antigen available so that the body can make its own antibody. In these situations, antibodies formed by another person or animal can be given. This is known as passive immunization. Gamma globulin is a form of passive immunization because it is the antibody portion of the blood of other people in concentrated form. Because we cannot produce active immunity against hepa-

titis (no antigen or vaccine is available to do so), gamma globulin is frequently given to patients to provide them with passive immunity.

For persons who have never been immunized against diphtheria and tetanus and who have developed the disease, or who are in danger of developing it, passive immunity can be produced by giving antitoxin (antibodies against the toxin), which has been produced in animals. Passive immunization is never as good as active immunization, however. In addition, such immunity only lasts about six weeks.

Today it is both the right and the privilege of every child to receive protection against such diseases as smallpox, diphtheria, tetanus, whooping cough, poliomyelitis, and measles. It is therefore the duty and responsibility of every parent to be certain that his child receives this protection. Vaccine cannot prevent disease if it remains in the doctor's office. It can protect the child only if it is given according to the recommended schedules. Your doctor or local health department is the best source of advice on such schedules. Every parent should keep an adequate record of immunizations for all members of the family. Both dates and type of vaccine given should be recorded.

Common Immunizations

There are at least five diseases (smallpox, diphtheria, whooping cough, tetanus, and poliomyelitis) against which most Americans are immunized in childhood, and it will not be long before most American children receive measles vaccine. In addition, there are two other diseases, influenza and typhoid fever, against which many are vaccinated, as well as several other vaccines which are recommended when one travels in some parts of the world. All important to any program of immunizations is careful planning so that the vaccines are given at the proper times and in the proper sequence. Listed below are the vaccines most commonly given in the United States today.

Smallpox

Smallpox vaccine is a living virus vaccine. It has been derived from the virus of cowpox over a period of many years. This virus is introduced by minute punctures into the skin. The virus then grows and multiplies at the site to form a round, scabbed, ulcer-like sore which appears in approximately one week and disappears during the following 10-day period.

This ulcerated, scabbed-over sore is called a primary vaccination. It occurs in persons who have no preexisting immunity to smallpox. A modified reaction develops in persons who have previously been vaccinated and have some remaining immunity. Within three days after vaccination, a small pimple appears at the site of vaccination. Along with this there may be some mild redness and itching, but this usually disappears within 7 to 10 days. If no reaction develops at the site of vaccination, it means either that the vaccine virus was dead or that the vaccine virus has not successfully entered the skin. Under such circumstances, the person should be revaccinated so that either a primary or modified vaccination reaction can develop.

Frequently at the time a primary vaccination reaction develops, the individual also develops fever and an aching feeling. In rare instances, the lymph nodes under the inoculated arm may swell up and become tender. The modified reactions that come with revaccination, however, do not include such symptoms. Generally, older individuals develop more symptoms from primary vaccination than do young children. For persons successfully vaccinated in childhood, revaccination has modified reactions with virtually no symptoms. No one need fear periodic revaccination.

There are relatively few reasons not to vaccinate against smallpox and almost all children should receive smallpox vaccination within their first year of life. However, if a child is receiving hormone treatment such as cortisone, or if a rare blood disorder such as agammaglobulinemia is present, vaccination should not be done. No child with eczema or other skin rashes should be vaccinated. In such instances, the vaccine virus may spread over the entire body, resulting in a condition known as generalized vaccinia.

A child recently vaccinated against smallpox may transfer the virus to his brother or sister who may happen to have eczema. Your physician is the best source of advice under such circumstances. A child who may have had

IMMUNIZATION SCHEDULE FOR CHILDREN*

Diseases		Age at Time of First Dosage	Material (Antigen)	No. Doses	Interval	Age at Time of Booster (Recall) Doses
Diphtheria Tetanus Whooping Cough		2 months	Triple Preparation	3	Not less than one month nor more than three months	12 months after third dose; again at 4 years and 8 years Tetanus and diphtheria toxoids (adult type) 12 years and 16 years Tetanus toxoid every 5 years thereafter
Poliomyelitis		2 months	Inactivated (Salk)	4	One month intervals; 4th at 15 months	Every 2 years after 4th dose
		2 months	Oral (Sabin) vaccine Type I Type III Type II	1 dose each	6-8 weeks	12-15 months, Types I-II-III combined
		2 months	Oral (Sabine) trivalent vaccine (3 vaccines combined)	3	6-8 weeks	4th dose 12-15 months
Smallpox		6-12 months	Cowpox virus	1		Every 5 years, when going overseas, or in presence of epidemic
Typhoid-paratyphoid-fevers		Only when needed	Typhoid—paratyphoid vaccine	3	1-4 weeks	Upon advice of physician or public health authorities
Measles (4 Plans)	1	9 months	live, attenuated vaccine	1		No recommendations; immunity may be permanent
	2	9 months	Same + gamma globulin	1		
Choice rests with physician	3	9 months	Inactivated vaccine	3	Monthly	One or more booster doses; intervals undetermined; not for routine use
	4	9 months	Same, followed by live attenuated vaccine			Recommendation pending

*Adapted from Table One, The Red Book, American Academy of Pediatrics, 1964, modified by Supplementary Statement October 25, 1964.

eczema during the first year of his life may be safely vaccinated after the skin condition has cleared and does not seem likely to return.

Once successfully vaccinated, everyone should be revaccinated at least every five years to maintain adequate immunity. Under special circumstances such as living abroad, one should be vaccinated as often as once a year, depending upon the part of the world in which he is living. A certificate proving smallpox vaccination within the past three years is required in order to enter or reenter the United States.

DPT Immunization

While one can be immunized against diphtheria, whooping cough, or tetanus separately, it is common practice today to give infants all three vaccines at one time. Such immunization is called the DPT, or triple shot. This vaccine contains inactivated diphtheria toxin called toxoid, killed whooping cough germs, and inactivated tetanus toxin or toxoid. Each of these is also available separately, or diphtheria and tetanus immunization can be combined without whooping cough. Then it is called DT or double toxoid. DPT, or triple vaccine, is usually given in three doses at monthly intervals beginning at about six weeks of age. A reinforcing dose is then given approximately one year later. Such a series of inoculations is termed the primary series.

The need for every child to receive DPT immunization is really quite obvious. Diphtheria still occurs in the United States. Every year between 50 and 75 children die from the disease. Invariably, these children had not received immunization; thus they therefore die, unnecessarily.

So long as some children remain unvaccinated, there will be danger from diphtheria, for the diphtheria germ can be carried by healthy persons. The adequately immunized child who picks up the diphtheria germ, will probably fight it off successfully. If, however, an unimmunized child picks it up, the results can be disastrous. Even if he remains well, he may expose enough children until one of them, not previously immunized, becomes seriously ill.

Diphtheria need not be a threat to your child, however. After the primary series of inoculations in infancy, booster doses of diphtheria toxoid should be given at least every three years until high school age. Special toxoids have been developed for older children and adults in the event that a diphtheria epidemic should make immunization of older age groups necessary.

Whooping cough is a serious illness among infants under the age of two because of complicating pneumonias. Under two, at least 1 out of every 10 infants developing whooping cough will die. Invariably, children at that age who develop whooping cough have not received their primary immunization. It is important that other young children in a family be immunized so that they will not bring the disease home to the newborn baby. Because the disease is so serious in the newborn period, immunization should not be delayed any longer than necessary, and preferably should begin at six weeks of age. After a child begins school at age five or six, booster shots against whooping cough are no longer given. Also, the physician may decide not to give whooping cough vaccine to certain children who have epilepsy or other nervous system diseases.

Tetanus, or lock-jaw as it is commonly known, is a disease which will always remain a threat unless a person is adequately immunized. Tetanus is caused by germs which lie dormant in the soil. After the dormant form (called spores) enters the body, the spores begin to multiply. As they do so, they form a very powerful toxin which paralyzes the muscles and causes them to twitch and convulse.

Anytime a person's skin is broken, particularly in areas such as the backyard, camping or picnic sites, swimming areas, and along the highways where automobile accidents may occur, there is danger of tetanus. The injury itself need not be major. About one-half of all cases of tetanus seen in American hospitals are the result of an injury so trivial as to go unnoticed until symptoms of tetanus occur.

The only real safeguard, therefore, is to keep your tetanus immunization up to date. After the primary series of inoculations in infancy, boosters should be given at the start of school and every three to five years thereafter. When injuries which are commonly associated with tetanus do occur, your physician will immediately give a booster shot.

Poliomyelitis

Today the incidence of poliomyelitis in the United States is at an all-time low. Since 1955, when the Salk vaccine was introduced, polio has occurred primarily in areas or neighborhoods where the vaccine has not been fully utilized. Each outbreak has occurred among groups with a much lower vaccination rate than nearby areas which remained free of the disease. In the United States today there are still a great many persons who either don't seem to care or who don't know the necessity for adequate immunization. So long as such attitudes exist, small and localized outbreaks of paralytic poliomyelitis will continue in the United States.

Two different poliomyelitis vaccines are presently in use. The Salk vaccine is a suspension of the three types of polio virus which have been killed. The Sabin or oral vaccine is live polio virus which has been changed sufficiently in the laboratory so that it will not cause disease. There is a separate oral vaccine for each of the three types of polio virus and also one oral vaccine containing all three types.

Salk vaccine is injected, beginning as early as six weeks of age, in three doses at one-month intervals. Some manufacturers combine the Salk vaccine with DPT to make a four-in-one shot. After the original three doses, an additional dose is recommended at approximately one year of age. Booster shots every two years thereafter are recommended in order to maintain immunity.

Sabin vaccine is given one type at a time, beginning as early as six weeks of age, at one-month intervals. This is given as a sweet, cherry-flavored syrup. A booster dose of trivalent oral vaccine is given at one year of age. Recommendations for booster doses for older children or adults have not been formulated as of this writing.

Measles Vaccine

Measles vaccine has only recently been licensed for use in the United States. Most parents will be thankful for this new advance in medicine because measles is quite severe and prolonged, particularly in the very young baby. Furthermore, the number and type of complications following measles has concerned everyone. This vaccine provides protection against the red measles (five-day measles, Rubeola) only, and not against the German (Rubella) measles.

One measles vaccine currently used is a live virus which has been modified in the laboratory. At the time of vaccination, an injection of gamma globulin is given in the opposite arm. This is to further modify the effect of the live virus. Following vaccination, most children will develop a mild fever about one week later. Some children (about 15 per cent) will de-

velop a high fever and a slight rash. This is usually short lived, however, and in all instances is much more mild than a case of the measles. Because of the use of gamma globulin, vaccination against measles is more expensive than most immunizations.

A killed virus vaccine which does not require the use of gamma globulin has also been developed. Not enough time has yet elapsed to ascertain the length of immunity conferred by this vaccine.

Measles vaccine is not recommended prior to nine months of age. Before that age, the baby still has sufficient protection from his mother (if she has immunity), and the vaccine might not take. Of course, if a baby should happen to develop measles before nine months of age, there would be no need to give him the vaccine. Such instances are relatively rare, however. At the present time, measles vaccine is not recommended for children over the age of five, because the rate of complications accompanying measles in older children is much less than in younger children.

Scheduling Immunizations

Because artificially acquired immunity is not permanent, periodic doses of vaccine are needed to provide continued protection against disease. Furthermore, some vaccines require more than one dose to provide initial protection. It is necessary, therefore, to follow certain vaccination schedules. The accompanying table gives a recommended schedule of immunizations beginning at birth. For children who have not received prior vaccinations, these may, of course, be begun at any time; but always remember, the sooner, the better! If a child has already passed the age of five, he will not usually receive measles or whooping cough vaccine. An adult would receive the special diphtheria-tetanus combined toxoid for adult use, but should receive smallpox and polio vaccines in the same schedule as children.

Many parents become confused when they realize that one of their children may have received only two of a series of three injections (such as DPT or Salk polio vaccine). "Do I need to start over?" is a frequent question. Often, if the time elapsed since the previous two is less than one year, the answer is no. Your physician or local health department is the best source of advice under such circumstances. The most important consideration is not to delay further.

Common Communicable Diseases

In this section are listed some of the commonly encountered communicable diseases with pertinent information regarding their cause and control. The diseases are listed in alphabetical order. The information is modified from the Report of the Committee on the Control of Infectious Diseases of the American Academy of Pediatrics.

Special attention should be called to the fact that state laws and local health department regulations regarding communicable disease vary. Therefore discrepancies may be observed between the information here set forth and the recommendations received from your local or state department of health. These differences will not be of serious importance. Your local or state recommendations and regulations must, of course, govern because they are specifically designed to meet local needs.

Chickenpox (Varicella)

Agent: A virus, closely related to, if not identical with, that causing herpes zoster (shingles).
Source: Human beings only.
Mode of transmission: Most often by direct contact with person ill with chickenpox or herpes zoster. Dry scabs are not infectious.
Incubation period: 14 to 16 days; occasionally as long as 3 weeks.
Period of communicability: Probably not earlier than 1 day before appearance of rash, and no longer than 6 days after appearance of first blisters.
Isolation of patient: Until 6 days after appearance of first blisters. No need to isolate until all crusts have dried or have fallen off.
Quarantine of contacts: None.
Care of exposed susceptibles: If exposed susceptible person is receiving cortisone or related hormones, a physician should be consulted as soon as possible.
Control measures:
   a) Immunization—None.
   b) Other—None practical.

Croup (Laryngitis)

Agent: May be bacteria or virus. Croup in most instances is a result directly or indirectly of a virus upper respiratory infection.
Source: Secretions from nose, throat, skin, and other lesions of infected persons or carriers.
Mode of transmission: Direct contact with patient or carrier; indirect contact with articles contaminated by infected persons or carrier.
Incubation period: Not uniform; varies with agent.
Period of communicability: Probably the duration of the acute illness.
Isolation of patient: Advisable.
Quarantine of contacts: None.
Care of exposed susceptibles: Close observation.

Control measures:
   a) Immunizations—None.
   b) Other—None practical.

Epidemic Diarrhea in Newborn Infants

Agent: Specific types of bacteria or viruses cause most of the outbreaks of diarrhea among newborn infants.
Source: So far as is known, all the agents are from human sources.
Mode of transmission: Because all agents are found in feces, transmission of disease by fecal contamination is most likely. Spread by infectious droplets via the air is also possible. Infection may be contracted from sick infants, from infected infants showing no symptoms, or from attendants of infants.
Incubation period: Usually 2 to 5 days.
Period of communicability: Presumably as long as the bacterium or virus is excreted in stool or is present in upper respiratory tract. This is variable with individual patient. For most types, the average period of communicability is about 2 weeks.
Isolation of patient: The infected infant should be removed from contact with other newborn infants.
Quarantine of contacts: Yes, if susceptible.
Care of exposed susceptibles: Exposed susceptible infants should be quarantined. Breast-fed infants are very rarely affected.
Control measures:
   a) Immunization—None.
   b) Other—Rigid aseptic technique in nursery. Reporting of diarrhea and other illness by nursery personnel, and thoughtful consideration of best method of dealing with each reported incident. Careful search for minor signs of infection among newborn infants in nursery, so that beginning of epidemic of diarrhea will not be overlooked. Program to encourage breast-feeding of all infants since breast-fed babies are not susceptible to this desease.

Diphtheria

Agent: Corynbacterium diphtheriae, a bacterium.
Source: Secretions from nose, throat, skin, and other lesions of infected persons or carriers.
Mode of transmission: Direct contact with patient or carrier; indirect contact with articles contaminated by infected persons or carriers.
Incubation period: 2 to 6 days; occasionally longer.
Period of communicability: Variable, usually 2 weeks or less, seldom more than 4 weeks.
Isolation of patient: Should be isolated until 3 consecutive bacterial nose and throat cultures, obtained at intervals of 24 hours or more, are all found to be free of germs.
Quarantine of contacts: Close child contacts should be quarantined until 2 successive nose and throat cultures have been obtained and 7 days have elapsed since last exposure.
Care of exposed susceptibles: Take nose and throat cultures; quarantine as above. Children in an

exposed household should receive a booster dose of toxoid immediately and be observed daily by a physician or a nurse.

Control Measures:
   a) Immunization—See previous section.
   b) Other—Distinction of articles possibly contaminated by the patient or discharges from the patient. When the disease has run its course disinfection by thorough cleaning and airing of sickroom.

Hepatitis (Infectious)

Agent: Infectious hepatis (hepatitis A) virus.
Source: Infected persons, including those undetected.
Mode of transmission: Largely via fecal contamination; possibly by secretions of nose and throat. May be spread by consumption of fecally contaminated water, food, or milk, or by blood and blood products obtained from persons carrying the hepatitis virus.
Incubation period: 10 to 50 days; average 25 days.
Period of communicability: Unknown. Virus has been detected in blood and feces 2 to 3 weeks before onset of disease, as well as during the acute stage. It is not known how long virus persists in these materials.
Isolation of patient: Recommended for first week.
Quarantine of contacts: Not feasible.
Care of exposed susceptibles: Passive immunization for approximately 6 weeks can be achieved by intramuscular injection of gamma globulin.
Control measures:
   a) Active immunization—None.
   b) Passive immunization—Gamma globulin.
   c) Other—Environmental sanitation (community, personal and hospital) may limit the spread of infectious hepatitis virus.

Hepatitis (Serum)

Agent: Serum hepatis (hepatitis B) virus.
Source: Infected persons, including those undetected.
Mode of transmission: Through transfusions of blood or plasma which have been obtained from carriers of the hepatitis B virus. Through the use of needles or syringes or equipment for inoculations which have not been thoroughly and adequately sterilized and which may have been contaminated with hepatitis B virus.
Incubation period: 60-160 days.
Period of communicability: Unknown.
Isolation of patient: Not necessary.
Quarantine of contacts: Not necessary.
Care of exposed susceptibles: Gamma globulin may be used depending upon the circumstances and the strength of the evidence that an individual has been exposed.
Control measures:
   a) Immunizations—None.
   b) Other—Adequate screening of blood donors to eliminate those who may be carriers of the virus. Persons who have been jaundiced or exposed to hepatitis should make this known when donating blood.

Influenza (Virus)

Agent: The influenza viruses, two types, A and B, have repeatedly been encountered in recent epidemics. Types A and B include numerous distinct strains.
Source: Discharges from the mouth and nose of infected persons.
Mode of transmission: By direct contact, through droplet infection, or by articles recently contaminated by infected persons; possibly airborne.
Incubation period: Usually 1 to 3 days.
Period of communicability: Probably briefly before onset and up to 1 week thereafter.
Isolation of patient: None required.
Quarantine of contacts: None.
Care of exposed susceptibles: None.
Control measures:
   a) Immunization—Vaccines are currently available and recommended for the elderly, or persons with chronic heart or lung diseases, as well as pregnant women. The components of the vaccine must be changed periodically and persons must be revaccinated each year. The Surgeon General of the U.S. Public Health Service announces recommendations each summer.
   b) Other—Avoiding of crowded areas for prolonged periods during the epidemic season.

Measles (Rubeola: Red Measles)

Agent: A Virus.
Source: Secretions of nose and throat of infected persons.
Mode of transmission: Droplet spread by coughs or sneezes or direct contact with infected persons; indirectly by articles freshly contaminated with nasal and oral secretions; airborne in some instances.
Incubation period: 7 to 14 days, usually 10 days; gamma globulin may extend incubation period to 21 days.
Period of communicability: Particularly infective during coughing stage; usually 5 to 9 days, from 4 days before to possibly 5 days after the rash appears.
Isolation of patient: From first appearance of early signs until 4 to 5 days following appearance of rash, or about 8 days in all; longer if period before rash exceeds 4 days.
Quarantine of contacts: During epidemics in large communities, quarantine of exposed children is of little value in control of spread. Where conditions warrant, quarantine from 7th to 14th day after known exposure.
Care of exposed susceptibles: Gamma globulin.
Control measures:
   a) Active Immunization—See previous section.
   b) Passive Immunization—Gamma globulin given early after exposure may modify the disease.
   c) Other—Concurrent disinfection of all articles soiled by nose and throat secretions. After disease has run its course, disinfection by thorough cleaning and airing.

Measles, German (Rubella, "3-Day Measles")

Agent: The virus of rubella.

Source: Secretions of nose and throat of infected persons.

Mode of transmission: Direct contact with or droplet spread from patient or indirect contact with freshly contaminated articles.

Incubation period: 14 to 25 days; usually about 18 days.

Period of communicability: During the period of early symptoms and at least 4 days thereafter.

Isolation of patient: Where warranted, isolation from first appearance of symptoms until 5 days following appearance of rash.

Quarantine of contacts: None (Girls should have rubella whenever possible before childbearing period.)

Care of exposed susceptibles: None.

Control measures:
    a) Immunization—None.
    b) Other—None.

Meningococcal Meningitis

Agent: The meningococcus, a bacterium.

Source: An infected person with symptoms of respiratory tract infection, septicemia or meningitis, or a healthy carrier.

Mode of transmission: Most often by direct contact, probably by inhalation of droplets containing meningococci.

Incubation period: Variable. In the majority of cases, 3 to 7 days, with range of 1 to 10 days.

Period of communicability: As long as meningococci are present in nose and throat. This period is greatly shortened by treatment with a sulfa drug, probably not exceeding 48 hours after beginning of therapy.

Isolation of patient: Patient isolated for 48 hours after start of sulfonamide therapy.

Quarantine of contacts: None.

Care of exposed susceptibles: Close observation. Sulfadiazine may be prescribed by the physician.

Control measures:
    a) Immunizations—None.
    b) Other—In an epidemic in a school or military establishment, it may be advisable to give all personnel drug prophylaxis.

Mononucleosis (Infectious)

Agent: Unknown, presumably a virus.

Source: Infected persons.

Mode of transmission: Probably by direct contact or droplets from nose and throat of infected persons.

Incubation period: Thought to be 4 to 14 days.

Period of communicability: Unknown.

Isolation of patient: None.

Quarantine of contacts: None.

Care of exposed susceptibles: None.

Control Measures:
    a) Immunizations—None.
    b) Other—None.

Mumps

Agent: A virus.

Source: Saliva of infected persons.

Mode of transmission: Direct contact with or droplet spread from an infected person or indirect contact with contaminated articles of such a person.

Incubation period: 14 to 28 days; average 18 days.

Period of communicability: Fairly well established; virus may be in saliva from 1 to 6 days before onset of swelling or other clinical symptoms and may persist until glandular swelling has disappeared. Unrecognized infection occurs in about 40 per cent of exposed individuals.

Isolation of patient: Until swelling is subsided.

Quarantine of contacts: None.

Care of exposed susceptibles: Except under unusual circumstances, children should be allowed to develop mumps.

Control measures:
    a) Immunizations—None.
    b) Other—Concurrent disinfection of articles soiled with secretions of nose and throat.

Poliomyelitis

Agent: A virus of which there are 3 distinct types, types 1, 2, and 3. Type 1 has most frequently been the cause of epidemic paralytic disease.

Source: Feces and material from nose and throat of patients and carriers. Man is the only known natural host.

Mode of transmission: Probably by direct intimate contact with patient or carrier.

Incubation period: Usually 7-14 days, but may be less than 7 days.

Period of communicability: Not known exactly, but presumably corresponds to the time during which virus is present in the throat or feces. Virus can be found in the throat for several days before the onset of symptoms and for approximately 5 days afterwards. Virus can be recovered from the feces of most patients during the first week of illness, becomes progressively more difficult to find thereafter, but may be present for a month or more.

Isolation of patient: Most communities require isolation for 1 week. As noted above, the patient is potentially infectious for a month or more.

Quarantine of contacts: Not feasible.

Care of exposed susceptibles: Should be vaccinated immediately.

Control measures:
    a) Immunization—See previous section.
    b) Other—None practical.

Staphylococcal Infections
(Sties, Boils, Furuncles, Carbuncles, Nail Infections)

Agent: Staphylococcus aureus, a bacterium; a few particular strains seem to be particularly pathogenic.

Source: Other human beings; either carriers or persons with actual infection.

Mode of transmission: Person to person by direct contact, or by articles contaminated by infected persons.

Incubation period: 1 or 2 days to many weeks. A person may be a carrier for many weeks before an infection develops.

Period of communicability: As long as the staphylococcus is present in the discharges of the infected person.

Isolation of patient: Not practical except in hospitals.

Quarantine of contacts: None.

Care of exposed susceptibles: Adequate personal hygiene, hand washing, regular change of clothing, etc.

Control measures:
a) Immunizations—None.
b) Other—Same as care of exposed.

Streptococcal Infections

Agent: Hemolytic streptococci, a group of bacteria.

Source: From infected persons or from articles contaminated with hemolytic streptococci.

Mode of transmission: Direct contact and droplet infection.

Incubation period: 2 to 5 days.

Period of communicability: Until recovered or for 24 hours after beginning of antibiotic therapy.

Isolation of patient: Unnecessary if properly treated with antibiotics.

Quarantine of contacts: None.

Care of exposed susceptibles: None recommended by most health departments. However, in certain circumstances it may be desirable to have cultures taken of the exposed individuals, especially intimate family and hospital contacts, and to treat those with positive cultures, especially if the original case developed nephritis. The importance of careful investigation and adequate treatment of any contact who has a history of rheumatic fever cannot be overestimated.

Control measures:
a) Immunizations—None.
b) Other—None.

Tetanus

Agent: Clostridium Tetani, a spore-forming bacterium.

Source: Soil, street dust, animal, or human feces; articles contaminated with organisms.

Mode of transmission: Direct or indirect contamination of an obvious or minor wound or scratch.

Incubation period: 3 days to 3 weeks, depending on circumstances; average 10 days, occasionally longer, especially when patient has received partial protection from tetanus antitoxin.

Period of communicability: None.

Isolation of patient: None except to minimize nervous stimulation.

Quarantine of contacts: None.

Care of exposed susceptibles: None.

Control measures:
a) Immunization—See previous section.
b) Other—In addition to appropriate administration of toxoid and/or antitoxin to a patient with a suspicious wound, the wound should be cleaned by a physician.

Tuberculosis

Agent: Mycobacterium tuberculosis, a bacterium.

Source: An infected individual or articles contaminated with the organism.

Mode of transmission: Direct contact or droplet spread from an infected person; indirectly by contact with freshly contaminated articles of such a person.

Incubation period: 2 to 10 weeks

Period of communicability: Children with uncomplicated primary tuberculosis are usually noninfectious. Children with lung cavities, reinfection type tuberculosis, or draining sinuses are infectious so long as bacteria are present.

Isolation of patient: Children with infectious complications should be isolated until laboratory studies are consistently negative. Care should be exercised to prevent contamination with infected pus or excreta from the patient. The patient with infectious pulmonary disease (positive sputum) should wear a nose and mouth mask.

Quarantine of contacts: None. Careful search for and examination (including chest x-ray) of contacts, particularly adults, should be carried out to determine source of the child's infection. This should apply to all members of household, including servants, nurses, and baby sitters, as well as frequent visitors to the home, neighbors, and others, if necessary.

Care of exposed susceptibles: Repeated physical examinations, tuberculin tests, chest films, and observation for a number of years.

Control measures:
a) Immunization—BCG vaccine under special circumstances as advised by the physician.
b) Other—Education about tuberculosis, its mode of spread and methods of control.

Typhoid Fever

Agent: Salmonella typhi, a bacterium.

Source: Feces and urine of patients and carriers.

Mode of transmission: Direct or indirect contact with patients or carriers, usually from hands. Principal vehicles are water and food, sometimes milk. Flies may spread the infection.

Incubation period: 7 to 21 days; average 14.

Period of communicability: As long as patients or carriers harbor organisms.

Isolation of patient: Required until 3 consecutive negative stool cultures are obtained, taken at least 24 hours apart and not earlier than 1 month after onset.

Quarantine of contacts: None. Family contacts should be excluded as food handlers until 3 successive negative stool and urine cultures from them have been obtained.

Care of exposed susceptibles: Remove from contact and inoculate with typhoid vaccine if risk of repeated exposure exists. Exposed food handlers should be excluded from work until negative cultures are obtained.

Control measures:
a) Immunization—Under special circumstances as advised by your physician.
b) Other—Proper sanitation of water, food, and disposal of human excretions.

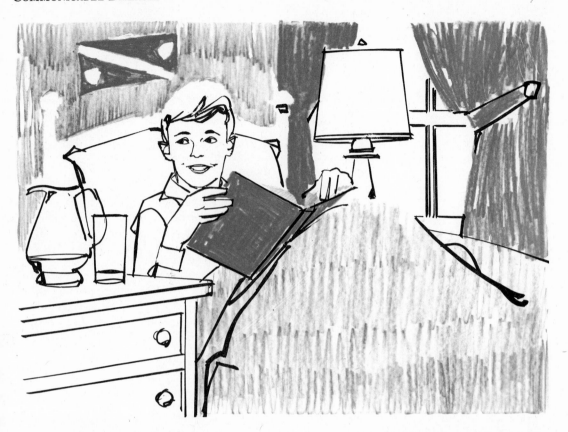

Whooping Cough (Pertussis)

Agent: Bordetella pertussis, a bacterium.

Source: Discharges from the respiratory mucous membranes of infected persons.

Mode of transmission: Direct contact or droplet spread from an infected person; indirectly by contact with freshly contaminated articles of such a person.

Incubation period: 5 to 21 days; almost uniformly within 10 days.

Period of communicability: Greatest in coughing stage before onset of whooping. The organism rarely can be found after the 4th week of the disease, and after 6 weeks patients may be considered non-infectious.

Isolation of patient: Should be isolated but not kept indoors for 3 weeks from onset of whooping.

Quarantine of contacts: Non-immunized children should be quarantined for 14 days following household exposure.

Care of exposed susceptibles: Gamma globulin for those under age 2 who have not been vaccinated formerly against the disease.

Control measures:

    a) Immunization—See previous section.

    b) Other—Concurrent disinfection of discharges from nose and throat and articles soiled thereby. Disinfection and thorough cleaning of the sickroom after the illness. Protection of very young infants is difficult since maternal antibody is not transmitted and the young infant's antibody response to active immunization may be retarded. The best protection for such young infants comes from avoiding household contacts with whooping cough, which is best assured by adequate immunization of all older brothers and sisters.

Disease Prevention

Most common infectious diseases of man are spread from person to person. When a person is infected, germs frequently are found on his body and clothing. Anyone who comes in contact with the patient or his clothing may carry away the germs. The patient, of course, may leave germs on articles he touches such as dishes, towels, bed clothing, or food, and a healthy person may pick up germs by using the contaminated article. Some diseases may be spread through the air. A sick person may release germs by coughing or sneezing, and a healthy person may inhale the contaminated air.

Other diseases are transferred from animals to man. Most of these are transmitted through the bites of insects such as mosquitos, ticks, mites, fleas, or lice. Adequate protection of the home from insects, particularly in areas where insect-borne diseases are common, is necessary to prevent their transmission. Adequate knowledge of the care of household pets and the potential dangers in the spread of disease by such pets should be obtained from a veterinarian before pets are brought into the home.

Because of the many factors which help cause disease, one can do many things to prevent infection in the family. As we have already seen, natural resistance is quite important in disease. Therefore, one should keep his body as healthy as possible. Good nutrition, plenty of rest, fresh air, and frequent exercise to maintain a high degree of natural resistance comprise the first step in preventing illness.

Good personal hygiene and body cleanliness reduce the number of germs on the body and clothing. Also, if one does come in contact with sick people, the number of germs carried away and the length of time you carry them may be reduced by frequent handwashing and bathing. Frequent changes of clothing with frequent laundering likewise reduce the number of germs which may eventually gain entrance to the body. Children should be taught at an early age to wash their hands with soap and water after using the toilet, after playing, and before eating and going to bed.

Since sick persons expel many more germs than healthy carriers or persons only mildly ill, protection of the family from persons with known communicable disease will reduce the degree of the exposure. The number of germs entering the body is one of the factors in causing disease. Thus, the fewer germs that enter the body, the less likelihood of developing illness, or if illness does develop, the less likelihood of that illness being a severe one. If it is necessary to visit a person ill with a communicable disease, the shorter the visit, the fewer will be the number of germs encountered. Under such circumstances, do not touch the ill person, his bed, or any of his personal articles. Immediately upon leaving his presence, wash your hands thoroughly with soap and water.

During epidemics of such common diseases as mumps, influenza, strep throat, or poliomyelitis, take care to avoid crowded, confined areas for long periods of time. Under such circumstances the air, dust, and clothing become filled with infectious particles from the nose and mouth of infected individuals. Close quarters greatly increase the opportunity for spread of such infection. Adequate ventilation and fresh air go a long way to reduce and disperse the number of such germs. Now that the water of most public swimming pools is adequately

safeguarded, the greatest danger in summer sports or camping activities during epidemic seasons is undue fatigue, which reduces one's natural resistance to infection.

If a person in the household becomes ill, he should remain in bed in a room by himself. Contact with other household members should be kept at a minimum and care taken in the disposal of bodily excretions. In the case of vomitus and diarrhea, these can be disposed of safely in a flush toilet. If such sewage facilities are not available, the excretions should be mixed thoroughly with chloride of lime for one hour before disposal. Disposable paper handkerchiefs should be used for nasal secretions and sputum then placed in a paper bag, and burned at periodic intervals. Any food that the patient does not consume should be discarded, and all dishes should be washed thoroughly with soap and hot water. Little is to be gained by boiling dishes if proper cleansing procedures are followed.

After the patient recovers, bed clothing and other washable items should be thoroughly laundered with soap and hot water. Here again, little is gained by boiling unless such clothing is unusually contaminated. The room and its contents should be thoroughly ventilated. It is no longer necessary to destroy valuable property, such as mattresses, pillows, or clothing; washing, dry cleaning, airing, and sunshine will make them safe to use again.

The Health Department's Role

Communicable diseases frequently occur as epidemics within the community. When the number of cases of a disease exceeds the usual and expected amount, it is termed an epidemic. Epidemics have certain characteristics which may give clues to their cause. These characteristics include, among others, the time of year in which they occur, the age of the people affected, and the patterns of transmission of the disease.

It is the responsibility of the local health department to keep adequate records of communicable diseases. These records may be used as a guide for community action against disease such as immunization campaigns, rodent control, and the like. Careful analysis of such records may detect impending epidemics or reveal patterns which explain their continued occurrence.

By law, it is the responsibility of every physician to report cases of certain communicable diseases to his local health department. It is the civic responsibility of every citizen to cooperate fully with his physician and health department in this important activity.

If a member of your family has a communicable disease, a representative of the health department may telephone or visit you to obtain details of the illness. By doing so, the health department may better understand how to prevent other household members or your neighbors from becoming ill. At the same time, the representatives of the health department will be a ready source of information or assistance to you in helping the patient recover and in protecting the rest of your family, as well as the rest of the community.

During epidemics, your health department, with the cooperation of the local medical society, will determine what community action, if any, should be taken. Their decisions will be based upon the analysis of records which they gather from many sources. They may issue warnings ahead of time of an impending influenza epidemic or the need for immunization of school children. They may decide to close a school (rarely) or a swimming pool, to begin mass inoculations, or they may decide not to interrupt normal community activities. Whatever the decision, the full cooperation of all citizens is essential. Every citizen should familiarize himself with the activities of his health department and should be alert for statements and advice which may come from it.

The health department does not provide medical care for communicable disease patients, except where they are hospitalized by the municipality. Medical care is the responsibility of the family and its physician.

CHAPTER FIVE

ANIMAL DISEASES AND HUMAN HEALTH

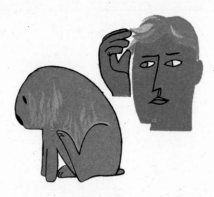

SINCE TIME IMMEMORIAL, man's search for fur, food, and fun has brought him into close contact with the lower animals, many of which he has domesticated. He has gained more than he has lost from these associations because animals have provided materials for clothing and food in the form of skins and furs and meat, milk, and eggs. They have done work for him and protected him. They have given him pleasure in the sports of hunting and racing. They have played an important role in medical research. Additionally, animals have served as friends and companions. A recent survey estimated that more than 75,000,000 dogs, cats, parakeets, canaries, finches, and other cage birds, turtles, monkeys, and skunks were being kept as pets in American homes. Every year their numbers increase.

An estimate furnished by the American Veterinary Medical Association showed the following number of pet and farm animals in the United States:

Dogs	24,130,000
Cats	22,050,000
Cattle	99,500,000
Hogs	56,982,000
Sheep	31,446,000
Goats	4,016,000
Horses, Mules	3,089,000

Understandably, man has also shared many of the diseases that afflict these animals. Of the 200 known communicable diseases of animals, the World Health Organization lists more than 100 as being potentially communicable to man. These diseases which are transmitted from animals to man and sometimes back again, are called zoonoses.

Fortunately, most of them do not cause a great deal of human illness; some, however, do. People catch most of their diseases from other people. While the zoonoses cause but a fraction of the total of human illnesses, public awareness of them has increased because of medical and veterinary progress. Unfortunately, many misleading articles and news stories have appeared about the diseases we contract from animals. Exaggeration and the "fear" approach promote readership, but often distort the facts.

Since Americans presumably will continue to own pets, raise livestock, and wander through forests, we will probably also continue to have zoonoses in the United States. Control and eradication of these diseases depend upon better knowledge of the problem and upon cooperative efforts with agencies and professions dealing with the prevention, control, and treatment of these diseases.

Significant Zoonoses

Brucellosis (malta fever, undulant fever, or Bang's disease) is one of the most common diseases transmitted from animals to man. In man it is usually a generalized infection characterized by either a sudden or slow onset. It may resemble the flu with such symptoms as headache, fatigue, chills, sweat, and loss of weight. The symptoms may persist for days or months. Repeated attacks may occur.

People contract the disease primarily by using unpasteurized milk and through direct contact with infected cattle, pigs, or goats. The disease organisms are found in the animal excretions and secretions (milk included), and especially in the afterbirth and vaginal discharges.

The germs may enter through either broken or unbroken skin, and through the mouth, eyes, and air passages. Animal products such as raw milk and other unpasteurized dairy products also serve as sources for human infection. Most human cases are seen among occupational groups that have contact with infected animals. These include farmers and their families, meat industry workers, veterinarians, and others who raise, handle, or market animals and animal products.

A recent report by the Public Health Service Committee on Brucellosis indicates that from 1957 to 1960 the percentage of human cases of brucellosis due to contact with infected hogs increased, while those from infected cattle decreased. The same report revealed that the probable source of nine per cent of the 1960 human cases was contaminated raw milk. Human cases have steadily declined in the United States since 1947, primarily through state and federal brucellosis eradication programs. Continued support of swine and cattle brucellosis eradication programs should result in further declines.

Pasteurization of milk and dairy products and wearing gloves when handling potentially diseased animal tissues will help control and prevent the disease in man. Immediate and proper disposal of infected fetuses and placentae is necessary. The disease will cease to occur in man only when we have eliminated the disease in animals.

Leptospirosis (lepto, swine herder's disease, infectious jaundice) causes more economic loss in domestic animals in the United States than does brucellosis. The disease in many animals ranges from a mild "flu-like" form to a severe or fatal form. Animals that spread the disease to man are cattle, pigs, dogs, rats, sheep, goats, cats, skunks, foxes, mice, and other wildlife. The most common symptom seen in cattle and swine is that of abortion. Farm persons handling the aborted material including the weak or dead pigs are apt to contract the disease.

The leptospirosis germ infects the kidneys and thus many infected animals continue to shed the germs in their urine for weeks or months. Many young children and adults have contracted the disease by swimming in farm ponds or slow-moving streams thus contaminated. Most people who catch leptospirosis are livestock farmers, agricultural, packinghouse,

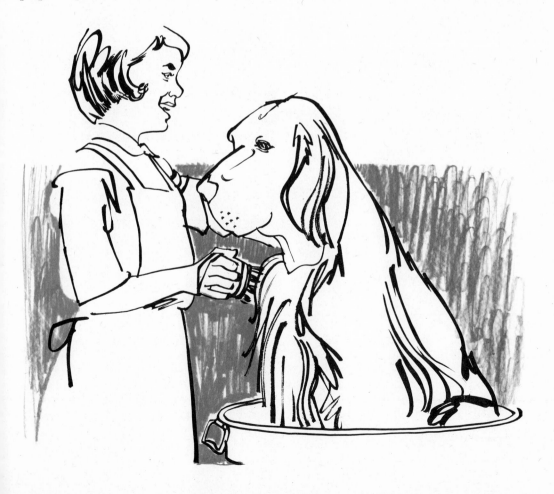

fishery, sewer, and dock workers, and persons who have considerable contact with damp or moist ground that has been contaminated by infected animals.

The germs usually enter the body through the eyes, nose, or mouth, or through a cut or break in the skin. Most human cases occur in the warm period from July through September, but cases do occur in other months of the year.

Proper diagnosis by a veterinarian of the condition in animals is essential. Vaccines are available for several of the animal species. Drinking water for animals and human beings should be protected from contamination. People should not swim in water (particularly farm ponds) frequented by infected animals. Rodent destruction is also helpful. Workers dealing with potentially contaminated materials should wear boots and gloves.

Viral Encephalitis (Eastern Encephalitis, St. Louis Encephalitis, Western Encephalitis) is most commonly called "sleeping sickness." Its characteristics are fever, confusion, and delirium or coma.

The three types of encephalitis are important mosquito-transmitted diseases seen primarily during the summer months. In the United States they are common infections among wild and domestic birds, horses, and occasionally mules and man. An outbreak of Eastern Encephalitis in an eastern state in 1959 caused 21 human deaths. An outbreak in a southeastern state involved more than 176 persons of whom 19 died. Birds appear to be the reservoir of infection, but mosquitoes pass the disease from birds to man and other animals. Man does not get the disease from horses. Vaccines are available for horses and mules, but similar vaccines have not been recommended for general use with people. Destruction of adult mosquitoes and larvae by sprays and the use of repellents is recommended. Other preventive measures include screening of sleeping and living quarters and the elimination of stagnant water pools where mosquitoes breed.

Psittacosis (Ornithosis, Parrot Fever) is caused by a virus and is widespread among all types of birds, both domestic and wild. People catch it by inhaling the virus. Birds do not usually show any symptoms of the disease and may shed the virus in droppings and nasal discharges for weeks or months. The persons who most commonly catch the disease are those who have direct contact with such psittacine birds as parrots and parakeets, as well as those who work in or around turkey and chicken pro-

cessing plants, pet shops, aviaries, and pigeon lofts.

The disease in man resembles pneumonia with fever and a headache. Regulations concerning the importation of birds, quarantine, and the use of medicated feeds have aided in reducing human cases. Pet birds should be purchased from reputable dealers. Local public health officials should know if particular dealers have had problems with this disease. The practice of feeding pet birds from the lips should be avoided. When cleaning cages, care should be taken to avoid inhaling dried droppings and to wash the hands afterward.

Q-Fever is caused by an organism that man contracts from infected cattle, sheep, and goats. Ticks may transmit the disease from animal to animal, and occasionally but rarely to man. Animals do not usually show symptoms. In man, vague symptoms with fever make diagnosis difficult.

Infected animals discharge large numbers of germs in birth materials. Raw milk has been considered a source in some instances. Man contracts the disease by inhaling the organism on dust particles contaminated by animal discharges.

Since this organism can be airborne, persons not directly involved with the raising, handling, or slaughtering of cattle, sheep, or goats may contract the disease. Thus mechanics who repair the trucks that haul these animals may contract the disease as well as barbers who inhale the organisms carried on the hair or clothing of clients.

Control of the infection is difficult since it causes no symptoms in animals and is contracted by inhalation of the organism. Vaccination of high-risk occupational groups is recommended. Proper disposal of infected animal tissues and pasteurization of milk will help reduce the disease in man, but it will not be eradicated until the disease is controlled in the animal population.

Rabies (Hydrophobia, Mad Rage) is an acute disease of the central nervous system caused by a virus. All warm-blooded animals are susceptible. The virus is transmitted to man by the bite of a rabid animal or, more rarely, by the saliva of an infected animal entering an open wound or scratch. Once the symptoms appear in man, death invariably follows. In terms of the number of human deaths each year in the United States, rabies is not of major concern. But in terms of anxiety for those bitten and economic losses of domestic animals for farmers, it is of paramount importance. The animals principally involved in spreading rabies vary from region to region in the United States. Since 1960, more cases of rabies have been reported in wildlife species than in domestic farm animals, dogs, or cats. Skunks, foxes, bats, and raccoons are the primary wildlife victims. Rabies is becoming increasingly common. In 1961, 186 cases of bat rabies were reported from 28 states as compared with 88 cases in 18 states in 1960. In 1963, 38 states reported cases of bat rabies. Between 1951 and 1960, six human deaths were attributed to the bite of rabid bats.

Rabies vaccination programs have helped reduce dog and cat rabies in urban areas, but more preventive measures are needed in rural areas where wildlife rabies is emerging as a major problem for farm families and their livestock. Each year, more than 30,000 persons find it necessary to take the lengthy, painful, and expensive antirabies treatment, because they were bitten by a suspected or known rabid animal.

Do's and don'ts for rabies control and prevention include:

1. If bitten by an animal, immediately wash the wound thoroughly and briskly with soap and water and then phone a physician and describe the circumstances surrounding the bite incident.

2. Identify and restrain if possible the animal that did the biting. Use care if the animal is wild. Do not shoot the animal through the head. Call a veterinarian for proper evaluation and diagnosis of the symptoms in the animal. Give him your physician's name. The veterinarian will know whether to quarantine the animal for observation or send the brain to a laboratory for testing. These steps are important to help your physician decide whether or not antirabies treatment should be started.

3. Have dogs or cats vaccinated with antirabies vaccine. Veterinarians can advise about types of vaccines and when they should be administered.

4. In caring for sick farm animals or pets, take care to avoid being bitten. Children should be warned not to handle strange-acting or sick wild animals, including bats.

5. Urge adequate laws controlling stray animals and insist on their enforcement.

6. Request additional information on rabies pertinent to your locality from your local or state health department.

Ringworm is a disease or group of diseases caused by a large number of species of fungi that affect the skin, hair, and nails. These infections are widespread in both man and many kinds of pets, domestic farm animals, and wildlife. The fungi grow on the skin and in the hair follicles. The hair often breaks and in many cases, the skin becomes inflamed. Exposed parts of the body such as the hands, face, arms, and neck are most commonly affected. Man becomes infected by direct contact with infected animals or indirectly by contact with contaminated bedding, straw, feed, horse halters and ropes, and animal hair in the environment.

In urban areas, most ringworm is caught from infected dogs and cats. In one family that had recently purchased a young kitten that had ringworm, four cases occurred in children. The oldest boy was affected most because he slept with the pet. Infected cattle, primarily young calves, appear to be the major source for human infection in rural areas.

Regular grooming of pets allows for early detection of infected areas. When ringworm is suspected in your pet, take him to your veterinarian for proper diagnosis and treatment. A drug called griseofulvin has been used with success in both man and animals.

Salmonella infection is a term used to cover a large group of infections common to man and many types of animals and birds. They are primarily intestinal infections that cause fever, diarrhea, and a wide range of symptoms. The symptoms observed depend upon age, resistance, type and numbers of organisms consumed, and species of salmonellae. Among the bacteria in this group are those causing typhoid fever, paratyphoid fever, bacillary dysentery, and some food infections. Newborn animals and young children are the most seriously affected. Following infection, many animals remain carriers of the organism for indefinite periods. Fowl, pigs, mice, and rats appear to play a major role in the spread of the organisms via their feces.

Many food infections are caused by salmonella germs. Almost all species of salmonella organisms grow rapidly in such foods as eggs, meat, and milk from infected animals. They can survive for long periods outside the animal body.

Flies and other insects may carry the organisms from animal discharges to food items. Since these organisms can grow in most foods, proper sanitation and keeping mice, rats, and flies out of the house are necessary. Proper cooking renders most foods safe. A good rule:

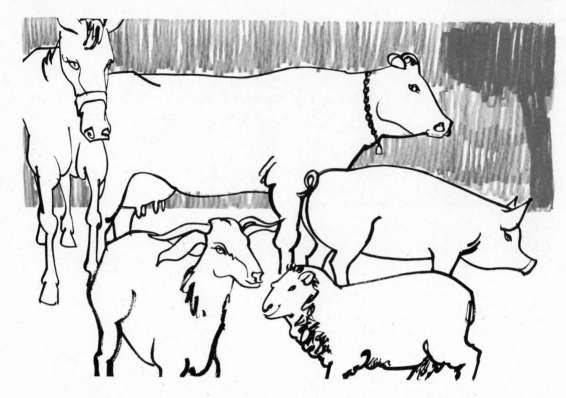

Always keep hot foods hot and cold foods cold prior to eating.

Trichinosis is a disease caused by eating raw or improperly cooked flesh of pigs or other meat-eating animals infected with the larvae of a roundworm, Trichinella spiralis. In the United States, pork and pork products are the major source of human infection. Symptoms in man include fever, muscle pain, sweat, chills, vomiting, and swollen eyelids. A midwestern state reported an outbreak of 18 cases among 25 members of 10 families who had eaten un-cooked, homemade smoked pork sausage. Seven persons who ate the sausage did not be-come ill. Trichinosis can be avoided if pork is always well-cooked or properly cured before it is eaten.

Tularemia (rabbit fever, deer fly fever) is primarily a disease of wild animals (principally rodents and rabbits) and some of their external parasites. People become infected with it by contact with infected animals while dressing them to eat. They may also contract the dis-ease as a result of a bite from an infected fly or tick that has previously fed on a tularemia-infected animal.

Human cases occur in the United States dur-ing every month of the year, but vary by region because of different hunting laws, animal species, and insect carriers. The cases are fre-quently unrecognized. A small sore occurs at the site of infection, followed by fever and symptoms mistaken for flu.

Control measures involve avoidance of bites and drinking raw stream water, the use of rub-ber gloves when dressing wild game, and proper cooking of such game meat.

Hunters should check with local or state health departments for the major sources of tularemia in their area. They will give ad-ditional information on prevention. Early di-agnosis and treatment by a physician is essential as this disease can be fatal without treatment.

Round worms, a chronic and usually mild infection caused by the larval stage of round-worm parasites, is carried by dogs and cats. Young children who frequently eat soil con-taminated with infective Toxocara eggs from infected dogs and cats are most often infected.

The true number of human cases each year is unknown because diagnosis of the disease is difficult. It depends on the discovery of the eggs in the feces of the patient. These preventive measures will help:

● Cover children's sandboxes when not in use to avoid frequenting by cats.

● Remove stools of dogs and cats from areas where children frequently play.

● Discourage children from eating dirt and

encourage them to wash their hands after playing in the soil.

• Have a veterinarian test a stool specimen from pet dogs or cats every six months or as needed to determine whether the pet is infected or not.

Periodic treatment by a veterinarian may be necessary. Do not rely on patent "shotgun" capsules that guarantee 100 per cent treatment for all types of worms. Money will be saved by first consulting a veterinarian.

Tips on Pet Care

Zoonoses will vary depending upon where you live, in an urban or rural area, and the pet involved. When a physician is consulted, he should be told of animal contacts in case the illness may be one of animal origin.

Animal care and feeding are complex sciences. As a trained medical man, the veterinarian has the modern techniques to help keep pets healthy and alive. The following tips may be useful for those with pets in the home.

1. Only persons who will take good care of pets should own them. Proper grooming, feeding, exercise, attention, discipline, and medical care are "musts."

2. Children should be taught not to tease or abuse pets, especially when the pet is eating.

3. Do not break up dog fights: you risk being bitten.

4. Place the telephone number of a veterinarian (along with the fire department number, police department number, and physician's number) next to your telephone. In case of an emergency, the babysitter or friend who is caring for pets should know whom to call.

5. Keep pet medicines separated from human medicines and keep both out of the reach of children.

6. Raw milk and candy do not cause worms in pets and garlic is not a worm remedy. Old wives' tales and "neighbor's helpful hints" regarding animal or human medical care are not substitutes for proper professional advice.

7. The indiscriminate use of antibiotics or "patent" animal drugs can be disastrous without proper veterinary advice. Many patent medicine advertisements state that they will "check" or "control" or "relieve" a multitude of conditions, but words such as these can often be misleading and guarantee little.

8. Many persons believe that a dog that scoots its rear end along the ground or over a floor has worms. In the majority of instances, the dog has impacted or full anal glands that do not empty properly. This condition may cause considerable irritation and can be relieved by having a veterinarian empty the glands periodically. Many pets have received needless worm treatments when, in fact, they have had full anal glands or some other condition such as allergic dermatitis.

9. In addition to controlling fleas on dogs or cats, you must also eliminate the fleas from the pet's bedding and home surroundings. Seek professional advice. When flea sprays or dips are purchased from sources other than a veterinarian, read the directions carefully. Some products cannot be used for both dogs and cats.

10. For additional information regarding public health aspects of animal diseases, consult a physician, veterinarian, public health nurse, local or state health department personnel, or county agricultural extension director.

CHAPTER SIX

DISASTER HEALTH CARE

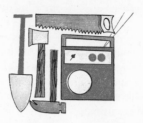

WHEN DISASTER STRIKES, how many people will be its victims and whether they die or are crippled will depend to a great extent on how well the community and its homes are prepared to meet such emergencies. Americans have traditionally worked together to combat disasters, as families and as communities. Pioneers fought hostile Indians from their wagon trains and from stockades. Groups of farmers rebuilt neighbors' barns or houses destroyed by fire. The hazards of pioneer life are gone, but the hazards of earthquake, hurricane, flood, epidemics, explosions, and fire are still with us.

Today, thermonuclear warfare is considered to be the ultimate type of disaster, but the local community stricken by storm, fire, earthquake, or explosion may well face almost as high casualty rates as would the nation in case of nuclear war. A village inundated by flood, with a loss of over 4,000 lives, is devastated as surely as if it were hit by a multimegaton bomb. The fact that a disaster is limited to a small area makes it no less horrifying for those who are within that area.

We live in a highly centralized and very convenient civilization. In the United States today we can obtain pure drinking water by merely turning on a tap and hot water by turning on another. Sewage disposal is seldom a problem because of our intricate systems of sewer pipes and sewage disposal plants. Electric power supplies us with light and often heat for cooking. It operates the sump pumps in our basements and supplies power for refrigeration and many other facilities which we have come to take for granted. We get our choice of food by merely going to the nearest market or by telephoning and ordering it sent to our homes. The telephone can also obtain for us, if necessary, medical care, fire and police protection, and almost every other conceivable service.

All these services make our lives easy in normal times. The fact that we depend so greatly on them, however, contributes to our weakness in case of a large-scale disaster. What happens to the average community or family in a disaster area? First of all, the electric power supply is impaired. Without electricity there are no lights, radios and television sets will no longer function, and refrigeration will last for only a short time. If the heating plant is operated electrically, it will cease to function.

The telephone lines may well be out of operation, making it difficult to summon help from the fire or police department or to contact the family physician or local hospital. Even if they can be contacted, the condition of the roads and streets may make it impossible for them to reach you. If the grocery stores survive the disaster, their contents may be so damaged as to be unsafe to use. Food stored at home in refrigerators or freezers will not keep from spoiling for longer than a day or two.

The water of many communities is pumped from a well, reservoir, or lake by electric pumps. If the pumping station is damaged, the water supply will quickly be exhausted. Or the disaster may damage water mains so badly that contamination makes the water no longer safe.

When we stop to consider how disaster can disrupt the modern, overcentralized American urban community hit by disaster, we come to realize that perhaps the safest place to be in a disaster would be far from the city, perhaps on a farm. Many farms have storage places for food. Their water supply comes from an individual well and is often pumped by hand. Many farms have stoves that can burn wood cut nearby and stored at the farm house. Sewage disposal on the farm may be primitive, but such methods will continue to function long after the intricate city sewer system becomes useless.

Despite this bleak picture, city dwellers can survive a major disaster provided they know some simple basic procedures to follow.

Disease Prevention

Disease thrives under disaster conditions. Prevention of disease involves sanitation, isolation, and immunization.

Sanitation involves the proper disposal of

waste, especially human waste, and the control of whatever may carry disease. Disease carriers include rodents, house flies, roaches, mosquitoes, and other insects.

Isolation refers to the process by which the individual with a communicable disease is kept separated from healthy individuals, as nearly as possible, to prevent the spread of his disease. Isolation is not always easy under disaster conditions, but may always be carried out to a certain degree. The person who covers his mouth while coughing is practicing isolation.

In the disruption of community facilities which follows a disaster, isolation becomes more difficult. It becomes doubly important, however, because infections spread more easily in such conditions. Thus, instruction and guidance should be sought as to how to care for a patient with a communicable disease with the least risk of infecting others.

Immunization is the best form of preventive medicine. It is an especially practical step in preparing for disaster situations because it can be taken in advance.

Those best prepared to weather limited or widespread disasters are the persons who have heeded the constantly repeated advice of medical and public health authorities to become properly immunized against disease. The subject of immunization is dealt with in Chapter Four of this section.

Seeking Safety

The home and place of employment should be examined in advance to decide where will be the safest place in case of a disaster. Whenever possible, this area should be distant from windows since ordinary glass presents a particular hazard in storms and explosions. Under most disaster circumstances, the safest place in a building will be the basement. If there is no basement, then the most central portion of the building, such as an interior corridor, will be the area of choice. Obviously a basement will provide protection only if it does not flood. In those disasters which involve flooding, it may not be possible to use any area of the house which is below ground level. Sump pumps cannot be relied upon to keep your basement dry, since the electric power may be nonexistent.

Utilities

All members of the family should know where to shut off the gas valves in case the disaster ruptures gas mains. Never hunt for a gas leak with any type of flame such as a candle or match. Since any disaster may cause shortcircuiting of wires within the building, everyone should also know where to turn off the main electrical switch in order to prevent fire.

Several flashlights should always be kept in reserve for an emergency created by electric or gas failure. If these are not available or if they are inadequate, candles, matches, or lanterns may be used only if there is definitely no danger of explosion. Avoid setting candles or lanterns near anything which can catch fire.

If the heating system of the home is not operating, various types of camp stoves and portable heaters may be used. However, any heater which uses oil, gas, or coal should be utilized only if there is an abundant supply of fresh air. Otherwise, there is grave danger of carbon monoxide poisoning or suffocation.

If the disaster occurs during the cold part of the year and the heating plant stops functioning, then obviously the main objective is to conserve body heat. This can be done by using heavy winter clothing or by improvising such clothing from materials about the house. Remember again, that the use of gasoline or kerosene heaters, or any type of heater which uses a fuel, may be dangerous unless there is enough air to prevent suffocation or carbon monoxide poisoning. Light will have to be furnished by either flashlights, candles, or lanterns. Occasionally a home will have a standby generator. This of course will solve many problems including that of lighting.

Water Supply

Water supply may be a serious problem in any disaster situation. The water mains may be damaged and the central pumping station stop working. Even if there is water in the mains, it may become contaminated.

Many simple methods of treating water can make it relatively safe for drinking purposes. If water is boiled for at least one full minute after being brought to a boil, it will usually be safe from a bacteriological standpoint. Water may also be treated by adding 10 drops of ordinary household bleach to 1 gallon of water and allowing this to stand for 30 minutes before using it. An alternate method is to use 20 drops of U.S.P. Tincture of Iodine to 1 gallon of water and again allowing it to stand for 30 minutes before using.

If someone has had the foresight to store

water, such water will be safe for an indefinite period of time even though it may have a somewhat unpleasant taste. The preferable method of storing water for emergencies is in tightly sealed plastic containers. The same containers in which household bleach is sold may be ideal for this purpose if they are plastic. The little residue of chlorine left in the containers will merely render the water that much safer.

There are several sources of water within the home even after the central water supply is disrupted The hot water heater usually holds 30 to 40 gallons and, while this may be murky, it is safe to drink. The pipes of any home contain several gallons of water and there may be water in the hot water heating system. The flush tanks contain safe drinking water even though it may have some sediment in it. Canned goods, especially fruit and fruit juices, are a source of fluids in an emergency.

Sanitation

Sewage disposal methods, if the sewers are not functioning, are likely to become primitive. Even if the sewer system should be intact, it may be impossible to use it because of the lack of water for flushing. If it is safe to go out of doors, sewage may be buried or burned. Otherwise, all sewage should be carefully disposed of in waxed paper or plastic bags which are tightly closed and then disposed of in covered metal cans. Powdered chlorinated lime may be added to this sewage to deodorize it and also to keep away insect pests.

Sealed cans of chlorinated lime are extremely useful items to have on hand in case of emergency. This is an antiseptic and may be used to treat sewage or water for drinking purposes. When storing materials in anticipation of disaster, it will be well to store some insecticides and spray guns or aerosol containers of insecticides. Insects thrive on disaster conditions and many are disease carriers. It is not safe, however, to use aerosol bombs or insect sprays in confined spaces. Some individuals will become seriously ill if they breathe these sprays in high concentration. Sealing food supplies and proper waste disposal are the best ways to control insects and rodents.

Disaster Equipment

The area of the home designated for shelter in case of disaster should also be provided with certain basic tools. These should include a shovel, ax, hammer, and saw. A crowbar may be useful to move debris under which someone is trapped.

A transistorized radio should be on hand and it is urgent that its batteries be maintained fresh. This radio may be the only means of communication with the outside world for hours or even days. Only through such a radio could one learn what the situation is elsewhere and what are the hazards which must be guarded against during the time of disaster. For example, a second storm may be approaching or citizens may be warned that the water is unsafe to drink.

If the disaster situation means confinement in a shelter area beyond an hour, some method will be needed to occupy the minds of all involved, especially the children. A few simple games, toys, and books should be stored to meet this contingency.

Because of the danger of flying pieces of glass, and because windows are often blown out during storms and explosions, it is also advisable to have pre-cut plywood or other sturdy material which can be fitted rapidly over a window opening. This will serve to keep out the weather and will make the shelter area far more comfortable and safe. It might also help keep out radioactive particles in case of fallout from a distant nuclear explosion.

Emergency Treatment

First aid and the care of injuries were covered in detail in Part XI, Chapter Two. Here we will only review briefly a few basic principles which you should always remember. There is a priority in the care of the injured. For example, a man may die in a few minutes if his breathing stops but he may die in less than a minute if blood is gushing from a major blood vessel. The priority of care of the injured is this:

First, control major bleeding. Remember this applies to only large amounts of blood and not to slow oozing. Slow oozing may be controlled later.

Second, restore breathing. Do this by one of the approved methods. Mouth to mouth respiration is the best; back pressure or arm lift is second best.

Third, prevent shock and treat shock.

Fourth, treat other injuries.

Fifth, with rare exceptions, a patient should not be moved until bleeding has been stopped, respiration restored, and injuries treated.

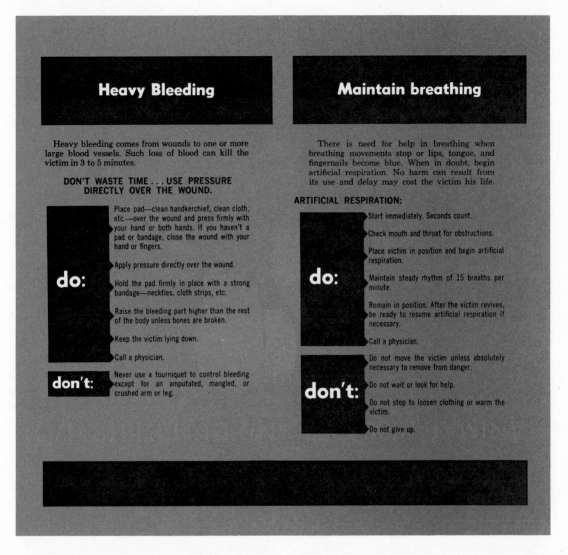

Large scale disaster may mean being cut off from medical supplies as well as medical help. For this reason, everyone should find out from his family doctor what medications he might advise keeping on hand in case of emergency. This is especially important for people who have chronic diseases such as heart disease or diabetes. An adequate supply of insulin must be on hand for diabetics; adequate means enough to last for about two months, if necessary. Oral drugs may be partial substitutes for insulin. The family physician can explain the use of these in conjunction with or in place of insulin. All diabetics should learn to administer insulin themselves since they may have to do this under disaster conditions.

Heart patients should also determine what medications they may need. The physician is best equipped to advise whether such patients need digitalis, nitroglycerin, or other drugs stored in case of disaster. He will also advise about how long these drugs will keep so that they can be replaced at proper intervals. Similarly, patients who have severe allergies should also consult their physician regarding storage of antihistamine drugs or other drugs needed to protect against severe reactions.

In some instances special foods should be stored, especially when there are infants in the home. Sometimes the very elderly also require special foods.

Nuclear Attack

Survival in nuclear disaster is possible, too. If one understands what he and his family can do to protect themselves, there is an excellent chance that the serious effects of nuclear bombing can be prevented or sharply decreased.

Survival in massive enemy attack means that everyone must be prepared to do what is necessary. Such a situation calls for a maximum civil defense effort.

The best way to protect against radiation is to provide adequate shelter. By far the greatest number of casualties from nuclear explosions would be produced by radioactive fallout. This particular effect goes far beyond the area of blast and can affect people hundreds of miles from the target area.

Radioactivity consists of rays from outer space (cosmic) and from chemicals like radium and from x-rays. It is something with which we all live every day of our lives since this effect occurs naturally from cosmic rays and mineral deposits. However, the amount of this normal radioactivity is so low that it produces no effects on people.

In a nuclear explosion the very nature of the event causes many substances to become radioactive in addition to the radioactive materials broadcast by the bomb itself. Wherever the bomb touches the earth's surface, radioactivity is created by the mixture of bomb products and earth. This material is then swept into the air by the pressure changes that take place. The material is drawn high into the atmosphere and is carried along by prevailing winds. Eventually this dust and debris settles out and falls back to the earth or is washed down by rain or snow. Where it reaches depends on the direction of the prevailing winds. Areas at varying distances from the target point could receive radioactive fallout. However, with the passage of time two things take place:

1. There is dispersal of the particles in the air which decreases their concentration.

2. The particles lose strength in a measurable and predictable way, and in time become harmless.

Until this decay of radioactivity occurs, people must be shielded against it, since living beings can tolerate only a limited dose and still survive.

Since all the effects of a nuclear bomb are known and have been studied, it has been determined that shielding—as provided by shelters—will be most effective against fallout. Brick, earth, or concrete make the best shielding materials.

The U.S. Civil Defense Administration has urged the development of community shelters. To this end it has been conducting an extensive survey of public buildings suitable for this pur-

pose. These are to be clearly marked and adequately stocked with food and medical supplies sufficient for a two-week period.

In many parts of the country, people will not be near a community shelter, or able to get to one. In such cases, families must prepare their own homes for protection. It is possible to construct a low-cost shelter in the basement of a home or in a cellar. Even if such a shelter is not constructed, every home has areas which will provide some sort of protection, and some protection is better than none.

To meet this family responsibility, one can obtain excellent information and plans together with cost estimates from one's local or state civil defense authorities. Since a home shelter must be provided with food and water, information on this important aspect is readily available from the same source.

It is conceivable that disaster may strike while the children are in school or parents at work. This, of course, would produce a situation which would result in anxiety. However, community planning and preparedness will go a long way toward alleviating this apprehension. It is to be expected that the schools will make adequate preparation for children's care during school hours. Each school should have a designated shelter area stocked with food, water, and medical supplies. Under certain conditions, particularly after an alert, it may be unwise to send the children home. Hence, parents should satisfy themselves that schools have a proper disaster plan and, where this is not so, exert necessary effort to see that one is promptly prepared.

Shelter provisions must also be made at places of work. Most office buildings in the country have been surveyed and shelters designated. Stocking these with supplies is now going on as part of a federal program. These places are to be used both by the workers in these buildings and passers-by in the event of an alert. Many factories have made provision for protecting their employees. This program should be adopted by every business establishment in the nation.

In the event of an alert, one should go to the nearest protective area. Running about aimlessly or trying to get home will, for obvious reasons, be extremely dangerous. If we plan well to take care of others, then we and our families must benefit from such preparedness. Children should be informed as to the preparations which are being made for them in case of emergency.

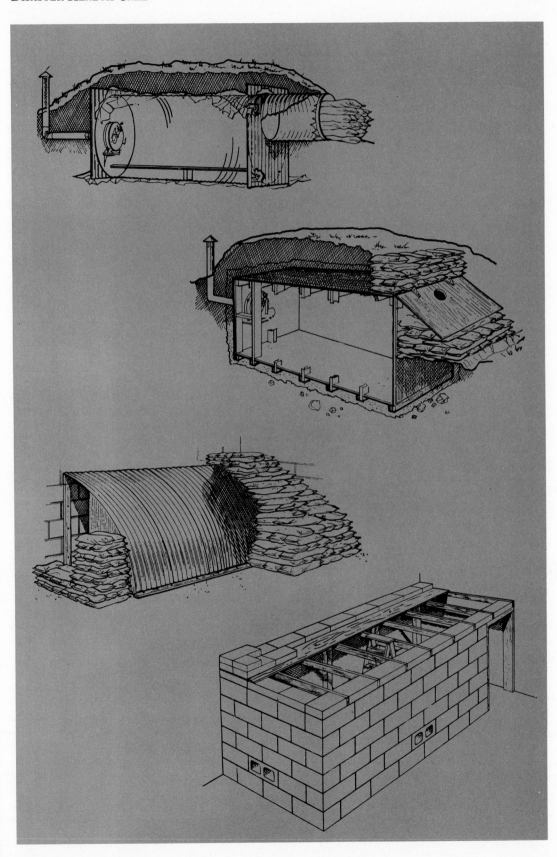

Another major effect of a nuclear bomb is that caused by the blast itself. It is known that in an area five miles around the point of explosion, most buildings would be destroyed. As one goes farther from this point the severity of destruction would decrease. Shelters would provide a degree of protection, not in the immediate vicinity of the explosion, but gradually as the distance from the center increases. Much experience was gained from a study of air raid shelter effectiveness in World War II that can be applied to the present.

Another effect is that produced by heat. This can create severe burns on the bare skin of people in the open for a distance of up to 18 miles. This suggests another important function of a shelter, if adequate warning is received of an impending attack.

Community Planning

Every community should have a civil defense plan and organization. This can be used not only for nuclear attack, but also for any other kind of disaster. In many communities in the country this has had to be used to augment the community's resources in emergencies such as floods.

In planning for civil defense one cannot know in advance whether his area will be affected or whether it will be a neighboring community that needs assistance. If we are all prepared to help each other, then we are prepared to help ourselves.

From a disaster medical care standpoint, it is essential that plans be developed to provide care after an attack has happened and a period of rebuilding sets in. It is necessary to take care of the injured so they may be restored to health and help restore the community and their homes. This is a responsibility of the uninjured survivors, not only in a given area, but in the entire country.

Only communitywide planning can accomplish this. If hospitals are destroyed, other facilities must be provided. This is to be done in part by using the 200 bed Civil Defense Emergency Hospitals of which the federal government has nearly 2,000 spread throughout the country at present. In addition, hospitals in unaffected areas will need to expand. Medical supplies in large quantity are stored in accessible locations throughout the nation. Medical facilities can be improvised where the emergency sites and supplies have been destroyed.

There will not be enough physicians to give needed care since many of them could be casualties. Therefore, it is necessary that members of the allied health professions, who in peacetime so ably assist the physician, become proficient in tasks they usually do not perform. The doctor can then devote himself to the more difficult and complex treatments required. The expanded capabilities of all of the allied health professions has been spelled out in the American Medical Association's Report on National Emergency Medical Care.

In addition to these, there is need for a great number of people to assist in the operation of the hospital system in every department from the supply room to the operating room. Further, people are required to rescue injured persons and to act as litter bearers, ambulance drivers, and members of first-aid teams. All of these people require training to carry out their jobs. Such training courses have been developed and are available. These are in addition to the Medical Self Help Training which provides an excellent base.

The average community has delegated responsibility for civil defense to specific persons from whom information can be obtained about these courses and other matters. Medical societies are actively cooperating in these programs, and may be consulted for information. There is usually an Office of Civil Defense with a director to plan for the community's needs. This stems in a direct line from the Department of Defense (Army) which has the federal responsibility, delegated by the President and the Congress. In turn, each state, through its governor and legislature, has the responsibility of preparing for its role in protecting its inhabitants. The counties and cities in turn carry out preparedness functions within their area. In those communities where little has been done, public interest will result in increased activity.

From a medical standpoint, health matters have been assigned to the United States Public Health Service by the President. State medical societies, with the guidance and assistance of the American Medical Association, have been developing plans for the care of people. At the local level, county medical societies have undertaken voluntarily to work with local civil defense authorities in planning for medical care. All of the allied health professional groups are engaged in working with medical societies in this vitally important area.

Information can be obtained from several sources. Within the community the local office of civil defense will be able to provide booklets on many subjects as well as to answer questions. The local health department and the county medical society will be able to provide health information. Of course, the U.S. Government Printing Office, Washington 25, D.C. can provide material on any phase of civil defense.

Many people are required to make good civil defense functional. People can volunteer in their communities by applying to their civil defense office, the health department and, in many places, the local medical society. Where necessary, residents should urge the community to present proper instruction on these vital subjects.

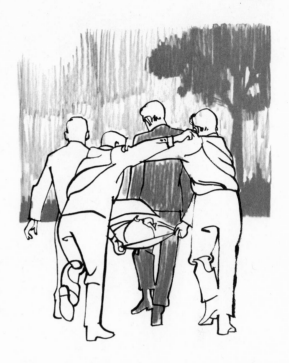

Medical Care

The threat of a large-scale enemy attack makes it necessary to know about environmental and personal health matters, as well as the care of the sick and injured. Under conditions which will require people to live in close quarters with limited facilities and food, disease is more than likely to develop. This can be combated by careful attention to commonsense measures which everyone can learn.

People in a shelter can suffer the same illnesses that they might under usual living conditions. For example, one can have a cold, an asthma attack, stomach upset, hernia, eye irritation, or heart emergency. Some people will have been ill with chronic conditions prior to entering a shelter. Childbirth or miscarriage can take place. Many people will have been injured during the bombing. Some will be in shelters; others will be rescued later. The early care of such injuries is important if these lives are to be saved.

Often, no physician or other professionally trained person will be available. Thus, it is essential that at least one member of each family know about these matters. Such knowledge can be obtained from the Medical Self Help Program developed by the United States Public Health Service with the active cooperation of the American Medical Association.

Medical Self Help is a training program which can be taught to everyone who will attend a total of 16 hours of very interesting instruction. It does not necessarily require only professional people to teach it. Its main emphasis is on a people-to-people approach. It provides knowledge and some skills in treating injuries and caring for the sick in case of nuclear attack or other disaster situations such as a flood or hurricane.

There have been many instances where people who have had this course have used the knowledge to save life. For example, a father saved the life of his son by knowing how to stop bleeding when the child poked his arm through a storm door, sending a glass splinter deep into his chest.

A mother found her two-year old son unconscious, still clutching a hairpin inserted in an electrical outlet. The mouth-to-mouth breathing she learned in medical self-help training enabled this mother to restore her child's breathing to normal.

There are other first-aid courses one can take, notably that given by the American Red Cross. This covers many of the things contained in medical self-help. Those which are not given can be added to the Red Cross course as a supplement which will then qualify the student for a Medical Self Help Certificate.

In facing the reality that so long as weapons of terrible potential exist they may be used, it is emphasized that much can be done to provide for healthful living during the period after disaster. Granted, it will not be that to which we are now accustomed. But it will be enough for survival. And the most important thing is survival. All of this can be accomplished by prudent planning, by participating in training, and by an attitude of confidence.

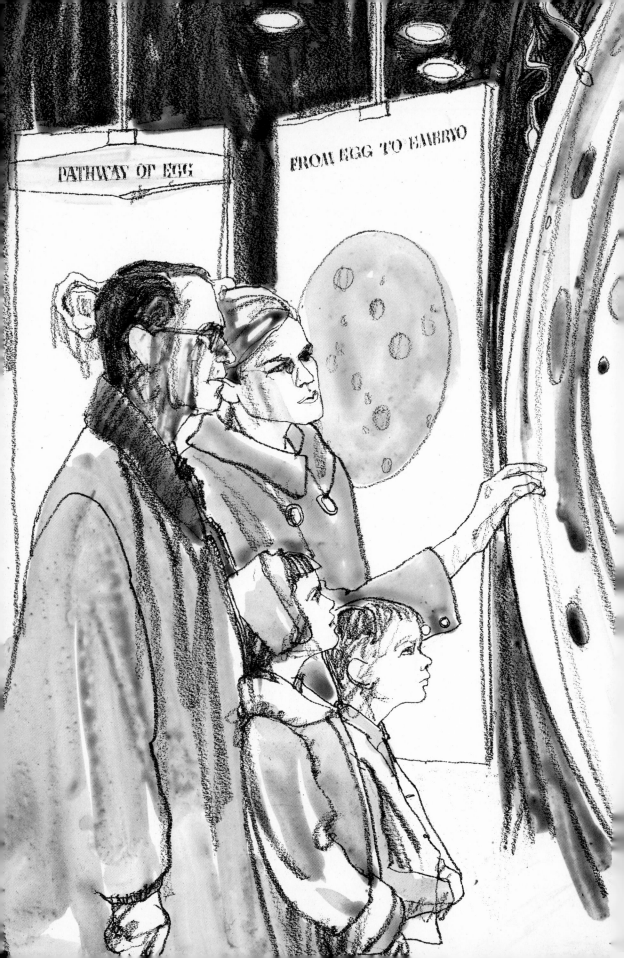

PART XV

Keeping Posted

Chapter One

MEDICAL PROGRESS

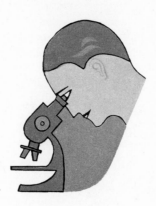

Medical history is a fascinating topic for study as a hobby. Along with the kings, warriors, and revolutionists who made history, the physicians were always close to the throne. Many took an active part in the making of history, entirely aside from their functions as physicians. Five doctors signed our Declaration of Independence.

Medical history goes back as far as 7,000 years before Christ, beginning with the dawn of the Sumerian, Egyptian, and Minoan civilizations. About 3,000 to 2,500 years before Christ came the age of the pyramid builders; surgical operations are depicted on these tombs of the Pharoahs. Set down in about 2,040 B.C., the Babylonian Code of Hammurabi contains one of the earliest statements of medical ethics and doctor-patient relationships.

The millenium of 2000 to 1000 B.C. produced some of the oldest of medical documents. These are mainly lists of prescriptions and descriptions of treatments of disease, such as the Ebers papyrus and the Berlin papyrus. The first Olympic games were held in Greece during this period and there was a beginning of medicine in the Brahmin culture of Asiatic India. The ancient Chinese practiced massage and the puncturing of the body with needles for the curing of disease.

A date well-known in medicine is 460 B.C. when Hippocrates, the legendary father of medicine, was born. Physicians still live by the principles of the Hippocratic oath. They have found that many of the so-called aphorisms of Hippocrates, which were descriptions of diseases and other statements of medical facts as he saw them, still hold true.

Athens suffered a great plague epidemic in about 400 B.C., and a little later Alexander the Great looked out from his throne and found no more worlds to conquer, but was himself soon overcome by what is believed to have been a combination of gall bladder disease and malaria.

This is only one of the many epidemics that pepper medical history. There was one at Orosius in 125 B.C., one at Antoninus, which lasted for 16 years, ending in 180 B.C., and another at Cyprian, which lasted 15 years, ending in 266 B.C.

In the Christian era, we find descriptions of great plagues following the eruption of Vesuvius in A.D. 78, as might be expected, because floods and earthquakes today still disrupt health facilities. At this time hospitals began to be erected, such as the one of St. Basil at Caesarea by Justinian and the plague hospital at Edessa in the fourth century. In the sixth century we find the first use of the word "variola," the modern term for smallpox, by the Bishop of Avenches, and a description of a smallpox epidemic by Gregory of Tours at that place. Late in this century occurred the famous epidemic of St. Anthony's fire in France, which was due to ergot (a fungus) poisoning.

Medical Historical Highlights

1214: The Italian City of Bologna first appointed a city physician, a forerunner of the modern public health officer. A medical school was founded at Salerno by Frederick II.

1250: The first description of scurvy in the troops of Louis IX at the siege of Cairo.

1266: First use and teaching of the antiseptic treatment of wounds by Theodore de Rico Borgognoni.

1348-1350: Great epidemic of Black Death (bubonic plague) swept over Europe.

1409-1410: "Insane asylums" established at Seville, Spain, and Padua, Italy.

1472: The first treatise on pediatrics was published.

1473: The first dictionary of medical terms was published.

1486: The "sweating sickness" (probably tuberculosis) broke out in England.

1500: The first authenticated caesarean section was performed on a living subject (Julius Caesar's manner of birth is legend).

1510: A worldwide epidemic of influenza occurred.

1515: First public dissection of human cadaver; created a tremendous ethical and religious controversy.

1518: Nuremberg, Germany, first regulated the sale of foods.

1530: Fracastorius wrote a poem from which was derived the name of the disease syphilis. Sarsaparilla was introduced to Europe from America as a drug and a flavoring.

1545: The first apothecary (drug) shop established in London. Ambroise Paré revolutionized the treatment of gunshot wounds and made numerous other contributions to surgery in succeeding years. He introduced the use of artificial eyes.

1547: Establishment of the famous London mental hospital St. Mary of Bethlehem, commonly known as "Bedlam."

1550: Paré introduced "version," the method of turning the unborn child to facilitate birth; he also demonstrated the reimplantation of teeth and pioneered in the surgical specialty of orthopedics.

1565: Tobacco was introduced into England by Sir Walter Raleigh and into France by John Nicolle.

1583-1600: An epidemic of diphtheria raged in Spain.

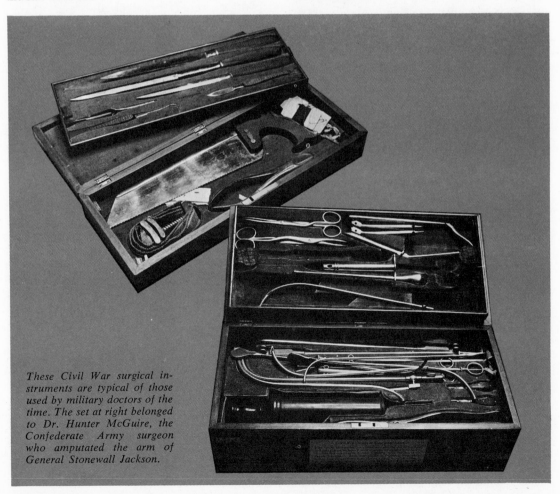

These Civil War surgical instruments are typical of those used by military doctors of the time. The set at right belonged to Dr. Hunter McGuire, the Confederate Army surgeon who amputated the arm of General Stonewall Jackson.

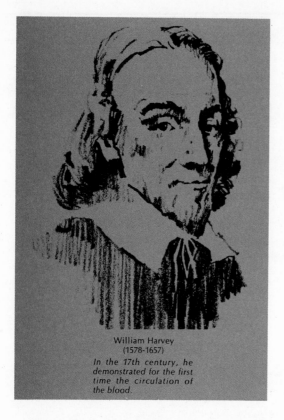

William Harvey
(1578-1657)

In the 17th century, he demonstrated for the first time the circulation of the blood.

1590: The compound microscope was invented by the two Dutch scientists, Hans and Zacharias Jensen.

1597: A treatise on plastic surgery was published.

1628: William Harvey published his researches on the circulation of the blood.

1633: The first book on emergency first-aid was published.

1640: Local anesthesia was first produced by using ice and snow.

1643: Malpighi in Italy demonstrated the blood capillaries, the only item missing from Harvey's description of the circulation of the blood.

1665: The first transfusion of blood from one dog to another.

1667: The first transfusion of blood performed on man.

1668: The importance of oxygen for combustion and respiration was first recognized.

1669: First discovery that blood takes up oxygen in the lungs.

1670: A physician first discovered the sweet taste in diabetic urine.

1675: Van Leeuwenhoek first observed "little animals" in drops of water under the microscope.

1683: Sydenham published the first treatise on gout.

1689: Van Leeuwenhoek discovered "rods" in the retina of the eye, and the finer anatomy of the cornea.

1690: The pulse was first counted by a watch. Yellow fever broke out in Boston.

1699: Massachusetts enacted a law for the control of communicable diseases.

1710: The first operation for an arterial aneurysm was performed. The muscles in the larynx were first demonstrated. The tuning fork was invented; later used as a diagnostic tool.

1717-1718: Inoculation by the Asiatic method (not vaccination) was first introduced into Europe for preventing smallpox.

1726: Stephen Hales demonstrated the mechanism of blood pressure.

1733: Hales produced artificial dropsy by injecting water into veins.

1739: A chair of midwifery (obstetrics) was established in the University of Edinburgh.

1746: Malocclusion (irregular teeth) and pyorrhea were first recognized.

1749: Patients with chest diseases, later identified as tuberculosis, were first sent to the mountains for treatment.

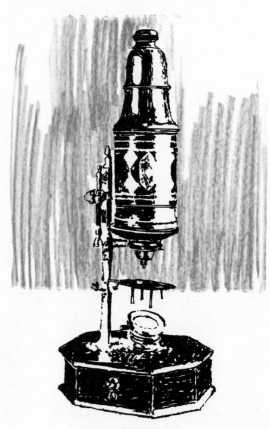

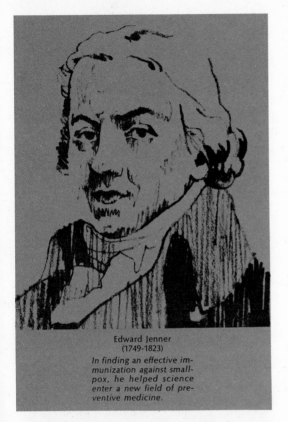

Edward Jenner
(1749-1823)

In finding an effective immunization against smallpox, he helped science enter a new field of preventive medicine.

1760: Medical practice was first regulated by law in New York City.

1770: King's College, Long Island, granted the first medical degree in the U.S. The State of Pennsylvania established the first quarantine act in America. A smallpox epidemic began which killed over 3,000,000 people in the East Indies.

1775-1800: Witnessed a succession of chemical discoveries: oxygen by Lavoisier; ammonia by Priestley; chlorine by Sheeley, and numerous others.

1776: First recognition that nerve fibers when cut will grow out if the cell is not injured. William Withering learned of dropsy "cures" by tea made from the leaves of foxglove (digitalis) and established its value as a drug in heart diseases.

1780: Benjamin Franklin invented bifocal spectacles.

1796: Edward Jenner vaccinated Edward Phipps with cowpox and succeeded in preventing smallpox.

1800: Smallpox vaccination introduced into America by Dr. Benjamin Waterhouse.

1809: Dr. Ephraim McDowell performed, and Jane Todd Crawford endured without anesthetic, the first removal of an ovarian tumor.

1817: Parkinson described the nervous disease now known by his name.

1823: Fingerprints were first described.

1833: Dr. William Beaumont took advantage of an unhealed gunshot wound which exposed the interior of the stomach to make fundamental contributions to the knowledge of digestion.

1840: Infantile paralysis and toxic goiter were first described.

1842: Crawford W. Long first used ether as an anesthetic but failed to report his discovery until 1846.

1846: Oliver Wendell Holmes pointed out the contagiousness of childbed fever. Morton, Jackson, and Wells made their contributions to the discovery of general anesthesia. Oliver Wendell Holmes coined the name for anesthesia. Claude Bernard discovered the digestive functions of the pancreas. Stokes described heart block for the first time.

1847: Semmelweiss in Vienna demonstrated clinically the contagiousness of childbed fever and reduced its mortality.

1850: Helmholtz measured the speed of the nerve impulse.

1859: Darwin published his controversial *Origin of Species.*

1860: Méniére described the combination of dizziness, deafness, and ear noises called by his name.

1865: Gregor Mendel published his report on hybridization of plants which has become the basis of our knowledge of genetics.

1867: Joseph Lister introduced antiseptic surgery. Helmholtz published important research on physiology of the eye.

1869: Virchow in Vienna proposed medical inspections of schools.

1870: Research begun in bacteriology including such discoveries as those by Pasteur in rabies, anthrax, silkworm, and wine fermentation problems, pasteurization as a sterilizing process, and many others; Koch's work in tuberculosis; von Behring's discoveries relating to diphtheria; Neisser's identification of the gonococcus; Eberth's researches in typhoid fever; and many, many others.

1884: Crédé introduced the instillation of silver nitrate into the eyes of the newborn to prevent gonorrheal infection.

1889: Von Mering and Minkowski produced experimental diabetes in dogs. Von Behring discovered antitoxins of diphtheria and of tetanus.

1890: Von Behring treated diphtheria with

antitoxin. Robert Koch introduced tuberculin for treating tuberculosis.

1894: Kitasato and Yersin discovered the bacillus of bubonic plague.

1895: Roentgen discovered the x-ray. The Nobel prizes were instituted.

1897: Sir Ronald Ross in India traced the spread of malaria to the Anopheles mosquito.

1898: Radium was discovered by Piérre and Marie Curie.

1899: Reed, Carroll, Lazear, and Agramonte discovered the mosquito which spreads yellow fever.

1905: Schaudinn discovered the spirillum which causes syphilis.

1918-1919: The great worldwide epidemic, known as Spanish influenza.

1922-1923: Banting, Best, and McCleod discovered insulin to be effective in the treatment of diabetes.

1924: Whipple, Minot, and Murphy discovered a principle contained in liver which would hold pernicious anemia in check. Willem Einthoven developed the electrocardiograph.

1928: Fleming and Florey discovered penicillin. Charles Nicolle published new information on typhus fever.

1929: Hopkins discovered growth-promoting vitamins. Eijkman discovered the antineuritic group of vitamins.

1930: Landsteiner developed a method for human blood grouping.

1932: Liebor pioneered the development of hearing aids. Adrian and Sherrington explained the function of the nerve fibre.

1933: Thomas Hunt Morgan described the hereditary functions of the chromosomes in the cell nucleus.

1939: Gerhard Domagk showed the antibacterial effect of a dye called prontosilate, which became the basis for the revolutionary sulfa drugs for fighting infections.

1940: Chevalier Jackson invented the bronchoscope, a device for inspecting the bronchi.

Progress In Recent Years

As we approach closer to the present day, it is more difficult to fix a discovery to a given date. Scientific research is carried on in many

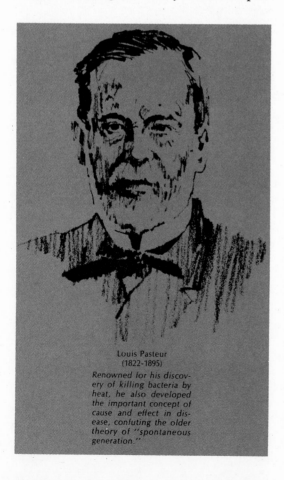

Louis Pasteur
(1822-1895)

Renowned for his discovery of killing bacteria by heat, he also developed the important concept of cause and effect in disease, confuting the older theory of "spontaneous generation."

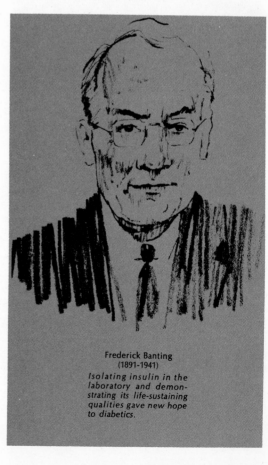

Frederick Banting
(1891-1941)

Isolating insulin in the laboratory and demonstrating its life-sustaining qualities gave new hope to diabetics.

quarters, and many persons contribute to progress. Discoveries which seem important today may be forgotten tomorrow, as were many in more remote times. The best we can do with the modern medical picture is to summarize in a general way the progress which is going forward at an accelerated tempo.

Culminating in the 1940's were the fruits of decades of research by Ludwig Hektoen in bacteriology, parasitology, immunology, and cancer. Further light was shed on vitamins by Hendrik Dam and Edward Doisy. Joslin and his associates, Woodyatt, and others advanced and refined the treatment of diabetes. Minot contributed further progress against pernicious anemia. Hench, Kendall, and Reichstein introduced cortisone and ACTH into the treatment of arthritis. Graham, Ochsner, and others advanced the surgery of the chest, especially the lungs.

Heart surgery was born as a specialty, advanced by Beck, Blalock, Taussig, Potts, Matas, and numerous others. Nonsurgical heart therapy was advanced by Herrick, Paul White, and others. Electrical timers for the

Alexander Fleming
(1881-1955)
Discovered penicillin, the
forerunner of modern
antibiotic drugs.

heart were used with success. New heart valves were implanted, and artificial arteries of synthetic materials replaced damaged vessels. Aneurysms, sacs formed by the dilatation of the walls of an artery or a vein, were successfully treated by surgery.

The 1950's saw the development and use of polio vaccines, oral and by injection. Progress against viruses is credited to Enders, Salk, and Sabin, and numerous other contributors. Spinal anesthesia was introduced into the United States by Wayne Babcock, and a variation of the same, caudal anesthesia, was used in obstetrics. DNA, an important acid found in cell nuclei, was first discovered and then chemically manufactured. The heart-lung machine was invented. A few kidney transplants were successful enough to offer hope for more in the future. X-ray treatment has been helpful in conditioning the recipient's tissues to be more receptive to the transplanted tissues and organs.

In at least one case a severed arm was sewn back on and functioned fairly well.

Methods have been devised to detect allergy to penicillin before giving the drug. Many modifications of the cortico-steroids (ACTH and cortisone) have widened their usefulness by reducing side-effects.

Cancer controls have been improved by hormone treatment, earlier discovery, more advanced surgery, use of lowered temperatures, and such preventive measures as smear tests, biopsies, and periodic examinations. Limited success with drugs against cancer gives hope for the future.

Leukemia patients survive longer and longer through more effective drug therapy.

Relationship of drugs given the expectant mother to deformities in the infant are better understood as a result of the thalidomide experience. Oral contraceptive pills command wide interest.

The part played by overeating, too much smoking, and too little exercise in heart and blood vessel diseases gains increasing recognition among researchers.

The thymus gland, long considered unimportant, is now being studied in connection with white blood cells.

Numerous advances are being made in understanding nervous diseases and mental health; PKU disease of infants in relation to retardation, and its dietary control; relationship of chromosomes to mongolism; development of a drug called Dopa for treatment of Parkinsonism; newer methods in group handling of mental patients; and an encouraging note, a steady decline in the mental hospital patient population.

Orthopedic surgery has helped victims of arthritis by straightening deformed fingers, loosening joints or stiffening them, and restoring the function of the hand through making thumb-and-finger function possible again.

Newer operations on the ear include fenestration—reopening the window into the inner ear when it is closed by bony growth, and freeing the chain of little bones in the ear to vibrate more normally when they have been fused by disease. Méniére's disease is being attacked by surgery of the nerve of hearing and by attempting to reduce pressure on the internal ear's organ of balance, the labyrinth. These delicate operations are made possible through the development of surgery under magnification. Efforts are under way to develop a transistor radio which can be implanted in the middle ear.

The nation's public health record is marked by a continued high level of health and freedom

from major epidemics. New attacks are being made on air pollution, and an alert watch is kept on evidence of nuclear fallout. The American Medical Association has created a Department of Environmental Medicine and is also active in all public health programs, especially immunizations against smallpox, polio, tetanus, and measles.

Medical schools, where the doctors who will care for the people in the years to come are educated, are under constant study with regard to their programs of undergraduate and postgraduate study, their contributions to research, and the problem of holding medical costs to a minimum consistent with adequate service. Similar consideration is being given to intern, residency, and advanced postgraduate study, to certification of specialists, and to maintaining the supply of general practitioners.

Similar attention is focused upon hospitals and their services and upon nursing homes. A commission has been created jointly by the American Medical Association, the American Nursing Home Association, and the American Hospital Association to deal with standards,

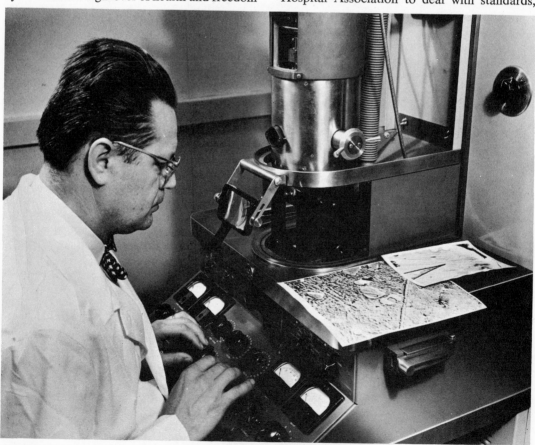

Instruments such as this electron microscope are helping medical scientists push research into important areas.

accreditation, and licensing of nursing homes. Hospitals are experimenting with gradations of medical and nursing care, providing intensive service for the seriously ill and gradually withdrawing services until the convalescents take care of themselves, thus cutting hospital costs and overcoming personnel shortages. Varieties of experimentation in such procedures are made possible by the private enterprise system, in cooperation with government.

The great strides made in health and hospitalization insurance, including coverage for the aging and for all with long-term (castastrophic) illness, is discussed fully in Part VIII, Chapter Five.

In terms of modern communication and transportation, the world is a shrinking globe. Events far removed in distance come closer and closer to us in time. A traveler can now touch four continents in one day by jet airplane, and in so doing can spread disease if he happens to be infected. World health and the organizations by which it is maintained therefore become of interest to every home. There is continuous activity the world around by the World Health Organization and in the western hemisphere by the Pan American Health Organization. These endeavor to control epidemic disease and to assist populations in less favored portions of the world to improve their general health and well-being. Since all of these factors influence international relationships and world peace, they are of vital interest to every American, and it is worthwhile, if not essential, to keep as well-informed as possible about health conditions in all parts of the world. Those who travel abroad are particularly interested in a personal way.

Medical progress has been compared to an iceberg, only a small fraction of which shows above the surface. A medical discovery credited to one individual is often the combined work of many who may never receive the credit to which they are entitled. An apparently small discovery may be the key to tremendous developments. For example, the modern vaccines which are weakened so that they produce immunity without producing disease are the result of an incident in Pasteur's laboratory in Paris. He developed a culture of bacteria for use in the study of a disease of chickens. He was distracted from the experiment and the culture stood around in the laboratory for some time. When he got back to the experiment and tried to use this old culture, which should have infected the experimental birds with disease, it

was found that nothing whatever happened. When a new culture was used, the birds did not become ill. These observations might have passed unnoticed, except for Pasteur's active, keen, and suspicious mind. He immediately began to wonder what happened to the culture that stood around and what, if anything, that culture did to the birds that they failed to become ill from the later injection?

Putting two and two together, he arrived at the conclusion that the first culture had grown weak through aging and that, although weakened, it might still have the ability to protect. Further experiments instituted to prove the point were the beginning of aging or otherwise weakening bacterial cultures to create immunizing agents.

In a similar fashion, penicillin was discovered because it was noticed that bacterial cultures sometimes failed to grow as expected but developed other types of growths. Examination of these under the microscope disclosed a well-known mold, the penicillium or ordinary bread mold. The secretion or product of penicillium produced an inhibiting effect on the growth of bacteria. This led to its clinical application. It was appropriately named penicillin.

Medical science as it exists today is not the result of chance. It is the outcome of centuries of progress, of innumerable hours of tedious, laborious work by devoted individuals with intense scientific curiosity. A knowledge of how medical science has developed should put at rest forever any feelings of confidence in the cults which have sprung up all along the way, each promoting without scientific support a theory for the cause and cure of disease, without going to the trouble of finding the facts. Anyone who has a faint concept of medical history will always want to know what and who are behind new discoveries, how they have been tested, how safe and how effective they are, and how reliable are the sources from which they spring.

Another fact about medical history is that it is never still. In a book which is printed and bound in a permanent form like this guide, there can be no up-to-date record of medical progress. This you will have to find in the daily press and other mass communications media, and you will have to learn how to interpret this news so that you will not be misled by premature publicity or overoptimistic estimates. The AMA magazine *Today's Health,* published monthly, is a reliable and interesting guide.

In reading scientific news of progress, it is

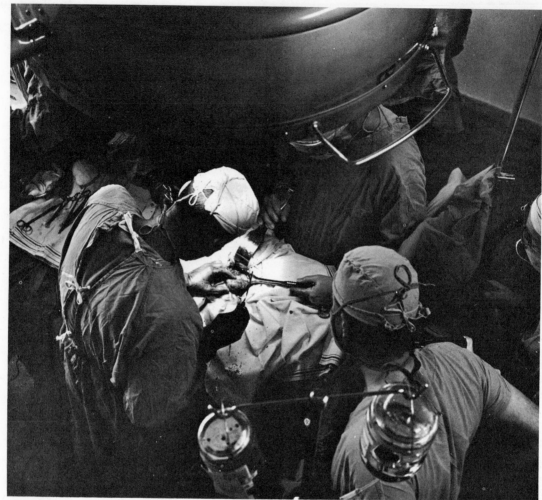

Operations performed today, such as this organ transplant, were hardly more than dreamed of fifty years ago.

important first to remember that headlines are not written by the writer of the article. Furthermore, they are limited by the available space and therefore are often not truly representative of the actual contents of the article. Another important caution is to read all of an article, and to note carefully the qualifying factors. Many an advance is reported with the comment that this opens the way to new research. Some readers immediately interpret this statement to be a claim that the problem is solved. Medical research means gaining a little here and a little there and ultimately putting all the parts together.

Before becoming over optimistic about what looks like a tremendous medical advance, it is well to check it with your family physician or with an authoritative source like your local medical society, the American Medical Association, your state or local health department, a medical school in a nearby college or university, or a scientific organization devoted to research, such as the Public Health Service, or the various voluntary agencies. Becoming familiar with quackery and the methods of quacks and cultists will also be helpful (Part VIII, Chapter Four.)

What of the Future?

It would require a high degree of boldness to attempt any specific forecasts of health and medical progress in the future. In a space age, when even the incredible is happening every day, one need not be too much surprised at anything. In general terms, here are some reasonable expectations:

1. More people will live longer, and there may be some extension of the upper limits.

2. Older people will live better and more

comfortably through constantly improving medical care.

3. Improvements and refinements in medical techniques will continue in the principal areas—diagnosis, medical treatment, surgery, the specialties, preventive medicine, and public health.

4. There will be continuous and accelerated use of electronics and other advanced techniques in improving medical methods.

5. Better understanding of heredity will follow cell and chromosome research.

6. Handling of nervous and mental diseases will improve.

7. Better understanding of handicaps and rehabilitation will occur.

8. More intelligent use of family planning seems inevitable.

9. Better control of the chronic diseases will come through long-range preventive methods, earlier recognition, more healthful patterns of living, and more widespread practice of preventive medicine.

10. Health education programs will be expanded for all ages.

11. Hospital, nursing home, out-patient, home, and office treatment of patients will be more effectively coordinated.

12. Health and hospital insurance coverage will expand until it provides for all major illness costs.

13. There will be relaxation of rigid age-retirement regulations and a broader policy of more gradual retirement for qualified persons.

14. Greater subtlety will emerge in medical quackery, demanding better information and greater discrimination on the part of the user.

15. Pressures will continue to involve government more deeply in local public health and medical affairs; and so will continued resistance on the part of the medical profession, in the best interests of the patient, except where government plainly has a proper role.

16. Continued increase may be expected in the costs of medical care as knowledge increases; greater values in medical services will more than offset costs.

17. Greater needs will develop for qualified young men and women to enter the healing professions with a service motivation.

18. Better and more widespread understanding of mental and emotional influences on individual health is imminent.

19. Better knowledge of child growth, development, and psychology will help in child rearing and guidance.

20. Better understanding and use of safety principles and practices must be achieved to offset the growing importance of accidents as causes of death and disability.

Progress will come only with mutual understanding and cooperation between professional groups such as doctors, nurses, and related health groups on the one hand, and the patients on the other. In this cooperation, the home and family group play a vital part.

CHAPTER TWO

SOURCES OF HEALTH INFORMATION

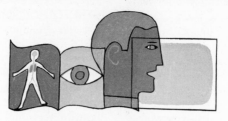

BEING ALERT to health advances which might help their family's health is a responsibility that most parents willingly accept, when they recognize its importance. For example, a new vaccine has recently proved to be effective against measles in field trials. This vaccine or an improved version of it may bring an end to a serious disease from which almost all children have suffered and some even died. Wiping out measles, however, depends upon how alert parents are to the availability of the vaccine and how promptly they obtain its benefits for their children.

A new type of oral immunization against polio was announced in 1963 which called for fewer doses, and afforded protection against all three types of the disease. Yet many young children remain unprotected and the initial immunizations against polio of others have lost their effectiveness. Because the threat of epidemics of paralytic polio has declined, some parents have become complacent. As a result, new outbreaks of the disease could easily occur. No parent can afford to be complacent about protecting his family's health. Parents must keep abreast of new protective procedures, understand the need for periodic strengthening or "booster" doses, and keep a proper record of immunizations for all family members so that they can be kept up to date.

The above illustrates the importance of reliable sources of health information for the family. It also points up the value of a health record in which the facts about family health can be recorded.

Health progress is so rapid today that knowing where sound health information can be obtained is invaluable. This is particularly true because of the vast amount of misinterpretation and misrepresentation that exists concerning health products and services.

Family Doctor Best Source

Your personal physician is your primary source of health information because he can fit the information he provides to the needs of a specific member of your family. You can obtain answers to your questions during visits to your physician's office for immunizations, health examinations, and other preventive services. The physician can sometimes answer questions relating to minor illnesses and accidents by telephone. However, since most doctors must serve many patients he must give a fair share of his time to each. Luckily, there are other reliable sources to which the family can turn for health information.

State and local medical societies publish or can procure leaflets and reprints covering a variety of health subjects. Community health departments usually have health education materials available, and voluntary health agencies generally publish information concerning the health problems with which they are concerned. These agencies also advise about the validity of information obtainable from other sources. Reading lists of acceptable current books and articles on health that can be found in libraries and bookstores are often available from these same sources.

Health columns and articles in newspapers and magazines written by medical authorities or the science writers who work with them are generally reliable and up-to-date. Some, unfortunately, are prone to oversimplify or oversensationalize and a few are more interested in how well their material sells than in its reliability.

Other sources of health information include farm, labor, and industrial associations which distribute health materials to their members or the general public, and private insurance companies with an interest in health education. Since materials distributed by these groups are sometimes colored or even highly slanted by their own special interests, they should be compared with materials from sources as free from bias as possible. The advice of the family physician, the public health department, or a medical society should be sought to evaluate their reliability.

Families who live in areas far from the usual sources given above can write to their national offices. National health agencies generally prefer to make their contacts with the public through their local affiliates, however.

Family health guides like this one which you are presently reading are being seen in increasing numbers on bookstore shelves. Some of these are medical encyclopedias. Those that are scientifically sound and confine their advice to preventive and emergency care that a non-medical person can safely carry out are good home references. Some, however, carry questionable material.

The Health Museum

Museums of health or health galleries in science museums are relatively new on the American scene. They do not deal with antiquities, displays of natural history, or the masterworks of art, but with human beings themselves. The health museum is a place where people can inform themselves about themselves for better health.

"To educate the public in matters of health"—so reads the first Article of Incorporation of the Cleveland Health Museum, which was incorporated in 1936 and opened its doors to the public in November, 1940. It was the first permanently established health museum for the public in the United States.

The American Medical Association in the same year urged its component societies "to give all possible support to such museums wherever they may be developed in the United States, in conjunction with local medical organizations." The American Medical Association especially through its loan exhibits has helped in the establishment of health fairs where hundreds of thousands of people gain a better understanding of how the human body works, the early signs of chronic diseases, and what to do and not to do in medical emergencies and home nursing.

Almost every county or state fair has health exhibits presented by either voluntary or governmental health organizations. The visitor often has a chance to participate in demonstrations to detect early cases of diabetes or glaucoma. He may have a vision or hearing test or a chest or dental x-ray.

With the increasing shortage of medical personnel of all kinds, Health Career Days are held annually in many communities to recruit doctors, dentists, nurses, and medical technicians. Exhibits play an important role in this recruitment process.

Health museums have the advantage over health fairs in that they make visual information available the whole year around. The Cleveland Health Museum, for example, is open 360 days a year. It is visited by nearly 100,000 annually and reaches many more through radio and television. There are regular instruction periods for students, mainly in family life, nutrition, and personal health.

Health museums can be visited at the State Fair grounds in Dallas, Texas, and in the Medical Arts Building in Hinsdale, Illinois, a suburb of Chicago. Chicago itself has had for many years extensive medical exhibits in the palatial halls of its Museum of Science and Industry. These exhibits were developed with the guidance of the American Medical Association during the years when Dr. Thomas Hull was the curator.

More and more hospitals are incorporating health museums into their activities. The first such was the Mayo Foundation Museum of Hygiene and Medicine, sponsored by the Mayo Clinic, in Rochester, Minnesota, which opened its doors in 1934.

The Lankenau Hospital, located in a suburb of Philadelphia, has had a Health Museum since 1953, and on Washington's Birthday in 1963, a Health Education Center opened at the Reading (Pennsylvania) Hospital. In Halstead, Kansas, the home of the famous "Horse and Buggy Doctor," Arthur E. Hertzler, a Health Museum opened early in 1964. Nebraska for many years has had well attended health galleries on its State University campus, located in the State Museum Building.

Whoever goes sightseeing in Washington, D.C., might very well include the Medical Museum of the Armed Forces Institute of Pathology, which has been in existence since Civil War days, next to the Smithsonian Institution. The Smithsonian Institution, itself, has in one of its galleries, a Hall of Health which has as its main attraction, like many other health museums, a transparent woman.

Many state historical societies are including health exhibits in their programs. One of these is the Museum of Medical Progress at Prairie du Chien (Wisconsin). The Stark County Historical Society of Canton, Ohio has a one-room health museum in its new Historical Center Building, located next to President McKinley's Monument. A similar establishment is in preparation for the Memorial Building of the Franklin County Historical Society at Columbus, Ohio.

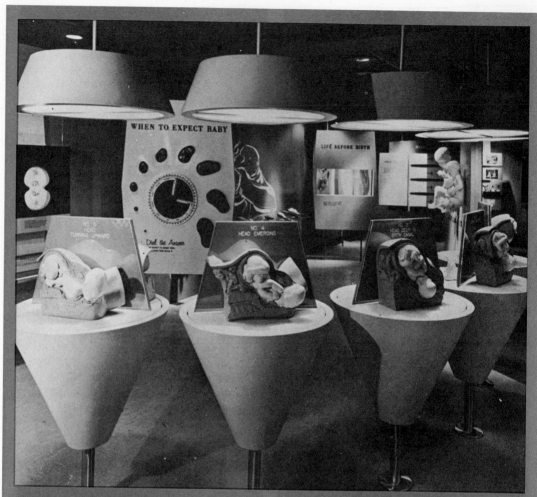

Exhibits, such as this one on birth from the Cleveland Health Museum and the AMA nutrition exhibit below, have done much to inform the American public in previously neglected areas of health education.

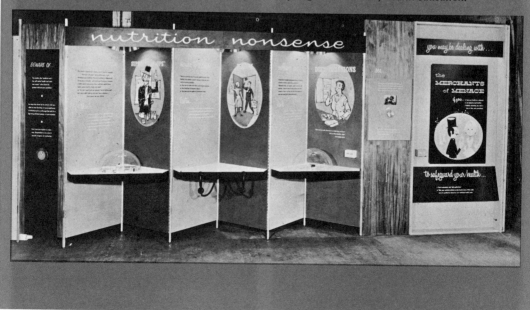

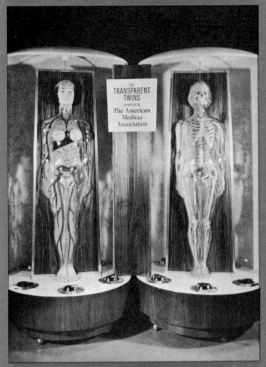

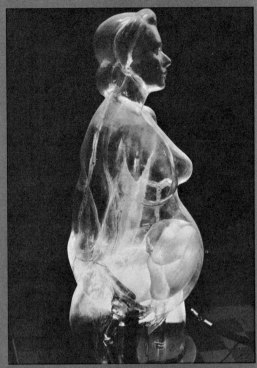

Museum of Science and Industry, Chicago

Other medical exhibits include three transparent woman models and a walk-through model of the human heart.

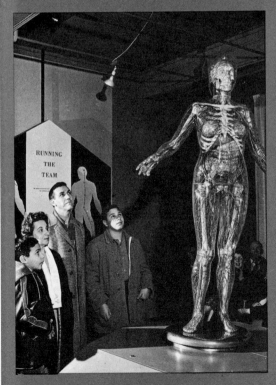

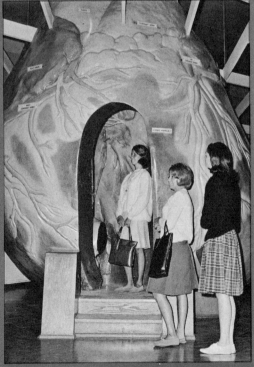

Museum of Science and Industry, Chicago

CHAPTER THREE

MEDICAL FOLKLORE

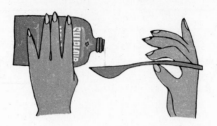

WHILE MUCH of medical folklore is now obsolete, it is unsafe to regard all of it as a mass of quaint misconceptions without foundation and without logic. American medical traditions stem from an age very different from the one in which we live. It was an age of pioneering, of isolated homesteads, of primitive settlements, and of relatively disorganized medical knowledge as compared with what we know today.

The settlers who developed the United States a hundred or more years ago were faced with the grim necessity of getting relief from their illnesses as best they could. Many of the niceties of medical diagnosis now in common use were unknown at the time, and those that were known were not available in the wilderness. So the early settlers turned to the country about them, to the tradition of their ancestral homelands, and to the methods of the Indians, and came up with a medical lore all their own.

The Greeks, Romans, and other ancient peoples personified their health ideas and attributed them to their mythical gods. Apollo, for example, was regarded as the originator of the healing art, but he was also credited with introducing disease, because when he was angry he was believed to send pestilence and death by his arrows. He was reputed to be quick to stop an epidemic when soothed by music and "songs that sweetly pleased." The real god of medicine was Aesculapius, who was said to have flourished some 1,300 years before Christ. He was described as the son of Apollo and the father of two goddesses, Hygeia, the Goddess of Health, and Panacea, the Goddess of Medicine. From the former we get our modern word *hygiene* and from the latter *panacea* (cure-all). Mercury, too, the messenger of the gods, was said to have something to do with health; his winged staff is now the official emblem of the medical departments of the United States armed forces. It is frequently mistaken for the true staff of Aesculapius which has a single

serpent on a branched staff and no wings.

Influences upon health or disease were attributed to the Babylonian god, Marduk, reputed to be "the expeller of all maladies." Another Babylonian god, Ea, was vested with the healing qualities of water. The catheaded Egyptian goddess, Bubastis, was credited with control of fertility in women, and another Egyptian goddess, Isis, was endowed with a broad, protective influence over all persons suffering illness, especially those with disturbed digestion. She was supposed to have originated the enema; so our gratitude to her may be somewhat tinged with reservation.

In later days, health and disease were attributed to evil spirits and to many other factors, supernatural and natural. In modern times, our ideas about disease and health are accepted and passed along in less personalized and less romantic forms, if not always with greater accuracy.

But let us make it clear: Grandma is not always wrong. Why, she has behind her the accumulated experience of the race. Her conclusions are not always correct, because they are based on incomplete or erroneous observations, but a good many of them have since been justified. We need only to point to Peruvian bark and to the digitalis leaves which grew in the gardens and roadsides of rural England to see that the observations of the pioneers were often shrewd and perceptive.

We now use refined quinine derived from the fever-curing Peruvian bark to treat malaria. Instead of teas made from the leaves or the flower of the foxglove, we use the drug digitalis refined from this plant. The modern drug ephedrine, useful in treating allergies and nose and throat conditions, came from the herb ma huang, known for generations to the Chinese. It has properties similar to epinephrine or adrenalin, derived from animal sources.

Coincidence played a large part in establishing the reputed effectiveness of traditional remedies. Warts, which come apparently from nowhere and often disappear for no apparent reason, gave undeserved reputations to innumerable remedies which happened to be used just preceding the spontaneous disappearance of a wart. The self-limiting character of many diseases, such as the milder sore throats and colds, also caused simple herbs and other home methods to gain a curative reputation which they did not merit.

Many traditional remedies are now known to be of little or no value. In Europe the mandrake was highly esteemed as a drug for the relief of pain. It was commonly reputed to be dragged shrieking from the ground under certain special conditions.

Old Wives' Tales

There is perhaps no more fruitful field for folklore than that of pregnancy and childbirth. This universal phenomenon, marvelous and spectacular as it must have been to the uninformed minds of a nonscientific generation, was sure to bring about innumerable misconceptions. There was the common belief that

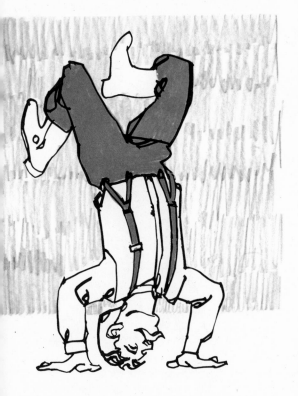

For backache, do somersaults as whippoorwill calls.

having a baby would cure menstrual cramps and would correct a poorly positioned uterus and overcome sexual frigidity. It was generally believed that bleeding in early pregnancy always meant an abortion or a possible defect in the embryo, whereas we know now that scant bleeding is a common occurrence in early pregnancy. An amusing and reasonably accurate old English superstition was that a pregnant woman had better be careful when her abdomen protruded farther than the tip of her nose.

Mothers used to be prohibited from doing any painting or decorating while pregnant. This was a real and useful warning, because paint in those days contained a great deal of white lead and turpentine. The white lead was truly dangerous and the turpentine was nauseating and unpleasant; so both were regarded as hazardous. Paints today contain very little of either white lead or turpentine and so the expectant mother, if physically able and ambitious, may amuse herself in repainting the baby's furniture. She may even paint walls because, contrary to general belief, there is no danger to the expectant mother in stretching. Women used to avoid hanging out their clothes, for fear of causing twists or tying knots in the umbilical cord or wrapping the cord around the baby's neck. Today's mothers to a great extent have put aside such fears as handling a rope during a pregnancy because it might cause twisting or knotting of the umbilical cord.

Sexual relationships during pregnancy were commonly believed to cause disastrous results to mother and baby. We know now that, within reason and moderation and with the exception of the last few weeks of pregnancy, these fears were unfounded. We know also that pennyroyal, tansy, and other herbs, formerly reputed to be effective in terminating unwanted pregnancies, are without effect.

The old fallacy that every baby requires the sacrifice of a tooth can now be abandoned. It was formerly believed that every mother must eat for two. It is true that she must consume the necessary nutrients for two, but this does not mean that she must eat twice as much.

Women used to fear pregnancy past the age of 35 or 40. While it is true that expectant mothers are safest between 20 and 24 years of age, there is so little margin of danger in pregnancy at any age that even older mothers may have babies with a 200-to-1 chance of surviving childbirth. Far from regarding pregnancy as a time of sickness, as in the past, it is now recognized that normal pregnancy at any age is usually beneficial rather than detrimental to health.

There is a persistent belief that the sex of the child can be determined in many ways; these ideas differ in various localities with changing times and cultures. There is no way to tell to which sex the infant belongs until it is observed at birth, nor is there any way in which the sex of the individual can be influenced at any stage of development.

It used to be considered essential for the expectant mother to be in bed for 10 days after delivery, and to be fairly inactive for another 2 or 3 weeks. Now we have almost returned to the primitive practice of getting the mother up and about promptly. This causes less trouble with bowel and bladder performance, helps the uterus to return to its normal condition more rapidly, and very greatly reduces the danger of blood clots. Fears of uterine prolapse, or so-called fallen womb, are entirely without foundation.

A woman can take a bath either in tub or shower just as safely immediately after childbirth as she does during menstruation. She can go up and down stairs without harm and she need not baby herself any more than she feels she ought to, unless the physician feels there are special problems.

Breast feeding is still the best way to nurse a baby, but it will not prevent pregnancy since nursing has little or no effect on ovulation.

Other Superstitions

General medical superstitions cover a wide range of subjects, materials, and methods. Sore throats are very common and have been treated in a number of ways. Because many of the old preparations contained honey for palatability, honey got a great reputation as a medicament. Actually it is only a solution of sugar with not enough vitamins or minerals to be nutritionally important.

Honey is described in the National Formulary, an official drug compendium, which gives its medical uses in three words: "A flavoring vehicle." The U.S. Department of Agriculture's description of honey states that it contains 80 per cent sugars and 16 per cent water, dextrin,

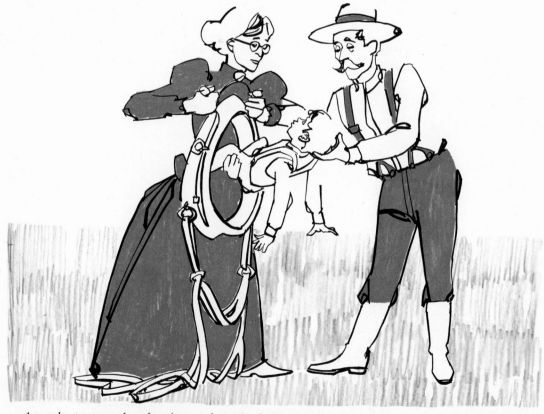

A popular treatment for whooping cough consisted of passing the patient through a horse collar three times.

and gums. The remaining 4 per cent includes flavoring and aromatic substances and "traces of vitamins . . . but none in amounts significant for human nutrition." Minerals are not mentioned. The *Journal of the American Medical Association* states that honey "has no known therapeutic value peculiar or specific only to itself." Honey, therefore, must be regarded as a useful and indeed delightful food, but not as a medicine. It contains sufficient pollen to cause allergic reactions in some people.

Kerosene has been applied internally and externally, or both; externally by rubbing and internally by swishing about in the throat. Gold or amber beads or a gold chain used to be worn around the neck to prevent sore throat. So was a dirty or used dark stocking worn around the neck to prevent colds "going down into the chest." The bandage of red flannel is still in use. Sometimes it is combined with thin slices of salt pork and onions and sprinkled with black pepper. Poultices of black pepper and lard were also used for treating asthma. So were poultices of boiled onions and the well-known mustard plaster. Goose grease and camphorated oil applied to the chest did little for the patient, but it helped keep the family happy.

An infusion of an herb known as goldthread used by the Indians was popular as a treatment for so-called canker, which meant any eruption in the mouth and throat. Sage tea or brakeroot was used for similar purposes. Chestnuts, dried bumblebees, and molasses or urine were popular for the treatment of croup. A combination of sugar with moss obtained from the north side of a maple tree was in common use as a cough medicine, as were syrups made of yellow or red clover or an infusion of sunflower seed.

Red clover had a reputation for special effectiveness in the treatment of whooping cough, as did a concoction of elderberries. For colds there was catnip, elderblossom, or peppermint leaf tea, and, of course, the ever popular camomile. These were administered on the general theory that whatever was wrong with a person, a good "physic" was always in order. Hard cider, as might be expected, was popular, especially when served with cayenne pepper. This was prepared by taking a mug of hard cider, sprinkling it with cayenne pepper, and then plunging a red-hot poker into it, causing it to bubble and foam.

An herb called boneset, more properly thoroughwort, was used in a severe form of influenza then called "breakbone fever," and so was elderflower tea. If these remedies did not work, it was generally conceded that they were not used early enough.

Perhaps the most fantastic of all ideas was one for the prevention of tuberculosis. When a man had died of this disease, his family, tired of harboring so many cases of tuberculosis, decided to put a stop to it. After the funeral they lingered in the cemetery, lifted the casket, and turned it over. By burying the victim face down, they were firmly convinced that they had ended consumption in that family. The record does not say whether the family had also ended with this patient.

Another remedy for consumption was carried out in the case of two sisters who both suffered from the disease. When one died, her parents were told that by burying her heart near a brook in the neighborhood, they would prevent the death of the other daughter. The record shows that she ultimately died of the same disease.

Greasing the patient was considered a sovereign remedy for any disease such as a cold in the chest, pneumonia, or tuberculosis. This is still a common practice although such old remedies as skunk's oil, camphorated oil, and goose grease are no longer as popular as formerly. These greasings only make the patient messy, smelly, and uncomfortable, but those who believe in them say that any fool knows that the greases strike straight through into the lungs and help to loosen the cough.

A lovely plant called pipsissewa or heartsease, which came to the United States from England, was used for diseases of the heart, and also for the "broken heart." Garlic was eaten then as it is still by some for its supposed influence in preventing high blood pressure and hardening of the arteries.

One old woman's sure cure for dropsy was reported by a physician in the following terms: "A little garden celandine, a little pipsissewa, a little ivy run over the ground, green of alder, and white of henna. Slowly simmered over a slow fire and taken in copious drafts, this will produce such slushes of water as ever your eyes have beheld."

Naturally, there were cures for fever, and among the most common of these were teas, made of such herbs as sage, catnip, or yarrow, or a combination of spirits of lavender with ether. Paradoxically, patients were warned against taking water when they had a fever, perhaps as a result of the old adage "stuff a cold and starve a fever." The so-called water cure was a method of treating illness by various

forms of bathing; this was rather unpopular in a day when bathing was much less routine than it is today.

To prevent nosebleed, wearing a length of red woolen yarn or a piece of nutmeg on a string around the neck was recommended. Bloodroot hung over the foot of the bed was supposed to stop nosebleeds in children. Fresh blossoms of red trillium were held to the nose for the same purpose. For bleeding from the nose or elsewhere, it was common practice to stuff the area with cobwebs or to use the fine powder from the puffball mushroom after it had gone to seed.

There is a record of a patient who states she knew someone who took red clover for a fibroid tumor. This treatment was supposed to render the tumor "benign." These people were not, of course, aware that fibroid tumors are always benign, allowing for the difference in the meaning of that word medically and in common use.

Naturally, stomach upsets because of their great frequency were the subject of many interesting ideas, beginning with the descriptive language used. The word "sick," for example, usually meant being nauseated or vomiting. It was not commonly used as it is today, to mean "ill" or "not well." This varied according to where one lived.

A family doctor book or guide to health published in 1844 advises: "Abstain from medicine and live upon a sixpence a day and earn it. Arise with the sun, saw wood for half an hour, and breakfast upon a crust of bread." However, people did not seem to take this advice, because measures for combating stomach upsets were in common use. To make one vomit, the so-called pukeweed or lobelia was used. It was supposed to "tear off the liver." Lobelia has more recently been used in an attempt to help people stop smoking.

The yellowing of the skin, commonly referred to as yellow jaundice or sometimes "jaunders," was treated with "turkey dung bitters warmed," and also by ironwood bark. The tendency to blame digestive disturbances on the liver is a good old English doctrine and came over with the colonists. The hepatica or liverwort, which supposedly resembles the lobes of the liver in its shape, was also used, naturally enough, as a remedy for liver troubles or supposed liver troubles.

The use of liverwort for the liver and heartsease for the heart was part of the general idea that through the mercy of Divine Providence, herbs were shaped with characteristics which would suggest their medicinal uses. A plant with a wormlike stem was used to treat intestinal worms. Baldness was treated with a plant that had hairy characteristics. This treatment of baldness was as successful as anything that we have today—in other words, it did no good whatsoever.

Aromatic weeds, such as spearmint, were naturals for the treatment of nausea, and for constipation rhubarb and senna were commonly employed, as were burroweed tea and a medicine prepared from the inner bark of the butternut tree. The bark of the willow tree, a source of wintergreen oil, was used in Austria, India, and Africa long before German chemists produced its derivative, aspirin. A widespread belief held that the bark of certain trees would have a laxative effect when it was stripped downward, but would cause vomiting when it was stripped upward.

Diarrhea received a number of common names, including dysentery, intestinal flu, the trots, the runs, the flux, and more recently the "tourist trot." Remedies for this condition were numerous, including blackberry roots, steepweed, steepleroot, hardtack, strawberry blossom, oak bark, sweetleaves, and smartweed. In children especially, diarrhea was called summer complaint and the second summer was considered the most important and most dangerous era in a child's life.

Even green apples were given to cure diarrhea, despite the common belief that they were often the cause of this symptom. Finely grated green apples, used in the Black Forest for treating diarrhea in children and adults, are still effective. Modern therapy now employs apple pectin to control diarrhea.

The contagious diseases were considered more dangerous if they "struck inward," that is, if they did not develop a rash. Naturally then there were measures for bringing out the rash. These included the drinking of hard cider and snakeroot and saffron tea or the nanny goat tea which was made from the droppings of goats, lambs, or sheep. Perhaps the best method for bringing out the rash was the hot bath. Of course, the passage of time worked to give this home remedy an unmerited reputation.

"Remedies" used to prevent mumps from "going down" and involving in boys the testicles and in girls the breasts or ovaries were logical though ineffective. Strands of flax around a girl's neck or a boy's waist were supposed to do the trick.

Reliance upon nature for medicine included employment of trees. A baby born with a physical defect it was said, could be cured by splitting an ash sapling near a brook so that the gap ran in a north and south direction. The child was then passed through the gap. The child so treated was supposed to outgrow his defect. A closely related idea is one for the prevention or cure of goiter; this consisted in taking a lock of the patient's hair, splitting a tree or bush at a height greater than the stature of the patient, putting the lock of hair in the cleft, and then letting the child grow up to that height, at which point the goiter was supposed to have disappeared. Sometimes it had!

Naturally there were blood medicines, of which the best known is sulphur and molasses. Molasses was generally credited with a great deal of value. It was also combined with sage. Rhubarb and dandelions, pepsissewa, wormwood and vinegar, sassafras tea, firewort, elder flowers, bloodroot, aloes, and poplar bark mixed with burdock have all been recommended as blood medicines. Dandelion wine was a great favorite, perhaps because of the alcohol which gave it a special uplift power.

Naturally rheumatism called for many sovereign remedies and preventives, beginning with the well-known buckeye or horse chestnut. Another alternative was to carry in the pocket the bone from a raccoon's penis. Various kinds of teas were popular for the relief of rheumatic joint pains, including the leaves of Canada thistle and, of course, the universal remedy camomile, which gave rise to the derisive couplet "How the doctor's brow should smile, crowned by wreaths of camomile."

Lard and other substances were heated and and mixed with cereal to make poultices. These ways of applying heat have some limited value for comfort and to give the family a satisfying sense of "doing something for the patient," but they are not curative. Mullein leaves boiled in vinegar were used for sprained ankles, and catnip was also supposed to relieve swellings when used as a poultice. One old recipe calls for "common ground worms, simmered in lard" for relaxing sinews which have contracted and drawn the limbs out of shape.

Somewhat more remote methods employed were treating cramps in the legs by turning the sufferer's shoes upside down under the bed. This is closely related in its reasoning to the idea of putting a sharp knife edge-upward under the bed during childbirth, in order "to cut the pains in two."

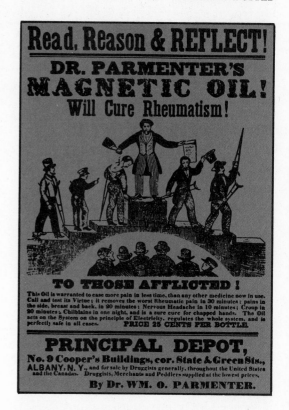

Miscellaneous ideas for various situations include warnings against wearing rubbers indoors for fear of injuring the eyesight. Gold earrings were supposed to help weak eyes. Sore eyes were bathed in rose petals; rose water preparations are still on the market today as eye washes. Warm milk directly from the mother's breast was supposed to help sore eyes in babies, and so was fresh urine.

Earache was treated by tobacco smoke blown into the aching ear, or by spitting tobacco juice into it. Warm pickerel juice was another common remedy, prepared by skinning a pickerel and hanging it in the window in the sun. This warmed the fat in the body of the fish, which was then drained into a bottle. Warm oil is used as a first-aid remedy for earaches today when no medical care is available. A hot baked potato or the "rusted" (heated or roasted) heart of an onion was sometimes held against the ear.

It was common practice to apply heat to the body by killing a chicken and applying the warm carcass of the bird to an area of pain or imflammation.

When children were too young to chew their own food, the parent or other adult relative would chew it before putting it into the baby's mouth. This was before modern concepts of sanitation were evolved, but the practice has not entirely disappeared.

Various kinds of charms or amulets were worn around the neck. Perhaps the most familiar was a bag of asafetida or camphor which was supposed to ward off communicable diseases.

Anyone who has ever had a good whiff of asefetida will realize that this was not such a stupid idea, because it most effectively kept people at a distance. We now know how diseases are spread by close personal contact. This is perhaps one of the best examples of how Grandma not only was not always wrong, but was likely to be right for the wrong reason.

Amber beads have already been mentioned in several connections, but other objects and substances were used as well, such as a string of Job's tears (seeds of an East Indian grass) which were famous for supposedly preventing fever. A white strap in a figure-eight design across the chest and the back of the child was regarded as a teething jacket.

Practically every grandmother remembers the day when grinding of the teeth at night was considered a sure sign of worms, for which the child would possibly receive a dose of beef gall or have a bag of tansy hung around his neck to keep the worms from coming up into his throat and choking him to death. Parenthetically, this idea of worms coming up into the throat is not a baseless notion; it happens. Starving a patient who had a tapeworm in order to starve the worm was a common procedure, and thereafter a bowl of steaming hot soup would be held at the patient's mouth so that the worms, smelling the good food, would come up and could be captured.

Skin diseases were common subjects for home remedies and a great deal of harm was done then as now by treatments which often prolonged the disease by irritating the skin. Sulphur and rum were used for boils. Gunpowder boiled in water or the "sweat" from a heated axe were recommended for ringworm. Yellow dock boiled in vinegar was used for athlete's foot and balm of Gilead buds fried in mutton tallow for bedsores. Wounds from rusty nails were bound with a piece of salt pork to draw out the infection. This bad practice still persists. Human urine was used for cuts and wounds.

For snake bites, snakeroot was the obvious remedy provided by nature. A poultice of squash was used for the bite of the water moccasin and the cut surface of an onion for the bite of a rattlesnake. An onion cut in half and applied to the soles of the feet was also supposed to be a remedy for pneumonia and bronchitis. Discoloration of a substance, such as an onion, was considered ample proof that it had "drawn out" the poison.

The use of available materials for the treatment of burns would make a long list, including the repulsive idea of "fresh" cow dressing, presumably cow dung.

Woodsmen ate the leaves of the poison ivy to prevent ivy poisoning; immunizing tablets supposedly preventing ivy poisoning have been marketed within the past few years. Neither procedure is recommended. For treatment of ivy poisoning celandine, pilewort, or jewel weed or sweet fern was rubbed on.

The wart gave rise to numerous remedies: rubbing with a bean and throwing the bean away; rubbing with salt pork and burying the pork; rubbing with a used dishcloth and hiding the cloth; rubbing with a penny and throwing the penny away; tying as many knots in a string as the individual had warts and leaving the string where someone would find it; the finder was supposed to get the warts. So-called ab-

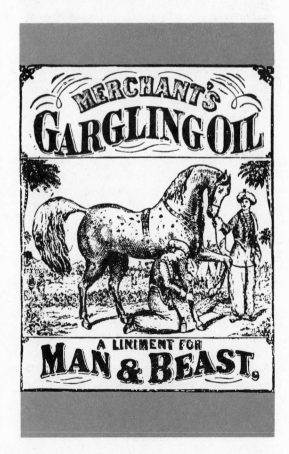

sent treatment by individuals who had or pretended to have occult power was also believed to be capable of getting rid of warts.

Chilblains or frostbite was prevented or treated by rubbing with kerosene, turpentine, or pig's foot oil, or painting with oil of lavender applied with a feather. Rubbing with snow or walking barefoot on a cold floor was also recommended and the inevitable onion salted on the cut surface and rubbed on the foot was popular.

The power of using and understanding herbs was commonly attributed to one or more persons in the community. These were frequently old women or old men with no medical training and little education of any kind. In spite of this, some of them became very successful quacks while making a great deal of trouble for the patient whom they failed to cure and sometimes even harmed with their unscientific treatments.

Dr. Harold D. Levine, from whose article in the *New England Journal of Medicine* many of the preceding ideas were gleaned, remarks:

"One may be amused at the faith that these people placed in the healing virtues of their herbs, but it is none the less true that modern research has substantiated many of the old ideas. After all, it was from English folklore that Dr. Withering (an English physician) culled the idea that digitalis was useful in dropsy."

Many misconceptions arise from the effort to explain commonly observed facts on a basis of inadequate information. This does not mean that people are stupid. It simply means that no one has yet been able to explain certain factors in health and disease. This may account for the tendency to ascribe phenomena of one kind or another to supernatural causes, probably a carryover from the association of the tribal priests with the medicine man in primitive cultures. This explains the faith which people had in the effectiveness of incantations, sacrifices, charms, and amulets.

Another source of error was the tradition that astronomic and weather phenomena may be associated with health factors. This is not as far fetched as it seems because we now know that barometric pressure affects allergies, that rheumatic joints really can foretell weather changes, and that many diseases occur seasonally. Such scientific knowledge, however, is quite different from the belief, for example, that the lungs of an ox, a long-winded animal, would be a good treatment for tuberculosis, or

that the fat of a bear, which was hairy, might be useful for baldness. Eating a lion's heart will not promote bravery, nor will rattlesnake or earthworm oil make the athlete more limber.

There is the outmoded theory of homeopathy which says in effect that like cures like. This is commonly practiced under the more popular title of "a hair of the dog who bit you," the favorite excuse of the alcoholic to have a quick one in the morning after a hard night of drinking.

People are prone to attribute either too much or too little power to the doctor. In either case they are disappointed and the doctor is embarrassed. Many people consider that drugs are the only way in which disease is treated, forgetting the importance of changes in living patterns and attention to nutrition and other factors.

There is the old superstition about maternal impressions affecting the unborn child, which has been proved again and again to be an anatomical and physiological impossibility. Most of the so-called birthmarks, which are supposedly due to maternal impressions, are actually present long before the occurrence which is supposed to be responsible for them. Yet a considerable percentage of readers will remain unimpressed because they think they have seen it happen.

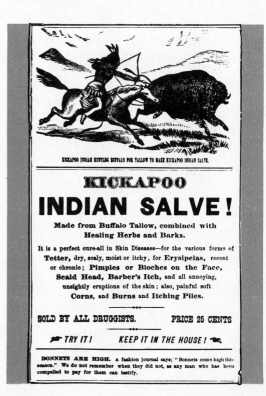

KICKAPOO INDIAN HUNTING BUFFALO FOR TALLOW TO MAKE KICKAPOO INDIAN SALVE.

KICKAPOO
INDIAN SALVE!

Made from Buffalo Tallow, combined with Healing Herbs and Barks.

It is a perfect cure-all in Skin Diseases—for the various forms of **Tetter,** dry, scaly, moist or itchy, for **Erysipelas,** recent or chronic; **Pimples or Blotches on the Face, Scald Head, Barber's Itch,** and all annoying, unsightly eruptions of the skin; also, painful soft **Corns,** and **Burns** and **Itching Piles.**

SOLD BY ALL DRUGGISTS.   **PRICE 25 CENTS**

☛ *TRY IT !*   *KEEP IT IN THE HOUSE !* 🐾

BONNETS ARE HIGH. A fashion journal says: "Bonnets come high this season." We do not remember when they did not, as any man who has been compelled to pay for them can testify.

Many people are afraid that they will damage their hearts by athletic exercise, whereas it is well established that normal or even strenous exercise will not damage a normal heart, because the muscles and wind fail before the heart can be hurt.

Biliousness, which is merely a symptom, continues to be accepted as a supposed explanation for disturbed liver function. A similarly outmoded term is catarrh, which is applied to many diseases of the nose and throat. This is simply a vague term for which the cause must be sought before it can be treated.

Many people are not satisfied with thirst to guide them as to the amount of water they should drink. Instead they adhere slavishly to rules about six glasses or eight glasses of water a day, depending on whose theories of hygiene they have been reading at the moment. It is possible to do harm by taking too much water and it is also possible to take too little, but ordinarily thirst is a good guide unless it becomes excessive, in which case medical advice should be sought.

A favorite old bogey is autointoxication, which means selfpoisoning and is usually attributed to infrequent bowel movements. The physiological fact that very little except water is absorbed into the rest of the body from the large intestine does not disturb people who cling to this mistaken idea.

Oxygen and carbon dioxide, contrary to popular belief, are not the major factors in room ventilation. Motion of the air is more important and so are the air's temperature and humidity.

Deep-breathing exercises are commonly relied upon as a guarantee of health. Certainly their benefits have been disputed and at best they are only a minor factor in healthful living.

Modern Misconceptions

Miscellaneous misconceptions include such ideas as:

Bad breath means disease (not so).

Masturbation causes insanity and other disasters (untrue).

Eating between meals is always harmful (incorrect).

Milk should not be taken at the same time as sour fruits (not so).

Proteins and carbohydrates should not be eaten at the same meal (not so).

Daily bowel movements are necessary for health (untrue).

Pain in the back must indicate kidney disease (incorrect).

Pain in the abdomen means an overloaded stomach (wrong).

A laxative is good for abdominal pain (it is dangerous).

Posture is important because it builds health (it is really a by-product of good health).

Food kept in an open tin can is necessarily poisonous (not if properly refrigerated).

Scales from scarlet fever and measles spread the disease (nose and throat secretions actually do so).

Sewer gas makes people sick (no—it's just unpleasant).

Pimples and boils indicate bad blood (they are due to outside infections).

Marriage of relatives necessarily produces degenerate children (only if heredity is bad or intermarriage is too frequent).

Laymen may safely diagnose and treat disease (they are not qualified).

Boric acid strengthens the eyes (it does not).

Fried and highly seasoned foods are harmful (not in moderation).

A cold can be broken up (it lasts a week no matter what is done).

You feed a cold and starve a fever (no).

Eye muscle exercises will eliminate the need for glasses (a dangerous fallacy).

Vegetarianism is good for health (it simply makes good nutrition more difficult).

Common Misconceptions

For those who would like to know the facts about other common misconceptions, here is a list, which doctors frequently meet:

Blood pressure of 100 plus the individual's age is *not* the normal value.

Red meats and alcohol are *not* necessarily harmful to those with high blood pressure.

Fish is *not* a brain food, it is simply a good food for *all* parts of the body.

Sweets, while possibly detrimental to the teeth, are *not* the sole cause of tooth decay.

There is no reason of health why one should *not* eat shell fish and ice cream at the same meal, providing neither one of them is spoiled.

Lemons, tomatoes, oranges, and grapefruit do *not* cause "acidity" of the body.

The old adage that fruit is golden in the morning, silver at noon, and lead at night *is without foundation.*

Fat people are *not* necessarily carefree and jolly.

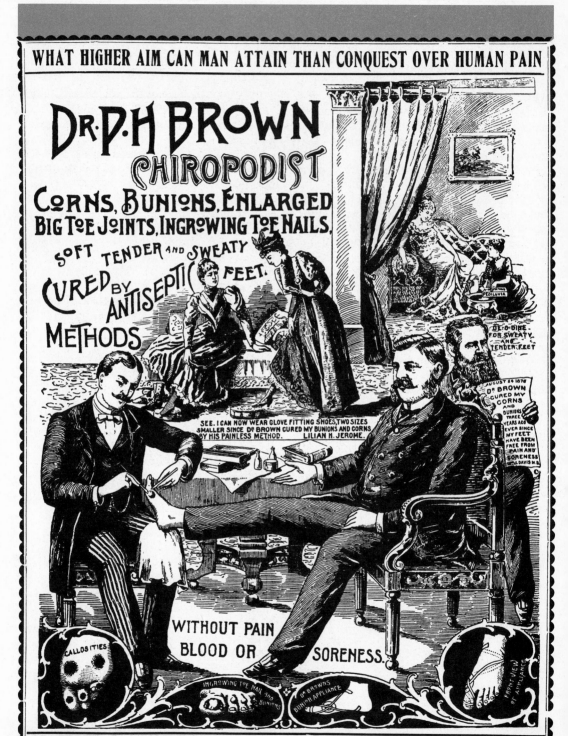

Being fat and 40 and feeling well does *not* constitute a good reason for declining to lose weight.

It is *not* necessarily unwise to drink water with your meals, if you don't gulp it.

The food value of broth or soup, so often given to invalids, is the food value of the rice, barley, or vegetables which it may contain; the broth alone has no nutritive value.

Gargles and mouthwashes do *not* kill the germs in the mouth or throat.

Boils are *not* due to impure blood.

Punctures from rusty nails are *no more dangerous* than punctures from clean shiny nails; the danger lies in the germs that either one may introduce.

Removing a mole properly will *not* result in cancer; cancer is more likely to result from *not* having it removed if it ought to be.

Night air is *not* unhealthful; it may even be more healthful than daytime air because it may be less polluted.

It is *not* necessary to open the windows of your bedroom wide or at all at night, especially when it is cold.

Whiskey with aspirin is *not* a good treatment for cold, even though the cold may improve in spite of it.

There is *no medicine* which can be taken by mouth to dissolve gallstones.

Heart disease is *not* necessarily a reason for refusing an operation or for being afraid to take an anesthetic.

Flowers absorb some oxygen but the principal reason they are removed from the sickroom at night is because they keep better in the open air.

Insulin does *not* cure diabetes but it substitutes for the insulin which the body is unable to provide and thus keeps the patient well.

If the eruption of shingles should entirely surround the chest, this does *not* mean that the patient will die as is commonly believed; in fact, nerves which are most commonly involved in shingles do not meet in front so it would be impossible for the eruption to surround the chest in any case.

Premature baldness in men is *not* caused by wearing hats; nobody knows what causes it, except that men are male.

Cancer has *not* been shown to be contagious.

It is *not* important to lie on the right side when sleeping to keep from interfering with the heart; the heart is in the middle of the chest and not on the left side.

Persons over 40 need *not* avoid strenuous exercise if they have been accustomed to it and if they are in good condition.

It is definitely *not* true that failure to pay the doctor's bill assures the patient that the doctor will not be available while the patient's name is on his books.

Old superstitions, unlike old soldiers, do not fade away. Unfortunately, they are replaced by new superstitions and new misconceptions. For example:

Today, we have the mistaken idea that necessary and harmless chemicals used in processing foodstuffs may cause mysterious diseases like cancer.

We see people afraid to cook with aluminum cooking utensils for fear of poisoning the food.

We observe people who refuse to wear glasses and others who shun much-needed hearing aids.

People oppose fluoridation of public water supplies because the same chemical has also been used for poisoning rats, overlooking the fact that the whole difference here lies in the matter of dosage.

Many people blame climatic changes on the atomic bomb; past generations attributed such changes to artillery fire, to the use of radio and television.

Countless mothers live in fear for their children's lives because a heart murmur had been reported. Most heart murmurs are harmless.

There is still active opposition to the use of immunizing procedures, such as vaccination and immunization, because of a superstitious dread of introducing poison into the system.

Food Fallacies

There is a modern cult of naturalism which holds that only "natural foods" are wholesome because foods grown with the aid of chemical fertilizers are inadequate.

Many harbor prejudices against canned or frozen or otherwise processed foods, and even advocate eating raw food exclusively.

Naturally, the interest of the individual in food would give rise to numerous food superstitions and misconceptions. In a report on food misinformation published by the American Dietetic Association, there are listings of almost 200 such misconceptions about food. Some of the more common and important ones are the following:

Never give milk to a patient with a fever.

Parsnips should be eaten often to cleanse the kidneys.

Beets build blood.

Pork is indigestible.

Sardines, frozen celery, and kelp are recommended every other day for better health.

Sour foods, such as lemon juice or sauerkraut, can cure diabetes.

Diabetes is caused by eating too many sweets.

For the treatment of arthritis, grapejuice, honey, dried poke berries, carrot juice, and tomatoes are recommended.

Celery is good for the nerves.

Cooked cereals heat the blood.

Asparagus is good for the kidneys.

Alfalfa tea cures rheumatism.

Warm bread may cause a stroke.

Sassafras, vinegar, and other substances are said to thin the blood.

Putting cream in coffee makes the coffee more harmful.

Ice water causes heart trouble.

Watermelon causes polio; cucumbers and soft drinks have also been blamed.

An egg a day is harmful.

A teaspoon of whiskey in which arborvitae has been soaked will cure cancer, if taken before eating.

Raw vegetable juice contains life-giving properties, but cooked foods are "dead."

Olives, oysters and raw eggs increase sexual potency.

Wine makes blood.

White sugar is not good for the health.

White bread is poisonous.

Children should not eat potatoes.

If you can foods while menstruating or during pregnancy, the jars will burst or the food will spoil.

If the expectant mother holds her weight down, the size of the baby will be reduced.

Raw foods are harmful to a nursing mother.

Raw cucumbers without salt are poisonous.

Dried currants are poisonous berries.

Ripe, sweet cherries destroy old age matter in the body.

Tomato juice causes heart disease.

Eat all you want until 4:00 p.m. in order to lose weight.

Enriched candy is good for reducing.

Calories don't count.

Honey is not fattening and can be substituted for sugar in diabetes.

Melba toast has no calories.

Aspirin will help to preserve canned apples.

Never eat rabbits because they are all disease carriers.

If a few vitamins are good, more must be better.

Sauerkraut must be made in the light of the moon or the brine won't rise.

Yogurt and brewer's yeast are requirements in a good diet.

Let us repeat: the list above represents beliefs *that are not so*. If you have just read the list, turn back and read the introductory paragraph again to be sure that you cannot accept this list as things that you ought to believe. They are representative of the kind of things that you ought *not* to believe. When you read or hear statements of this nature, check them carefully with people who know about foods, medicines, and the human body.

Behind all these errors in belief, there lies an underlying cause, namely a strong tendency to believe a plausible error and to reject the truth. This may rise out of deep-rooted suspicion in the mind of man who rejects what he does not understand. The results are often deplorable, especially when mistaken and misguided adults pass on their ideas about health to children for whose welfare they are responsible. In extreme cases the courts have intervened to order operations for children whose parents were fanatically opposed to surgery. However, millions of cases do not come to such a dramatic conclusion. For these people who reject the light of truth and live in the darkness of superstition, health can never be at its best, nor can life bring them its full rewards.

Let us repeat here that this chapter is not intended merely to ridicule false beliefs, but to explain them, and where necessary, to help correct them. Adherence to false and mistaken ideas is by no means a sign of stupidity, although it may be an indication of stubbornness. In order to interpret situations correctly, one must have a background of factual knowledge and experience. Thus the doctor who would attempt to build a bridge would make numerous mistakes, not because he is stupid but because he is out of his field. By the same token, the engineer in medicine, the scientist in literature, the artist in mechanics, or anyone outside his own field is almost certain to make mistakes. We should now have outgrown the era of unfounded conclusions and entered into an age when it is possible to bring scientific proof to bear on traditional beliefs. Sometimes this justifies them, but often for reasons other than those which prompted their growth.

Take the matter of an asafetida amulet worn around the neck to prevent communicable dis-

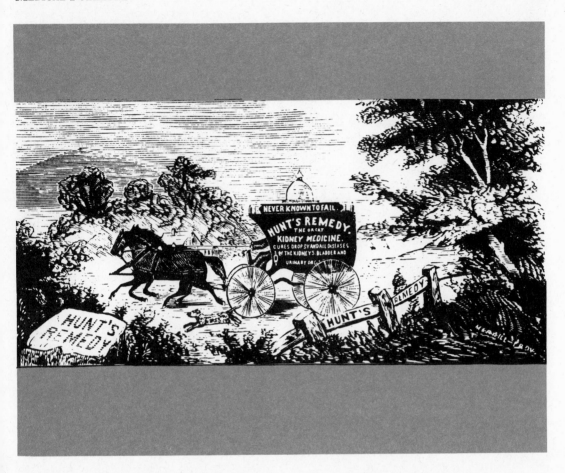

eases. This does not work by magic nor through any physical action of the asafetida. Any other substances equally offensive in odor would be just as good, because what effectiveness this preventive measure has lies in the fact that communicable diseases are passed on by close personal contact. Obviously, an amulet of asafetida does not encourage such contact, but we now have ways to prevent most major communicable diseases that are far superior to the amulet of asafetida. As a shrewd if not well-founded approach to a difficult problem, it was worthy of respect in its day. That day has passed and we should put belief in the amulet of asafetida back into its proper time and lay it to rest once and for all.

The same reasoning may be applied to many other measures which may have had a limited usefulness and certain justification in their day.

This chapter contains a formidable list of fallacies and misconceptions. The list is by no means complete. It would take practically an encyclopedia of medical fallacies to provide a complete list. So far as we are aware, no such encyclopedia is available. Thus, when you run across a bit of medical folklore or a medical opinion that looks as if it might be traditional in nature, it would be wise to check it with your physician before you allow it to influence your thinking and your pattern of living.

GLOSSARY

A

AA: Alcoholics Anonymous, a group of alcoholics that helps other alcoholics.

abortion: the premature termination of pregnancy, either intentional for medical reasons, or accidental; when performed intentionally without medical necessity, it is a criminal act.

abortive: interrupted before the normal course is finished.

abrasion: a scraped or scratched skin wound.

acceptance: in the psychological sense, a favorable attitude toward a person.

Achilles tendon: thickest and strongest tendon of the human body (heel tendon).

acidosis: a reduction in the normal alkaline reaction of body tissues.

acne: an inflammatory disease of the sebaceous glands, occurring mostly about the face, chest, or back.

actinomycosis: a fungus infection acquired from animal contacts.

action: as of a drug, the expected result from taking it (see also *reaction*).

acute: lasting a short time.

addict: one who is habituated to some practice, especially the use of a narcotic drug (Blakiston).

addiction: the habitual use of and dependence upon a narcotic drug by one who has no illness or legitimate reason for such practice.

adenocarcinoma: a cancer arising from glandular tissue, as in the breast, stomach, etc.

adipose: fat, or fatty tissue.

adrenal: a gland of internal secretion; there is one on top of each kidney.

adrenalin: see epinepthrin.

aggression; aggressive: exaggeration of drive toward a personal goal.

albino: an individual with skin in which there is an absence of pigment from birth; the hair is white, and the iris of the eye is pink.

albumin: a protein constituent of the blood serum, found in urine in certain forms of kidney diseases.

algae: chlorophyll-containing water plants, living in both sea and fresh water, varying in size from microscopic to many feet in length.

allergen: a substance capable of producing allergy (see allergy).

allergy: a sensitivity of the body to substances which in themselves are not irritating to the normal body.

alveoli: air sacs in the lung at which the blood exchanges carbon dioxide for a fresh supply of oxygen to carry to the body tissues.

alveolus: the small breathing chambers in the lungs.

amnesia: loss of memory.

amphetamine: a stimulating drug contained in so-called "pep pills."

amyotrophis lateral sclerosis: a deterioration of nerve pathways in the spinal cord, causing muscle deterioration.

analgesic: a preparation or method for relieving pain.

androgens: a group of hormones characteristic of the male.

anesthesia: literally "without feeling"; insensibility to pain, with or without loss of conciousness; anesthesia may be general, local, or regional (block); it may be induced by inhalation, by introduction of the agent into a vein, or into the spine by hypodermic injection or injection into a nerve trunk.

anesthesiology: the medical specialty concerned with anesthesia.

aneurysm: an enlargement in an artery due to weakened walls, sometimes compared with weakening of a tire wall before a blowout.

angina pectoris: literally, pain in the chest; usually refers to pain caused by heart weakness.

aniline: a coal tar ingredient which is the basis for many drugs.

antacid: a drug to overcome excess acidity of stomach secretions, or to render the urine alkaline.

antibiotic: literally "opposed to growth"; substances which check the growth of bacteria (but not viruses) and help the body to overcome infections more rapidly.

antibodies: substances existing in the blood, either naturally or through deliberate immunization procedures, which counteract bacteria or bacterial poisons in the system.

anticoagulants: drugs which help keep the blood from clotting in the vessels.

antigen: any stimulus that produces defensive reactions in the body, creating antibodies (see antibodies).

antihistamines: drugs which tend to neutralize effects of histamine, a substance active in allergic reactions.

antiperspirants: preparations which reduce the amount of perspiration.

antiseptic: a drug that tends to overcome bacterial infection.

antitoxin: a chemical substance in cells and blood serum produced as a defense reaction to a poisonous substance (toxin).

appendicitis: inflammation of the vermiform appendix.

appendicular skeleton: the arms and hands, legs and feet, shoulder, and pelvic bones.

arteries: the largest class of vessels carrying blood away from the heart; arterioles are next in size, and capillaries are the smallest.

arteriosclerosis: hardening of the arteries through deterioration of the elastic tissue components in their walls.

artificial respiration: methods to keep the patient breathing when this normal function has ceased.

ascorbic acid: chemical name for vitamin C.

asthma: difficulty in breathing, due to allergy to food or to substances breathed in; also colloquially used for any kind of breathlessness.

atherosclerosis: a disease affecting the lining membranes of the arteries.

"Athlete's foot": a widely prevalent infection of the skin on the feet, by no means limited to athletes.

atomic: referring to the atom, the unit of chemical entity.

atresia: a blocking of a canal or passage, as of the ear.

571

atropine: a drug derived from the deadly nightshade plant; used medicinally, especially in anesthesia.

audiologist: a person professionally trained in ear testing and choice of hearing aids.

audiometer: an instrument for testing hearing.

autonomic: a term describing the portion of the brain and nervous system which functions automatically to control digestion and other activities which sustain life.

autonomic nervous system: nerves which control the smooth (involuntary) muscle tissue of the internal organs.

auxiliaries: organizations, usually of women, who act as cooperators and helpers in the work of a hospital or health agency.

axial skeleton: those bones including the spinal column and rib cage.

axon: the fiber extending from the neuron which is longer than the other fibers.

B

bacillus: any of a large group of rod-shaped germs.

balloon technique: the use of inflated balloons to apply medication or to change the temperature in hollow organs such as the stomach or bladder.

Bang's disease: Malta fever; brucellosis; an infection causing abortion in animals and a feverish disease in man.

barbiturate: a class of sedative drugs based on barbituric acid; may be habituating.

BGG: a vaccine made from a living but weakened strain of tuberculosis bacilli, used under certain conditions for immunization where tuberculosis is common.

biliousness: an obsolete term formerly applied to all sorts of digestive disturbances.

bismuth: a metal whose salts may be found in hair dyes; also used medicinally.

bituminous: asphalt or blacktop.

blood fractions: separated chemical portions of the blood used for purposes other than transfusion.

blood grouping: the classification of human blood according to four main types.

blood platelets: small grayish discs in the blood which collect at the site of any wound and appear to assist in forming clots.

blood pressure: the pressure of blood against the inner walls of the blood vessels as it is being pumped through the circulatory system.

blood typing: the identification of blood with respect to the group in which it belongs.

Blue Cross: the title and emblem of plans organized to insure the costs of hospital care.

Blue Shield: the title and emblem of medically organized plans to insure the costs of medical and surgical treatment.

boils: germ infections of the skin, usually due to the staphylococcus.

brain waves: tiny, but recordable, electrical impulses reflecting activity in the brain.

Bright's disease: a common form of kidney disease first described by Dr. Richard Bright and named for him.

bronchi: the two cartilaginous branches of the trachea (windpipe) which go to the right and left lung respectively.

bronchial: referring to the branching system of breathing tubes leading to and into the lungs.

bronchioles: tiniest branches of the bronchi, which have walls of muscle instead of cartilage and which terminate in the alveoli.

brucellosis: Malta fever; Bang's disease; an infection causing abortion in animals and a feverish disease in man.

burning tongue: painful burning sensations in the tongue.

bursitis: an inflammation of a pocket (bursa) lined with smooth lubricating membrane (serous).

C

callus: new growth of bone tissue that surrounds a break during the process of repair; also, a hard, thickened area on the skin.

calorie: in nutrition, a unit used to express the fuel or energy value of a given quantity of food.

cancellous: resembling lattice-work; the spongy tissue in bones.

cancer: the Latin for crab; the name of a group of diseases which have the common characteristic of wild and uncontrolled cell growth.

"Candy-striper": adolescent girls who help in hospitals, so named after their pink and white striped uniforms.

canker sores: sores in the mouth of unknown cause.

capillaries: minutest branches of the arterial system, which diffuse blood to the tissues and eventually link up with the smallest branches of the venous system.

carbohydrate: one of the major classes of necessary foods, belonging to the class of compounds represented by the sugars, starches, and cellulose.

carbuncle: multiple boils which tend to undermine the skin.

carcinoma: a cancer that arises from the cells of the skin or the lining cells of the inner organs.

cardiac sphincter: muscle surrounding the entrance to the stomach which permits food to enter and retains it after it has been admitted.

cardiovascular-renal: referring to disease involving two main organ systems at one time; cardio(heart)-vascular (blood vessel)-renal(kidney).

cartilage: a tissue less hard and more elastic than bone, found in joints and elsewhere; commonly called gristle.

catalyst: substance which induces or speeds up a reaction by its presence but itself remains intact.

cataract: a clouding of the crystalline lens in the eye.

cathartic: a drug that stimulates bowel action.

catheter: a flexible rubber tube used for draining bladder or other cavities.

central nervous system: the brain and spinal cord.

cerebral: referring to the brain, or more specifically the forebrain, where conscious controls center.

cerebrospinal: pertaining to the brain and spinal cord.

cerumen: the wax in the outer ear canal.

cesarean section: surgical removal of the baby from the uterus.

chemotherapy: treatment with chemical means; drug treatment.

chiggers: small biting and burrowing insects common in many areas where vegetation occurs.

chiropractor: a practitioner of a "healing" cult based on unscientific theory and unproved assumptions.

chloramphenicol: an antibiotic drug.

chloroform: a liquid anesthetic which evaporates readily and is inhaled.

chloroquin: a drug useful in the treatment of arthritis.

chlorpromazine: a tranquilizing drug.

chlorpropamide: (Diabinese) a drug used for the oral treatment of certain diabetics (see also tolbutamide).

choriocarcinoma: a rare form of cancer found in women after pregnancy.

chronic: lasting a long time.

cobalt: a metal capable of radioactivity, useful in treating cancer.

cocaine: a drug derived from coca leaves, used as a local anesthetic; also a habit forming narcotic.

codeine: a pain-dulling drug derived from opium.

colic: abdominal distress due to spasms or obstructions of intestines, gall bladder, or ureter.

colitis: inflammation or spasm of large bowel, often due to emotional causes.

collagen: a general term referring to the structural tissues of the body other than bone; cartilage, membranes, tendons.

colloid: a special type of chemical solution; an oatmeal bath.

colonic irrigation: high enemas promoted by cults and quacks; of limited usefulness and potentially dangerous unless carefully administered under medical supervision.

coma: deep and continuous unconsciousness formerly common in diabetes.

common cold: a virus infection of the upper breathing organs.

compatible blood: blood from individuals of the same blood group or type, that can be safely given in transfusion.

compensation, workmen's: indemnities paid by employers through insurance or otherwise, to workers injured on the job.

compulsion: the necessity for repeated actions, such as washing the hands repeatedly, or checking up again and again on whether all the lights have been turned out at night.

concussion: an injury, usually to the brain, produced by the shock of an explosion or of violent blows without external signs of injury.

cones: specialized cells in the retina of the eye which are able to distinguish colors.

confusion: medically used to indicate symptoms more severe than ordinary status of being mixed up.

conjunctiva: the membrane which covers the eyeball and lines the eyelids.

conjunctivitis: inflammation of the eye membrane.

connective tissue: the binding tissue of the body holding other tissues together or in proper relation to each other.

constipation: inability to perform normal bowel elimination functions.

contact receptors: nerves which transmit stimuli only on contact, as touch.

contraindication: circumstances which suggest avoidance of certain medical or surgical procedures.

contrast bath: use of alternating hot and cold water, usually as a spray.

convolution: twist or coil of any organ; especially one of the prominent convex parts of the brain.

convulsions: unconsciousness accompanied by muscular twitching.

cornea: the clear window at the front of the eye.

coronary: "crownlike," describing the arteries which supply blood to the heart muscle, and are concerned in (coronary) heart attacks.

cortex: the outer layer of cells of an organ such as the adrenal gland or kidney.

cortisone: a hormone of the adrenal cortex; useful in certain forms of rheumatism and many other diseases.

Coxsackie virus: a virus causing various types of infection.

cranial nerves: those nerves arising directly from the brain and exiting through an opening in the skull.

cranium: the cavity that contains the brain; the skull.

croup: a closing of the voice-box due to infection or spasm.

cusps: component parts of heart valves.

cystitis: inflammation of the urinary bladder.

cystoscope: an electrically illuminated instrument by which the bladder and the kidneys can be visually examined.

D

dander: the skin particles of animals which may cause allergy when breathed.

dandruff: castoff cells from the outer layer of skin, mainly noted in the scalp.

deafness: loss of hearing.

deafness, conductive: hearing loss due to inability of the ear to transmit sounds to the nerve ending in the inner ear.

deafness, nerve: inability of the hearing nerve to transmit sound stimuli to the brain.

death rates: the number of deaths per unit of population or other frame of reference, usually stated as deaths per thousand.

deciduous teeth: the 20 baby teeth.

decongestant: a drug that will reduce tissue swelling.

deerfly fever: see tularemia.

delusions: belief in non-existent circumstances.

dementia: loss of mental capacity due to changes in the brain.

dendrites: fibers extending from the nerve cell (neuron); other than the axon.

dentifrice: a preparation useful in cleaning the teeth.

denture: a fixed or removal device for replacement of lost teeth.

deodorants: preparations which mask or diminish body odor.

Department of Investigation, AMA: repository of information about quacks and quackery.

dependence: the body's need for a narcotic drug.

depilatory: a preparation for the removal of unwanted hair.

depressant: a drug or other influence that lowers the level of body activity.

depression: a mental state of deep sadness and self-accusation beyond the normal reaction to grief or other adverse circumstances.

dermabrasion: removing outer skin layers by friction in order to remove or improve scars, especially those of acne.

dermatology: the medical specialty dealing with the skin.

dermis: the corium, or true skin, lying just below the epidermis or surface skin.

detergents: cleansing agents derived from petroleum and other sources, which are used in place of soap; most are mild but some may irritate some skins.

diabetes mellitus: commonly called sugar diabetes; the inability of the body to utilize starches and sugars by reason of a deficiency in insulin.

diagnosis: the doctor's identification of the disease or abnormality; a necessary preliminary to treatment.

diaphragm: main muscle of breathing; separates chest cavity from abdominal cavity.

diarrhea: frequent loose watery stools.

diastole: relaxation of the heart muscles after contraction.

diathermy: an electronic method for producing heat in body tissues.

dietitians: persons trained in nutrition, found in hospitals, nursing homes, and other institutions.

digestive juices: secretions of the digestive tract which act chemically to help convert food to forms the body can use.

digitalis: the botanical name for the fox-glove; also a basic drug for use in certain types of heart disease.

dislocation: an injury where the bones of a joint are wrenched out of place, usually tearing the joint capsule.

disorientation: confusion as to time and place where the person finds himself.

distance receptors: nerves which receive stimuli transmitted over a distance, as the eye and ear.

diuretics: drugs which increase the amount of urine secreted by the kidneys.

donor: one who gives blood for transfusion.

dope: the common term for narcotic habit-forming drugs.

DPT: the combined immunization against Diphtheria, Pertussis (whooping cough), and Tetanus (lockjaw); commonly called "triple shot."

dropsy: the common term for waterlogging of the tissues when too much fluid is retained in the body.

drowning: suffocation due to inhalation of water into the lungs.

drug: a substance used in the treatment of disease or the promotion of better health.

duodenum: the portion of the small intestine immediately adjacent to the stomach.

dysentery: two specific diseases caused respectively by bacteria and by amebae; also used colloquially to mean diarrhea from any cause.

dystrophy: faulty development.

E

Echo virus: a virus related to influenza which causes obscure types of infection.

eczema: a chronic skin condition of allergic origin.

edema: tissue swelling due to retained fluid; commonly called dropsy.

elastic fibers: fibers capable of returning to their original form after being stretched or compressed; can accommodate change in shape.

electrocardiograph: an electronic instrument for recording the action of the heart as it discharges minute electrical impulses in the course of its muscular and valve action; the record itself is a tracing called an electrocardiogram (ECG).

electrolysis: the removal of unwanted hair by use of a negative galvanic current.

electron microscope: an instrument capable of enlarging extremely minute objects such as viruses.

embryo: an organism in the earliest stages of its development; in the human, before four months.

embolism: a blood clot loose in the circulation, lodging in a small vessel and wholly or partially blocking it.

emollient: a preparation for softening the skin.

emotional climate: the atmosphere of loving care, or the lack of it, which surrounds a child as he grows up.

emphysema: a stretching or inflation of the lungs, causing breathing difficulties.

encephalitis: inflammation of the brain and its coverings due to a virus spread by mosquitoes; popularly called "sleeping sickness."

endocarditis: inflammation of the lining membranes of the heart.

endolymph: fluid in the inner ear.

energy deficit: insufficient energy for ordinary demands of living.

enuresis: wetting the bed during sleeping.

enzymes: substances created by living cells whose presence aids another process within the body or speeds it to completion.

epidermis: the outer, non-vascular, non-sensitive layer of horny cells that protects the "true skin" or dermis.

epiglottis: a flap-like structure that lies over the opening to the larynx and aids in keeping food and other foreign matter out of the air passage.

epilation: removal of hair.

epilepsy: a disease of the brain and nervous system characterized by unconsciousness and convulsions, (grand mal) or short partial blackouts (petit mal).

epinepthrin: a drug prepared from the inner portion of the adrenal gland, more familiarly known as adrenalin.

epistaxis: a nosebleed.

erythema: abnormal redness of the skin due to local congestion, as in inflammation, sunburn, etc.

esophageal speech: speech learned by persons whose larynx has been removed in which the stomach and esophagus are used in place of the windpipe.

esophagus: musculo-membranous canal about nine inches long extending from the pharynx to the stomach.

estrogen(s): a group of hormones characteristic of the female.

ether: a liquid anesthetic which evaporates readily and is inhaled.

ethmoid: a bone in the base of the skull and the sinuses it contains; the latter located between the eyes.

ethyl chloride: a liquid anesthetic which evaporates very rapidly; this gives a cooling and local anesthetic effect.

eustachian tube: a partially collapsible canal which admits air from the throat into the middle ear and equalizes pressures on the ear drum.

excretions: wastes expelled from the body.

expiration: expelling of breath from the lungs.

extension: straightening, as an arm, leg, or back.

elliptical: oval in shape.

external respiration: breathing, i.e., the visible act of inhaling and expelling breath.

external skeleton: a bony framework carried on the outside of the body; as the crayfish.

F

fat: an oily substance found in meats, fish, cheese, milk, and some vegetables; useful for energy and certain essential nutrients required by the body.

fat-soluble: capable of being dissolved in body fat.

feces: the waste products of digestion; excreted by the lower bowel.

Federal Food, Drug and Cosmetic Act of 1938: the legislation and its amendments under which the Federal Government helps to protect the consumer against dangerous products and services.

Federal Register: a periodic publication by the National Archives and Records Service, a branch of the Federal Government, containing important news from the Congress and the Governmental Departments.

Federal Trade Commission: a body charged with enforcement of fair competition in business, including medical claims for commercially promoted medications.

feeblemindedness: lowered mental capacity; mental deficiency.

fenestration: the operation opening the obstructed window (fenestra) between the middle and inner ear.

fenugreek: a hay-like plant whose seeds are used for condiments; promoted as a tea by food faddists.

fertility: the ability to become a parent.

fertilization: the union of sperm and ovum in conception.

fever: elevation of body temperature above the normal; also a part of the name of certain diseases, as typhoid *fever.*

fibrillation: an irregular, usually rapid, rate of excitation of the heart muscle.

fibrositis: inflammation of any fibrous tissue.

flammable: likely to burn.

flexion: bending, as an arm, leg, or back.

flexor: the muscle which bends a joint; extensor: the muscle which straightens a joint once it is bent.

fluoride, fluoridation: fluorides are desirable constituents of some natural water supplies; where the amount present is lacking, adding minute amounts of fluorides supplies the deficiency.

Food and Drug Administration (U.S. Department of Health, Education and Welfare): charged with protection of the public against dangerous, mislabeled, misrepresented, or contaminated food, drugs, and cosmetics.

fovea: a pit or depression, usually applied to the center of the retina (the nervecoat of the eye) where the optic nerve leaves the eye for the brain; the fovea is a blind spot.

fracture: a broken bone; *compound* fracture, one where the bone is exposed; *simple* fracture, where the bone does not penetrate the skin; *comminuted* fracture, where the bone is shattered; *greenstick,* where the bone is bent and splintered on one side.

frigidity: literally "coldness," especially sexual indifference.

frontal: in front, as the forehead; the sinus or hollow in the frontal bone of the skull.

frostbite: devitalized skin or deeper areas due to exposure to cold.

frustration: inability to achieve personal goals.

fulcrum: the fixed point against which a lever operates.

functional: a disease not accompanied by demonstrable changes in the body.

fungus: a microscopic plant growth; some fungi are capable of producing diseases, others like penicillium, of helping to overcome them.

furuncle: a staphylococcus infection commonly called a boil.

G

galactosemia: a birth defect which causes some babies to show mental retardation if they drink milk.

gamma globulin: a protein substance in blood serum, concerned with immunity against infections.

ganglion: a collection of neurons and fibers forming a subsidiary nerve center within a main nerve system.

gas: a substance in the form of vapor; many are poisonous.

gastrointestinal: referring to the stomach and the intestines.

gingivitis: inflammation of the gums.

glaucoma: a hardening of the eyeball due to interference with normal circulation of the eye fluids.

globulins: a group of proteins found in animal tissues which differ from the albumins in that they are soluble in pure water.

glomerule: the important functioning unit of the kidney.

glomerulonephritis: disease affecting the glomerules which perform the principal kidney functions.

glucose: grape sugar; one of the simpler chemicals belonging to the general class of sugars.

glycerin: a chemical of the alcohol group.

glycogen: starch stored in the body to be converted as needed into sugar (glucose).

gout: a general disease due to inability of the body to handle protein foods containing purin bodies; its principal symptoms involve the joints.

gray matter (cortex): the substance forming the outer part of the brain and the inner part of the cord, containing the specialized cells of these parts.

greenstick fracture: like breaking a green twig, where cracking will occur but not complete severance of the parts.

griseofulvin: a drug used in the treatment of ringworm infection of the skin.

group health insurance: purchase of health insurance through organized groups in industry, lodges, or associations.

gumboil: an infection at the root of a tooth which drains through the gum.

gynecology: the medical specialty concerned with the diseases of women.

H

habituation: becoming accustomed to the use of a drug, such as a laxative, to an extent which affects the normal functioning.

halitosis: unpleasant breath.

hallucination: seeing or hearing things that are not there.

hallucinogen: a drug that gives a false sense of well-being (see peyote, jimson weed, LSD-25).

Harrison Act: a law controlling the sale, possession, and prescribing of habit-forming drugs, intended to combat drug addiction.

Haversian canals: openings running through the compact substance of the bone in a longitudinal direction and connecting with one another by transverse branches.

hay fever: the form of allergy affecting the nose and eyes, and prevalent mainly in the Fall.

health foods: a term used by faddists and promoters; there are no health foods as such.

health insurance: insurance against some of the costs of medical, surgical, and hospital care, and sometimes nursing home care.

heat exhaustion: collapse due to excessive exposure to heat.

hemaglobin: an iron-containing pigment in the red blood cells which carries oxygen to the tissues.

hematoma: a circumscribed collection of blood in the tissues.

hemisphere (of the brain): either lateral half of the brain.

hemoglobin: the coloring matter of the red corpuscles which has a strong affinity for oxygen and is used to carry it to the body tissues.

hemorrhoids: varicose veins about the anus, commonly called "piles."

hepatitis: infection of the liver, formerly called infectious jaundice.

hernia: an imperfection in body structure permitting organs to be pushed into areas where they do not belong; commonly called "rupture."

heroin: a drug derived from opium; outlawed in the United States.

hiccups: spasms of the diaphragm usually due to irritations in the upper abdominal area, such as overeating.

histamine: a substance released in the body during allergic reactions.

history, medical: the record of past illness, operations, accidents, and other pertinent experiences of the patient and of his forebears insofar as the latter facts are available.

hives: itching bumps in the skin which come and go; due to allergic reactions, often toward foodstuffs; also caused by emotional upsets.

horny layer: the epidermis, or non-sensitive outer skin layer which protects the true skin, or dermis.

house dust: the mixed dusts which accumulate in the air of dwellings and cause allergic reactions in some persons.

humectant: a preparation intended to preserve moisture in the skin.

humerus: bone of the upper arm.

hydrochloroquine: a drug useful in the treatment of arthritis.

hydrophobia: See rabies.

hygienist: a person technically trained in the principles of healthful living or as an assistant to a professionally qualified person; for example, industrial hygienist, dental hygienist.

hyperplasia: overgrowth in numbers of tissue cells.

hypertension: high blood pressure.

hypertrophy: enlargement, as of a muscle.

hypnosis: a state of suspended consciousness accompanied by a dependence upon the hypnotist.

hypnotic: something, usually a drug, that induces sleep.

hypochondriac: a person obsessed with real or imaginary disease in himself.

hysteria: the conversion of mental or emotional illness into physical symptoms such as blindness, paralysis, etc.; not to be confused with the common term "hysterical."

I

immunity: the capacity of the body to resist infection.

immunize: to protect against a communicable disease by having it and recovering, or by taking vaccine or other protective agents which stimulate natural body resistance.

impetigo: a superficial, highly-contagious skin infection.

impotence: absence or failure of the sexual function in the male.

indigestion: digestive distress or upset due to many different causes.

infarction: an area of tissue death or injury due to blocking off of its blood supply; usually referred to the heart.

infection: invasion of the body by germs, viruses, or parasites.

infertility: the inability to become a parent.

influenza: a group of virus infections commonly called "flu."

infra-red: the rays beyond the red end of the light spectrum; useful as heat sources in medicinal treatment.

insect repellent: a preparation to be applied to skin for the purpose of discouraging biting insects.

insertion (of a muscle): the point where it is attached to produce a motion.

inspiration: intake of breath.

insulin: the internal secretion of the islands of Langerhans, situated within the substance of the pancreas; its deficiency causes diabetes mellitus.

intern: a young physician, graduated from medical school who is gaining experience in a hospital.

internal medicine: the medical specialty concerned with illnesses of a non-surgical nature, mainly in adults.

internal respiration: that portion of the respiration process which takes place inside the organism.

internal skeleton: bony framework on the inside of the body which grows with the body, as in man.

involuntary (smooth) muscle: unstriated muscle tissue which acts independently of the will to govern automatic physical functions.

iris: the colored layer of the eye, surrounding the pupil; especially that part of it which is visible behind the cornea; also called uvea.

islands of Langerhans: clusters of cells in the pancreas which supply the body with insulin.

isoniazid (INH): a drug useful in the treatment of tuberculosis.

isotopes, radioactive: common chemicals "tagged" with a radioactive charge; useful in diagnosis and treatment, especially of malignant disease.

J

jaundice: bile pigment in the blood and tissues giving them a yellow appearance.

jimson weed: a weed from which a drug is derived which gives a false sense of well-being.

K

kelp: seaweed; promoted far beyond its limited usefulness as a source of iodine in the diet.

keratolytic: capable of dissolving keratin, the hard substance of the hair and nails.

L

lactose: a sugar found in milk.

laryngectomee: a person who has had his voice box removed.

laryngectomy: removal of the voice box because of cancer.

larynx: the organ of voice situated at the front of the neck, beginning below the base of the tongue and being continuous with the windpipe; the air breathed passes through it.

laughing gas: an anesthetic gas, nitrous oxide.

lead: a dangerous chemical producing poisoning when swallowed; found in some hair dyes.

leptospirosis: swine-herder's disease, infectious jaundice; an infection of swine transmitted to man and causing illness with fever, jaundice, and kidney disease.

leukemia: a disease in which white blood cells become too numerous in the blood stream; due to disease of the bone marrow, probably cancerous.

leukoplakia: white patches in the mouth, also called smokers' patches.

life jacket: an inflated garment intended to keep a person afloat in the water.

lobotomy: an operation on the brain.

longevity: the length of life.

LSD-25: a drug which creates a false sense of well-being.

lymph: a clear, yellowish fluid which bathes all cells and is returned to the blood stream from the tissues by the lymphatic vessels.

lymph nodes: small glandular organs inserted in the lymph vessels at strategic points where they can filter out infection and so protect the remainder of the body; also called lymph *glands.*

lymphatic system: a circulatory network of vessels and filter glands which drain and distribute the lymph (body fluids).

lymphocytes: also called lymph cells; a leucocyte (white cell) formed in the lymph nodes.

lymphoma: a tumor arising from the lymphoid tissue in the body.

M

Mae West: a nautical term for a certain design of life jacket.

malady: an illness, discomfort, or disability.

malocclusion: a state where teeth do not meet properly and there is an abnormal "bite."

malingering: the intentional faking of disease.

Malta fever: Bang's disease, brucellosis; an infection causing abortion in animals and a feverish disease in man.

Mantoux test: a form of tuberculin test that injects the test material between the layers of the skin.

maple sugar urine disease: a birth defect in body chemistry.

marijuana: a common weed which has exhilarating effects when smoked, often leading to troublesome conduct.

massage: stroking, kneading, or pressure scientifically applied by trained persons for the relief of pain or muscular stiffness.

mastoid: the heavy bone at the rear of the base of the skull, and the sinuses it contains.

maté: a South American herb used as a tea; a folk medicine of no special value; Paraguay tea.

matrix: a mold; the cavity in which anything is formed.

maxillary: referring to the upper jawbone and the hollow or sinus in that bone.

medical social workers: trained persons who assist in solving the financial and social problems of the sick, in hospital or out.

medication: drugs taken internally or applied externally, as distinguished from other forms of medical treatment.

melancholy: a state of sadness.

melanin: a dark pigment occurring naturally, though in varying amounts, in skin or in body parts such as the eye, hair, etc., or from "suntanning."

melanoma: a malignant growth arising from pigmented tissue, usually a certain type of skin mole.

mellitus: a derivative from the Latin for honey; applied to the sweet taste of urine in diabetes mellitus.

membrane: thin layer of fibrous tissue surrounding a part, or separating adjacent cavities.

membrane, serous: a connective tissue sheet lubricated with slippery serum.

Meniere's disease (or syndrome): disturbed hearing and balance due to disease of the inner ear.

meningitis: inflammation of the covering membranes of the brain and the spinal cord.

mental deficiency: lowered mental capacity; feeblemindedness.

meprobamate: a tranquilizing drug.

metabolism: the process of transforming foodstuffs into tissue elements and into energy for use in body growth, repair, and general function.

metastasis: the wandering of malignant tumor cells through circulatory channels to remote areas, where a secondary tumor may start growing.

microorganism: a general term covering microscopic forms such as germs, viruses, etc.

migraine: a severe type of headache, often one-sided and sometimes accompanied by visual disturbances.

miliary: a term describing generalized tuberculosis infection.

mineral: a metallic substance found in nature; many minerals are essential for human and animal nutrition.

molds: fungi which produce spores; some may cause allergies.

mononucleosis: an infectious disease of young adults and adolescents sometimes called the "kissing disease."

morphine: a pain-dulling drug derived from opium.

motion sickness: an illness due to motion in trains, automobiles, ships, planes, buses, or swings.

motor nerve: concerned in, causing, or pertaining to, motion.

mouthstick: a device for use by persons who have no functioning hands.

mouthwash: a pleasant preparation useful for rinsing the mouth, but of no medicinal value.

multiple sclerosis: a nervous system disease of many symptoms, due to deterioration and hardening (sclerosis) of brain and nerve tissues.

mumps: a virus infection of the salivary glands; sometimes affecting the sex glands, the female breasts, and the pancreas.

muscoloskeletal: referring to the framework of the body, including muscles and skeleton.

muscular dystrophy: a disease in which muscle tissue gradually wastes away.

mutilation: the loss of a member or portion of the body.

myasthenia gravis: severe muscle weakness of a specific type.

myositis: inflammation of muscular tissue.

N

NA: Narcotics Anonymous, a group fashioned after Alcoholics Anonymous to help former narcotic addicts.

narcotics: drugs which induce sleep or depress body functions.

nasopharnygoscope: an electrically-lighted instrument for examining the throat and larynx.

nasopharnyx: the upper part of the throat, behind the nose.

naturopath: a practitioner of a healing cult which relies on so-called natural methods—diet, air, sun, and water—to treat disease; naturopaths do not have a medical education.

nephritis: literally an inflammation of the kidney but loosely used to cover other kidney diseases.

nervousness: an inaccurate term covering almost anything for which no other cause can be found.

neuresthenia: an out-moded term for chronic fatigue and weakness; the cause of these symptoms is now sought in concealed disease conditions.

neurology: the medical specialty concerned with the physical diseases of the brain and nerves.

neuron: a nerve cell.

neurosis: an abnormal way of meeting a situation; an emotional disorder.

nitroglycerine: a drug which reduces spasm in the arteries.

nitrous oxide: an anesthetic gas commonly called laughing gas.

non-striated (smooth) muscles: the involuntary muscles controlling actions of the internal organs.

norm, normal: as it ought to be.

nostrum: literally "our"; a quack or secret medicine.

nurse, practical: a trained person capable of performing limited nursing services under supervision.

nurse, registered: a hospital graduate, often with some college education, registered as a nurse by the state.

nurses' aide: trained women employed in hospitals to perform non-medical services such as making beds, serving meals, etc.

O

obesity: overweight, usually applied to weights more than 15 per cent above normal, and due mainly to fat rather than bone and muscle.

obstetrics: the medical specialty concerned with the care of the pregnant woman and her delivery.

occipital lobe: one of the sections, or lobes, of the cerebrum; located toward the back.

occlusion: the closing of a tube or duct, such as a blood vessel.

oculist: an eye physician or ophthalmologist.

ophthalmologist: a doctor of medicine specializing in eye diseases, also called an oculist and eye physician.

ophthalmology: the medical specialty concerned with diseases of the eye and conservation of vision.

opiates: the group of drugs obtained from opium; also sometimes used loosely to refer to all sedatives.

optician: a maker of lenses and optical instruments.

optimum: the most desirable state of affairs.

optometrist: a technician trained in the behavior of light, and in fitting glasses, but not in diagnosing nor treating eye diseases; not a doctor of medicine.

oral surgery: surgery in and about the mouth.

orderlies: men who care for maintenance needs and do some of the heavier work around hospitals.

origin (of a muscle): the point where it can be said to "begin."

organic: a disease accompanied by demonstrable changes in the body structure.

ornithosis: disease acquired through birds; also, "parrot" fever, a virus disease transmitted by parrots and related to birds.

orthodontic: referring to corrective dental work beyond the filling of cavities or extraction of teeth.

orthodontist: a dentist who corrects irregularities of the teeth and poor "bite."

orthopedics: the medical specialty concerned with the bones, joints, and other supporting tissues.

osteo-arthritis: the common, usually non-crippling form of arthritis due to aging.

osteoblast: cell concerned with forming new bone material and repairing old.

osteoclast: cell which eliminates bone tissue not needed for skeletal strength and efficiency, as after injury or fracture has healed and left superfluous bony ridges.

osteocyte: a bone cell carrying on continuous maintenance activity within the bone.

osteopath: a practitioner of a system of treatment based originally on a faulty theory of vertebral displacement; most osteopaths no longer hold this theory; some are qualifying as doctors of medicine.

otologic: referring to the ear (*otology, otologist* are derivatives).

otosclerosis: deafness due to obstruction of the opening (window) between the middle and inner ear.

out-patient service: care of patients in hospital clinics without admitting them to a hospital bed.

oxidation: the chemical process of uniting with oxygen, or burning; in the body this takes place in many ways.

P

Pacinian corpuscles: elliptical, semitransparent bodies that occur along the nerves supplying the skin, especially of the hands and feet, and record deep pressure stimuli.

pain receptors: bare nerve endings in the tissue cells of skin and other organs, though not present everywhere in the body.

paired organs: organs of which the body has a pair: eyes, kidneys, sex glands, lungs, etc.

palliation: treatment which improves the patient's feelings without curing his disease.

palpitation: excessive consciousness of the heart beat.

palsy: the popular term for paralysis, especially if there is shaking or trembling associated with it.

pancreas: the principal digestive gland, situated behind the stomach; also the location of the islands of Langerhans, which furnish the internal secretion *insulin,* by virtue of which the body is able to make use of sugars and starches.

Pap test: short for Papaniculao test, named after the discoverer; it consists of examining smear specimens of body secretions for the early detection of cancers.

Paraguay tea: a decoction made from the South American herb maté; of no special medicinal value.

paralysis: loss of nervous function, especially loss of motion.

paramedical: services related to medicine and performed by technically trained persons.

paraminosalicylic acid (PAS): a drug useful in the treatment of tuberculosis.

paranoid: pertaining to type of mental illness in which suspicion plays an important part.

parasympathetic nerves: those nerves which reverse the action of the sympathetic nerves; also a part of the autonomic nervous system.

Parkinson's disease, parkinsonism: a brain disease affecting the nerves and through them the muscles, with stiffness and trembling.

parrot fever: a virus infection transmitted by bird, especially parrots and related species.

pasteurization: the heating of milk to destroy disease-causing germs; named after Louis Pasteur, its originator.

patch test: a means of determining skin sensitivity or general allergy, used in diagnosis and as a test for safety of hair dyes.

"patent" medicine: a commercially-promoted drug preparation of secret composition, NOT patented, since patenting would require disclosure of its composition, which usually consists of common and well-known drugs or of largely worthless and outmoded herbs and other substances.

pathological: abnormal tissue conditions, characteristic of disease.

pathology: the identification of abnormal tissues and processes.

pediatric: the medical specialty concerned with the diseases of children, up to 18 years of age.

pediatrician: a medical specialist who treats children, primarily up to the age of 18 years.

pedodontics: treating the teeth of children.

peer: an associate of about equal age; contemporary.

pelvic girdle: the ring of bones which form the hips and lower abdominal area.

pemphigus: a skin disease which affects the general health; it causes blisters.

penicillin: the first and most widely used antibiotic; a product of the bread-mold penicillium.

pep pills: stimulating drugs used to keep the person from falling asleep; they are dangerous and may be habit forming.

peptic ulcers: ulcers in the stomach and the duodenum.

perfusion: isolating the circulation in a limited portion of the body for the purpose of treating cancer in that area with highly potent drugs.

periodontics: treatment of disease in tissues around the teeth.

peridontitis: inflammation of tissues surrounding the teeth, sometimes causing loosening of the teeth.

periodontosis: wasting away of the bone surrounding the teeth, with consequent looseness of the teeth.

periosteum: membrane covering surfaces of bone, except where ligaments are attached or where bone becomes cartilaginous.

peripheral: away from the center, as the nerves and blood vessels in the arms and legs.

peripheral nervous system: continuing on from the central nervous system, and including nerves running to the sense organs, heart, and internal organs, and the skeletal muscles.

peristalsis: wave-like motion of esophagus, stomach, and intestines which keeps the food material moving.

peyote: a stimulating drug derived from the mescal weed, used by the Indians in religious ceremonials; misused for "kicks."

phagocyte: a white blood cell which destroys bacteria and tissue debris.

pharmaceutical: pertaining to drugs and pharmacy; a drug.

pharmacist: a person trained in the handling of drugs and the compounding of prescriptions, and licensed by the state.

pharynx: the space at the back of the mouth, generally called the "throat," which extends upward to meet the nasal cavities and is continuous with the esophagus and the larynx going downward.

phobia: a morbid fear, with or without foundation; in relation to disease, cancerphobia for example.

photosynthesis: the process by which green plants use light to form carbohydrates from the carbon dioxide and water in the air.

physical medicine: the use of physical agents in treating disease; light, heat, water, massage, and exercise.

physiotherapy: treatment based on physical agents—light, heat, electricity, massage, vibration, water, and exercise.

pigment: coloring matter in the skin, hair, and eyes.

pitchman: a promoter, usually posing as a health lecturer, for food fads or other forms of quackery.

pituitary: the principal gland of internal secretion, located under the middle of the lower surface of the brain.

PKU (Phenylketonuria) disease: a birth defect in body chemistry causing retardation unless discovered.

placenta: the special organ which nourishes the unborn; the "afterbirth."

plasma: the serum or liquid portion of the blood.

plastic: pliable; also a synthetic substance adaptable to many purposes, such as nylon, orlon, vinyl, etc.

plastic surgery: surgery aimed at restoring lost function and in some instances improving personal appearance.

poison ivy: skin irritations due to toxic oils in this common wild plant.

poison oak: skin irritations due to toxic oils in this common wild plant.

polarization: referring to light, a condition in which the vibrations all take place in one plane; it reduces glare in glasses and mirrors.

pollen: the male cell of certain plants, distributed by the wind; some pollens cause allergies in certain persons.

pollution: the spoiling of a natural resource such as air or water by noxious or dangerous contaminants.

polyp: an abnormal growth from a mucous membrane, usually not cancerous, but occasionally malignant.

pox: any eruptive disease: smallpox, greatpox (syphilis), chickenpox.

precancerous: referring to body conditions which might favor the development of cancers, such as chronic sores, irritations, and exposure to substances known to cause cancer.

preventive medicine: efforts to avoid the development of illness, practiced by all physicians.

proctoscope: an electrically lighted instrument by which the larger bowel can be examined and treatment performed.

prognosis: the doctor's forecast of the probable future course of illness.

prostate: the gland which surrounds the bladder opening in the male; commonly miscalled prostrate.

prosthodontics: the creation of special appliances to compensate for oral malformations.

protein: a food substance based on compounds of nitrogen, essential for body growth and maintenance; found mainly in meats, fish, eggs, poultry, cheese, and the leguminous vegetables.

protoplasm: the living matter of cells and tissues.

pseudohypertrophic: giving a false appearance of enlargement.

psittacosis: "parrot" fever; a virus disease spread by parrots and related birds.

psoriasis: a chronic disfiguring skin disease.

psychiatrist: a doctor of medicine with advanced training and experience in the diseases of the mind and disturbances in the emotions.

psychiatry: the medical specialty concerned with diseases of the mind and problems of emotional character.

psychoanalysis: a division of the specialty of psychiatry, involves prolonged exploration of the patient's personality.

psychologist: a person, not a physician, who has been trained in the study of human behavior and psychology.

psychosis: a specific mental illness.

psychotherapy: treatment aimed at helping the patient solve his psychic and emotional problems.

psychosomatic: a term describing a disease in which mental or emotional (psycho) influences produce or aggravate physical (soma) changes.

puberty: the time of maturing of the sexes.

pulp, dental: the inner substance of a tooth including the nerve.

pupil: the opening in the colored layer of the eye.

purin bodies: constituents of proteins most common in red meats, and internal glandular organs such as sweetbreads; important in cases of gout.

purpura: a blood condition which causes bleeding under the skin and into other tissues, such as joints.

pusher: a seller of illegal narcotic drugs.

pustule: a pimple.

pyelonephritis: inflammation of the body of the kidney.

pyloric sphincter: muscle surrounding the opening at the lower end of the stomach.

Q

Q-fever: an infectious fever transmitted from cattle, sheep, and goats by ticks or carried by air and breathed in.

quack: a person, usually not a physician, who pretends to have medical knowledge and experience which he does not possess, for the purpose of defrauding patients for his own profit.

quacksalver: one who "quacks" (sells) his salves; a medical huckster; usually shortened to *quack.*

quarantine: the period of isolation for preventing the spread of communicable disease; gradually being used less and less as better methods become available.

R

rabbit fever: See tularemia.

rabies: a serious virus infection transmitted from many wild and domesticated animals to man.

radiation: the invisible energy rays given off by x-ray, radium, and other chemicals when exposed to radioactive sources.

radiology: the medical specialty concerned with use of radiation in diagnosis and treatment of disease.

radium: a source of radiation useful in treating disease.

ragweed: a common inconspicuous weed whose wind-blown pollen is one of the main causes of autumn hay fever.

reaction: a term indicating undesired and unpleasant effects from a drug or other medical procedure.

receptor cells: specialized cells that collect information for the organism.

receptors: peripheral nerve endings in the skin and the special sense organs which enable the human organism to detect stimuli.

red blood cells: minute, circular discs floating in the blood which carry oxygen to the tissues and carbon dioxide away from them; also called red corpuscles.

red marrow: found in the interstices of cancellous bones.

reflex: an involuntary response in which a stimulus is received by a nerve, transmitted, and finally translated into muscular activity—all in a fraction of a second.

reflex arc: the mechanism necessary for a reflex action.

refraction: the behavior of light rays passing from a medium of one density to one of another; also the process of testing the eyes for fitting spectacles or contact lenses.

regimen: a program of healthful living and medical care.

rehabilitation: restoration to the best possible functioning state after serious illness or injury.

rejection phenomenon: the tendency of the living body, animal or human, to destroy tissues from another individual or animal when transplanted.

rejuvenators: preparations or methods supposedly capable of returning lost youth; they are worthless.

reserpine: a tranquilizing drug derived from the Indian snakeroot.

resident physician: a senior physician-in-training in a hospital or an employed physician who lives in the hospital.

residual: remaining after a disease or injury, as "residual" disability.

respiration: the total process by which oxygen is absorbed into the system and the oxidation products, e.g., carbon dioxide and water vapor, are given off; the outward signs of this process are the inhaling and exhaling of air.

respirator: a device using alternate pressure and vacuum to help patients breathe when they have had a paralyzing illness or injury.

respiratory: referring to the breathing organs.

retina: the layer of light-sensitive nervous cells at the back of the inner surface of the eyeball which makes vision possible.

Rh factor: a characteristic of blood which is of importance in pregnancy.

rheumatic fever: an acute, severe illness usually following a severe sore throat; not the same as rheumatism.

rheumatoid: a severe and often crippling form of arthritis.

rhythm: family spacing by limiting sexual intercourse to the relatively infertile phases of the menstrual cycle.

ringworm: a fungus infection of the skin, hair, and nails.

rods: specialized cells in the retina of the eye that are sensitive to fine degrees of light and dark.

rose hips: the fruit or seed of a rose, used in pharmacy and promoted by food faddists.

roundworms: intestinal worms which infest children usually through contact with infested pets, especially dogs and cats.

rubella: German measles, one-day measles.

rubeola: "red" measles, five-day measles.

rupture: see hernia.

S

salivary glands: six in number and located three on each side of the mouth, they secrete the saliva which moistens the food during chewing and begins the digestive process.

salmonella: an organism related to that of typhoid fever which produces intestinal upsets.

sanatorium: a special hospital for the treatment of tuberculosis patients (see also sanitarium).

sanitarium: an older term for a mental disease hospital.

sanitation: the proper disposal of all wastes and noxious matters and proper cleanliness in regard to environment, especially foodstuffs.

sarcoma: a malignant (cancerous) tumor arising from bone, muscle, or other framework tissue in the body.

schistosome: a parasite present in fresh water, which causes swimmers' itch.

sclerosis: a hardening of a tissue, as in a scar.

scopolamine: a drug derived from the deadly nightshade, related to atropine; commonly called "truth serum."

screening: rapid superficial examination of groups of persons to identify those most in need of medical care.

Scuba: Self-Contained-Underwater-Breathing Apparatus; also used to refer to the sport of underwater diving and swimming.

seborrhea: a disturbance of the oil glands in the skin.

sebum: the oily secretion from sebaceous glands in the skin.

secretions: the products of glandular organs.

sedative: a calming effect, often induced by a drug.

sedentary: literally "seated," used to indicate insufficient physical activity.

sensitization: changes in the body due to exposure to a drug or a protein substance which cause the body to react violently to subsequent contacts with the same.

sensory nerve: a nerve which conveys sensations from the periphery of the organism to the centers.

septum: a dividing wall of tissue such as that between the two sides of the nose or the right and left sides of the heart.

septum (of the heart): wall of muscle separating left and right portions of the heart.

septum (nasal): the partition between the two nostrils.

serum: the clear, yellowish fluid of the blood which is left after blood clots in a test tube.

sheath: a membrane covering or "wrapping" an organ, muscle, or other structure.

shock treatment: electric current passed through the brain; also induced by injections.

shot: a vernacular term for an injection; used also to denote a dose of a narcotic.

sibling: a brother or sister.

sign: an evidence of disease or abnormality observable by the physician, as distinguished from a symptom felt by the patient.

signal: instruction or direction sent from the brain.

sinus: a space or cavity, such as the hollows in the bones of the head; or a similar space elsewhere in the body.

skeleton: the bony framework of the body.

smallpox: a serious and highly contagious virus disease.

socialization: adaptation of an individual toward getting along with others.

sodium bicarbonate: baking soda.

sodium chloride: ordinary table salt.

soft palate: the rear portion of the roof of the mouth.

solar energy: the light or heat from the sun which is capable, when properly harnessed, of doing work, providing fuel, etc.

soluble: capable of being dissolved; water-soluble, in water; fat-soluble, in fats or oils, etc.

solvent: a substance capable of dissolving other substances; water, alcohol, and oils are solvents.

sorbitol: an alcohol; a sugar solution used in treatment of patients whose skin is retaining too little water.

sound: sensation produced in the ear when certain vibrations (sound waves) are caused in the sourrounding air.

spectrum: the breakdown of white light into colored bands; also indicating the range of effectiveness of drugs.

sphenoid: a bone in the skull and the sinuses it contains, located behind the nose in the center of the head.

sphincters: muscles surrounding certain parts of intestinal tract; these widen or narrow the lumen as required.

spinal cord: the nerve structure running within the spinal canal of the spinal column.

splint: a rigid device for holding broken bones in place or easing pain in certain rheumatic diseases.

spores: seed-bodies of fungi, often the cause of allergic symptoms.

sprain: an injury to ligaments around a joint, often including small fractures.

staphylococcus: a pus forming germ concerned in many ordinary infections.

staples: one of the three tiny bones in the middle ear which transmit sound vibrations.

sterile: free from germs or viruses; also, incapable of procreating.

sterility: the condition of infertility.

stethoscope: a simple instrument used to carry sounds from within the chest or other parts of the body to the ears of the physician.

stimulant: a drug or other influence that raises the level of body activity.

stimuli: goads to incite action, exertion, or response from an organism.

stomatitis: inflammation of the mouth.

strabismus: squint, more commonly called crossed eye; also "wall" eyes.

stratum lucidum: translucent layer of the epidermis.

streptomycin: an antibiotic useful in treating tuberculosis and other conditions.

"strep" throat: a severe sore throat due to infection with the streptococcus organism.

stress: circumstances which put a person under pressures which may have unfavorable influence on his mental or emotional health.

striated muscles: striped or voluntary muscles which are subject to control by the will.

stroke: brain injury from rupture, blocking or spasm of an artery; also applied to similar tissue elsewhere, as in the heart (coronary) or other organs.

stuttering: a speech habit that is normal in small children and is usually outgrown if not emphasized by parents.

stye: an inflammatory condition of an eyelash follicle.

subarachnoid: the space between the brain and its innermost covering membrane.

sucrose: a complex sugar; common table sugar.

sulfa drugs: properly called sulfonamides; drugs derived from a dye substance; they help control certain types of bacterial infection.

sulfonamide: a class of drugs based on a dyestuff, effective against certain germ infections.

sunstroke: injury to the brain from excessive exposure to sun.

suture (cranial): line of joining or closure.

sympathetic nerves: that portion of the autonomic nervous system which stimulates the involuntary (smooth) muscles of the body to activity.

symptom: something abnormal that the patient feels, as distinguished from evidences observable by the physician (See also "sign").

synapse: the intertwining of terminal branches of neurons so that nerve impulses may pass from one to the other.

syndrome: a commonly observed combination of symptoms.

syphilis: an infection with a spiral-shaped germ, spread by sexual and other personal contact.

systemic: influencing or affecting the body as a whole.

systole: contraction of the heart muscles to squeeze blood out.

T

taste buds: nerve organs on the tongue which enable the person to distinguish tastes.

technician: a person skilled in procedures requiring special knowledge and training and which are applied under medical supervision; x-ray and laboratory technicians are two examples.

tendon: band of dense, fibrous tissue forming the end of a muscle and attaching the muscle to the bone.

tenomyositis: inflammation of a muscle or muscles and their tendon.

tenositis: inflammation of a tendon.

tenosynovitis: inflammation of a tendon and sheath.

testimonial: a written or spoken endorsement of a drug or other medical treatment by a patient, usually one not qualified to judge.

therapist: a person trained to give therapy (treatment) by physical means (heat, light, water, massage, and exercise) or by teaching the patient to use his muscles in performing occupational exercises incidental to the making of some object or performing some useful service.

therapist, occupational: one who directs rehabilitation through constructive occupations which help overcome physical or mental disabilities.

therapist, physical: one who uses physical means: light, water, heat, massage, exercise.

therapist, speech: one who deals with speech problems.

therapy: the medical word for treatment.

thermal: pertaining to heat.

thermostat: a device, usually electronic, which controls temperature of air or water.

thoracic surgery: surgery involving the organs in the chest.

thrombosis: the complete or partial blocking of a blood vessel by clot formation.

thymus gland: a structure lying beneath the breast bone, which normally disappears at or about birth.

thyroid: a gland of internal secretion situated in the lower front region of the neck.

thyroid gland: a butterfly-shaped gland in the front of the neck which regulates the body chemistry and helps control growth and maturing.

tic: a twitching muscle.

tick: a skin parasite common in wooded and brushy areas, which infests animals and man; some cause tick fever.

tinnitus: ringing in the ears, or other ear noises.

tolbutamide: (Orinase) a drug used for the oral treatment of certain diabetics (see also chlorpropamide, Diabinese).

tolerance: the ability to take increasing doses of a drug by reason of the diminishing effect which occurs with use.

tolerance test: observation of the ability of a person to take a large dose of sugar and utilize it effectively.

tonsils: lymphoid structures in the throat, behind the nose (adenoids), and on the base of the tongue which protect against breathed or swallowed infection until they themselves become infected.

tourniquet: a constricting band about a limb to control severe bleeding.

toxic: poisonous.

toxoid: a toxin that has been deprived of power to injure but which still stimulates immunity formation.

trachea: the windpipe; air from the nose or mouth passes into it via the larynx.

trampoline: an apparatus for tumbling consisting of a frame on which a sheet or web of canvas is stretched by means of elastic ropes or springs.

tranquilizers: drugs which calm disturbed nervous reactions.

transfusion: the transfer of blood plasma or blood with matching type and characteristics to a patient from another individual or a blood bank.

transplantation: the replacement of a diseased organ with a similar organ from another person; now largely experimental.

tremor: trembling.

tuberculin test: a skin test which shows whether or not an individual has received tubercle bacilli in his body.

tuberculosis: any infection with the tubercle bacillus.

tularemia: a disease of wild animals which infects man through breaks in the skin.

tumbling: a gymnastic exercise best described by its name.

turbinates: baffles in the nose which increase its mucous surface.

tympanum: the ear drum.

typhoid fever: a generalized infection with an organism of the salmonella group.

U

ulcer: a sore; either on the skin or on the mucous membrane of any internal organ; in the stomach and intestine such a sore is called a peptic ulcer.

unsaturated fats: fats which have a lower content of hydrogen than saturated fats; unsaturated fats are vegetable in their origin.

uremia: a disease state due to accumulation of wastes in the blood and tissues consequent upon kidney failure.

uric acid: end result of body use of proteins rich in purin bodies; gout is the only form of arthritis which involves uric acid.

urinary disinfectant: a drug that tends to clear the urine of bacteria.

urology, urologist: the medical specialty and the specialist concerned with diseases of the urinary tract.

urticaria: hives.

"used" blood: blood that has traveled through the body and exchanged its supply of oxgyen for carbon dioxide.

uvea: the pigmented (colored) layer of the eyeball.

V

vaccination: any immunization by means of a vaccine; commonly applied to smallpox vaccination.

vaccine: a preparation of living, weakened, or killed microorganisms or viruses, used in prevention of disease through immunizing of persons likely to be exposed.

valve: a device permitting control of an opening so as to allow free passage one way, but not in the other.

varicella: chickenpox.

varicose: a dilated portion of a vein.

variola: smallpox.

vasodilator: a drug that causes the smaller blood vessels to grow larger.

vasomotor nervous system: the nerves which control the size of blood vessels without conscious effort on the part of the person.

veins: largest category of vessels carrying blood to the heart; next in size are venules and capillaries.

venereal: an adjective applied to certain diseases spread largely though not entirely through sexual contacts.

venom: the poisonous substance injected in bites by snakes, certain spiders, bees, wasps, and hornets.

vertigo: dizziness.

vibrations: the motion of the particles of a mass of air in a wave-like manner and at different speeds, usually with enough force to be picked up as "sound" by a receiving unit such as the human ear.

Vincent's infection: an inflammation of the mouth caused by two specific germs acting together.

virus: an entity which grows only in living tissue, is too small to be seen by ordinary microscopes, and is the cause of many diseases.

vitamin: a nutrient substance supplying no calories but essential to health and good nutrition, amply supplied to normal persons by a well-chosen diet.

vocal cords: two transverse parallel folds of mucous membrane at the upper end of the larynx which can either be relaxed toward the sides of the larynx during soundless breathing, or tightened and pulled toward each other to vibrate and produce sound.

voluntary (striped, striated) muscle: sometimes called skeletal muscle because of attachment to the skeleton; it is voluntary muscle tissue, i.e., subject to the will.

W

wantedness: making a person feel wanted in his group or family.

wart: a virus infection of the skin.

water soluble: capable of being dissolved in water.

white cells (leucocytes): minute bodies in the blood, about one-third larger than the red cells, which war against infection; also called white corpuscles.

whorl: circular arrangement of like parts around a point on an axis; as in leaves, flowers or skin ridges (fingerprint).

withdrawal: abnormal shyness and unwillingness to mingle with others; taking drugs away from an addict.

"Wonder" drugs: see sulphonamides.

XYZ

yellow marrow: found in the hollow center shaft of bones.

zoonose: a disease transmitted from animals to man and sometimes back again.

APPENDIX I

QUESTIONS and ANSWERS ON HEALTH

The following pages contain questions on health and medical science that have been directed to American Medical Association publications in the past. The answers given here have been prepared by competent medical and scientific authorities.

APPENDIX II

FAMILY HISTORY

QUESTION: *What is seven-year itch, and does it really last that long?*

ANSWER: No, it only seems that long. Many persons who have not suffered from persistent itching do not realize that this experience can be more trying than pain. Itching is not funny. So-called seven-year itch is properly called scabies. It is caused by a mite, a small parasite related to the spider family. The mite burrows into the skin, leaving a trail of its excreta and eggs. This can be followed by examining the area involved, which is often on the wrists and the hands. The condition is contagious and can pass from person to person. Members of families can infect and reinfect each other, for a long period of time, giving scabies its common name. It is also called ship itch, jail itch and camp itch, for fairly obvious reasons. The condition is often made worse by amateur home treatment. Some of the drugs used may cure the scabies and substitute an irritated dermatitis that is worse than the original itch. With this, as with many other apparently minor conditions, the quickest and cheapest way to take care of it, and the one with the least wear and tear, is to get competent medical treatment right from the start.

QUESTION: *For several years I have used cream type "facial depilatories" with no ill effect; however, several people recently have told me that this could induce skin cancer. Is this so?*

ANSWER: A great many people have used cream-type facial depilatories for many years; they need not be regarded as dangerous from the standpoint of inducing skin cancers. They do sometimes cause the skin to darken, but even this is not the usual result. The main objection to them is that their effects are temporary and some of them have an unpleasant odor.

QUESTION: *I have soft warts about my face and on the eyelids. What causes them? Am I deficient in some sort of vitamin?*

ANSWER: Any vitamin deficiencies you might have would have no connection with warts. Warts are virus infections of the skin. They can be removed by medical treatment, but you should not try to remove them yourself, especially those on the eyelids.

QUESTION: *I have a boy 14 years of age. His face is full of pimples. I have made him try different soaps and a few other things, but they don't seem to help. Do you think it is the changing of his blood or could you recommend something?*

ANSWER: It is quite common for a boy to have pimples. Trying various soaps is no remedy. He needs to go to a physician for appropriate treatment. In most cases, this condition can be helped and it should be because it seriously embarrasses a boy to have a pimply face. You should take your boy to a physician immediately.

QUESTION: *I have had a bad case of alopecia areata, losing practically all my hair. Now most of it is back, except for a few spots on my head. Why should my hair be very oily, and what can be done about it?*

What is the best type of pins or curlers for setting my hair? How soon may I get a permanent? What are the chances of a return of the patchy baldness? My doctor hasn't answered these questions for me, even though I asked him.

ANSWER: We don't have a crystal ball either. These questions are not easy to answer. Some people have oily scalps, others do not; the only thing to do is keep them clean and get medical help if they become inflamed. Pins and curlers should be of a type that do not irritate the scalp or pull on the hair—the last is important. Your own doctor is the only one who can tell you when a permanent would be advisable. And finally—will you have another experience with alopecia areata? No one knows.

QUESTION: *I have a lump as big as a small egg on the right side of my back, next to the shoulder blade. My doctor says it is a fatty tumor and is doing no harm and need not be removed, but it is embarrassing. Should I have it removed?*

ANSWER: Your doctor is probably right. On the other hand, if it bothers you as you say it does, the removal should be a minor matter, easily and simply accomplished.

QUESTION: *I have an obstruction in a gland under the lower lid in both eyes, which makes a lump that doesn't hurt, but I am afraid it will get bigger and bigger. I have been told that it is filling up with secretion and will not burst. It there anything I can do to avoid being cut?*

ANSWER: No, there is nothing you can do. If your description is correct, you probably have some small wens, and these usually have to be "cut" as you put it, but it isn't much of a cut. We would warn you especially not to try any homespun treatment so close to your eyes. You might make things much worse than they are.

QUESTION: *I sleep eight hours at night, but still I have dark circles under my eyes, and bags. What can I do? I am 43 years old.*

ANSWER: These may be family characteristics, assuming that you are in good health. If they are, you can only groan and bear it—unless you can also learn to grin. It would be possible to cover the circles with a special covering preparation available at most cosmetic counters, but the bags are another matter.

QUESTION: *What can you tell us about boils? Do they normally follow removal of a gall bladder, which my husband had done two years ago, or an operation for kidney stone, such as I had several months ago? We have both been having boils. Is something lacking in our diet, or is our resistance low?*

ANSWER: Boils have nothing to do with diet. They are an infection from germs commonly found on the skin, the staphylococcus aureus. They tend to spread by infecting the skin through the discharges of the boils that burst or are opened. They can be passed from one person to another, particularly on the hands. Low resistance may have an influence, but external infection and its spread through unskilled dressing of the boils is the main cause for their spread. You should be under medical care, and should have demonstrations about how to care for boils to keep them from spreading. The Visiting Nurse Association, listed in your telephone book, can send a nurse at small expense to show you the proper technique.

QUESTION: *What causes small, brown or liver-colored spots to appear on the skin?*

ANSWER: Spots appearing on the skin, especially as one grows older, are of various kinds. They are often called liver spots, but actually have nothing to do with the liver. They may be accumulations of skin pigment. Usually they are of little importance except as they mar the appearance, but on occasion one may have considerable significance. It would do no harm to have your doctor look at them.

QUESTION: *The skin on my heel has a tendency to crack. How may it be cured?*

ANSWER: If simple lubrication of the skin with a cream or oil does not prevent it, a physician should be consulted for diagnosis and treatment.

QUESTION: *I have had some superfluous hair removed by electrolysis and I find that one has to have it removed again very often. The operator tells me this is due to "regrowths." How many such regrowths can there be?*

ANSWER: If there is a regrowth of hair after electrolysis, it means that the hair follicle or root was not destroyed.

QUESTION: *.I am four months pregnant, and I menstruate from time to time. My neighbor says this is normal. What do you say?*

ANSWER: We don't say. We ask, is your neighbor a doctor? Good neighbors are wonderful, but their medical advice should be disregarded. A woman who is four months pregnant should be under medical care, and should ask her doctor about her bleeding. Bleeding from the vagina may be due to causes other than menstruation.

QUESTION: *Since otosclerosis is caused by a calcium deposit, is it then advisable to abstain from drinking milk and also eliminate the vitamins that are high in calcium? Thousands of hard-of-hearing people would like to know.*

ANSWER: No. Your conclusion involves three misconceptions: First: otosclerosis is by no means the most important cause of loss of hearing. Second: otosclerosis is a hereditary bone disease in the ear for which the cause resides in the patient, not in his diet. Third: no vitamin contains any calcium; vitamin D influences the use of calcium but does not supply any. For these reasons it would be futile to attempt to prevent loss of hearing, even that due to otosclerosis, by eliminating from the diet the only good source of cal-

cium. The body requires a normal supply of calcium to maintain the blood, muscles and nerves, as well as bones and teeth, in good condition.

QUESTION: *Each spring I have·trouble with itching of my eyes, but I never have it in fall or winter. The itching causes the eyes to burn and there is a stringy secretion which scratches the eyeball. My eyes are very sensitive to light, and I wear sunglasses. I am 30 years old and have had this trouble since I was 14. I am a housewife on a budget and do not feel that I can afford an allergist.*

ANSWER: Maybe you don't need an allergist, but you do need a physician, an ophthalmologist. A budget should provide for necessary medical treatment, since few people escape the need for it; if you really are unable to pay for medical service, it can be provided without cost to you through health and medical agencies in your state. The limitation of your trouble to spring suggests a connection with something in the air at that time; in other words, a possible allergy. What this may be might take some investigation to discover.

QUESTION: *My husband is 53 and he complains of specks or floaters before the eyes, and he can't read or do anything for any length of time without his vision becoming blurred and he has to quit. Isn't there anything that can be done?*

ANSWER: Floaters or specks before the eyes are a nuisance, but they do no harm, and nothing can be done for them. The blurring is something else. At your husband's age, he should have his eyes examined by an oculist, and should be sure to have a pressure test to be certain that his internal eye pressure is not too high. For this, something can and should be done.

QUESTION: *Are kidney stones the same as gravel? My husband is troubled with gravel, which he can't pass, and the pain is terrific—he can't eat or sleep. Does diet have anything to do with it? He likes ice cream before he goes to bed.*

ANSWER: It is assumed that your husband is under medical care. He should ask his doctor about the ice cream, and do not be surprised if he says "no" to it. Ice cream is a fine food, based on milk, which is also a fine food. But it contains more calcium than any other food, and must usually be restricted in the diet when there is a tendency to stone formation. The "difference" between kidney stones and gravel is merely one of size and location.

QUESTION: *After a patient has had a kidney infection and recovered, can he eat liver? What kind of a diet should he have?*

ANSWER: Since you say he has recovered, and make no mention of any permanent injury to the kidneys, he should be able to eat liver, if he likes it, or anything else within reason. Acute kidney infections which leave no permanent effects should not affect future dietary practices. If in doubt, the physician should be consulted, since advice about diet is as important in medical treatment as medication or surgery.

QUESTION: I have gallstones. Please give me a list of foods that I can eat. Must they be strained? Is it better to eat five small meals a day or three regular meals? After I have my gall bladder removed, do I have to eat a bland, low-fat diet the rest of my life to prevent the formation of stones in the billiary passageway? I am always constipated; what can I do to overcome this? Do gallstones make one feel tired and weak, nervous, underweight, constipated, veins protruding, bitter taste in the mouth, snapping joints, and several other symptoms? Should I undergo an operation for the removal of the gall bladder if I feel weak, faint, tired and am underweight?

ANSWER: If you have gallstones, the only person who can give you a list of foods suitable for you is your family doctor, after he finds out what foods you can tolerate. This means that your own experience enters into the selection of such a list. There is no general list of foods applicable to all persons with gallstones. In general, such persons should avoid too much fatty food, especially fried food, too much roughage in fruits and vegetables, especially those which experience teaches them to avoid, and any food that causes distress when taken. Constipation is likely with a diet restricted in fats and in roughage. It is important to realize that with such a diet there will necessarily be fewer and smaller eliminations; it is not abnormal under the circumstances. The common impression that one must have a bowel movement every day is without foundation. Use of laxatives to force action merely makes matters worse. You should be guided by your doctor with regard to this whole problem. You may have to be more careful about your diet after removal of the gall bladder. Patients differ in this regard, and you will have to feel your way, guided by experience and your doctor's advice. The symptoms you mention may or may not be due in part to your gall bladder condition and accompanying digestive upset; your doctor will have to evaluate your entire condition to answer that question. No doctor can advise you by mail whether to have an operation or not; your own physician must be the judge.

QUESTION: My husband had his gall bladder removed almost a year ago, and was told not to eat any pork gravy or ham or raw vegetables or fruits. Now all he will eat is soup, meat, milk and dessert and I claim that this is not a balanced diet. What can I do?

ANSWER: When there is gall bladder disease it is usually necessary to restrict the patient's consumption of fats and sometimes raw vegetables. As a rule the restriction is not so drastic as your husband seems to have imposed upon himself. Ask him to return to his physician for a new evaluation of his condition, which he should have anyway, and a reconsideration of his diet.

QUESTION: What do you recommend for diarrhea in older people?

ANSWER: The first thing to recommend is a thorough examination of the digestive tract for abnormalities which may be causing the diarrhea. Giving medicine for such a symptom as diarrhea without a prior diagnosis is like shooting in a dark cellar at a black cat that isn't there. Diarrhea, or any change in bowel habits in an elderly person, is one of the seven signs of possible cancer. It should call for immediate diagnosis by a physician, possibly with the aid of x-rays and other laboratory tests.

QUESTION: What can be done for a rumbling stomach? It is most embarrassing in church when everything is quiet and I have even declined to go on a trip because of it. I am 46 and in good health. I eat a snack before I go to bed, and I am awakened in the morning by the churning discomfort in my stomach.

ANSWER: There are so many possible causes which might be operating in the abdominal organs, that all one could do on the basis of information furnished would be to guess. You need to see a physician. He may wish to have x-rays of your digestive tract and make other examinations before coming to a conclusion and giving you the relief you desire.

QUESTION: Could an abundance of gas in the stomach, which affects the heart action and causes a light-headed feeling, be a symptom of ulcers? Does the presence of an ulcer in the mouth indicate that there is one in the stomach, too?

ANSWER: The presence of too much gas in the stomach merely indicates that something is wrong—either in the diet or in the digestive process. It does not necessarily suggest an ulcer; it does suggest the advisability of making the necessary medical investigations to ascertain the cause, which may be dietetic, physical or emotional. The presence of an ulcer in the mouth does not necessarily suggest the presence of one in the stomach.

QUESTION: What is the difference between an enlarged liver and cirrhosis of the liver? Can either be cured? Are any operations performed on the liver? Is there a special diet? How long does a person convalesce or live with either of these ailments?

ANSWER: The liver may become enlarged as a result of inflammation abscess, impaired circulation or tumor. Inflammations, such as acute hepatitis, may be overcome. Abscesses may be drained surgically. Circulation can often be improved. Tumors are often inoperable, especially if they are secondary cancers from the stomach or bowels. Cirrhosis is a hardening due to scar tissue from repeated or chronic infections or from the actions of poisons, of which alcohol is one. For many years liver surgery, like heart surgery, was mainly limited to emergency repairs following injury, often with indifferent success. More recently, it has been found possible to perform surgery on the liver for cancer, and to remove consideration portions of diseased liver. New methods are also being used to deal with the accumulations of fluid in the abdomen when liver disease blocks circulation in this area. Operative deaths are not excessively high, but the postoperative history may be difficult, depending on the basic condition for which surgery was done. After operation, the remaining liver tissue has strong regenerative capacities.

QUESTION: What is emphysema? Where does it come from? Is it an old disease? Is there a cure?

ANSWER: Emphysema is most simply described as an overinflation of tissues with air or gas. The term is used mainly in connection with overinflated lungs. It is commonly found among persons who either have difficulty with their breathing, as in asthma, or have one of the lung diseases which used to go with dusty occupations like mining, milling or grinding. It may also occur in persons who use their breathing occupationally, such as musicians playing wind instruments, or glass blowers. If the disease is of long standing, it is not likely that there will be a cure, though there may be improvement if the underlying cause can be eliminated and medical treatment begun. Long-term emphysema causes permanent replacement of the elastic tissues in the lungs with scars, and this process cannot be reversed.

QUESTION: I am 13 years old and 5 feet 5 inches tall and weigh only 109 pounds. I have read about a new liquid or pill to put weight on people. My mother says it is not good for me; my father disagrees with her. I don't think it would hurt me.

ANSWER: This is one time when father doesn't know best. Your mother is right. The only way you can gain weight is through proper eating, enough rest and sleep and plenty of exercise and activity. First, you should have a medical examination to be sure that no medical causes are keeping you thin. And don't say you can't afford it—you were all ready to waste your money on something that would have done you no good.

QUESTION: What is the cause for white spots on the tonsils; they come and go without making my throat sore? I am 17 years old and am having these spots now for the seventh time this year.

ANSWERS: The tonsils are spongy masses of tissue rich in blood supply and filled with lymph cells. They are catchers or filters of infection introduced into the mouth and throat. Some infecting organisms make whitish membranous films or membranes over the linings of the mouth and throat, including the tonsils. Usually these make the throat sore. Since your condition keeps returning we suggest you call it to the attention of your physician.

QUESTION: I had a skull fracture a year ago, and now I have ringing in my ears and am dizzy; also deaf and slightly mentally confused. What do you advise?

ANSWER: The only way you can be helped is to place yourself at once under medical care; if the doctors who treated you at the time of the fracture are available, you may wish to return to them.

QUESTION: I had a cold or flu or something, and now I have lost my sense of smell and taste. I can taste sour, sweet and salt, but no flavors. My doctor says there is nothing to do but wait until my taster comes back, and he seems to think it will. Should I consult a specialist; there is none where I live and the nearest city is quite a way off?

ANSWER: Loss of smell following a cold is not uncommon, and since the finer flavors are perceived mainly through smell rather than taste, these will be lost too. Usually the sense of smell returns, but not always. There is little that a doctor can do to hasten this process, so it is in order for you either to wait and see, or consult a specialist, whichever you prefer.

QUESTION: Will you tell me about silicosis? My doctor said my husband must have had it at one time because he found a chest scar. The TB test was all right.

ANSWER: Silicosis is a condition affecting the lungs as the result of the breathing of dust. It used to be very common among miners, quarry workers and others in dusty occupations. Modern industry has contrived means of preventing dust inhalations, and silicosis is less common than formerly, except among older workers who have been exposed for a long time. The symptoms of many chest diseases, including both silicosis and tuberculosis, are very much the same since they tend to cause a cough, with expectoration and ultimately shortness of breath. The severity of silicosis varies greatly from mild to extremely severe, depending upon the length and degree of exposure.

QUESTION: I had shingles for five months (over one breast towards the back) and still feel it in certain spots on and off. The pains were terrific; I never knew what pains could be. I have no scabs. So many people had the shingles this winter. What is the cause of shingles? I am 73 years of age, never sick—hardly a cold or headache (knock on wood).

ANSWER: Shingles certainly are terrifically painful. They are a virus infection closely related to cold sores and probably to colds and influenza. The only thing you can do is to wait for the pain to go away, and have your physician prescribe relief in the meantime.

QUESTION: Is there any way to stop postnasal drip?

ANSWER: Some of the nasal secretions normally drain into the throat; this becomes a problem only when it is excessive. In such cases, much relief can be had by local medical treatment; often this must be repeated from time to time, especially in the "drippy" weather so common in cold, damp, changeable climates.

QUESTION: Could salt deficiency in the body cause dizziness? I have never eaten much salty food. What can I do for the unsteadiness?

ANSWER: Salt content of the body is normally controlled automatically. Even if you do not eat salty food or use extra salt, you still take in the constituents of salt in your other foods, and your body does the rest. Disturbance of salt metabolism causes weakness, which may include dizziness or unsteadiness, but these symptoms can come from so many other causes that it is unsafe to conclude that salt deficiency is responsible. The only way to find out why you are weak and dizzy is to have a thorough medical examination.

QUESTION: I am suffering what I call sinus headache. It starts above the left eye and behind the eye, over a portion of the left side of the head. There is soreness in the gland or muscle in the left side of the neck and across the shoulder. Is there any way I can obtain permanent relief? I have had my eyes checked and wear glasses.

ANSWER: It would be interesting to know what your doctor calls the headache which you call a sinus headache, and to which of the nasal sinuses he attributes it. Or does he think it might be a tension headache, or a migraine, or one due to your teeth, to an infection somewhere, to your blood pressure, or to any other of a myriad causes of headaches? There is no way to obtain relief, except possibly temporarily, without finding the cause and overcoming that. And that's why you, too, should like to know what your doctor calls your headache, and what HE proposes to do about it.

QUESTION: I am 70 years old and in good health. I have head noises or humming in the ears. For quite a few years, I spent a fortune just trying to get relief, which I did for a while. It is so bad I can't take it much longer. I will go out of my mind. I don't know where to go. How is it no doctor can give something to relieve it? Some medicines I take make the noises worse. I don't know what a good night sleep is. The doctors say you have to live with it. But they should have it one night; they would not say that.

ANSWER: Noises in your ears are extremely annoying, but your doctor is right when he says there is nothing to do in some cases except to learn to live with them. This may sound unsympathetic, but there is nothing else the doctor can do when relief is impossible. Your experience is the same as that of many other persons who have these head noises and can do nothing about them except to learn to endure them. The only possible recommendation is that you consult a specialist in diseases of the ear. If you are being treated by such a person, then you are doing the best that you can for yourself.

QUESTION: I have become positively friendless because of an offensive breath. Please tell me what can be done about halitosis. And don't recommend . . . . . .

ANSWER: It's an easy guess what the lady told us not to recommend—mouthwashes and toothpaste. She had tried them without success. It is undoubtedly true that a clean mouth is a safeguard against offensive breath arising from that source. Toothpastes and mouthwashes are helpful in this regard, if there is no disease condition in the teeth or gums which such preparations cannot remedy. But breath odors can arise from the nose and sinuses, the tonsils or adenoids, or the lungs. They can also come from the stomach, and from the blood—as in the case of garlic, eaten, absorbed into the blood, and excreted through the lungs. Where there is a genuine bad-breath problem, it often takes an extensive job of medical and dental detective work to ferret out its cause. Some persons, too, are superconscious of the "halitosis complex," in which romance always fades out at the crucial moment.

QUESTION: I have had enamelware pots and pans for over ten years and now they are chipped and must be replaced. I want aluminum, but my friends tell me that aluminum utensils are poisonous to cook with. I shall not buy anything until I hear from you.

ANSWER: You go right ahead and buy your aluminum cooking utensils, if that is the kind you prefer. Good—safe—cooking utensils are made of iron, enamelware (until it chips), glass, steel and copper. The story about poisoning from aluminum cooking utensils has more lives than a cat, and not a bit of truth. To begin with, there is aluminum in human tissues. The small amount of aluminum that certain foods may dissolve off the surface of the cooking utensils is in a form that does not dissolve in the body, and so it is eliminated without ever being absorbed. Let your friends use what kind of cooking utensils they please, and you do the same.

QUESTION: Is it true that a blood sugar test is more important than testing kidneys for diabetes?

ANSWER: The earliest best diagnosis of diabetes is made through testing the level of sugar in the blood. This is a far more sensitive test than a urine test and abnormalities appear sooner.

QUESTION: I have diabetes and am taking orinase. I have cold feet, even in bed. I attribute it to poor circulation. What can I do for it? I fear gangrene.

ANSWER: Poor circulation often accompanies diabetes. Since you are taking orinase, it is assumed that you are under medical supervision, which means that you should be seeing your doctor regularly. You should report your symptoms to him, so that he can check up on the effectiveness of the diabetes control with orinase. He may wish to change the drug or your diet, or both, or take other measures toward improving the circulation in your feet.

QUESTION: I know a woman who has diabetes and she says she got it from an auto accident, but I think she had it before that. How long can a person live with diabetes, and can it be cured after one gets blind from it?

ANSWER: Diabetes is not caused by accidents, but a severe accident might so upset the body functions as to bring an existing diabetes which has been unrecognized to the attention of physicians as they care for the patient. When this disease has been severe enough to cause blindness, it is pretty far advanced. However mild or serious it is, diabetes is never cured; it can, however, usually be controlled by proper treatment, and many patients live a long time with it.

QUESTION: I have been trying to find out what colic in an infant is like. How does a colicky baby behave?

ANSWER: He pulls his legs up against his tummy, squirms and twists, and screams as loud as he can. He may do this for an hour or more unless relieved. Colic usually occurs in well-nourished babies and, though they appear to suffer severely, they gain weight and thrive, while the parents suffer. Colic is often said to be an instinctive reaction by the baby to tensions in the home atmosphere, though this view is not universally accepted. Whatever the cause, the colic is an intestinal spasm, with accumulation of much gas. It is usually relieved by a small enema or by passing a soft catheter into the rectum; the latter is a job for a physician or a nurse.

QUESTION: Having had a baby girl who was a mongolian with a defective heart, and who died of pneumonia at the age of five months, I have become interested in the term "mongolian." I have learned quite a few of the characteristics, but I would like to know how a mongolian compares with an ordinary retarded child, physically and mentally. I have been informed that whatever causes the condition is present at the time of conception. So what happens to cause an ordinary retarded child? What percentage of retarded children are mongolian? I had four normal children prior to the last baby. I am now 31 years old. Would you consider it probable that I might have another mongolian?

ANSWER: I will answer your last question first by saying that no one can tell whether you will have another mongolian child or whether additional children will be normal. The probabilities are in favor of normal children, since mongolian children are rare, but no one can be sure, and certainly no one can promise you that this will be the case. Mongolism is now regarded as a defect due to the absence of certain genes at the time of conception. Retardation is a broad term and probably there will be many types of retardation due to many causes as our knowledge develops.

QUESTION: What can I do to cure the following; every few days I have a series of belches from my stomach; then for some time I have none, and then it starts over again?

ANSWER: If you lived in certain parts of the Orient, your belches would be counted as good manners. If they came after a meal, they would be considered a compliment to the cook. In Western countries attitudes are different. Many persons troubled with excessive belching are unconscious air swallowers. Their habit is a nervous reaction like nail-biting, and thus constitutes a signal for seeking an emotional cause. Your doctor should be able to help you, or you may wish to consult a psychiatrist. Everyone belches, of course, as a result of eating too fast or too much, or from taking an effervescent drink.

QUESTION: I am having trouble with my 13-year-old son wetting the bed—sometimes three and four nights out of the week. This has gone on since he was little and he has never seemed to outgrow it. He is a strong, healthy, active boy and enjoys all outdoor sports. Limiting the amount of liquids doesn't always seem to help. Could adding salt to food (in addition to the amount the rest of the family uses) make any difference? Any suggestions would be deeply appreciated.

ANSWER: If your boy has been wetting the bed since he was small and is still doing so at the age of 13, you are probably wasting your time trying to solve the problem by physical means, such as restricting fluids or adding salt to his diet. Bed-wetting is almost always a psychological problem, and the solution for it must be found in the relationships between your son and his parents, teachers, playmates, etc. You do not say whether there are other children. If there are, these relationships too must be looked into. When bed-wetting has been established for as long a time as it has in the case of your son, it can only be suggested that you get professional help, namely a pediatrician, or child guidance counselor or both. Your own physician can advise you as to how to get in touch with such qualified personnel.

QUESTION: Why should a person feel so depressed when first waking up in the morning; I feel so down and out but after I'm up for a while I commence to feel better.

ANSWER: Feeling depressed in the morning is quite a common experience. As long as you feel better later in the day, it is nothing to worry about. A good many people are sometimes called "slow starters," but once they get going they are all right.

QUESTION: My problem is my 15-year-old son, who worries me by bottling up his emotions, such as hurt, anger, fear, etc. His father died three months ago and he has never shed a tear. Most of the time he acts bemused, shows signs of extreme confusion, worry, and plays 18 to 27 holes of golf a day with a close friend, listens to the hi-fi and converses little. He likes to be left alone, except for his close friend. I've tried to get him to talk to me in a nonchalant manner, but he procrastinates. Neither his father nor I have ever tried to keep him from crying. What can I do to help him?

ANSWER: We are not close enough to this situation to know whether the boy needs to be helped, or whether he simply is of a retiring disposition who does not care to share his feelings with others. Dealing with personalities is a ticklish business, requiring the expert understanding and experienced touch of a professional. You should either do nothing or seek professional counsel. Why not talk the matter over with the family doctor; consult the boy's teachers; and in the meantime do not try to intrude upon his privacy. As a mother, you are too emotionally involved in the matter to have an unbiased judgment.

QUESTION: I have been biting my nails since I was three years old and I am now 12. My mother says I will get an infection if I don't stop biting my nails. The skin around them often bleeds. What can I do about it?

ANSWER: One can try not to bite one's nails but most people who do need help. Biting the nails is only a symptom of a deeper problem that can be helped only with medical advice. Parents should be asked to take the patient to a pediatrician who can find out WHY he bites his nails, and so help him to overcome the habit. He might get an infection, as his mother says, but that is the least important part of the problem.

QUESTION: Recently I fell down three steps and broke some ribs and hurt my spine, and now can only walk with a cane. But what bothers me is that I do not gain any strength, though I used to be very active *and raised nine children. I have been alone for 15 years. My children are very good to me, but I often wish I were out of their way. I lost one son suddenly a year ago. Could grieving keep me from getting better?*

ANSWER: An accident frequently does more injury than is immediately apparent. In addition to your rib and spine injuries you were probably considerably shaken up. Your letter does not say how long it has been since your accident, so it is impossible to suggest how long your recovery might be expected to take. The fact that your children are good to you shows that they appreciate you, and you should not be wishing yourself "out of their way." That is undoubtedly the last thing they want. It is too bad that you lost a son, but you still have the living ones to think of. Grieving can indeed act as an unfavorable influence on your physical progress, beside being bad for you in other ways. Try looking ahead and making the most of the present, instead of grieving over the past.

QUESTION: I am 39 and I have trouble with my joints cracking. This began two years ago in my knees, and now it affects my wrists and ankles too. I have been told this is the forerunner of arthritis. Is this true?

ANSWER: Cracking sounds in the joints do indicate arthritic changes, but for the most part these are not of the serious crippling type. It would nevertheless be a good idea to see a physician about what might be done to prevent further progression. Treatment might include weight control to protect the knees and ankles, also gentle exercises and perhaps heat to avoid stiffening, plus such drugs as the doctor might suggest, plus nutritious diet.

QUESTION: My husband seems to have hard lumps above his knuckles on a few fingers. What is the cause of it? Don't suggest a family doctor because I can't get him to go and see one.

ANSWER: Lots of people have hard lumps near the knuckles, especially as they grow older. The most common are what are called Heberden's nodes, which are the beginnings of osteoarthritis. The only possible recommendation is that he see a doctor, since there is no other way to find out the answer to your question.

QUESTION: Is cancer inherited?

ANSWER: Present views about the inheritability of cancer are negative in the sense that evidence now available does not indicate that cancers in human beings are inherited as such. Even those in newborn babies are not necessarily hereditary. Whether cancer tendencies are hereditary is difficult to determine in a long-lived species like man. Some cancers in mice have been shown to be hereditary. Statistical evidence relating to human cancers seems to indicate that individuals whose line of descent includes persons with cancers are not significantly more liable to cancers than those in the general population. The only possible exceptions are some of the rarer forms of cancer. Please note that the plural, cancers, is used rather than the singular, because cancer is a group of many diseases with significant differences.

QUESTION: Often while I am working in the office my face becomes very flushed and stings. This lasts a little over an hour but it never happens in the summer. I regularly take one vitamin pill a day and I discovered that two B-complex pills taken in the morning have eliminated my trouble. I take thyroid pills for an underactive gland. I am in my mid-twenties. Am I taking too many pills? Is my trouble due to my thyroid or my nerves?

ANSWER: There may be many reasons why your face becomes flushed, and no physician could tell why without seeing or examining you. You are experimenting too much with medications that you do not understand. Neither thyroid pills nor large doses of B-complex should be used without medical advice. All your questions can be answered by your own doctor, and by no one else.

QUESTION: I would like to know about lemon juice, pure lemon juice. Does it destroy the white and red corpuscles of the blood? Does it cause impotence? Does it increase the hydrochloric acid in the stomach? Or does it cure 174 diseases including leprosy, as a Spanish naturalist claims? I think it is good for cholesterol and reduces fat in the body. I am a lemon juice drinker, of course in small quantities.

ANSWER: There is no reason why you should not drink lemon juice, if you like it, even if it will not cure 174 diseases including leprosy. It will cure and prevent just one disease, scurvy, because of its vitamin C content. And you can rest assured that it will not destroy the blood cells, nor cause impotence, nor make the stomach more acid than it normally is. The lemon, of course, is useful in cooking and garnishing foods; ladies like to rinse their hair with its aid and they also like to think it bleaches freckles, although it doesn't really do that, either.

QUESTION: My neighbor has a fungus infection and she has seen her general practitioner rather than a dermatologist. Should I advise her to see a specialist?

ANSWER: Certainly not, for two reasons. First, the general practitioner can undoubtedly take care of her, and will refer her to a specialist if necessary. Second, trading medical advice is the poorest form of neighborliness.

QUESTION: What is the one-shot treatment for hay fever, and where can I get it? Is it really something new?

ANSWER: The so-called one-shot treatment for hay fever is not entirely new. It is a modification of the established method of immunizing a patient against hay fever or other allergies by a series of injections. These are time-consuming and expensive. By injecting the immunizing (anti-allergic) agent in oil instead of in water solution or suspension, the absorption is slowed, and the number of calls to the doctor's offices is reduced and the interval between is lengthened. The term "one-shot" is not strictly accurate, since it is not a one-shot cure. It must be repeated, but not so often as the ordinary injections. It should be available through any physician.

QUESTION: *My father had four strokes four years ago, when he was 65 years old. At first we thought he would die, but he has slowly improved, and now has some movement in his arms and legs. His mind was not affected; his voice is strong and we can distinguish some words. He sits up in a chair and enjoys TV. His doctors say he may live a long time, and they know of nothing more to do for him. Is there anyone who can help him?*

ANSWER: There is no one who could do more than your doctors appear to have done. Recovery from a stroke is a long and tedious process, and only recently has it been found possible to do more for strokes than formerly. However, a condition that has existed almost four years is not amenable to such effective treatment as in the case of a fresh stroke.

QUESTION: *I have just been in a hospital with a virus infection but I am fine now. Still, the doctor tells me I have a heart murmur, and that I must have had rheumatic fever as a child. Will you please explain this to me; we did not have a doctor when I was a child, the way people do now.*

ANSWER: A good many cases of rheumatic fever used to go without treatment, and as a result the heart was damaged. Rheumatic fever often does injury to the heart valves, which operate to keep the blood flowing in the right direction when the heart pumps—just as do valves in a mechanical pump. The disturbed blood flow makes a sound which differs from normal heart sounds, and because of the character of this sound it is called a murmur. Some heart murmurs are indications of serious heart disturbances; others are not. Only your own doctor can tell you about the murmur in your heart.

QUESTION: *I have been told I have a sluggish heart, and at times I awake from my sleep with shortness of breath and have to get up from my bed to get relief. My blood pressure runs from 100 to 112. Could this be the reason for a sluggish heart? I have heard that blood accumulates in the lungs and that is the reason for the shortness of breath. I have had an electrocardiogram which shows OK. Can you shed some light on this? My age is 50. Should I take exercises?*

ANSWER: Low blood pressure is one of the conditions which is more annoying than serious. Most persons with low blood pressure have a long expectation of life. It is better to have low blood pressure than to have high blood pressure, but it may be unpleasant, as you have found it. Whether the low blood pressure is responsible for the sluggish heart or the sluggish heart for the low blood pressure is a question similar to the one about which came first, the chicken or the egg. It is all part of the same picture, namely, a constitution which is, so to speak, in low gear. A doctor would not recommend any exercises for a man of 50 without preliminary medical examination. Unless you have kept yourself in good physical trim continuously since your youth, you might find that suddenly em-barking on a course of exercise would do you more harm than good.

QUESTION: *I am 60 years old and am troubled at night with leg cramps. They usually act up about 4 to 5 o'clock in the morning. I have tried taking a quinine capsule each night before retiring but they do not seem to help.*

ANSWER: Leg cramps may be due to many different causes and what to do for them depends on what causes them. A possible treatment is to lie in a tub of warm water—not hot—for about 15 minutes before going to bed, and raising the foot of your bed about 10 inches. You should not be taking any drugs without medical advice. If these simple suggestions do not help, then you should consult a physician.

QUESTION: *Under what conditions may the heart become enlarged? Is this due to defective structure? Once enlarged, can the heart ever return to normal size?*

ANSWER: Enlargement of the heart may occur under two principal sets of conditions: If an extra load of work is thrown upon the heart muscle by defective valves, heavy labor or strenuous athletic effort, the heart reacts like any other muscle. It enlarges to meet its requirements. Within limits, this is wholesome and is not an indication of weakness or disease. When, however, the load becomes too heavy, the heart may be unable to adjust to it, and the weakened muscle may dilate, creating an enlargement due to weakness. When the heart has enlarged within normal limits, it tends to remain that way. A dilated heart may, however, return to some degree to its proper size under rest and appropriate medical treatment.

QUESTION: *What does a doctor mean when he speaks of myocarditis? Is it serious?*

ANSWER: Myocarditis comes from MYO (muscle)-CARD (heart)-ITIS (inflammation). Hence the word means inflammation, or perhaps better, injury, to the heart muscle. This may be temporary, as during fevers or such toxic diseases as diphtheria in which the heart muscle is affected by the toxin or poison produced by the organism. If it is severe, the weakening effects may be permanent. Weakening of the heart muscle may also occur as a result of long-continued overwork, due to defective valves which allow the blood to seep backward and make the heart muscle work harder to keep the blood moving in the right direction. Whether the condition is serious or not depends upon the nature and extent of the injury and how long it has been present. Many persons with mild damage to their hearts live a long time if they are careful in following medical advice.

QUESTION: *What are the more obvious symptoms of hypertension? Is an elevated blood pressure necessarily one of them, or can there be a hypertensive condition without high blood pressure?*

ANSWER: It all depends on how you use the words. Medically speaking, hypertension MEANS high blood pressure, so obviously there can be no hypertension without elevation of the blood pressure. In non-medical language, there may be a state of enhanced nervous tension without high blood pressure, but it is very likely sooner or later to result in high blood pressure.

QUESTION: *Recently my husband (age 49) was told by his doctor that he has high blood pressure—180. He was told to omit all fattening foods, plus salt. Just how serious can this condition become? Is there anything you could recommend in addition to this diet?*

ANSWER: Some individuals have elevated blood pressure for quite a time without apparently serious results, while in others the condition progresses rapidly, damages the heart, and otherwise destroys their health. The only way your husband can find out what his future is likely to be is to remain under medical care and give his doctor time and opportunity to estimate his progress.

QUESTION: *What are the symptoms and treatment of anemia of the brain?*

ANSWER: Anemia of the brain is usually characterized by a sleepiness, sluggishness, or in extreme cases, disorientation and coma. The best example of anemia of the brain is ordinary fainting for which the treatment is to lay the patient on the floor, keep the head low, loosen the clothing and keep meddlers with good intentions from "doing something."

QUESTION: *Is allergy to certain foods due to a digestive weakness for those foods? Would improper function of either the adrenal glands or the pancreas be responsible? If so, which?*

ANSWER: Allergy is not a digestive disturbance. Food allergies are but one class of allergy; substances breathed in and substances making contact with the skin are other classes. The two latter have nothing to do with digestion. Allergy is a reaction by certain persons to substances which in themselves may be harmless to most persons. The air is full of ragweed pollens every fall, but only a limited number of persons suffer with hay fever. Millions eat strawberries and sea foods: only a few suffer allergies. Millions use cosmetics; a few have allergic reactions. The pancreas is not involved in allergies; neither is the adrenal gland, except insofar as the hormone epinephrine, a product of the adrenal gland commonly called adrenalin, is useful in treating allergic symptoms. Adrenalin is, however, not a cure.

QUESTION: *What can you tell me about swollen ankles? Has it anything to do with diet, coffee or tea?*

ANSWER: Swollen ankles ordinarily cannot be explained on any such simple basis as diet, coffee, or tea, as suggested in your letter. Ankles usually swell as a result of changes in the circulation, and these may be due to many causes which can be identified by medical examination only. The person so afflicted should consult a physician for a full explanation.

QUESTION: *What kind of lenses are especially helpful to a patient suffering partial blindness as a result of glaucoma?*

ANSWER: Unfortunately no lens can substitute for loss of vision due to nerve damage such as occurs in glaucoma; the remaining visual capacity may be helped by enlarging lenses such as are used in microscopes. The adaptation of the lens to your eyes is an exacting job and one for your oculist.

QUESTION: *I have valvular heart disease, and I have to have some teeth extracted. Is this dangerous? What anesthetic would be used?*

ANSWER: It is not nearly so dangerous as it would have been a few years ago. If your heart action is normal despite the injured valves, you can be protected against infection and further injury to the valves by penicillin or another antibiotic selected by your physician or dentist. Local anesthesia is usually employed, unless the extractions are numerous or difficult. In some instances the patient is hospitalized as a further precaution. The exact procedure in your case must be determined, of course, by your dentist in consultation with your physician.

QUESTION: *We have a boy 13 years old who has flat feet. He is not my own son but I would like to help if I can. Please tell me if there is any cure for it.*

ANSWER: Flat feet are not always a disadvantage. Doctors no longer speak of flat feet; they speak of weak feet. A strong, flat foot is better than a weak one with a "perfectly good arch." Your boy should, therefore, have his feet examined by an orthopedic surgeon to find out whether anything needs to be done for them. Weak feet are usually treated by muscle exercises and sometimes with supports. Simply buying supports at a shoe store may, however, make a weak foot worse because the muscles then are not required to develop strength.

FAMILY HISTORY

	birth date	if deceased—cause and date	pertinent medical facts (enter chronic diseases, illnesses—such as cancer, diabetes, epilepsy)
HUSBAND			
father			
mother			
brothers and/or sisters			
WIFE			
father			
mother			
brothers and/or sisters			

Individual Birth Record

name	date	city	hospital	comments

Illness

name	nature of illness, injury, or surgery	physician	hospital	date	length of illness	comments (e.g., if surgery, what was removed?)

Checklist of Diseases

name	chicken pox	measles	german measles	mumps	whooping cough	scarlet fever	diphtheria	mono- nucleosis	other

Dates of Immunization

name	whooping cough vaccine first	booster	diphtheria toxoid first	booster	tetanus toxoid first	booster	smallpox vaccine first	revaccinations

polio vaccine

Salk vaccine				Sabin (oral) vaccine			
dose 1	dose 2	dose 3	booster	type I	type III	type II	booster

other immunizations

Physical Examination

name	date	physician	advice or instructions

Health and Accident Insurance Information

name	policy number	date issued	company	type of coverage	premium

Records of Insurance Payments Received

_____
_____
_____
_____
_____
_____
_____
_____
_____
_____
_____
_____
_____
_____
_____

Additional Information

name	comments

INDEX

A

abnormalities. *See* heart; mental illness; sexual abnormalities.
abortion, 21
accidents. *See* safety
"acid stomach," 453
acne, 175
addiction
    alcoholism, 459
    narcotics, 466, 490
    smoking, 457
adenoids
    nightmares, 220
    throat, 183
adolescence
    acne, 174
    dating, 58
    sexual development, 56
advertising (of drugs), 323
aging
    automobile safety, 278
    eye degeneration, 169
    grief, 202
    health examination, 128
    home care, 68
    menopause, 63
    nursing homes, 317
    nutrition, 140
    senile dementia, 189
    skin, 81
    skin care, 174
aggression, 210
air
    respiratory system, 102
    ventilation, 8
air conditioning, 8
air pollution, 488
albino, 87
Alcoholics Anonymous
    alcoholism, 463
    mental health, 198
alcoholism
    automobile safety, 279
    calling doctor, 355
    community health resources, 489
    diseases, 459
    mental illness, 191
    National Council on Alcoholism, 501
    quackery, 325
alkalizer, 453
allergies
    alcoholism, 459
    disabling diseases, 423
    drugs, 374, 448
    emergency identification, 338
    hair dyes, 180
    insect stings, 350
    nose and throat care, 181
    skin rash, 360
    smoking, 455
Allergy Foundation of America, 501
amblyopia, 169
American Association for Maternal
    and Infant Health, 505
American Cancer Society
    cancer, 489
    voluntary health agencies, 502

American Diabetes Association, 505
American Epilepsy Federation, 507
American Foundation for the Blind, 505
American Hearing Society, 503
American Heart Association, 503
American Medical Association
    civil defense, 536
    doctors, 307
    emergency medical identification, 339
    emergency medical services, 363
    health insurance, 331
    health museums, 551
    quackery, 322
    smoking, 457
American Red Cross, 498, 506
American Rehabilitation Committee, 505
American Rheumatism Association, 501
American Social Health Association, 504
amulets, 561
analgesics, *See* pain
anatomy, 73
    blood circulation, 95
    digestive system, 107
    ear, 157
    hair, 86
    muscles, 88
    nervous system, 113
    nose, 181
    respiratory system, 102
    sense organs, 120
    sex education, 47
    skeleton, 74
    skin, 81
anemia
    blood, 101
    diagnosis, 320
anesthesia, 437
    alcohol, 459
    childbirth, 24
anesthesiology, 312
    aneurysm, 407
angina pectoris, 381
animals, diseases of, 524
    farms, 14
antibiotics, 447
antibodies, 442
anticoagulants, 447
antigen, 512
antihistamines
    allergy, 426
    drugs, 448
antiperspirants, 175
antiseptics, 447
anxiety, 197
    bedwetting, 218
    obesity, 142
    psychoneurosis, 190
apartments, 10
appendicitis, 319
artery, 95
arthritis, 389
    birth defects, 479
    quackery, 324
Arthritis and Rheumatism Foundation, 501
artificial respiration, 343
asefedita, 561
aspirin
    headaches, 395

X Y Z

CALORIES IN COMMON FOODS

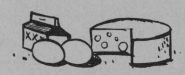

DAIRY FOODS

	SERVING	CALORIES
Butter	1 tbsp	95
Cheese		
American	1 ounce	110
cottage	½ cup	100
cream	1 ounce	105
Swiss	1 ounce	100
Cream		
coffee	2 tbsp	65
heavy	2 tbsp	120
whipped	2 tbsp	60
Half and half	¼ cup	80
Milk (8 oz.)		
whole	1 glass	170
skim	1 glass	85
buttermilk	1 glass	85
Ice Cream		
vanilla	⅙ qt	205
chocolate	⅙ qt	240
lemon sherbet	⅙ qt	265

VEGETABLES (raw)

Cabbage	½ cup	15
Carrot	1 medium	25
Celery	2 stalks	10
Cucumber	½ med	10
Lettuce	¼ head	10
Lettuce, green	1 lg. leaf	2
Onion, green	1 medium	5
Radish	1 medium	2
Tomato	1 medium	25

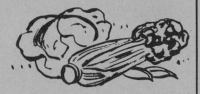

GREEN VEGETABLES
(cooked)

Asparagus	6, 4" stalks	15
Broccoli	½ cup	25
Cabbage	½ cup	20
Green Beans	½ cup	40
Greens	½ cup	30
Peas	½ cup	70
Pepper, green	1 medium	30

OTHER VEGETABLES
(cooked)

	SERVING	CALORIES
Beets	½ cup	40
Carrots	½ cup	25
Cauliflower	½ cup	25
Corn	1 med. ear	100
Onions	1 large	50
Potatoes		
plain	1 small	85
mashed	½ cup	150
creamed	½ cup	160
French fried	10 pieces	160
Squash, winter	½ cup	40
Sweet Potato	½ large	100
Tomatoes	½ cup	20

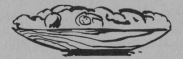

SALADS

Chicken-celery (mayonnaise)	½ cup	170
Cole slaw (cream dressing)	½ cup	85
Banana-nut (mayonnaise)	½ cup	260
Combination (lemon juice)	1 med	40
Perfection (no dressing)	½ cup	40
Potato (mayonnaise)	½ cup	200
Dressing		
boiled	1 tbsp	30
French	1 tbsp	70
mayonnaise	1 tbsp	100
Thousand Is'd	1 tbsp	65

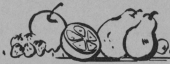

FRUITS AND FRUIT JUICES

Apple, fresh	1 large	100
baked	1 large	260
sauce	½ cup	80
Apricots, fresh	3 med	60
dried	5 halves	90
canned	6 halves	90
Avocado	½ pear	265
Banana	1 med	100
Cantaloupe	½ med	35

	SERVING	CALORIES
Cherries, sweet	15 large	80
Dates, dried	3-4	95
Fruit cocktail canned	½ cup	80
Grapefruit	½ small	45
juice	½ cup	45
Grapes, American	22 av	80
juice	½ cup	75
Lemon juice	1 tbsp	5
Olives	1 med	15
Orange	1 med	65
juice	½ cup	50
Peach, fresh	1 med	50
canned	2 halves	75
Pear, fresh	1 med	70
canned	2 halves	75
Pineapple	¾" slice	60
Prunes	4-5 med	150
Raisins	¼ cup	90
Raspberries	½ cup	45
Rhubarb sauce	½ cup	175
Strawberries	10 large	40
Watermelon	med. serv	100

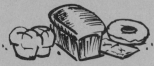

BREADS AND CEREALS

Biscuit	2 small	100
Bread, av	1 oz. sl	75
	thin sl	50
Cereals, average		
cooked	½ cup	75
ready prep'd	1 c., 1 oz.	100
Cornbread	2" square	130
Crackers	2" square	20
Doughnut, yeast	1, 3"	125
Muffin, av	1 med	100
Roll, av	1 med	100
sweet, iced	1 small	185
Ry-Krisp	1 piece	25
Waffle	1, 6"	225

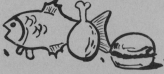

MEAT, POULTRY, FISH, EGGS

Meat and Poultry cooked, med. serving		
lean	3½ oz	175
medium fat	3½ oz	270